Histories of Fetal Knowledge Production in Sweden

Clio Medica

STUDIES IN THE HISTORY OF MEDICINE AND HEALTH

VOLUME 107

The titles published in this series are listed at *brill.com/clio*

Histories of Fetal Knowledge Production in Sweden

Medicine, Politics, and Public Controversy, 1530–2020

Edited by

Solveig Jülich

BRILL

LEIDEN | BOSTON

This book is published with support from the Swedish Research Council, Magnus Bergvall Foundation, Vilhelm Ekman Foundation, King Gustaf VI Adolf's Fund for Swedish Culture, Sten Lindroth Memorial Fund, and Åke Wiberg Foundation.

Cover illustration: Photograph by Lennart Nilsson of a sex education lesson in a Stockholm school in the mid-1960s. Courtesy of Lennart Nilsson Photography/SPL. Also included as Figure 0.16.

Library of Congress Cataloging-in-Publication Data

Names: Jülich, Solveig, 1966- editor
Title: Histories of fetal knowledge production in Sweden : medicine, politics, and public controversy, 1530-2020 / Solveig Jülich.
Other titles: Medicine, politics, and public controversy, 1530-2020
Description: Leiden ; Boston : Brill, [2025] | Series: Clio medica: studies in the history of medicine and health, 0045-7183 ; volume 107 | Includes bibliographical references and index.
Identifiers: LCCN 2024033677 (print) | LCCN 2024033678 (ebook) | ISBN 9789004536739 (hardback) | ISBN 9789004703759 (ebook)
Subjects: LCSH: Fetus–Research–Sweden–History. | Human experimentation in medicine–Sweden–Moral and ethical aspects. | Fetal death–Political aspects–Sweden. | Fetal tissues–Research–Sweden–Moral and ethical aspects.
Classification: LCC R853.H8 H56 2025 (print) | LCC R853.H8 (ebook) | DDC 174.2/8–dc23/eng/20240808
LC record available at https://lccn.loc.gov/2024033677
LC ebook record available at https://lccn.loc.gov/2024033678

Typeface for the Latin, Greek, and Cyrillic scripts: "Brill". See and download: brill.com/brill-typeface.

ISSN 0045-7183
ISBN 978-90-04-53673-9 (hardback)
ISBN 978-90-04-70375-9 (e-book)
DOI 10.1163/9789004703759

This book is printed on acid-free paper and produced in a sustainable manner.

Contents

Acknowledgments

This book is the result of work within the research program 'Medicine at the Borders of Life: Fetal Research and the Emergence of Ethical Controversy in Sweden,' hosted by the Department of History of Science and Ideas at Uppsala University between 2015–2021. It has been an immense pleasure to collaborate with the members of the 'MBL' research team and I am grateful for their contributions to this volume: Eva Åhrén, Annika Berg, Elisabet Björklund, Maria Björkman, Maja Bondestam, Isa Dussauge, Helena Franzén, Francis Lee, Helena Tinnerholm Ljungberg, and Morag Ramsey. I am also very happy that Tove Paulsson Holmberg, Anton Runesson, and Anna Tunlid joined us in our collective effort to grasp 500 years of the history of the fetus and reproduction in Sweden.

During the seminars, workshops, conferences, and other events that the research program organized, we have learnt so much from colleagues and visitors. For their inspiring talks and insightful commentaries, we would particularly like to thank Barbara Duden, Sunniva Engh, Birgitta Essén, Jameson Garland, Lisa Guntram, Adam Hedgecoe, Nick Hopwood, Noortje Jacobs, Susanne M. Klausen, Lene Koch, Lena Lennerhed, Christer Nordlund, Jesse Olszynko-Gryn, Manon Parry, Leslie Reagan, Michael Sappol, Mette Nordahl Svendsen, and Kristin Zeiler. A warm thanks to the film collective Don't Stop the Motion that produced the animated short film *Icon: A Visual History of the Fetus* (2019) in collaboration with the research team.[1]

We are deeply indebted to the two anonymous reviewers of the manuscript for their careful readings and constructive suggestions on how to improve the book. Jonathan Reinarz, series editor of Clio Medica at Brill, was very helpful in the process. As editor, I am especially grateful to Sven Widmalm, Andrus Ers, and Lena Lennerhed who read and gave valuable comments of earlier versions of the introduction and epilogue. Sven supported this project from the very start and deserves a special thank you.

We would like to thank the artists, photographers, and other rightsholders of the images included in this book for giving approval to publish their work: the family of Edward Lindahl, the family of Margareta Sylwan, and Malin Thomas Nilsson. Extra thanks to Anne Fjellström at Lennart Nilsson Photography for her kind permission to use several photographs by Lennart Nilsson, including the cover image of the volume. Several cultural heritage institutions and private collectors and archives have generously provided us with reproductions of

1 https://www.youtube.com/watch?v=cer3CNvC9zk&t=3s.

images in the book: Dagens Bild, Olof Edlund, the EWK Archive of the Museum of Work, the Hagströmer Library of the Karolinska Institute, KvinnSam at Gothenburg University Library, the Museum of Drawings in Laholm, the Museum of Medical History at Uppsala University, the Nordic Museum, Skokloster Castle, the Swedish National Library, and the Wellcome Collection. Malin Thomas Nilsson provided excellent service with preparing many of the volume's images for print.

'Medicine at the Borders of Life' was funded by the Swedish Research Council (registration number 2014–1749). Sincere thanks to Ragnhild Blomqvist Fund for supporting six international workshops and conferences that took place between 2015–2019 at Uppsala University. We are grateful to the Bergman Estate on Fårö as well as the Kavala Guesthouse, run by the Swedish Institute at Athens, for hosting writing retreats in 2016 and 2018, respectively. Funding for the publication of this volume, copyediting, and image permissions were generously provided by Magnus Bergvall Foundation, Vilhelm Ekman Foundation, King Gustaf VI Adolf's Fund for Swedish Culture, Sten Lindroth Memorial Fund, and Åke Wiberg Foundation.

Figures

Abbreviations

The following abbreviations are used in the notes and chapter bibliographies.

AACC	American Association for the Aid of Crippled Children
CHS	Center for History of Science, Royal Swedish Academy of Sciences, Stockholm
FCD	Foundation for Child Development records (FA019), Online Collections and Catalogue of Rockefeller Archive Center, Sleepy Hollow, NY
GUA	Gothenburg University Archive, Gothenburg
KI	The Karolinska Institute, Stockholm
KIREC	Archives of the Karolinska Institute's research ethics committees, 1967–2003, Karolinska Institute, Solna
LUH	Archive of Lund University Hospital, Regional Archives of Skåne, Archive Centre South, Lund
LUL	Lund University Library, Lund
MHSA	Ministry of Health and Social Affairs, Main Archive 1975–1996, National Archives of Sweden, Stockholm
MI	Archives of the Ministry of the Interior, National Archives of Sweden, Stockholm
MRC	Archive of the Medical Research Council, National Archives of Sweden, Täby
NA	National Archives, Kew
NAS	National Archives of Sweden, Stockholm and Täby
NBL	Archive of the National Bacteriological Laboratory, National Archives of Sweden, Täby
NBM	Archive of the National Board of Medicine, National Archives of Sweden, Stockholm
NBM-AB	The Apothecary Bureau of the National Board of Medicine 1920–1967, Archives of the National Board of Medicine, National Archives of Sweden, Stockholm
NCN	Archive of the National Counsellor for the Neurosedyn issue 1947–1967, National Board of Health and Welfare, National Archives of Sweden, Täby
NIH	The National Institutes of Health, Bethesda
NPL	Archive of the National Pharmaceutical Laboratory, National Archives of Sweden, Täby
SCA	Stockholm City Archive, Liljeholmen/Stockholm
SHM	South Swedish Society for the History of Medicine, Lund
SOU	Swedish Government Commission Official Reports
SRA	Document archive, Swedish Radio Administration, Stockholm
SRCA	Skåne Regional Council Archive, Archive Center South, Lund
SSM	Archive of the Swedish Society of Medicine, TAM Archives, Stockholm

Notes on Contributors

Eva Åhrén
is director of medical history and heritage at the Karolinska Institute in Stockholm since 2013. Specializing in visual and material aspects of medical knowledge production and communication, Åhrén has studied epistemic authority and image production in the anatomical sciences of the nineteenth century; the role of specimens and anatomy museum collections in research and pedagogy; and wax moulages in venereology and dermatology. After receiving her PhD in 2002, Åhrén was a postdoctoral fellow at Yale University, head of research at the Nobel Museum, and a research fellow at Uppsala University and the US National Institutes of Health. Åhrén is the author of *Death, Modernity, and the Body: Sweden 1870–1930* (University of Rochester Press, 2009).

Annika Berg
is associate professor of history of ideas at Stockholm University. Her research focuses mainly on social, cultural, and political aspects of twentieth-century medicine and health care, including psychiatry and public health. She recently (with coauthors Urban Lundberg and Mattias Tydén) published a book on the first decades of Swedish development aid, contributing, for example, several chapters on Sweden's first bilateral family-planning projects, and is currently concluding her work in a transdisciplinary research project on suffrage restrictions in Sweden after the 1921 democratic 'breakthrough.'

Elisabet Björklund
is associate professor of film studies at Lund University, where her research focuses on sexuality and reproduction in Swedish film and television history. She is coeditor, with Mariah Larsson, of *A Visual History of HIV/AIDS: Exploring the Face of AIDS Film Archive* (Routledge, 2019) and, with Solveig Jülich, of *Rethinking the Public Fetus: Historical Perspectives on the Visual Culture of Pregnancy* (University of Rochester Press, 2024). Currently, she is working on a research project on reproduction in Swedish television in the 1950s, 1960s, and 1970s.

Maria Björkman
is associate professor of history of science and ideas at Uppsala University. She holds a position as senior lecturer in history in the Department of Culture and Society, and is also a member of the Center for Medical Humanities and Bioethics, both at Linköping University. Her research focuses mainly on early twentieth-century medicine, including the history of eugenics, genetics, urology, and disability.

Maja Bondestam
is professor of history of science and ideas at Uppsala University. Her academic interests are focused on the human body during the shift from the early modern to the modern period and on history of medicine and natural philosophy. Bondestam has published books and articles on themes including the politics of the maturing body, the history of hermaphroditism and monstrosity, the language of Carl Linnaeus, and gendered norms in medical advice literature. She recently edited the book *Exceptional Bodies in Early Modern Culture: Concepts of Monstrosity before the Advent of the Normal* (Amsterdam University Press, 2020).

Isa Dussauge
is a researcher at the Tyrili Foundation. Dussauge's academic interests in the social and historical studies of medicine encompass the history of ethics and activism, critical drug studies, gender and sexuality studies, and the studies of valuation and conflicting values in knowledge production. Dussauge coedited the volume *Value Practices in Medicine and the Life Sciences* (Oxford University Press, 2015).

Helena Franzén
received her PhD in the history of science and ideas at Uppsala University in 2022. In her doctoral dissertation, she examined the formation and uses of obstetrical and embryological collections at Uppsala University around 1830–1930, and explored their relations to the wider society. Her research investigates the dynamics of medical knowledge production, focusing on practices of collecting and using specimens in various contexts related to medicine and reproduction. Franzén has contributed articles to journals such as *Lychnos*, *Scandinavian Journal of History*, and *Scandia*.

Solveig Jülich
is professor of history of science and ideas at Uppsala University. Her research deals with media history of medicine and historical perspectives on medicine, ethics, and democracy. Between 2015 and 2021 she directed the research program 'Medicine at the Borders of Life: Fetal Research and the Emergence of Ethical Controversy in Sweden,' funded by the Swedish Research Council. She has published articles in journals such as the *Bulletin of the History of Medicine* and *Social History of Medicine* and is coeditor of several volumes, including *Communicating the History of Medicine: Perspectives on Audiences and Impact* (Manchester University Press, 2019) and *Rethinking the Public Fetus: Historical Perspectives on the Visual Culture of Pregnancy* (University of Rochester Press, 2024).

Francis Lee
is associate professor and senior researcher at the division for science, technology, and society at Chalmers University of Technology. His research deals broadly with how technology shapes society. One of his main research interests is how information infrastructures shape knowledge production. He has published in *Science, Technology & Human Values*; *Science as Culture*, *Valuation Studies*, and *History and Technology*. He coedited the volume *Value Practices in the Life Sciences* (Oxford University Press, 2015) and is currently directing the research program 'A New Scientific Revolution? Big Data and AI in the Biosciences' (https://francislee.org).

Tove Paulsson Holmberg
is a researcher in history of science and ideas at Lund University. Her PhD thesis (2017) analyzed early modern Swedish birth manuals and emergency obstetric practices. Her research focuses on early modern medical practices, birth and death rites, medicine and religion, and medical rhetoric. In 2020, she published a study on early modern Swedish birth practices and perinatal loss, 'Ambiguous and Transitional Bodies: Stillbirth in Stockholm, 1691–1724' in *Exceptional Bodies in Early Modern Culture: Concepts of Monstrosity before the Advent of the Normal*, edited by Maja Bondestam (Amsterdam University Press, 2020).

Morag Ramsey
is a researcher in the history of science and ideas at Uppsala University. Her doctoral dissertation traced the development of abortion pills in Sweden, and her research interests include the history of medicine and reproduction, and science and technology studies. Her current research project, funded by Riksbankens Jubileumsfond, focuses on the first uses of the modern intrauterine device in Sweden.

Anton Runesson
is a postdoctoral researcher at Stockholm University. In his doctoral dissertation, he investigated how ordinary people in early modern Sweden understood the body to function, with regard to principles of life, sickness and health, and religious influences. He is currently studying human-animal relations within early modern households, focusing in particular on notions of health and productivity.

Helena Tinnerholm Ljungberg
(PhD in political science) is assistant professor at the Institute of Environmental Medicine, Karolinska Institute, Stockholm, where she currently studies gendered aspects of sickness absence. She held a postdoctoral position within

the research program 'Medicine at the Borders Life' at Uppsala University in 2017–19. Her work has focused on the governance of reproductive research and the origins and development of research ethics committees. She acted as guest editor for a special issue of the *European Journal for the History of Medicine and Health* on the latter topic in 2021.

Anna Tunlid
is associate professor and researcher at the Department of Arts and Cultural Sciences and affiliated with the Birgit Rausing Centre for Medical Humanities at Lund University. Her research deals with the history of modern life sciences and medicine, specifically the history of genetics. A particular focus has been the relation between the development and use of knowledge and various societal, political, and institutional interests. Currently, she is working on a research project on the care of people with intellectual disabilities in Sweden, 1935–63.

INTRODUCTION

Historicizing Fetal Knowledge Production, Reproductive Politics, and Conflicted Values

Solveig Jülich

On April 10, 1973, the front page of the *Washington Post* featured the story 'Live-Fetus Research Debated.' The story revealed that the National Institutes of Health (NIH) supported human fetal research both in the United States and abroad, including studies on living fetuses obtained from abortion operations. National press coverage followed, pushing NIH officials to issue denials and clarifications. Repeatedly, Sweden was mentioned as a permissive country for fetal research where American scientists went to access human material that was highly limited at home. According to one source, the NIH had in fact funded studies at the famous Karolinska Institute (KI) in Stockholm in which aborted fetuses were kept alive for several hours by artificial means. Geneticist Kurt Hirschhorn of New York's Mount Sinai School of Medicine told a reporter that such investigations were not unethical because a 'nonviable' fetus is 'nothing more than a piece of tissue.' Cardinal John Crol, on the other hand, spoke of 'using victims of abortions as living human guinea pigs.' He was backed up by two hundred Roman Catholic high school students who protested in front of the NIH offices to call for a total ban on fetal research.[1]

Thus by the early 1970s, the Swedish context was closely interrelated with reproductive research and politics in other countries. This book demonstrates for the first time how Sweden came to occupy a central place in international and transnational scientific research that involved the use of aborted human embryos and fetuses. Our studies also highlight the particular historical circumstances that made this possible and show that specifically Swedish conditions were linked to international anti-abortion activism. But looking back to the 1970s is insufficient for understanding these developments. Instead, we

All translations in the chapters are by the authors, unless stated otherwise.

1 Cohn, 'Live-Fetus Research Debate' (quotation from Hirschhorn); Cohn, 'NIH Vows Not to Fund Fetus Work' (quotation from Crol); Cohn, 'Scientists and Fetus Research.' Other countries were mentioned, including Britain and Finland. However, as discussed below and in chapter 8, it was Sweden that continued to play a prominent role in the US media coverage; it also figured as a bad example when fetal research became a topic of heated public debate in Britain in the early 1970s.

 | DOI:10.1163/9789004703759_002

employ a long term perspective and fresh analytical approaches to bring to light the complex and multifaceted history of fetal knowledge production and public controversy in Sweden.

Public policy and bioethics scholars have discussed how research scandals and scientific breakthroughs in the late twentieth century sparked ethical and political debates on the use of human embryos and fetuses in science.[2] In particular they have pointed to research on early embryos, including surplus IVF embryos, embryonic stem cells, and cloned embryos as an important backdrop to ethical debate.[3] Authors have often framed these scandals and disputes in terms of the historical legacy of Nazism and eugenics, as well as linking them to a number of horrific clinical research studies including the Tuskegee syphilis study. Moreover, they have also stressed that what characterized the debate in the United States was the close connections made between embryo/fetal research and battles surrounding abortion. In this literature, today's bioethical definitions, policies, and regulations concerning research on embryos and fetuses are seen as the outcome of these public outrages and controversies.[4]

Our book approaches these questions in a different way. Drawing on international historical research on reproduction, our aim is to explore a variety of meanings, values, norms, and policies surrounding the uses of fetuses for medical knowledge production, including the development of vaccines and pharmaceuticals, in Sweden over a long historical period.[5] We understand 'the fetus' or 'pregnancy' not as stable entities but as created, materialized, and negotiated in shifting historical settings. By interrogating the conflicted views

2 On debates about embryo and fetal research as part of the rise of bioethics, see Jonsen, *Birth of Bioethics*, chap. 4. Scholarship that provides historical mappings of these debates as well as the role of bioethics includes Banchoff, *Embryo Politics*, and Hurlbut, *Experiments in Democracy*. For an early attempt at an overview of policy debates on fetal research that includes some pre-1970s examples, see Maynard-Moody, *Dilemma of the Fetus*. See also Ramsey, *Ethics of Fetal Research*.

3 Key events are usually said to be the first successful fertilization of a human egg outside the womb in 1969, the birth of Louise Brown through IVF a decade later, the isolation of human embryonic stem cells in 1998, and the first verified cloning of a human embryo in 2008. See, e.g., Banchoff, *Embryo Politics*, 1.

4 The role of national legacies in shaping ethical controversies about embryo research is discussed in Banchoff, 14–19. Rothman's *Strangers at the Bedside* is the classic account of how the field of bioethics emerged as a response to research scandals and other events. For a discussion of historical research that has challenged bioethicists' historiography, see Jacobs, *Ethics by Committee*, 8–11.

5 On the need for and challenges of long-term perspectives on reproductive history, see Hopwood, Flemming, and Kassell, 'Reproduction in History,' 13–14; Bock von Wülfingen et al., 'Temporalities of Reproduction.'

of a multitude of actors, including physicians, scientists, legal officials, policymakers, media teams, disability organizations, and women's movements, and observing how sensitive issues were defined at various times, we demonstrate how the uses of aborted fetuses for research became regulated in Swedish legislation in the late twentieth century. The institutionalization of ethics and bioethics, especially the launching of research ethics committees, certainly played a part in this historical process, but there is much more to the story.[6]

The volume then differs in three main ways from other valuable histories of public controversies around fetal knowledge production. First, the adoption of a long-term perspective, covering five hundred years of reproductive history. Most historical work on fetal knowledge production that has examined the period before the Second World War tends to be restricted to shorter time frames or does not address the issue of controversy.[7] To grasp both change and continuity, we need to reach further back in time. Our story begins in the mid-sixteenth century, at the time of Sweden's founding as a modern nation-state with imperial aspirations. It concludes in the present period, which is marked by ongoing conflicts over abortion and reproductive rights in numerous countries. Nevertheless, the focus is on the decades following the Second World War, during which Sweden emerged as a leading actor in the international field of human fetal research. We emphasize the 1990s, when the legal framework for fetal research was established, but also address the historiographical discussions that have taken place in public discourse up to recent years. Along the way, we highlight a variety of changing and conflicting understandings of fetuses and fetal experimentation. In this fashion, we strive to provide both context for more limited studies and details that can inform more general histories.

Second, our geographical focus is on Sweden, a country located on the Scandinavian Peninsula in northern Europe, often characterized as a highly secular and developed welfare state, promoting gender equality, sexual freedom, and women's rights. More national histories like this one can help reveal how reproductive and biomedical research as well as legal and ethical frameworks emerged in specific ways in different places. The established historiography is to a large extent based on an American narrative, even if the perspective has broadened in recent years to include the experiences of several European

6 For a recent account of the history of research ethics, using the Netherlands as a case study, see Jacobs, *Ethics by Committee*.

7 However, see Buklijas and Hopwood, *Making Visible Embryos*, and Hopwood, *Haeckel's Embryos*. For a long-term perspective on visualizations of fetal knowledge from an ethical perspective, see also Hornuff and Fangerau, *Visualisierung des Ungeborenen*.

countries.[8] Furthermore, there is a tendency to conflate the Nordic countries into one homogenous region. This is especially problematic when it comes to issues related to abortion. For historical and other reasons, abortion legislation and practices vary between Denmark, Finland, Iceland, Norway, and Sweden much more than is generally expected.[9] At the same time, as emphasized in this volume, international and transnational approaches are crucial, not least in order to map the landscape of research funding, professional networks, and ethics codes.

Third, we use a broad definition of the domain under study—fetal knowledge production—to allow for a historical investigation into different discursive and material practices across contexts. The empirical areas of study range from natural philosophy, medical science, and health care to religion, law, politics, and visual culture. Earlier scholarship's focus on embryo/fetal-research controversy as a route to bioethics is in itself limiting since it effectively rules out past meanings of ethics and how it should be practiced. For instance, a focus on past debates concerning medical confidentiality and abortion may reveal complex negotiations between states, physicians, lawyers, patients, and the wider public on the boundaries of medical secrecy.[10] Moreover, historically, medical ethics has competed with other cultural criteria for measuring value, most notably religious, scientific, and economic ones. Thus, it is important to study fetal research in relation to a wider set of colliding criteria, values, concepts, meanings, and technologies, as well as in terms of bioethicalization.[11]

The book brings together a multidisciplinary group of scholars working within areas such as the history of science, medicine, and technology, as well as political science and film studies. The fourteen chapters are chronologically organized and each focuses on one or several themes of fetal and reproductive knowledge production that relate to concepts and classifications; material and visual dimensions; the notion of controversy and value conflicts; and policies, politics, and regulations. Using a broad range of sources, including sermons,

8 Jacobs and Tinnerholm Ljungberg, 'How Ethics Travels.'

9 For a discussion of the idea of a Nordic model, see Andersson and Hilson, 'Images of Sweden and the Nordic Countries.' On abortion history in individual Nordic countries, see Elvbakken, *Abortspørsmålets politiske historie 1900–2020*; Lennerhed, 'No Backlash for Swedish Women?'; Nexø, *Det rette valg*; Takala and Häyry, 'Physicians Controlling Women's Reproductive Choices.'

10 Maehle, *Contesting Medical Confidentiality*, chap. 3.

11 The term 'bioethicalization' refers to the tendency to frame scientific and technological issues as bio/ethical and to call for bio/ethics expertise to resolve dilemmas and controversies. See Lee, Jülich, and Dussauge, 'The Politics of Valuation'; Hedlund, 'Ethicisation and Reliance.'

documentation from court cases, medical publications, parliamentary records, patient journals, and media material, the authors all share a historicizing approach to their respective empirical domains. The epilogue draws together and discusses the central theme of fetal research and public controversy in light of recent academic and popular literature. Throughout the book a number of images and documents have been included to highlight arguments and provide historical evidence of Sweden's reproductive history, from early modern artists' creative copying of international anatomical masterpieces to the world-famous photographer Lennart Nilsson's pictures of human development in the twentieth century.

We demonstrate that the 'unborn' has been imbued with a multitude of conflicting meanings and values since early modern times. This also leads us to confirm Lynn Morgan's observation that embryos and fetuses need not be automatically or naturally associated with abortion. Rather, they have been materialized, mobilized, and negotiated over time in response to particular social and political issues and concerns.[12] And, crucially, abortion history differs between countries. In this book, we illuminate the historically specific conditions and interests—including relatively liberal abortion legislation and support from US funding—that promoted the emergence of research on living fetuses in the Swedish postwar period. The repercussions of this research were felt internationally in the early 1970s, as anti-abortion groups in several countries prepared for battle. Taken as a whole, our book highlights both continuities and discontinuities in the *longue durée* of the Swedish history of reproductive politics. Until now, no such broad study has existed.[13]

1 Histories of Fetal Knowledge Production

This volume builds on and engages with international historical research on reproduction, most of which focuses on western Europe and North America. This extensive literature examines pregnancy and the human fetus across the fields of history and also includes other disciplines such as sociology, anthropology, and archaeology.[14] Early on, feminist scholars set the agenda

12 Morgan, *Icons of Life*, 160.

13 Two source books with valuable introductions and commentaries (only available in Swedish) are Arnberg, Laskar, and Sundevall, *Sexualpolitiska nyckeltexter*, and Arnberg, Sundevall, and Tjeder, *Könspolitiska nyckeltexter*.

14 Recent collections include Hopwood, Flemming, and Kassell, *Reproduction*, and Han, Betsinger, and Scott, *Anthropology of the Fetus*.

for exploring reproductive politics, including the construction of fetal personhood and fetal rights at sites beyond anti-abortion propaganda, for instance ultrasound imagery and fetal surgery.[15] The authors of this book present key references in their respective chapters; this section provides a brief overview of historical narratives of the rise of human fetuses as objects of knowledge and research material for medical science—that is, fetal knowledge production.

The conventional history of midwifery in early modern European culture described a shift in authority concerning the maternal-fetal relationship, from the experiences and understanding of the pregnant woman to the definition and control of medical men. More recent scholarship has nuanced this story of the disempowerment of the birthing woman and the professional struggles over childbirth between female midwives and male obstetricians.[16] Importantly, as Rebecca Whiteley has demonstrated, midwives of both genders used printed manuals and images to introduce and communicate new modes of knowing, approaching, and treating pregnancy.[17] This knowledge was often adopted from anatomy to lend authority to their own professional status. However, anatomy was not always seen as an ideal point of reference, since it was associated with death and dissection, and primarily gave visual access to the interior, including the reproductive organs such as the uterus and the placenta. Midwifery, on the other hand, relied heavily on haptic knowledge of the living, pregnant body.[18]

We have several histories about the collecting of human fetuses for research, education, and display. A common starting point is the seventeenth-century Dutch anatomist Frederik Ruysch's ground-breaking technique for preparing and preserving infant and fetal bodies.[19] By the late eighteenth century, evidence shows that human fetal and infant cadavers were considered a valuable and unique source of knowledge about normal anatomical development as well as congenital abnormalities.[20] 'Beaded babies,' preparations of human

15 For historiographic discussions, see Morgan, *Icons of Life*, 24–28, and Olszynko-Gryn and Rusterholz, 'Reproductive Politics'; on the visual history, also see Björklund and Jülich, *Rethinking the Public Fetus*.

16 For historiographic discussions, see Al-Gailani and Davis, 'Introduction to "Transforming Pregnancy,"' Fissell, 'Man-Midwifery Revisited,' and Kosmin, *Authority, Gender, and Midwifery*, 4–6.

17 Whiteley, in *Birth Figures*, is instructive in relating her historical analysis to earlier scholarship.

18 Whiteley, 'Limits of Seeing,' 112–13. See also Park, *Secrets of Women*, and Donaghy, 'Secrets of the Placenta.'

19 For a recent account, see Ray, 'Monsters of Peter and Wolff.'

20 Dittmar and Piers, 'From Cradle to Grave.'

fetuses decorated with trading beads, were collected in the context of early Dutch colonial anatomy.[21] As demonstrated by Nick Hopwood and Lynn Morgan, nineteenth- and early twentieth-century German and American anatomists assembled collections of embryos and fetuses in order to study human development, evolutionary theory, and the relationship of humans to other species. These collections contained whole embryos and fetuses preserved in alcohol as well as sectioned specimens.[22]

Adele Clarke has shown how the reproductive sciences took off in the United States after 1910, including reproductive physiology, reproductive endocrinology, and gynecological and obstetric research. Britain made early contributions, and several major research centers were established in the interwar period.[23] Experimental methods spread across disciplines, and a few systematic studies of a larger number of human embryos and fetuses were conducted. Emily Watson has described the work of American neuroanatomist Davenport Hooker, who, between 1932 and 1958, produced film recordings of neurological tests on aborted fetuses.[24] The same abortion technique that Hooker used, small cesarean section through the vagina or abdomen, was employed by National Socialist scientists conducting coercive experiments on pregnant women and their fetuses, which were surgically removed from the uterus during abortions and sterilizations.[25]

From the beginning of the twentieth century, attempts were also made to use fetuses not as an object of study in itself but as material for the growth of living human tissues. In 1949 the American virologist John Enders and his research group managed to keep the polio virus alive and replicating in cultures of skin and muscle from aborted fetuses and other materials. As Hannah Landecker has demonstrated, human cell culture technologies became a standardized technique in biological research.[26] In addition, HeLa, the first human cell line, was established in the United States in 1951, when the Johns Hopkins researcher George Gey cultivated samples of a cervical tumor from Henrietta Lacks, without patient consent. Among other scientific achievements, these technologies provided scientists with means to develop a vaccine against polio.[27] Several scholars have explored how fetal tissues and cells have continued to be used for research and therapy in various national and international contexts. In

21 Hendriksen, 'Fate of the Beaded Babies.'

22 Hopwood, 'Producing Development'; Hopwood, *Haeckel's Embryos*; Morgan, *Icons of Life.*

23 Clarke, *Disciplining Reproduction*, 9, 69–74; Clarke, 'Research Materials,' 334–35.

24 Wilson, 'Ex Utero.'

25 Czarnowski and Hildebrandt, 'Research on the Boundary.'

26 Landecker, *Culturing Life*, 121–25.

27 Landecker, 161–62.

particular they have highlighted controversies surrounding the use of pre-implantation embryos from in vitro fertilization clinics in stem cell research since 1998.[28] Less work has been focused on aborted fetuses as another source for stem cell research. However, research conducted in the United Kingdom suggests that there exist important differences between 'embryonic economies' and 'fetal tissue economies,' for instance in the way women who undergo abortion are viewed as a different kind of donor—compensating for their risky sexual behavior—than couples undergoing IVF treatment.[29]

After World War II new strands of fetal experimentation developed, as the relationship between science, medicine, and public health was profoundly transformed. Research funding was one crucial agent that contributed to the growth of the 'biomedical complex' and the emergence of international fetal research.[30] According to Clarke, the postwar period experienced a shift in US sponsorship of reproductive and contraceptive research: from a landscape composed primarily of private and corporate philanthropy to one that included governmental as well as industrial funding.[31] Crucially, these funding agencies promoted international collaboration across disciplines, including endocrinology, gynecology, pediatrics, embryology, and genetics. First, they sponsored foreign fellowship programs that allowed researchers from all parts of the world to spend time at federal and private research locations. Second, they supported US scientists wishing to access training opportunities overseas that were not available within the United States. Third, they financed multidisciplinary conferences that stimulated the development of new research areas and specialized fields; for instance, prenatal research. Fourth, they funded reproductive and fetal research programs and centers in countries that were considered to have more favorable conditions for conducting this research.[32]

This postwar context is essential for understanding the emergence of specific strands of research on human fetuses and how this research provoked public controversy. Indeed, it was not until this period that the term 'fetal research' started to be used in official documents and in the media. According to the American public policy researcher Steven Maynard-Moody, fetal research emerged as an 'exciting field' in the 1960s, and by the early 1970s it was 'a hot scientific area' that included drug testing and the development of

28 Waldby and Mitchell, *Tissue Economies;* Gottweis, Salter, and Waldby, *Global Politics*; Svendsen and Koch, 'Unpacking the "Spare Embryo."'

29 Pfeffer and Kent, 'Framing Women, Framing Fetuses'; Kent, *Regenerating Bodies*, 119–22.

30 For discussions on this general transformation, see Quirke and Gaudillière, 'Era of Biomedicine,' and Löwy, 'Historiography of Biomedicine.'

31 Clarke, *Disciplining Reproduction*, 225–29.

32 Clarke. See also Dron, *Teratology Transformed.*

prenatal diagnosis as well as attempts to invent 'artificial placentas.' Researchers entered the field expecting that their careers would be distinguished by discoveries and major contributions to prenatal health. In 1973, after the *Roe v. Wade* ruling had stirred up abortion opposition, 'fetal research became controversial, federal funding withered and scientific excitement soured.'[33] Building on Maynard-Moody's discussion as well as official reports, Joanna Schoen gave a similar account in her book on US abortion practices and anti-abortion activism in the three following decades.[34]

The postwar period also saw the development of prenatal diagnosis. Historians have traced the rise of various biomedical technologies that made the living fetus an object of study. In the 1960s the genetic analysis of human cells, the improvement of amniocentesis, the detection of biochemical markers of fetal anomalies in maternal blood, and the invention of obstetric ultrasound paved the way for routine testing for birth defects during pregnancy. From the 1970s and onward, fetoscopy became available.[35] In the 1980s, as scholarship has also detailed, the new field of fetology, concerned with fetal surgery, started to define the 'fetal patient.' Together with other medical specialties such as perinatal medicine (the study of the fetus and the newborn), this development contributed to perceptions of the fetus as a vulnerable organism in need of protection, a theme that echoed in abortion debates.[36]

Despite this wealth of historical writing on fetal knowledge production, we still lack long-term perspectives and geographical diversity. Analyses of shorter periods dominate, as do perspectives from the major Atlantic democracies. We are also left wondering precisely when and how human fetal research stopped being 'hot' and became controversial. Duncan Wilson, in his book on the history of tissue culture in twentieth-century Britain, states that the practices for obtaining and using human tissues were seen by both professionals and the public as unproblematic for most of the period. It was not until the 1970s that controversy emerged, reflecting opposition against the liberalization of abortion laws. Moreover, Wilson argues that demands for informed consent were often raised by the scientists themselves.[37] This is a bold claim that I will revisit in the epilogue of this book.

33 Maynard-Moody, *Dilemma of the Fetus*, 6, 13. On the typology of fetal research, see also Ramsey, *Ethics of Fetal Research*, 21–25.

34 Schoen, *Abortion after* Roe, chap. 2.

35 Löwy, *Imperfect Pregnancies*. See also Blizzard, *Looking Within;* de Chadarevian, *Heredity under the Microscope*; Nicolson and Fleming, *Imaging and Imagining the Fetus*.

36 Casper, *Making of the Unborn Patient*; Dron, *Teratology Transformed*, 222–28. For fetal physiology, see Buklijas and Al-Gailani, 'Fetus in the World.'

37 Wilson, *Tissue Culture in Science and Society*.

2 The Book's Approaches and Themes

In this volume we use 'fetal knowledge production' as an umbrella term for various ways of coming to understand the 'unborn,' utilizing material from fetuses for scientific research or, more broadly, fabricating visions of fetal life and death. Our focus is on the human side of the story because we are especially interested in the historical links between medical frameworks, abortion, and controversy.[38] We highlight knowledge production that involved not only pregnant women and their fetuses but also entities that we know of today as gametes, zygotes, and embryos, as well as miscarriages and stillborn or newborn with fetal damages. This approach contributes to a fuller historical picture. However, we have not included the more recent history of in vitro fertilization and human embryo research, from the 1960s and onward, as this would have taken us on a slightly different route to public controversy.[39]

An overarching aim of this volume is then to historicize fetal knowledge production, reproductive politics, and conflicted values in Sweden. The authors have adopted diverse analytical strategies to achieve this goal. Even so, four themes consistently emerge in a number of chapters: conceptual issues, material and visual dimensions, the notion of controversy and value conflicts, and perspectives on policies, politics, and regulation.

A first theme that is common to several of the chapters is the historical contingency of meanings around pregnant bodies, fetuses, and newborn. In processes where 'the beginning of life' is at stake, it is likely that boundaries are established but also contested and negotiated.[40] As interdisciplinary scholarship has demonstrated, definitions of 'pregnancy,' 'humanness,' and 'personhood' vary between cultures and across time. Lynn Morgan, among others, has emphasized that in some cultures the unborn is deemed to become an infant not through biological attributes but rather through processes

38 See Svärd and Tinnerholm Ljungberg, 'Fetal and Animal Research,' for an analysis of the intersection of Swedish debates about animal and human fetal research in the 1960s and 1970s.

39 Current debates about national laws and guidelines that restrict this research extend well beyond the use of human embryos for generation of embryonic stem cells and genome editing of human embryos. The development of technologies for culturing human embryos in vitro up to fourteen days and the creation of 'embryoids' (stem cell–based embryo models) have led scientists and other actors to question the so-called fourteen-day limit, a rule which restricts research on human embryos after they reach a key point of complexity—the formation of the primitive streak. On this new policy landscape, including Swedish regulations, see Matthews and Moralí, 'National Human Embryo.'

40 Bauer and Wahlberg, *Contested Categories*.

of social recognition. Notions of who or what is considered to be 'human' or 'non-human' have also been open to change and contestation, as have definitions of normal or deviant, abled or disabled bodies.[41] Following this line of inquiry, this volume interrogates how concepts and classifications of human fetal life and death have been produced, reproduced, and questioned over a long period of time.

A second theme underlines that reproductive concepts, categories, and values are always linked to material and visual dimensions of pregnant and fetal bodies. As many studies in the wake of the material turn have shown, discourse cannot be detached from the world of concrete objects and mundane practices.[42] Bodies matter as well as the technologies and images used to materialize and communicate knowledge of fertility, pregnancy, delivery, and birth. In particular, we are interested in how the availability of human fetuses and fetal material conditioned the formation of academic disciplines, infrastructures, and networks as well as new scientific conceptions of pregnancy and reproductive health technologies.[43] In addition, building on earlier scholarship on medicine's visual culture, we are interested in how representations of fetuses and other reproductive phenomena were made, circulated, and used by multiple actors over the course of several centuries. In intricate ways, these activities contributed to the rise of 'the public fetus.'[44]

Third, a central theme deals with the role of controversies and value conflicts over fetal knowledge production. Following Adele Clarke, the reproductive area is viewed as especially exposed to political and moral disputes and claims of illegitimacy. Therefore, some authors trace scientists' strategies for managing their controversial status and addressing audiences and stakeholders. Full-fledged controversy—when social worlds collide, to use Clarke's phrase—may not always arise.[45] Some authors examine ignorance production and secrecy as a way of handling sensitive information in specific historical contexts.[46] Drawing on valuation studies, a new interdisciplinary field, several chapters stress the conflicting yardsticks or criteria used in

41 Lupton, *Social Worlds*, chap. 1; Morgan, 'When Does Life Begin?'

42 For an overview and discussion of this literature, see Guerrini, 'Material Turn.' Recent contributions include Ankele, and Majerus, *Material Cultures of Psychiatry*, and Nott and Harris, *Making Sense of Medicine*.

43 For conceptual discussions: Clarke, 'Research Materials'; Creager and Landecker, 'Technical Matters.'

44 See, among others, Björklund and Jülich, *Rethinking the Public Fetus*; Hopwood et al., 'Communicating Reproduction'; Olszynko-Gryn, Ellis, and Gainty, 'Reproduction on Film.'

45 Clarke, *Disciplining Reproduction*, 233–36.

46 Topçu and Maffi, 'Rethinking Ignorance Production.'

classifying pregnant bodies, miscarriages, and fetuses. Moreover, it is shown that researchers and authorities involved in fetal research tried to shift the focus from contested values around abortion to neutral scientific values and justify their activities in terms of the good of mankind. These efforts have affinities with what has been described as a 'moral economy,' a term that also crops up in the book.[47]

A fourth theme that is addressed in this volume revolves around the politics, policies, and regulations that shaped and were shaped by fetal knowledge production. The concept of biopolitics is used to chart a long view of Swedish reproductive history, from the population concerns of the early modern nation-state to the modern welfare state's support and care for all people.[48] In particular, we are interested in historical questions related to the ethical and legal regulation of the uses of aborted fetuses for research, vaccine production, and drug development. General path dependency has been shown to play an essential role in regulatory regimes. However, there are considerable differences between national approaches to the regulation of fetal research. These differences need to be understood in light of varying historical, political, religious, social, and cultural conditions.[49]

One last consideration unites the chapters that follow. As historians we need to make decisions concerning the use of historical terminology. This is especially difficult when it comes to words that are interwoven with highly politicized issues such as pregnancy, abortion, and fetal research. The authors of this book have chosen the vocabulary that they consider appropriate for their specific cases and source material. As editor I have encouraged them to be attentive to how concepts are defined historically in order to avoid anachronisms. We largely adopt the historical actors' language, even when this implies the use of terms that today are considered unacceptable, such as 'monsters,' or disputed, such as 'pregnant women' and 'she/he.' Terms like 'birth defects' and 'congenital malformations,' although by no means unproblematic, are still used in medical practice today.[50]

The historical terminology in the area of reproduction is indeed rich and varied. Swedish has borrowed many words from German, French, and English,

47 For an introduction to valuation studies, see Dussauge et al., 'On the Omnipresence.' On the notion of moral economy and its use by scholars in the history of science, see pp. 17–18.

48 For a helpful introduction, see Lemke, *Biopolitics*.

49 For this argument, see Jacobs and Tinnerholm Ljungberg, 'How Ethics Travels.'

50 For a similar discussion, see Björklund and Jülich, 'Rethinking the Public Fetus,' 20–21.

and shares a history of Latin usage.[51] A common term during early modern times was 'life fruit' (*livsfrukt*), which could mean 'fetus' as well as 'child' and 'offspring.' The word 'egg' (*ägg*) can also be traced far back in time, and it was sometimes used in combination with another word, meaning 'blighted ovum' (*ofostrigt ägg*), when a fertilized egg implants in the uterus but does not develop into an embryo. The first known use of 'embryo' (*embryonem, embryo*) is from 1578, whereas 'fetus' (*foster*) has been employed at least since 1613. Even if 'fetus' was used with increasing frequency, 'child' seems to be the more familiar term in early midwifery books. For centuries 'embryo' and 'fetus' were used interchangeably.[52] In his work on Swedish criminal law, published in 1906, the Swedish lawyer and member of a legislative commission Johan Hagströmer stated that in medical terminology, a distinction was often made between 'embryo' and 'fetus,' in that the latter term was considered applicable only when the human forms became distinguishable, but that this distinction was foreign to legislative language.[53]

Yet even embryologists were not always strict in their terminology. August Hammar repeatedly used 'fetus' for all stages of development, whereas Ivar Broman, in his embryological textbook of 1927, emphasized that some authors preferred to employ 'embryo for younger fetuses (before the 25–30-mm stage).'[54] Much later, the 1991 Governmental Commission report on the medical uses of tissues from aborted fetuses indicated that from the eighth week of gestation there was strong growth and a further development of tissues and organs; in effect 'the embryo has become a fetus.' Nonetheless, the members of the commission stated that 'fetus' was to be used for all stages of human development in the report.[55] This may have been done for practical reasons, but imprecise language could also be used for political purposes. The Swedish anti-abortion movements, following their US and British counterparts, insisted that embryos and fetuses were 'unborn children.'[56]

51 For a helpful history of important terms, see Hopwood, 'Keywords "Generation" and "Reproduction."'

52 For the etymology of these words, see *Svenska Akademiens ordbok*, and the chapters in this book.

53 Thornstedt, 'The Beginning and the End,' 230. In fact, current Swedish legislation does not define 'embryo' but instead uses the term 'fertilized egg.' Since this characterization does not apply to 'embryoids,' research on them is permitted. See Matthews and Moralí, 'National Human Embryo,' 1910–11.

54 Hammar, *Några huvuddrag av fosterutvecklingen;* Broman, *Människans utveckling före födelsen*, 112.

55 Swedish Ministry of Health and Social Affairs, *Aborterade foster*, 25.

56 See Björklund's chapter in this volume, and her 'Contested Pictures of Persuasion.'

3 Population Policies and Concerns

This volume's fourteen chapters and the epilogue address more than 500 years of Swedish reproductive history. It starts with a chapter on early modern birth intervention strategies and ends with a chapter that deals with the regulation of prenatal diagnosis in the late twentieth century. In between, we have contributions showcasing the activities of many actors and various aspects involved in the uses and definitions of fetuses, stillborn, reproductive organs, and pregnant bodies. Although we engage with the long-term of fetal knowledge production, the emphasis is on the period after World War II. Therefore, the remaining part of the introduction will provide historical context for the volume as a whole, along the way highlighting and synthesizing the individual chapters as well as contributors' work published elsewhere. The current section gives a brief overview of Swedish population concerns and issues from the Lutheran Reformation to the welfare state.

Sweden was founded as a modern nation-state in the sixteenth century. Gustav Vasa initiated the Reformation that made it a Lutheran Protestant country. From 1560 wars were fought repeatedly with Denmark to gain control over the Baltic region. In the middle of the seventeenth century Sweden rose to the status of a great power in northern Europe, after the intervention of Gustav II Adolf on the side of the German Protestants in the Thirty Years' War. Following years of constant conflict, disease, and famine, the country lost its preeminence at the end of the Great Northern War in 1721. As a result of the outcome of the Finnish war in 1809, the eastern third of Sweden was established as the Grand Duchy of Finland within the Russian empire. As compensation for this loss, Norway was forced into a union with Sweden in 1814. This union was peacefully dissolved in 1905.[57]

During the reforms of the sixteenth century, Gustav Vasa confiscated the estates of the church, including care facilities and charitable institutions. Thereafter, the overall responsibility for health care lay with the royal administration. An important step toward a central authority occurred in 1663, when a group of university-trained physicians based in Stockholm founded the Collegium Medicum. This private corporation was engaged by the royal administration to tighten up the regulation of health services and exert some control over other health occupations. Its authority was not accepted without protests from the surgeons' guild. The conflict between physicians and surgeons was finally settled when in 1796 the Surgical Society merged with the Collegium Medicum,

57 Kent, *A Concise History of Sweden*, chap. 3–4, 153.

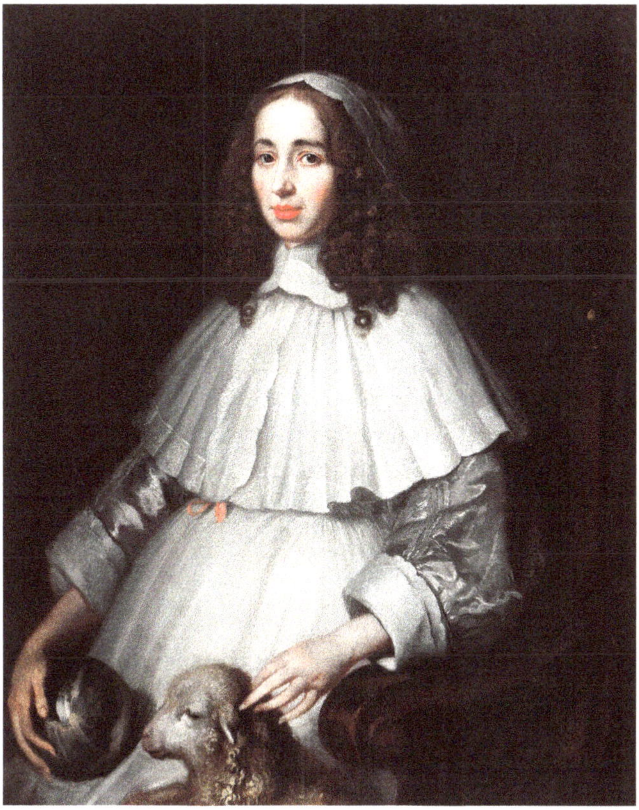

FIGURE 0.1
Portraits of pregnant women in early modern Sweden were quite rare. This image portrays Anna Margareta von Haugwitz, who was married to Carl Gustaf Wrangel, a statesman and field marshal who commanded Swedish forces in the Thirty Years' War, among others. They had eleven children together, of whom six died very young. She is holding the lamb and globe, which were symbols of Christian devotion and eternity. Oil painting by the Swiss artist Matthaeus Merian the Younger around 1650. Skokloster Castle.

further strengthening the collegium's position and influence within the state and in health care. In 1813 it became an administrative government agency under the name of the College of Health (later National Board of Medicine and National Board of Health and Welfare). Around the same time, the Swedish Medical Association and the KI, which took over responsibility for medical education from the Collegium Medicum, were established.[58]

During the seventeenth and eighteenth centuries, as elsewhere in Europe, mercantilism became the dominant economic policy of the Swedish state, and several initiatives were launched for stimulating export trade and domestic production. A growing population was considered of vital importance for the wealth of the nation, although the primary concern was not for the people themselves but for the work they performed. To regain Sweden's strength and increase its population, the state and the Collegium Medicum took measures

58 Carlhed, 'Rise of the Professional Field,' 3–5.

to expand health care, build lying-in hospitals and orphanages, and invest in training physicians, obstetric surgeons, and midwives. In addition, information about infant care, infection control, and preventive health care was distributed to audiences through printed media and other channels.[59]

In the eighteenth century the penalties for infanticide and abortion were tightened. Sweden, like many other countries in Europe, introduced a presumption—a reversed burden of proof—whereby an unmarried woman whose newborn died was suspected of having killed her child. If she had been alone at the time of birth, hid the child, and it was then found dead, the woman would be sentenced for infanticide and executed unless she could prove that the child was stillborn or had died a natural death. For a long time, abortion had been considered a less severe crime or not a crime at all if it happened before quickening, when the first movements of the fetus were felt. However, in 1688, a medicinal order forbade apothecaries and grocers to sell

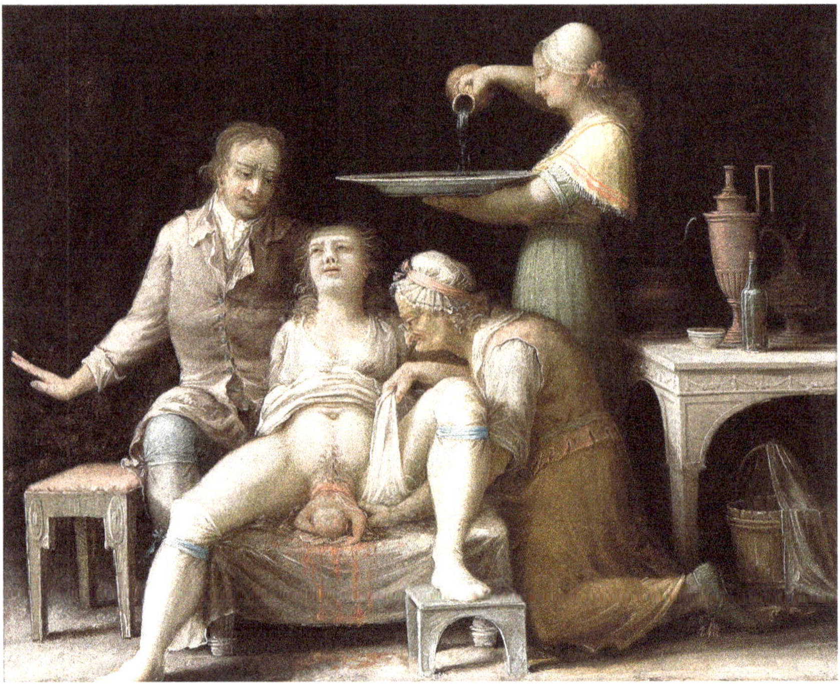

FIGURE 0.2 An extraordinary birth scene presumably in Åbo, Sweden (subsequently Turku in Finland) around 1800. On the left of the woman giving birth is the father, to the right a caricature of a midwife. The figure pouring water into a bowl may be a maid preparing to wash the child or perhaps the personification of the goddess Hygeia. Oil painting by unknown artist. CC BY-NC 4.0. Wellcome Collection.

59 Johannisson, 'The People's Health.'

abortifacients except to physicians. Similarly, midwives had to take an oath to never contribute to 'miscarriage.' Through the Civil Code of 1734, the first to apply to all of Sweden, the death penalty was introduced for abortion. No consideration was given to the length of the pregnancy or to the presence or absence of signs that the fetus was alive. The law was based on the opinion of a member of the Collegium Medicum that the 'fetus' was alive immediately after conception. Thus Protestant Sweden adopted stricter abortion legislation than several other parts of Europe, including Catholic countries.[60]

In practice, however, the laws were not strictly implemented. Moreover, the penalties for both infanticide and abortion were lightened from the late eighteenth century onward. Wanting to rule as an enlightened despot, Gustav III also issued the Infanticide Act of 1778, which made it possible for women to give birth anonymously and without public disgrace. In 1864 the death penalty for abortion was replaced with penal labor for two to six years, for both the woman seeking to terminate a pregnancy and the abortion provider. A reform in 1921 replaced the penal labor with a shorter term in prison for the woman, but kept the original penalty for the provider.[61]

In 1749, as part of Sweden's mercantilist policy, a system for national population statistics (the Office for Tabulation) was founded on the initiative of the Royal Swedish Academy of Sciences. As described in Maja Bondestam's chapter in this volume, the ground had already been prepared through the Church Law of 1686, which ordered parishes across the country to start keeping records on the population. This law had also made the clergy responsible for annual tax registration, and the church's existing organizational structure facilitated the collection of population data. Every parish had to register the members of all families, and the records were to cover births, including 'monstrous birth' and stillbirths, baptisms, marriages, deaths, and migration. The clergy compiled parish records and sent them to Stockholm for further statistical compilation. After a few years, in 1756, the Tabulation Commission, the first statistical agency in the world and the predecessor of today's Statistics Sweden, was established.[62] Bondestam argues that this interest in the lives and deaths of the population signaled the rise of Swedish biopolitics.

In the early nineteenth century, the population theory of Thomas Robert Malthus was introduced in Sweden. He argued that population growth, especially among the poor, would surpass a nation's available resources unless

---

60 Kumlien, *Finns det ett kristet synsätt*, 21–25. The member of the Collegium Medicum was the physician and anatomist Magnus von Bromell. See Bergenlöv, *Skuld och oskuld*, 396.

61 Kumlien, *Finns det ett kristet synsätt*, 26–27.

62 In addition to Bondestam's chapter, see Sköld, 'Birth of Population Statistics.'

kept down by either positive or preventive checks. Positive (nonfavorable) checks included death by disease, starvation, and war, which was the fate of many of the European populations in the eighteenth and nineteenth centuries. Preventive checks included celibacy and chastity, but also contraception, which Malthus condemned as morally indefensible along with infanticide, abortion, and adultery. Malthus used Norway and Sweden as two different models, drawing on observations and personal interviews from a Scandinavian trip as well as Swedish population statistics. He praised Norway's management of its population and natural resources. Sweden, on the other hand, was prone to positive population checks due to an efficient system of agriculture and the state's tendency to waste money on promoting public health. Unsurprisingly, not everyone accepted Malthus's claims, but few seem to have questioned the statistical evidence.[63]

In contrast to Malthus, neo-Malthusians in the late nineteenth and early twentieth centuries supported the use of contraception. The Uppsala student Knut Wicksell, later a well-known economist, argued in the 1880s that overpopulation in Sweden was the cause of poverty, alcoholism, a declining marriage rate, many illegitimate children, prostitution, and infanticide. Extensive emigration was associated with this problematic picture, since it meant the loss of able-bodied individuals. The solution that Wicksell proposed was that society, primarily physicians, should educate women so that they would have no more than two or three children.[64] But sexuality and sexual morals were a controversial topic at the time, discussed in newspapers, magazines, novels, and theatrical plays. The early women's movement did not have a unified position in this public debate.[65] Between 1910 and 1937 it was illegal to provide knowledge publicly about—but not to use—contraceptives. By 1937 the Swedish Association for Sexuality Education had spent several years campaigning for the right to contraception and sex education. Sweden became the first country in the world to make sex education compulsory in schools in 1955.[66]

Eugenic ideas were introduced in the Scandinavian countries during the decades around 1900, drawing on German, British, and US sources. Sweden, Denmark, and Norway went through a period of rapid modernization, with expanding industries, urban growth, and political democratization. Increasingly, class tensions, urban slums, and poverty were matters of concern. Birth rates declined dramatically, as the middle and upper classes shrank and the numbers of poor residents grew. This phenomenon was often interpreted as a

63 Dolan, 'Malthus's Political Economy of Health,' 13, 21–27.
64 Hedenborg, 'En alltför stor befolkning.'
65 Tjeder, 'Mellan utlevelse och kyskhet.'
66 Lennerhed, 'Taking the Middle Way,' 55–70.

sign of degeneration, caused by racial mixing as well as environmental factors. Across the political spectrum and among leading archaeologists, anatomists, and geneticists, eugenics was regarded as a solution to these complex societal problems. Moreover, Nordic nationalism promoted racial concepts such as the 'pure Nordic race.' In 1922, the State Institute for Race Biology was founded, following a decision by the Swedish Parliament. Initially, research projects charted racial traits of the Swedish population, especially the Sami minority in northern Sweden, measuring and photographing adults as well as children.[67] Racial studies persisted, but from the mid-1930s population genetics came into focus. The State Institute for Race Biology was reorganized and became the Department of Medical Genetics at Uppsala University in 1959.[68]

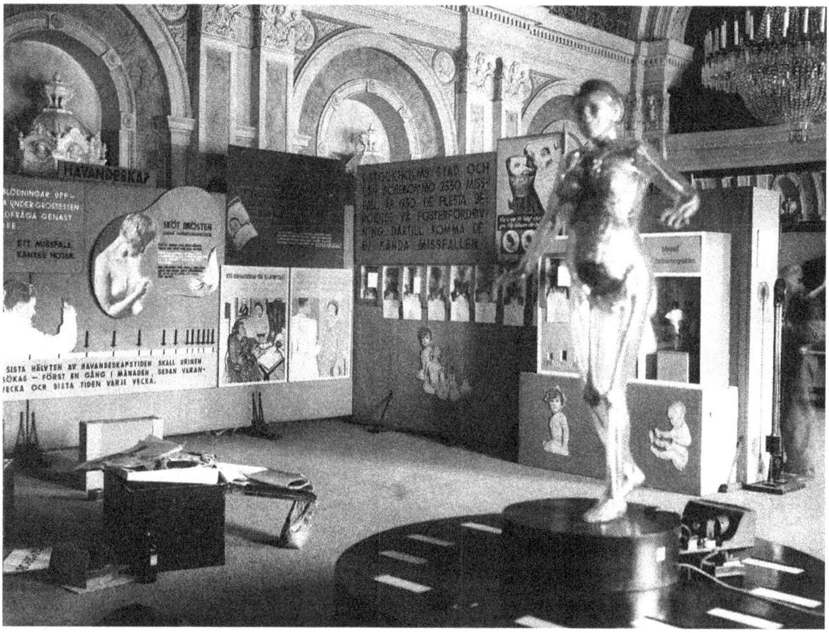
HAVANDESKAP
SKÖT BRÖSTEN
SISTA HÄLVTEN AV HAVANDESKAPSTIDEN SKALL URINEN
SÖKAS — FÖRST EN GÅNG I MÅNADEN, SEDAN VARAN-
VECKA OCH SISTA TIDEN VARJE VECKA.

FIGURE 0.3 The *Mother and Child* exhibition at Malmö City Hall (in southern Sweden) in 1936. This traveling exhibition was organized by the Swedish Red Cross and revolved around the 'population issue,' promoting the popularization of eugenics. To the right, the 'Transparent Woman,' a counterpart to the 'Transparent Man,' illuminated anatomical models built at the German Hygiene Museum in Dresden. In the background are exhibits on the importance of breastfeeding (*left*) and the severe risks associated with illegal abortion operations (*right*). Photo: Otto Ohm. Copyright Historisk Bildbyrå.

67 Björkman and Widmalm, 'Selling Eugenics'; Tydén, 'Scandinavian States.'

68 Tydén, 'Scandinavian States'; Ericsson, 'What Happened to "Race."'

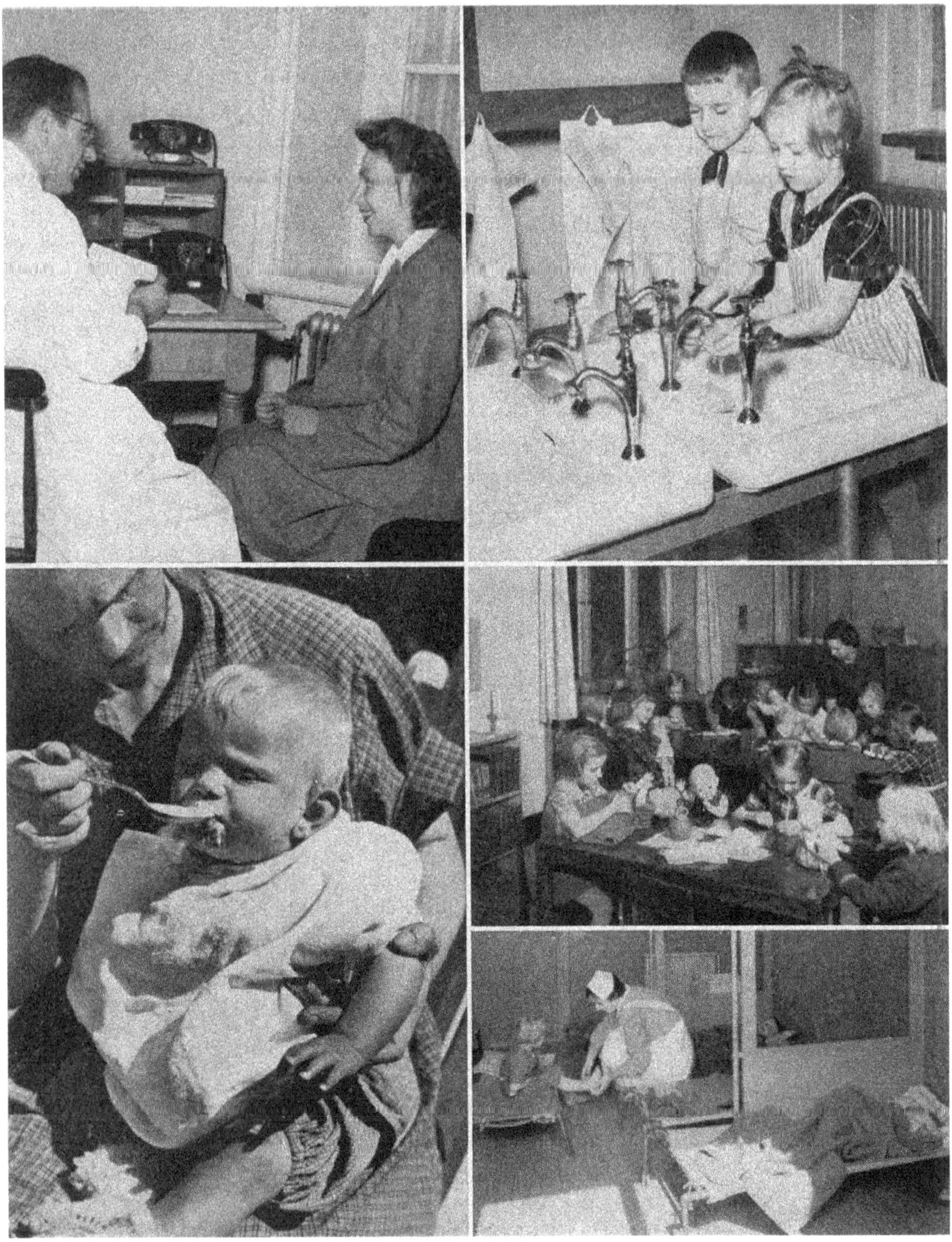

FIGURE 0.4 Page from a propaganda brochure about abortion and pregnancy demonstrating the welfare state's support of women who decide to give birth to children. *Top left:* the mother to be on a free visit to the maternity care center. The other images show scenes from a day-care center that has been established to help working women. Unknown photographer. From Asklund and Lundberg, *Havandeskap, samhällets hjälp, abort*, 12–13. Published with permission from the National Board of Health and Welfare.

The Social Democratic party came to dominate Swedish politics from 1932. In the following decades, they initiated a series of social and economic welfare reforms, including social security, general health insurance, and expanding the pension system. The 1930s and 1940s are considered the beginning of the Swedish welfare state (see figure 0.4). The state's approach to reproductive issues also changed. A law that allowed sterilization of the 'insane' was pushed through in 1934 and was significantly expanded in a few years. Abortion was a central concern, as many women died after seeking illegal abortion. In 1938 an Abortion Act was introduced, which permitted abortion on medical, eugenic, and humanitarian grounds: if the woman's life was in danger, if there was risk of hereditary disease, or if the pregnancy was the result of rape or incest. An abortion granted on eugenic grounds was to be combined with sterilization. This measure resulted in a substantial number of women being sterilized during the 1940s and 1950s. The Abortion Act was amended less than a decade later, in 1946, to allow abortions on socio-medical grounds. This meant that if the birth of a child was expected to negatively impact a woman, physically or mentally, an abortion could be permitted.[69]

Throughout this period, controversy surrounded the abortion issue. Opposition often came from conservatives but did not always align with party-political patterns. It could also be a matter of religious belief. Many Christians—members of the dominant Evangelical Lutheran state church as well as minor Protestant denominations—reacted against the socio-medical indication, even though they accepted eugenic abortion and medical abortion when pregnancy threatened a woman's life. Bishops and priests mobilized in the battle against abortion, and they were joined by some prominent physicians, using visual propaganda. As Solveig Jülich has shown elsewhere, photographer Lennart Nilsson contributed photographs of aborted fetuses to anti-abortion campaigns in 1950s Sweden (figure 0.5). A decade later, in 1965, he won international acclaim for his story 'Drama of Life before Birth' in the American magazine *Life*. By then Nilsson's images had started to be used as sex-education aids in Swedish schools, and he no longer expressed negative views of abortion.[70]

Sweden maintained an image of neutral politics during the Second World War, and thereafter neutrality became a foundation of Swedish foreign policy. This 'myth of neutrality' was also used as a way of positioning and legitimizing government-sponsored high-tech industry in Sweden in an international

69 Ramsey, *Swedish Abortion Pill*, 42–45. Compulsory sterilizations in connection with abortion operations were carried out until 1975.

70 Jülich, 'Picturing Abortion Opposition.'

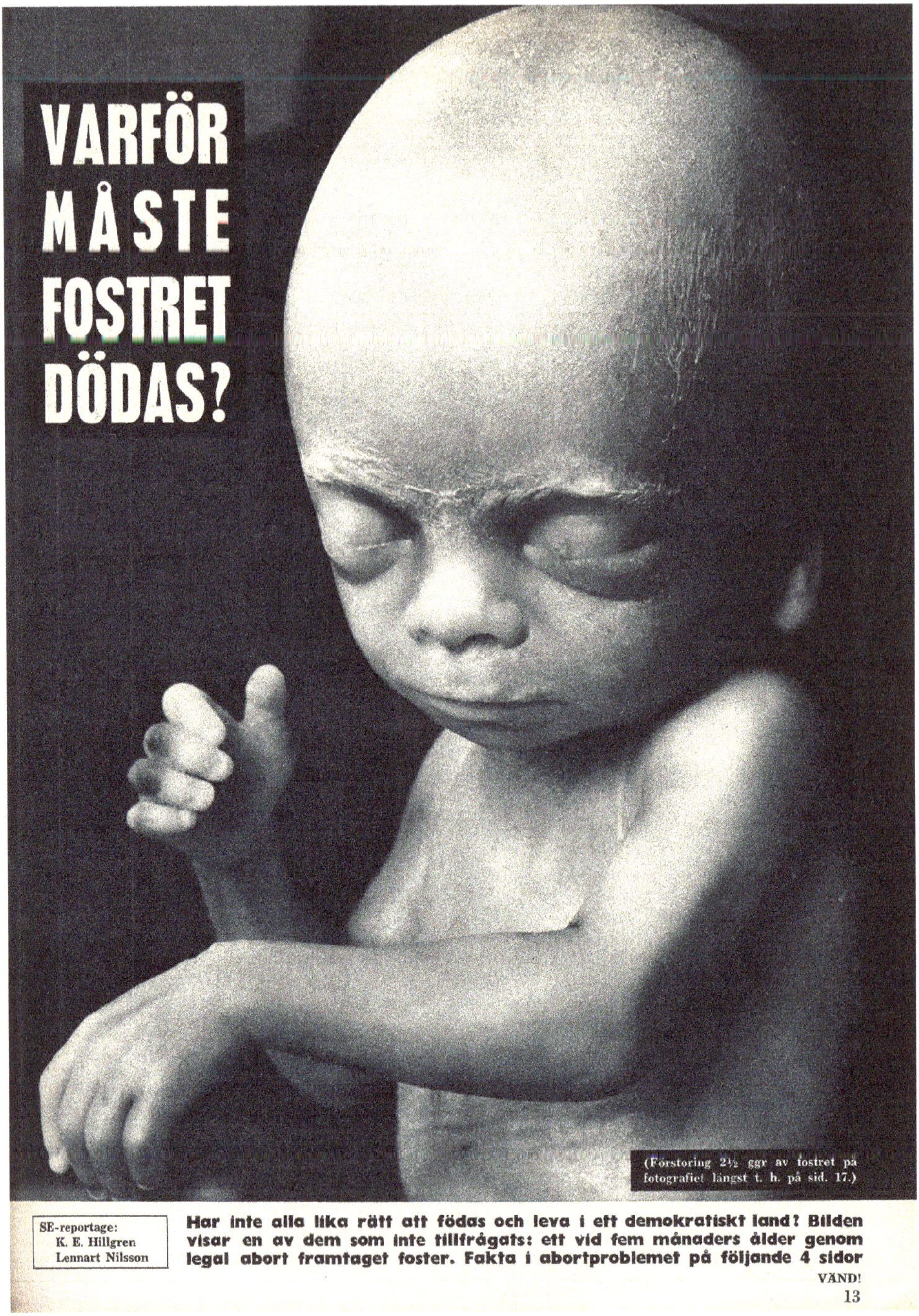

FIGURE 0.5 Photograph by Lennart Nilsson in an abortion-critical report in the popular magazine *Se* (See) in 1952. The caption reads: 'Does not everyone have the same right to be born and live in a democratic country? The picture shows one of those who was not asked: a fetus extracted during legal abortion at the age of five months.' From Hillgren and Nilsson, 'Varför måste fostret dödas?,' 13. Courtesy of Lennart Nilsson Photography/SPL.

context (e.g., research in atomic energy).[71] In the same vein, medical research was strengthened by the government's decision to establish the Medical Research Council in 1945 as well as by extensive economic support from the Rockefeller Foundation, the Ford Foundation, and other US funding agencies. The KI in Stockholm, the medical university and home of the medical Nobel assembly, was a major beneficiary of these grants.[72] During the 1950s the media promoted a strong faith in science, medicine, and technology, emphasizing the role of breakthroughs and individual heroic achievements. As time went by this approach would change, even if journalists' dependence on medical sources still limited their ability to offer criticism or independent analyses concerning the risks and negative effects of medical research, therapeutics, and drugs.[73]

In 1962, a public outcry followed media reports that women who had taken the drug thalidomide (in Swedish, Neurosedyn) during pregnancy had later given birth to children with severe deformities of limbs and other organs. It was revealed that the National Board of Medicine (from 1968 the National Board of Health and Welfare) already had information about the risks in November 1961 and stopped the sale of the drug but did not launch a campaign to warn the public; doing so would have stirred anxiety in pregnant women, according to the director general. After the fact, a number of measures were taken, including an amendment of the Abortion Act in 1963 that added fetal damage as grounds for abortion, as well as the establishment of a new regulatory framework for the clinical testing of new drugs.[74] As explored by Francis Lee in this volume, the scandal also stimulated the emergence of 'surveillance medicine' in Sweden. To prevent a new medically induced tragedy, the Swedish Register of Congenital Malformations was founded as an early warning system in the mid-1960s. Housed at the Tornblad Institute of Comparative Embryology at Lund University, this institution built on Sweden's long tradition of registering the population and joined a new international movement toward the surveillance of birth defects. In her chapter, Maria Björkman addresses tensions in the rehabilitation program launched by Swedish authorities in the years following the scandal. It aimed at normalization—expecting that the affected children should be able to live as normally as possible with the help of prosthetic technology. Nonetheless, it gradually became evident that existing devices were

71 Lundin and Stenlås, 'Technology, State Initiative,' 3, 8.

72 Ramsey, *Swedish Abortion Pill*, 53, 59.

73 Nordlund, *Hormones of Life*, 124; Jülich, 'Fosterexperimentens produktiva hemlighet,' 14.

74 Björkman's chapter in this volume.

inadequate for this goal. Björkman argues that the conflict between what constituted a normal body and thalidomide-affected people's 'own normal' was characteristic of the biopolitics of the Swedish welfare state.[75]

The thalidomide scandal and the shocking images of 'thalidomide babies' circulated by the media in the 1960s may have created public mistrust in pharmaceutical science and medicine. But it was also used as an argument to legitimize more scientific research on female reproductive and fetal bodies. Science continued to be an essential component of the Swedish welfare state's approach to governance, as did strategies for controlling sensitive information and maintaining ignorance. But before diving into the specificities of postwar fetal research, the next section will probe into the emergence of the fetus as an object of study along with the establishment of obstetrics, embryology, and teratology as scientific fields.

4 The Emergence of the Fetus as an Object of Knowledge

During the early modern period a shared academic culture emerged in Europe, as anatomists, physicians, and midwives disseminated knowledge in letters and printed works. Obstetrical and embryological images were an important part of this knowledge production. The womb was portrayed as a hidden and mysterious place containing the secrets of life before birth. Birth figures, showing fetuses in various positions and movements, had been produced before but became increasingly important in vernacular midwifery manuals as well as surgeons' treatises. From the last decades of the seventeenth century, a naturalistic and highly detailed style of representing the fetus *in utero* was developed in anatomical illustrations commissioned by authors versed in scholarly knowledge. Through physical circulation and processes of translation and copying, many of these printed texts and images, which were originally produced in Germany, Britain, France, Italy, Spain, and the Netherlands, enabled individuals in these countries to contribute to each other's culture of pregnancy and childbirth.[76]

Sweden, which had few formally educated medical practitioners and sent its limited group of students abroad, had little to offer to this transnational academic culture. Most medical books in Swedish were translations, and the images copied from foreign works. Yet these processes brought new elements

75 See also Björkman, 'Cost of Normalization.'

76 Whiteley, 'Limits of Seeing,' 95–97. For the fuller argument, see also Whiteley, *Birth Figures*.

to the representation and framing of medical knowledge. For instance, in 1578 Benedictus Olai, who had (possibly) acquired a medical doctorate at Wittenburg and was court physician to Erik XIV and later Johan III, published a medical handbook largely based on German and Danish sources, including Henrik Smid's popular *Laegebok* (1557).[77] In the preface Olai nonetheless emphasized that the selection of advice and treatments, many dealing with diseases of women and small children, was especially fitted for the Nordic country.[78] Moreover, the book included a woodcut of Sweden's national coat of arms with a wild man and a wild woman as supporters. A similar woodcut, itself resembling the central motif of rival Denmark's coat of arms, had appeared in the Gustav Vasa Bible, the first complete Swedish translation of the Scriptures.

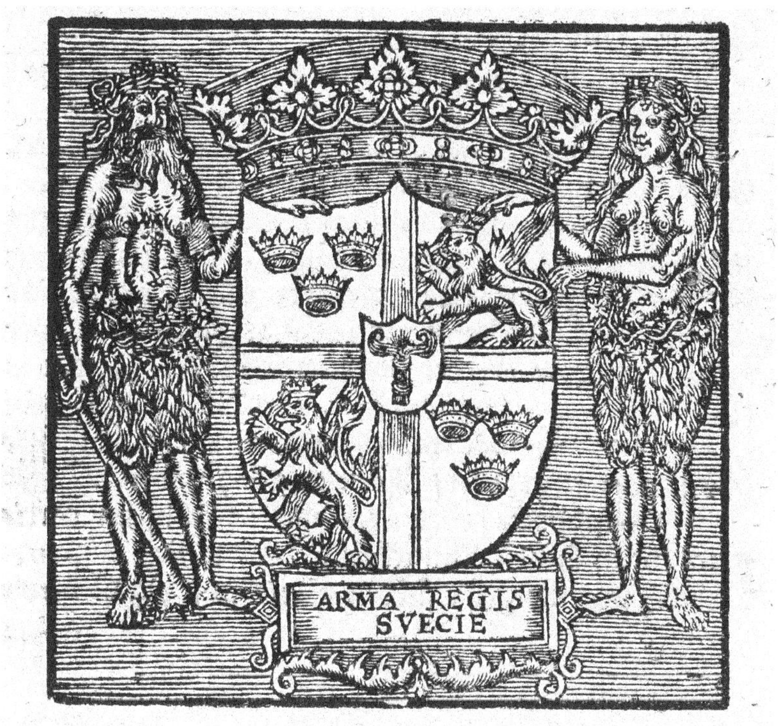

FIGURE 0.6 The wild couple, perhaps Adam and Eve in Gothic disguise, holding the royal coat of arms in the first medical book published in Swedish—a complex symbol of fecundity, descent, and territorial power. Woodcut by unknown artist. From Olai, *Een Nyttigh Läkere Book*, n.p. Uppsala University Library.

77 Håkansson, 'Den lärda världen,' 135–39. On Olai, see also Hult, 'Benedictus Olai.'
78 Olai, *Een Nyttigh Läkere Book*.

Commonly interpreted as a symbol or even a talisman of fecundity, the wild couple in Olai's book also alluded to the popular historiography of Sweden as the origin of the Goths. Building on this myth, the Vasa monarchs held that their reign could be traced back to Magog in the Old Testament. In this way, medicine and the emergent national state were symbolically aligned with each other during Sweden's great-power period.[79]

In the late seventeenth and eighteenth centuries academic medicine started to develop in Sweden. What remained constant, however, was the lack of dead human bodies for medical education and knowledge production. As elsewhere, anatomical study through dissection was fraught with ambiguity. In popular and Christian beliefs, the practice of dissection was a desecration of the dead body. Authorities, on the other hand, justified it as a means of advancing medical and surgical training for the benefit of all people in society. The ever-increasing demand for cadavers for use in anatomical investigations and study at universities, medical schools, and private courses exceeded the supply. Over time, new categories of dead bodies were made available by legislation, including those of executed criminals and members of socially vulnerable groups. Anatomists' access to fetuses that had died during pregnancy or stillbirth was, however, not regulated in law.[80]

In Stockholm around 1700, the Collegium Medicum organized anatomical demonstrations, some of which were open to the public. One of its members was the obstetrical surgeon Johan von Hoorn, who had studied medicine abroad in Leiden, Amsterdam (with the anatomist Frederik Ruysch), and Paris. He regularly performed dissections of the bodies of deceased pregnant women, as well as forensic examinations of dead and stillborn infants. Materials from these dissections formed the basis of a collection of anatomical specimens and models that he used in lectures and the private teaching of midwives.[81] Given the strong opposition toward human dissection at the time, it was no doubt of crucial importance to actively hide certain aspects of this activity and emphasize others. In addition, the female reproductive organs and childbearing were highly sensitive topics.

Feelings of shame and modesty often required male physicians to secure permission from their patients before undertaking physical examination, and these emotions and attitudes also affected writings about pregnancy and childbirth.[82]

79 Olai, n.p. On the woodcut in Gustav Vasa's Bible, see Collijn, 'Postscript,' 13–14; on wild men in Scandinavian heraldry, see Bartholdy, 'De danske kongers skjoldholdere'; on Gothicism, see Håkansson, 'Den lärda världen,' 120–24.

80 Åhrén, *Death, Modernity and the Body*, 19–24; Paulsson Holmberg, *Onaturlig födelse*, 152–55.

81 Paulsson Holmberg, *Onaturlig födelse*, 84–87, 156–61.

82 Paulsson Holmberg, 156, 171–73.

As elaborated by Tove Paulsson Holmberg elsewhere, von Hoorn used several strategies to steer the processes of reading and communication. First, several of his books begin with a preface, an epigram, or tribute poem, in which the disinterested and respectable character of the author is stressed. For instance, his colleague Johan Linder ascribes to the author of *Anatomes Publicae* (von Hoorn's work on embryology; 1709) 'a mind as pure as the snow of the northern mountains.'[83] Second, he is cautious when it comes to language. Publishing *Anatomes Publicae* in Latin was a strategic choice. It narrowed the audience to his peers, and von Hoorn could be more extensive in his descriptions, owing to the fact that the Latin names of the genitals were already accepted, while the corresponding Swedish words would appear 'ugly' or 'not recommended through any use by decently speaking people.' Third, the books were sparsely illustrated, not only for economic reasons. One plate in the obstetric manual *Den Swenska Wäl-öfvade Jord-Gumman* shows the uterus in cross-section with the cervix and vagina but, 'to escape annoyance as much as possible,' the author refrained from describing the external female genitalia. Like most engravings in printed medical books at this time, it had been copied from foreign sources.[84]

Contrasting views of how to understand the life and death of the unborn were held in early modern theology, medicine, and law. The clergy, on the one hand, assumed that the fetus was alive and ensouled at the moment of conception. Unlike Catholicism, which demanded that the fetus be born and baptized in order to be saved, Lutheranism held that it was possible to save the fetus through intercession prayers. The scientific position on the beginning of life was in flux. Many physicians claimed that the crucial time was when the pregnant woman felt the fetus move inside, 'quickening.'[85] Around 1700, the increasing success of the theory that a preformed embryo simply started to grow after fecundation bolstered supporters of early ensoulment. While the tradition of late ensoulment in the Catholic Church supported tolerance toward abortive practices, the Lutheran doctrine was harsher. As mentioned earlier, with the Civil Code of 1734, Protestant Sweden adopted the conception theory and introduced the death penalty for abortion at any stage of pregnancy.[86]

Yet, as suggested by Tove Paulsson Holmberg in this volume, the complex interplay between religion and medicine could foster a more utilitarian stance. The emphasis in Lutheran contexts on the significance of securing (at least)

---

83 Paulsson Holmberg, 176–77. In fact, von Hoorn was not the sole author of *Anatomes Publicae*, since at least some editions contain a section by Lars Roberg at the end.

84 Paulsson Holmberg, *Onaturlig födelse*, 177–79. The engraved plate originated from Siegemund, *Die Chur-Brandenburgische*.

85 See the chapters by Paulsson Holmberg and Runesson in this volume.

86 Kumlien, *Finns det ett kristet synsätt*, 21–26.

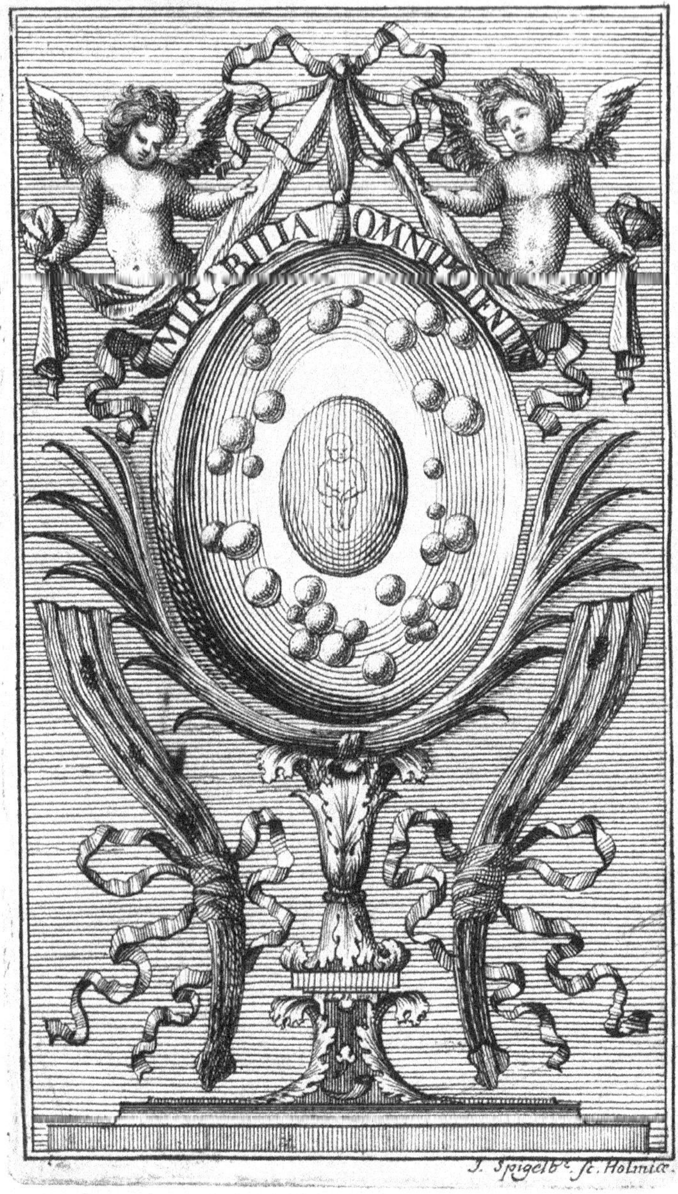

FIGURE 0.7 Preformationism visualized in a Swedish treatise on embryology. The homunculus inside the human egg had been copied from Portal, *La pratique des accouchemens*, 367. Frontispiece engraved by Johan Spiegelberg in von Hoorn, *Anatomes Publicae*. Hagströmer Library, KI.

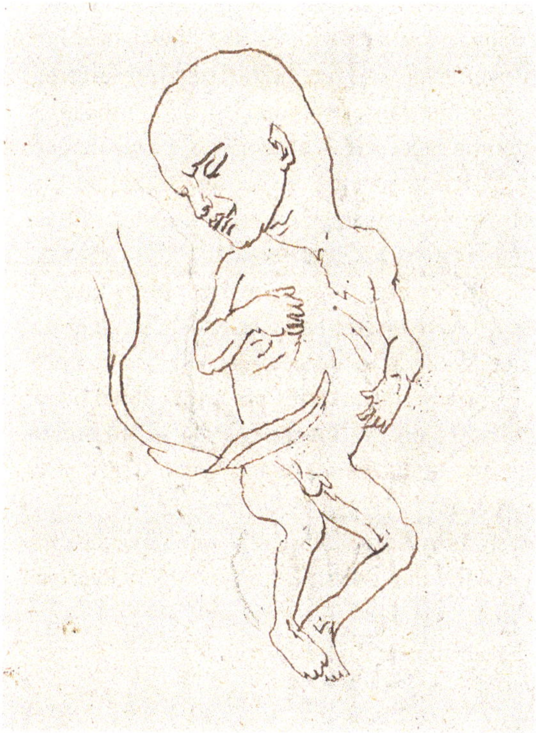

FIGURE 0.8
A picture of a male fetus with umbilical cord that often has been attributed to the Uppsala anatomy professor Lars Roberg, the teacher of Carl Linnaeus, but was sketched from Bidloo, *Anatomia Humani Corporis*, Pl. 57. The more naturalistic style that characterized Bidloo's atlas sheds light on the fact that this fetus is very dissimilar to Portal's homunculus in *Anatomes Publicae*, a treatise that Roberg contributed to. The drawing is preserved in the special collections of Uppsala University Library. Digital Source: Alvin, http://urn.kb.se/resolve?urn=urn:nbn:se:alvin:portal:record-100176 (accessed 2024-01-18).

temporary survival for newborns, and the simultaneous acceptance of the prospect of divine intervention in cases of unavoidable perinatal loss, contributed to a mental framework that encouraged the pragmatic termination of dangerous pregnancies when the life of the woman was in peril. Moreover, by drawing on court cases of suspected infanticides, Anton Runesson's contribution to this volume highlights the conflicting standards of valuation that underpinned definitions and practices of miscarriage and prematurely born children between 1600 and 1750. These sources show that fetuses were often classified as ensouled at a later stage of gestation than has been presumed in historical scholarship on 'quickening.' According to Runesson, this demonstrates that women who miscarried and handled the products of miscarriage, as well as honorable women serving as expert witnesses at the courts, embraced conceptions of the unborn that differed from those of legal, theological, and medical men.

Increasingly, physicians and obstetric surgeons such as von Hoorn were called in to assist lawyers and judges at the courts, and forensic medicine was established as a field of knowledge. Monstrous births posed a particular challenge in defining what constituted humanness, as discussed by Bondestam in this volume. For some eighteenth-century naturalists and physicians, fetuses and newborn with an excess or shortage of limbs, an animal's head, or other unexpected features were seen as wondrous and rare bodies that transgressed boundaries between the species. As in the court cases described in Runesson's chapter, these observations created the need for definitions. The well-shaped head was considered to be the physical mark of the soul and therefore the distinguishing sign of humanness. Around 1800, as Bondestam demonstrates, the category of monster disappeared from forensic medicine and civil law. Instead, viability, the capacity of the newborn to live on, was foregrounded in the emergent Swedish biopolitics. What had been a scientific fascination with monstrous births became the new field teratology (literally, 'the science of monsters'), producing new categories and standards of the dis/abled body. This history is echoed in Lee's chapter on the practical struggles to create standardized medical knowledge and statistics for the Swedish Register of Congenital Malformations in the 1960s.

Modeled on German forerunners, embryology, along with teratology, emerged as a specialized field of research in early nineteenth-century Sweden. Even so,

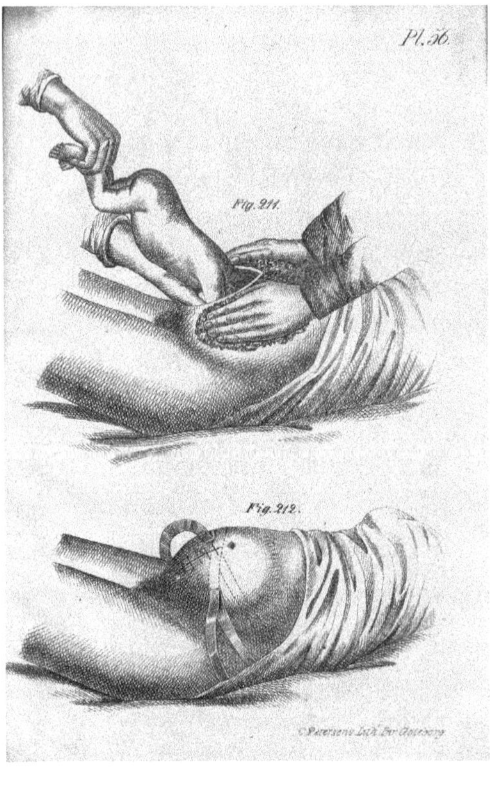

FIGURE 0.9
Cesarean section in the mid-nineteenth century, a surgery that was potentially deadly for the woman, but that might save the life of the fetus. This image was compiled along with others, most from foreign sources, in an atlas by a physician who trained midwives at Gothenburg Maternity Hospital in order to compensate for the 'complete lack' of obstetrical illustrations in Swedish medical literature. The original images in the plate were published in Busch, *Atlas geburtshülflicher Abbildungen,* Pl. 48. From Carlson, *Afbildningar till förlossningsläran:* 'Förord' and Pl. 56. Hagströmer Library, KI.

this field never became an independent subject. As shown by Eva Åhrén in her chapter in this volume, comparative embryology—based on the collection, preparation, and study of microscopic specimens—was introduced by anatomist Anders Retzius at the KI, the medical school in Stockholm. His son Gustaf Retzius later expanded this line of research, including morphological studies of gametes and fetal brains. This inherently visual and material work contributed to the knowledge of the development of individuals from fertilization to birth as well as the understanding of the evolution of all species over the course of history. By the early 1900s, Åhrén suggests, the embryo had become the all-encompassing model of development, unifying Swedish scientists in a progressive view of culture and society that advanced from the primitive to perfection.

In nineteenth-century obstetrics, bodies and fetuses from dead women were collected, prepared, and studied for similar yet distinct purposes. Whereas Anders Retzius assembled 'race skulls' for comparative analysis, his brother and colleague Magnus Retzius established a collection of 'race pelves' from numerous colonial contexts. Helena Franzén demonstrates in this volume that Magnus Retzius's obstetrical collection emerged within Sweden's

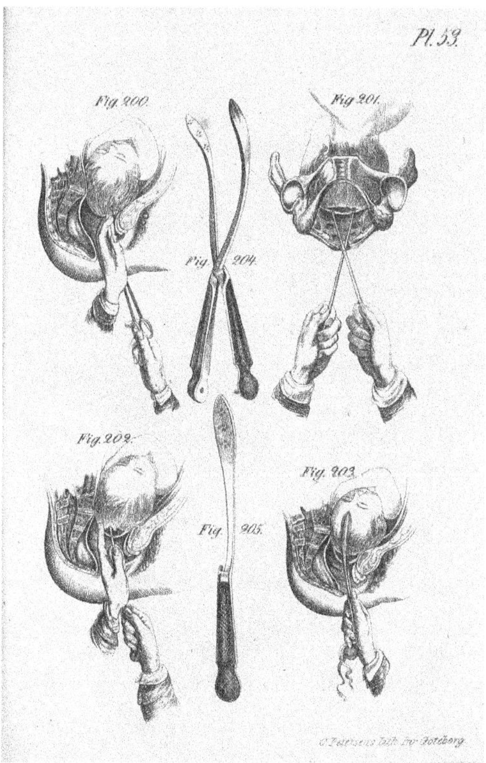

FIGURE 0.10
Craniotomy or, more broadly, embryotomy was a surgical intervention performed in severely obstructed labor when the woman's life was at stake. Various instruments could be used to reduce the volume of the fetal head, which prevented vaginal delivery. The original images in this plate were published in Churchill, *On the Theory and Practice of Midwifery*, Pl. 96–99. From Carlson, *Afbildningar till förlossningsläran*, Pl. 53. Hagströmer Library, KI.

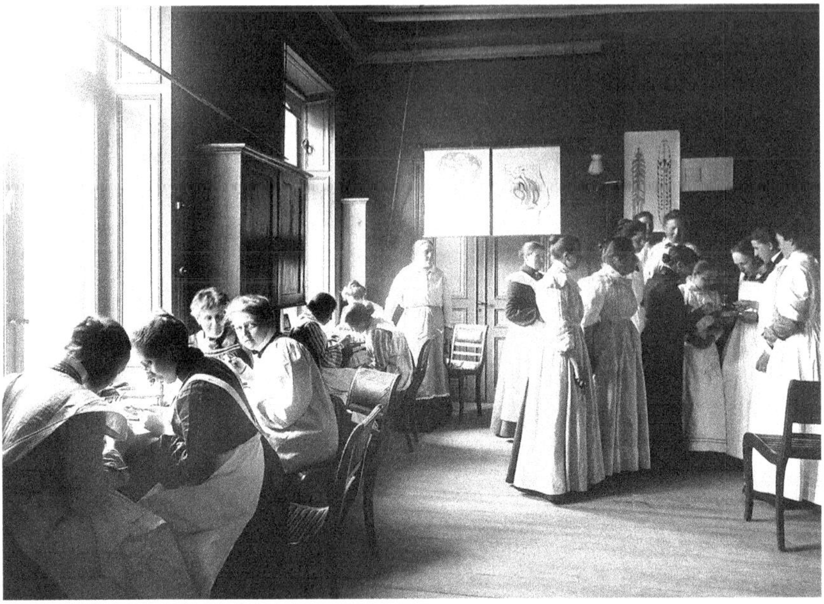

FIGURE 0.11 Animal dissection class in Stockholm around 1900. Karolina Widerström (dressed in black), Sweden's first female physician with a university degree, is supervising a group of student teachers. At the back are some of Widerström's anatomical posters. KvinnSam, Gothenburg University, A131.

nation-building efforts, and that his pelvis specimens materialized intersecting concepts of sex and race. These concepts, in turn, were used to construct the notion of a 'Swedish people' with a shared past, reminiscent of the Gothic mania that took hold during the great-power period.

Additionally, Magnus Retzius collected female pelves with pathological conditions. In several instances, as Franzén has shown elsewhere, these body parts came from radical surgeries—such as the cesarean section—on women in severely obstructed labor. Physicians faced a critical dilemma when the woman's pelvis was too narrow or deformed by disease, so that the fetus could not be delivered manually or with forceps. A decision had to be made either to dismember a living fetus through craniotomy in the hope of saving the woman, or to risk the patient's life by daring to perform a cesarean section. In Protestant Sweden, Franzén suggests, most physicians stressed that the ultimate decision should be made by the woman alone. Yet what this consent meant, and whether it was free from coercion by the medical practitioner, is impossible to know. The skeletonized pelves of the women who did not survive were

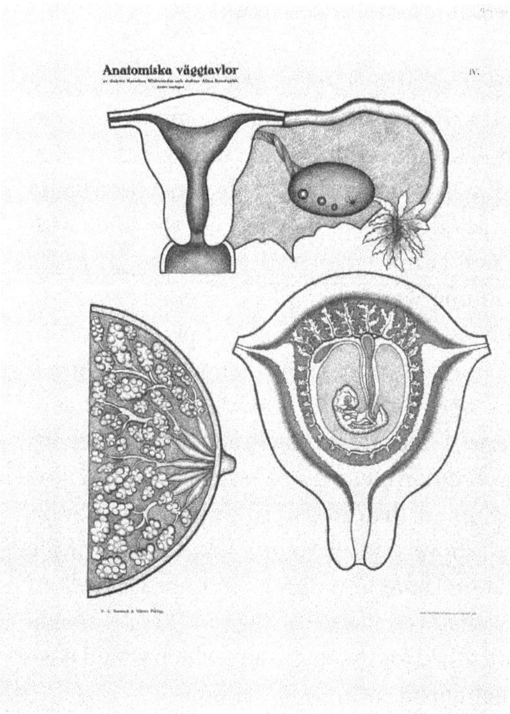

FIGURE 0.12
One of the anatomical posters of female organs and embryonic development that Karolina Widerström and fellow gynecologist and sex educator Alma Sundquist produced as teaching aids for schools. Widerström and Sundquist, *Anatomiska väggtavlor*, Pl. 4. National Library of Sweden.

used to train medical students to judge pathological conditions and decide when to intervene in obstructed labors.[87]

In these contexts—science, medicine, theology, law—the bodies of dead pregnant women, fetuses, and newborn were handled in different ways, imbued with meanings, and used as evidence for various purposes. Through the practices of anatomy and embryology, their bodies were sliced into pieces and then given new materiality through reconstructive technologies such as drawings and wax models that were brought into the public domain (or rather presented to select audiences). Embryos stood in for evolution and were increasingly asked to support theories concerning race and heredity. They became accessible owing to deliveries that went wrong and interrupted pregnancies, including induced abortions, but they did not primarily signal abortion. This interpretation began to change in early twentieth-century Sweden, as the next section will discuss.

87 Franzén, 'From Patient to Specimen.'

5 From Medical Waste to Valuable Scientific Material

In the decades around 1900, embryological specimens and illustrations were used in medical research and education as well as in training courses for teachers in primary and secondary schools. Pioneering female physicians created anatomical posters of fetal development and reproduction to educate girls and young women in 'sexual hygiene' (see figures 0.11 and 0.12). Collections with human and animal material, kept first at university institutions and gradually at schools' museums and biology rooms, were crucial for this enterprise.[88] To establish these collections, leading researchers and medical practitioners in Sweden, as elsewhere, established a reproductive bioeconomy in which products from interrupted pregnancies were defined as medical waste and converted into valuable scientific material.[89] Like Johan von Hoorn and the Retzius brothers before him, anatomist Ivar Broman created a collegial network of physicians and midwives that provided him with dead embryos and fetuses for his collection at Lund University. Jülich shows (in this volume) that several of the preserved specimens in this collection came from legal abortions carried out in the late 1930s and 1940s at the women's clinics in the region. There is no evidence that the female patients were asked for their consent, which would have been unlikely given physicians' paternalistic attitude at the time.

In scientific and pedagogic publications intended for a Swedish audience, Broman was careful not to expose his collecting practices, let alone mention the names of contributing colleagues. Historical sources are scarce, Jülich ascertains, but a probable reason for this secrecy was the delicate nature of reproductive research (reminiscent of von Hoorn's dilemma). Sexuality—especially that of women—was surrounded by strong norms and rules, and scientific fields that related to sexual and reproductive issues were particularly vulnerable to criticism and questioning from lay people. Above all, abortion was controversial. At the same time, the silence may have had to do with patient confidentiality.

After World War II, the heyday of Broman's comparative embryology was at an end. Still, the newly established Medical Research Council worked actively to enable researchers to utilize legally aborted fetuses for scientific purposes. According to the research council, animal studies were in many

88 Franzén, 'Att lära sig se'; Lennerhed, 'Taking the Middle Way,' 55–56; Thorsén, 'Karolina Widerström.'

89 On the classification of fetal remains as 'medical waste,' see Morgan, "'Properly Disposed of.'" On the concept of 'reproductive bioeconomy,' see Waldby, 'Production and Reproduction'; Jülich and Tinnerholm Ljungberg, 'Från medicinskt avfall till rättighetsinnehavare.'

ways inadequate for understanding human conditions. Therefore, the fetuses obtained from abortions were too valuable as research material to be thrown away:

> We do not know how long the current abortion law will last. It would be a remarkable waste of a unique scientific material if this was not used for extensive studies of chemical and physiological problems for which similar conditions probably exist nowhere in the world.[90]

Legal abortions offered a unique opportunity to conduct studies on human fetuses that were unauthorized or heavily regulated in other countries. This advantage was emphasized over and over again in official policy documents describing the conditions for medical research and vaccine development in postwar Sweden. Yet this interest in acquiring aborted fetuses for research did not automatically mean that the researchers and physicians approved of the Swedish abortion law. Quite the opposite; many of them were explicitly against abortion. A 'moral economy' was thus established on the basis of instrumental motivations. Since the damage had already been done, it seemed better to use the abortion material to save lives or improve the human condition. At least this is the reasoning that was communicated to the public.[91]

As Jülich and Isa Dussauge discuss in their chapter in this book, access to tissues from aborted human fetuses was essential for developing the Swedish polio vaccine in the early 1950s. A new supply infrastructure was created in Stockholm, linking state and municipal laboratories with women's clinics and gynecological wards at hospitals in the region. Organs from aborted fetuses were used by virologists to provide a substrate in which the polio virus could grow, testing the antigenicity of vaccines. This connection to legal abortion made the vaccine development controversial, and the state, as provider of abortions, was now the target for anti-abortion groups and campaigns. To counter criticism the leading virologist Sven Gard introduced the metaphor of 'the abortion medal' in interviews with the daily press. On the flip side of the medal there were abortions, the taking of human lives. But on the front side, these abortions could be used to save lives, especially those of children, the nation's future. Journalists happily adopted this metaphor.

This policy aligned with the promotion of Sweden as a modern country, upholding a neutral position in the Cold War and building its welfare on scientific expertise and technological development. However, in the late 1950s a more ambivalent image of Sweden emerged in an international, especially

90 Cited in Jülich, 'Fosterexperimentens produktiva hemlighet,' 17.
91 Jülich, 16–19.

SEXUALPROFET PÅ NÖJESFÄLTET

"Autodidakt på könslivets område!"

Sexualundervisning är ämnet för dagen. Dess vara eller icke vara i skolorna diskuteras av läkare, lärare, präster och lekmän. Olika former och förslag ventileras — och man kommer ingen vart. Under tiden tjänar sexualprofeter grova pengar på sexualundervisning ...

Den senast uppdykta profeten heter *Gustav Nyberg*, som på frågan om vilka medicinska kvalifikationer han har för att offentligt hålla föredrag om så svårbehandlade ämnen som genitalorganens funktioner och de veneriska sjukdomarnas diagnostisering, förlopp och bekämpande svarar, att han »är autodidakt på könslivets område»! Det är ute på Nöjesfältet han håller till; kanske den ungdomliga skara, som dväljes på detta nöjesetablissemang är speciellt lämplig som publik, men frågan är om det är så lämpligt att blanda sexualundervisning med swing, radiobilar och lustiga hus ...

»Anatomisk utställning — MÄNNISKAN — Propaganda för sexuell upplysning och Könssjukdomarnas bekämpande» står det i stora bokstäver utanför ingången till »utställningen», som består av en massa f. d. danska preparat i vax, preparat, som saknar beskrivande text. Frågar man herr autodidakten vad det eller det föreställer, svarar han antingen med de mest befängda galenskaper eller

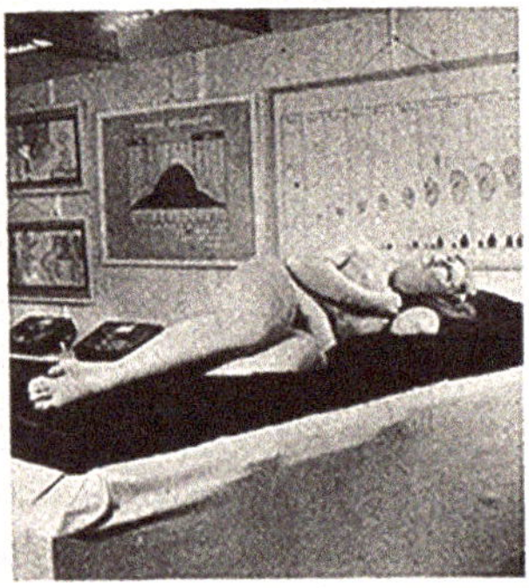

Det första man ser när man kommer in på »utställningen» är en liggande, realistiskt gjord kvinnofigur av vax — som saknar varje funktion! »Endast för damer» står det på en skylt in till Nybergs allra heligaste, men vänder man skylten, står där »Endast för herrar»... Skylten vändes vid behov!

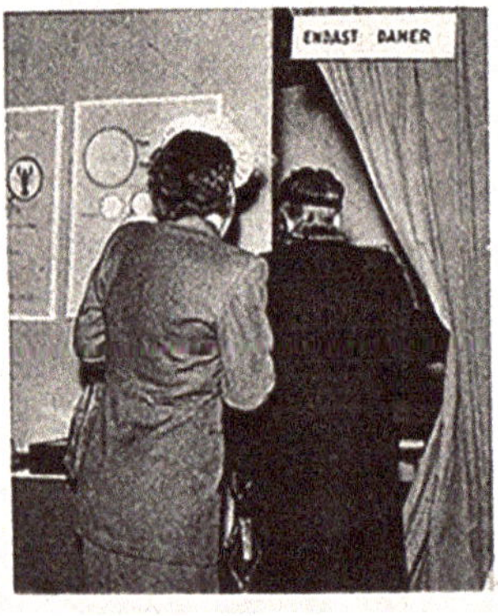

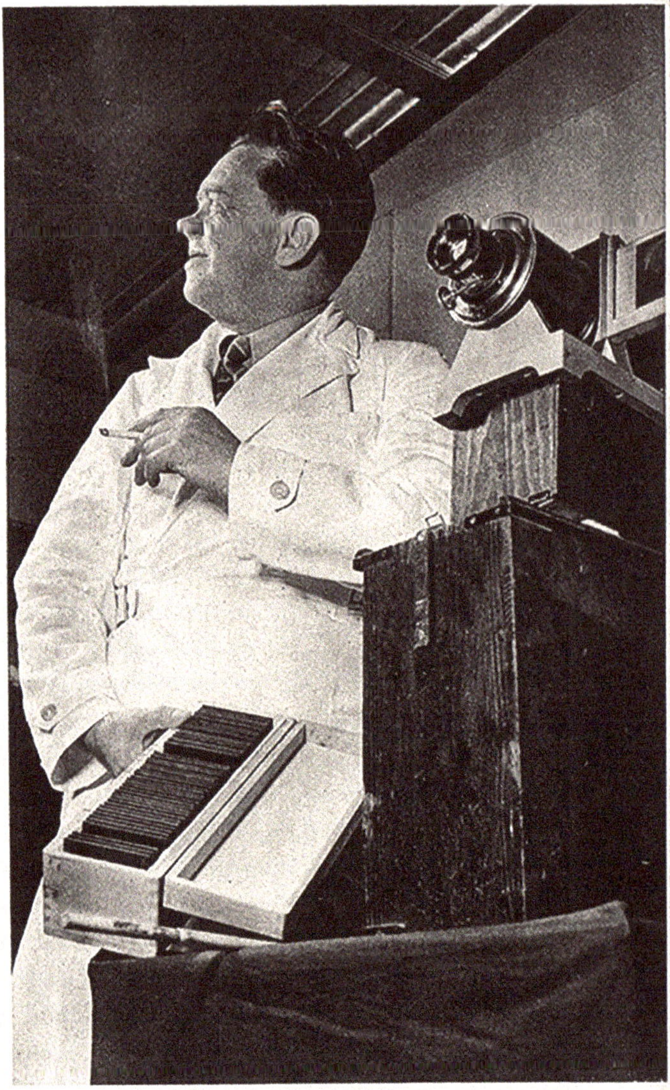

Med hjälp av en skioptikonapparat håller Nyberg sina »föreläsningar» och ådagalägger en praktfull beskäftighet. Att han hyser ett oerhört stort patos för »sexualupplysning» är det ingen som helst tvekan om, men han saknar varje spår av kompetens som föreläsare i dylika ömtåliga ämnen.

(FORTS. NÄSTA SIDA.)

5

FIGURE 0.13 Scientific interest in embryological specimens and models started to wane during the 1940s, but they were still used as attractions at amusement parks. To create legitimacy, they were presented a sex education (even if this too was associated with controversy). The magazine *Se* (See) mocked th "sex prophet" and "autodidact" Gustav Nyberg in one of its issues while at the same time presentin a series of titillating pictures from his show. Photo: 'Gey'. From 'Sexualprofet på nöjesfältet,' 5–6. Copyright Dagens Bild.

(FORTS.)

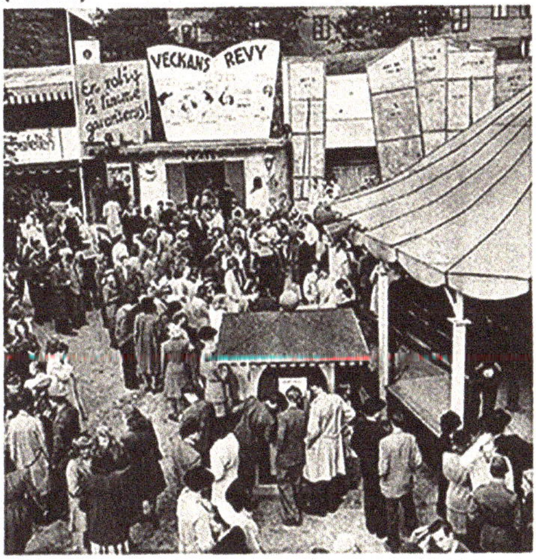

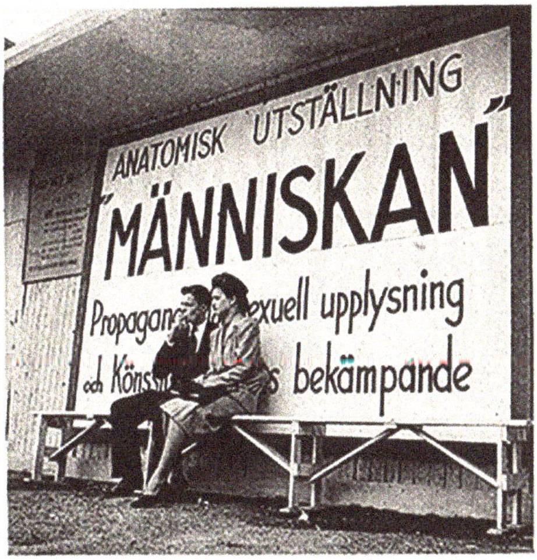

Dansbanan och tivolinöjena drar givetvis mer än hr Nybergs föredrag, men det är inte så få nöjesfältsbesökare, som tittat in till sexualprofeten och blivit »upplysta». Genom att förlägga en dylik »utställning» just på denna plats, bidrar man knappast till att få bort sensation kring sexualundervisningen.

också beklagar han, att han tyvärr inte riktigt tagit reda på den eller den »detaljen». Som ett exempel på hr Nybergs — han är f. d. tivoliarbetare och har f. n. en dansbana söder om Stockholm — medicinska kunskaper kan nämnas, att han förklarar att blödarsjukan beror på »brist på ett ämne i blodet som heter hämoglobin. Men numera kan man framställa hämoglobin syntetiskt och spruta in i 'paschänten', som visserligen inte blir botad men som kan leva ett prima liv»!! Blodets färgämne hämoglobin har intet med koaguleringen att skaffa och kan icke syntetiseras. Under de föredrag om syfilis och gonorré, som hr Nyberg håller med en till extas gränsande förtjusning, kommer de felaktiga och vilseledande uppgifterna med jämna mellanrum. Han talar t. ex. om dosering av sulfa-preparat vid gonorré, och förklarar att »varje paschänt behöver sin dos. Om man ger för mycket kapslar bakterierna in sig och blir motståndskraftiga». Förmodligen är det uppgiften om, att gonokockstammarna vid otillräcklig dosering lätt blir resistenta, som spökar i hr Nybergs hjärna.

Trots att denne Nöjesfältets sexualprofet saknar varje spår av kompetens att offentligt orda om så svårartade sociala och medicinska spörsmål som könssjukdomar och sexualundervisning, och trots att flera av de preparat och planscher, som visas på »utställningen» är enligt läkareutlåtande direkt missvisande, måste man ge honom den elogen, att han visar en klar respekt för läkare och den medicinska vetenskapen samt att han i fråga om könssjukdomar inte har ord nog starka för att råda sitt auditorium att uppsöka läkare så fort man misstänker sig blivit smittad. Det finns dock två beklagansvärda förhållanden i denna sorglustiga historia — att Nöjesfältet upplåtit plats åt gycklet, samt att hr Nyberg inte håller sina »sexualföredrag» för den trängre bekantskapskretsen.

(SE-foto: Gey, Dagens Bild.)

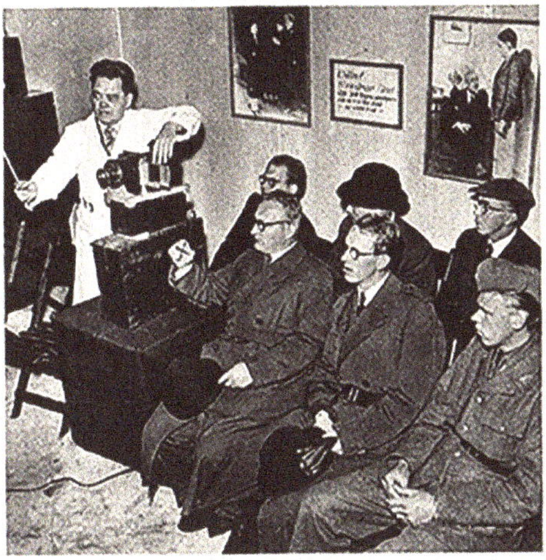

Inne i det »allra heligaste» håller Nyberg med förtjusning sina föredrag med beskäftig »sakkunskap». Föredragen hålles antingen för män eller för kvinnor.

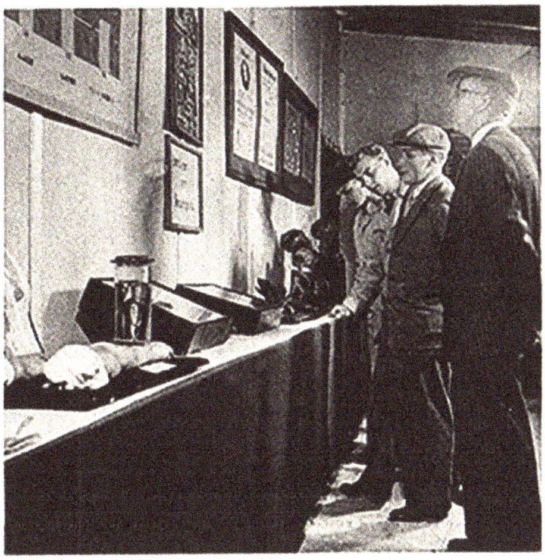

De flesta av utställningens preparat saknar förklarande texter, och många av de på väggarna hängande tavlorna och tabläerna är direkt missvisande.

American, context. Drawing on film and other cultural expressions, critics in other countries argued that 'Swedish sin' was a consequence of the secularized welfare state. Depictions of Sweden acquired more positive connotations in the 1960s, as the official Swedish view of sex stressed progressive values and equality between the sexes.[92]

Importantly, international research-funding agencies were attracted by the sexual politics and climate for medical research in Sweden. With the identification of global overpopulation as a social problem in the 1950s, several new sponsors took the lead. Swedish reproductive researchers became recipients of major grants from US federal and philanthropic funders, including the Ford Foundation and the American Association for the Aid of Crippled Children.[93] In addition, the international pharmaceutical industry supported endocrinological research directed toward the development of contraceptives.[94] All this contributed to making Sweden a global hub for reproductive research and training.

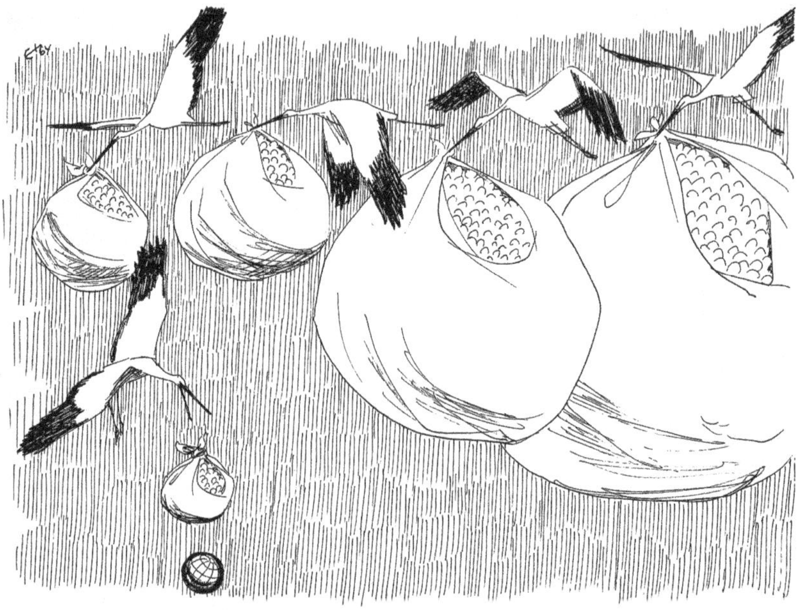

FIGURE 0.14 A drawing interpreting the debates about the global overpopulation crisis by Swedish artist Edward Lindahl, 1964. 'The child bomb' was a common metaphor in these debates. The Museum of Drawings in Laholm. Courtesy of the Edward Lindahl family.

92 For an overview of historical research on this theme, see Björklund, *Most Delicate Subject*, 16–19.

93 Jülich, 'Fosterexperimentens produktiva hemlighet'; Ramsey, *Swedish Abortion Pill*, 144–45; Tinnerholm Ljungberg in this volume.

94 Ramsey, *Swedish Abortion Pill*, 144–45.

It was not only access to an infrastructure of aborted fetuses that made Swedish medical research and vaccine development unique in an international context. Crucially, the fetuses obtained from abortions often were from mid-term pregnancies and well preserved.[95] In part this was because getting a legal abortion in 1950s and 1960s Sweden was by no means a simple procedure. The application process usually took considerable time since it involved visiting and getting the approval of two physicians and a social worker (otherwise the decision rested with the social-psychiatric committee at the National Board of Medicine). Many women who underwent abortion were between the thirteenth and eighteenth weeks of pregnancy.[96] For these abortions the most common method used was vaginal and abdominal hysterotomy (sometimes referred to as vaginal cesarean section and abdominal cesarean section). This was also the case for abortions performed on eugenic indication in combination with sterilization. By the 1960s, vacuum aspiration and injection-based methods gained popularity, which meant that the aborted embryo or fetus was extracted in pieces through the cervix.[97] These destructive techniques made the abortion material useless for the kind of investigations and methodologies that interested many reproductive researchers and virologists at the time.[98]

As described by Helena Tinnerholm Ljungberg in this book, several lines of reproductive research were developed in 1950s and 1960s Sweden that took advantage of access to mid-term aborted fetuses. For instance, pediatricians at the KI in Stockholm created a collection of whole fetal specimens and tissues that was part of an international, collaborative research program. The overall aim of the program was to advance knowledge of the factors causing prenatal mortality and miscarriage. In an earlier publication, Jülich has shown that endocrinologists at the KI also conducted research on whole fetuses from legal abortions. Led by Egon Diczfalusy, a so-called perfusion technique was developed that made it possible to keep human fetuses alive for a short period of time after the abortion operation (see figure 0.15). Above all, the researchers were interested in acquiring basic knowledge about the interaction between the fetus, placenta, and 'mother,' a system that was conceptualized as 'the fetoplacental unit.' It was anticipated that a new 'thalidomide catastrophe' could be prevented by

95 Tinnerholm Ljungberg in this volume. Mid-term pregnancy comprises weeks thirteen to twenty-six.

96 Ramsey, *Swedish Abortion Pill*, 73, 80–81.

97 Ramsey, 49–50.

98 Jülich and Dussauge (in this volume) highlight how the production chain of polio vaccine shifted to a substrate of animal tissues when the supply of aborted human fetuses diminished in 1955, owing to a decline in the number of abortions and of those conducted by hysterotomy. In turn, this trend was connected with women's opposition to hysterotomy, after the publicity created by a medical report showing that this procedure was riskier than others.

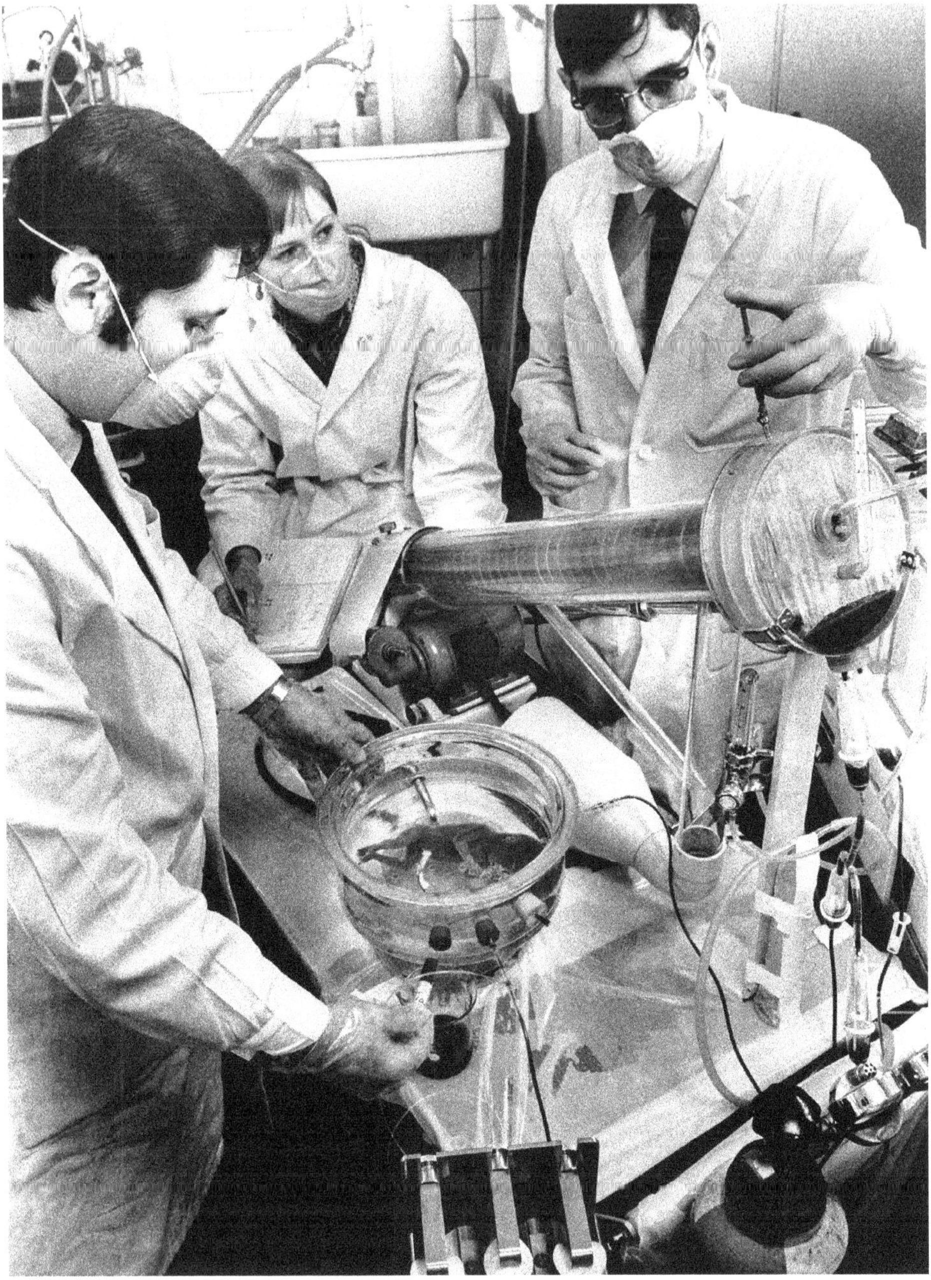

FIGURE 0.15 Researchers at the KI perfusing an aborted human fetus around 1970. In the center, a glass container (the 'perfusion chamber') filled with glucose solution ('artificial amniotic fluid') is enclosing the fetus. It ensured a constant temperature and blood volume. The cylinder (the 'oxygenator') served the purpose of oxygenating the blood. This apparatus made it possible to keep the fetus alive for several hours under conditions similar to those *in utero*. Photograph by Lennart Nilsson. Courtesy of Lennart Nilsson Photography/SPL.

investigating how and with what effects drugs were transferred from the pregnant woman to the fetus.[99]

Research on pregnant women and fetuses was not only motivated by arguments that the resulting knowledge would protect future individuals from damage, malformations, and death. Using cells from aborted fetuses, geneticists Joe Hin Tjio and Albert Levan at Lund University made the discovery in 1956 that humans have forty-six chromosomes, which led to the chromosome analysis for diagnosing Down syndrome.[100] Also at Lund, gynecologist Bertil Sundén evaluated the risks as well as the potential of obstetrical ultrasound by testing this new imaging technology on women who were waiting for legal abortions in the early 1960s. As investigated by Annika Berg in this volume, the availability of such women helped create a favorable milieu for innovation, placing Lund after Glasgow in the front line of ultrasound pioneers. Since the pregnancies were to be aborted, the experiments were not considered problematic, but it is uncertain to what extent the women were informed about possible risks, which were still under evaluation via rat studies.[101] Anna Tunlid's chapter in this volume highlights that, from a societal point of view, as various medical experts asserted, the development of prenatal diagnosis was essential to reduce costs for the care and rehabilitation of children with disabilities. For these actors, the focus was not on fetal cells or abortion patients, but on the larger collective good and the lives of normal children.

Moreover, 1960s and 1970s Swedish reproductive research seemed to provide a tool for solving the perceived global overpopulation problem. Through collaboration between medical researchers and pharmaceutical companies a new abortion method—abortion pills—was developed at the KI. Women who had been granted abortion were included in clinical trials of a specific compound that was seen as a promising abortifacient. As explained by Morag Ramsey in this volume, these mid-1960s trials were unsuccessful but led to new legislation that opened up possibilities for prostaglandin research, which supported the development of the more successful RU486, today used for medical abortion. But first a bill had to be passed to allow it. Several members of the Parliament who felt uneasy about this research positioned it against their own concern for protecting fetuses. Proponents stressed the potential humanitarian value of such work for controlling overpopulation by means of family

99 Jülich, 'Fosterexperimentens produktiva hemlighet.'
100 de Chadarevian, *Heredity under the Microscope*, 6.
101 See also Berg, 'Rays of Death.'

planning. Thus, what mattered most in this context was humanity as such, and less the fetuses and women in the clinical trials.

Postwar fetal research in Sweden was not conducted in secrecy. Researchers reported on their activities in international scientific publications and shared their results with colleagues at conferences. Yet the research was not altogether open either. The Medical Research Council asked grant recipients to keep a low profile and restrict public transparency.[102] Although the Freedom of the Press Act of 1766 stipulated that the media, indeed all citizens, had the right to access official documents, the Government and authorities could refer to provisions on secrecy to protect public interests.[103] As Jülich and Dussauge discuss in this book, newspapers repeatedly complained over the secrecy around the development of the polio vaccine and their lack of access to vital information about what was actually happening in the laboratories. Direct criticism was not to be expected, since 1950s media was highly dependent on good relations with physicians and institutions for medical reporting. In addition, news coverage often used technical language, and it is uncertain what the nonmedical reader would understand from the brief descriptions of scientific research offered in the media.[104]

At the same time, we may be historically insensitive or even ignorant to look for controversy here. What has been deemed controversial has changed across time and place. Either way, the debates in question were not about the personified fetus with moral or legal rights that we are familiar with from today's abortion wars. The development of the polio vaccine was indeed provocative because of its connection to abortion, but the aborted fetuses used by virologists were not discussed as vulnerable creatures worthy of protection or persons with autonomous lives.

Nonetheless, a tendency to present embryological specimens and pictures as evidence against abortion was already manifest in Broman's publications. In the 1930s, he used a photograph of an embryo showing the early formation of the heart to argue that abortion was unacceptable in all cases except when the life of the woman was in danger. This picture had been photographed against

---

102 Jülich, 'Fosterexperimentens produktiva hemlighet,' 18–19.

103 The Swedish Freedom of the Press Act of 1766 has been regarded as the world's first law supporting the freedom of the press and of information. It abolished censorship and stated that Swedish citizens have the right to access official documents. A revision was made in 1949, but its main principles remained the same. There were, however provisions on secrecy that restricted the right to access official documents—for instance, those that were considered to have exceptional importance for national security or whose circulation could in any other way severely harm the nation. For a report on the rules of the Freedom of the Press Act, see Swedish Ministry of Justice, *Public Access to Information.*

104 See also Jülich, 'Fosterexperimentens produktiva hemlighet,' 40–41.

a black background to achieve contrast and had a rather cold, scientific look.[105] Lennart Nilsson's earliest images of human development were similarly arranged. These specimen photographs, which encouraged the personification of embryos and fetuses, were produced in collaboration with physicians opposed to abortion (see figure 0.5).[106] In the 1960s, however, they were quickly superseded by Nilsson's spectacular color photographs of fetuses taken during abortions, as will be discussed below.

6 Fetal Research in Dispute

From 1960 until 1974, when the new Act on Abortion was passed by the Parliament, the view of embryos and fetuses as waste persisted and remained a prerequisite for fetal research—but it also faced growing resistance. At the same time, the fetus gained a new visibility outside medical contexts, not least through Lennart Nilsson's widely circulated photographs. Nilsson's work can be said to have influenced the visual culture of pregnancy in a paradoxical way. On the one hand, his images contributed to the individualization of the fetus by presenting it as an autonomous individual, separate from the pregnant woman. On the other hand, they have come to stand for the universal fetus, symbolizing the human collectivity. In any case, the Swedish photographer has been credited with an enormous impact on the rise of 'the public fetus.'[107]

As Jülich has discussed elsewhere, Nilsson's early photographs of the beginning of human life were produced in close collaboration with KI researchers who conducted experiments on fetuses obtained from legal abortions. From the late 1950s, Nilsson kept photographic and technical equipment in an office close to the operating room at Sabbatsberg's women's clinic in Stockholm. Placing aborted fetuses in saline-containing vessels (similar to the method Davenport Hooker had used for his fetal experiments), he tried various technical arrangements and color film to make the objects look as 'natural' as possible. These attempts were the basis for the production of photographs for the story 'Drama of Life before Birth' in *Life* as well as the advice book *Ett barn blir till* (*A Child Is Born*), both of which were published in 1965 and made Nilsson an international celebrity.[108] His images were soon promoted as first-rate

105 See Jülich's chapter in this volume.

106 See also the chapter by Jülich and Dussauge.

107 For a historical discussion on the paradox of embryo and fetus imagery today, see Morgan, *Icons of Life*, 213–17. On the concept of the 'public fetus,' see Jülich and Björklund, 'Public Fetus.'

108 Jülich, 'Drama of the Fetoplacental'; Jülich, 'Making of a Best-Selling.'

sex education material that would help stimulate young people to talk freely and participate in discussions on various aspects of sexuality. A book oriented toward the American audience, *Sex and Society in Sweden* (1967), included pictures by Nilsson that showed school children and students studying his famous story of fetal development. Commentators have repeatedly made such associations between the photographer and Sweden's progressive society over the years.[109]

In 1960, the newspapers reported that Diczfalusy had received a larger research grant from the American NIH; in conjunction with this story, his fetal experiments were also described. This was the starting point for debates that would be held in both public and political contexts over more than a decade. The crucial question was whether the aborted fetus should be considered 'viable' or not, and what this determination meant in terms of rights and protection. New legislation also drew attention to fetal research. This was the case with the population registration law, which provided that every fetus that breathed at birth and showed a heartbeat or pulsations in the umbilical cord

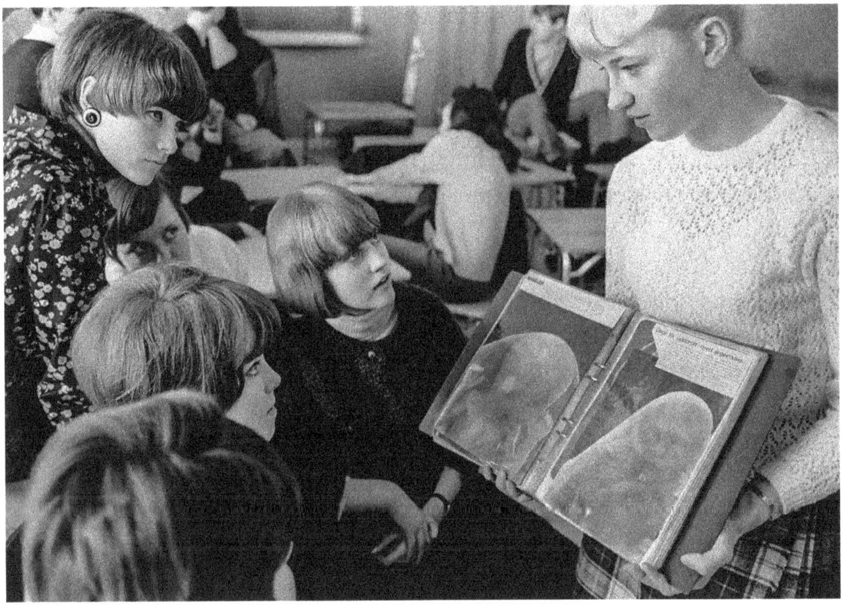

FIGURE 0.16 Photograph by Lennart Nilsson of a sex education lesson in a Stockholm school in the mid-1960s. The school students are being shown a folder containing his world-famous fetal pictures from *Life* magazine. Courtesy of Lennart Nilsson Photography/SPL.

109 Jülich, 'Fetal Photography'; Linnér, *Sex and Society in Sweden*.

should be recorded as a live birth, regardless of its size and degree of development. Second, a law had been introduced in 1958 that allowed tissues and other biological material from deceased persons to be used for transplants. These laws came to affect the debates, even though the legal texts did not refer to aborted fetuses.[110]

Reports in the daily press drew a response from the (liberal) People's Party member and pastor Axel Gustafsson. He demanded clarification from Herman Kling, minister of justice in the Social Democratic government, on the question of whether scientific studies in which aborted fetuses were kept alive could be compatible with the new population registration law's definition of life. Kling's response was evasive; he emphasized that the fetuses in question were so undeveloped that they had no chance of surviving. He also referred to medical expertise which, in light of the new Transplant Act, equated fetuses with surgically removed organs or tissues. The experiments therefore did not contravene current legislation, even though they were 'less appealing from an ethical point of view.'[111]

The debate continued in different media and political contexts with varying degrees of intensity throughout the 1960s. The voices that were critical of fetal experiments were found above all in the Church of Sweden and the free churches. Christian politicians and commentators, not the women's movement, were the earliest to express the view that abortion patients should be asked for their consent to use their fetuses for research. The Society for the Neurosedyn [Thalidomide] Affected was also active and demanded information: Did abortions occur on suspicion of birth defects and, if so, were the aborted fetuses used for medical research? A former member of the Parliament, from the Conservative Party, asked for the legal status of fetuses to be clarified and requested that the authorities investigate whether Sweden had violated the United Nations Charter on Human Rights.[112]

From the mid-1960s, journalist Eskil Block tried to mobilize opinion against fetal experiments. The truth was, he argued, that medical researchers used 'living' aborted fetuses—these fetuses had independent lives and should be accorded human dignity and rights. Were abortion applications deliberately delayed so that researchers could get larger fetuses for their experiments? Was hysterotomy chosen as an abortion method so that the fetuses were whole and intact after the abortion, which served research interests? Nilsson's photographs and his collaboration with fetal researchers were also criticized. The

110 Jülich, 'Fosterexperimentens produktiva hemlighet,' 19–20.

111 Jülich, 21–22

112 Jülich, 29, 31–32.

famous pictures of embryos and fetuses, Block stated, did not portray 'the drama of the beginning of life' but rather a manipulated, beautified version of what the fetus looked like after a small cesarean section. In 1969 he filed a complaint with the Parliamentary Ombudsman, who investigated but took no further action.[113]

In the early 1970s, two motions regarding concerns over fetal research were submitted by members of the Swedish Parliament. The 1974 Parliamentary Committee on Education dealt with the motions and conducted a comprehensive investigation, in order to find out whether 'still living,' aborted fetuses were used in research. The committee demanded answers from key medical institutions. Nevertheless, its conclusion was that research on fetuses obtained through abortion procedures was to be equated with studies on dead organs and tissues. When used in research and teaching, such surgically removed organs and tissues did not require the consent of the patient, and therefore consent from the woman undergoing the abortion was not needed either. With the new Abortion Act that came into force the following year—and which set a sharp limit for late abortions after the end of the eighteenth week of pregnancy—the conditions for research on viable fetuses were in any case considered to have been eliminated.[114]

This growing concern over fetal research in Sweden can be seen in light of international debates, as discussed by Tinnerholm Ljungberg in her chapter in this book. In fact, Sweden played a central role in these debates. For some time, allegations that living aborted fetuses were sold for medical experiments had been circulating in the UK press. The Peel Advisory Group, appointed in 1970 to investigate fetal research and named after its chair, Sir John Peel, learned about Diczfalusy's perfusion studies and internally described them as very sensitive. Although it did not mention Sweden explicitly, the so-called Peel Report concluded that research on 'nonviable' fetuses had occurred outside the United Kingdom, then proposed a set of guidelines for British fetal research.

Tinnerholm Ljungberg also discusses the heated US public debate that took off in 1973, after coverage of fetal research in the *Washington Post*. As already mentioned, these articles revealed NIH-funded research on living aborted fetuses in Sweden and US researchers' frequent travel to the KI to participate in such research. Other scholars have highlighted the publicity related to Agneta Philipson, a visiting researcher on leave from Karolinska Hospital. She was one of four physicians affiliated with Boston City Hospital who in 1974 were convicted for 'violation of sepulture,' the 1814 'grave-robbing' statute. The four of them had been collaborating on a study of the effects of antibiotics on

113 Jülich, 26–28.
114 Jülich, 34–39.

the fetus, using aborted fetuses from the pathology department. A fifth physician, Kenneth Edelin, was convicted of manslaughter under the same statute for performing a second-trimester abortion using hysterotomy. These controversies had a direct effect on national regulation.[115]

In 1974, president Nixon signed into law the National Research Act, establishing the National Commission for the Protection of Human Subjects of Biomedical and Behavioral Research and imposing a temporary moratorium on all fetal research. The commission consisted of physicians, lawyers, ethicists, biomedical researchers, and one public representative, who were tasked with investigating research on living fetuses and recommending whether such research should be supported by federal authorities. Their report, entitled *Research on the Fetus*, included a review of the scientific literature on research involving the fetus inside and outside the uterus, primarily from the 1960s to the early 1970s. Research on the nonviable fetus *ex utero* was found to be limited, comprising fewer than twenty articles (this estimate was inaccurate). Only one principal investigator had conducted research in the United States, as part of a study involving attempts to develop an artificial life-support system. All other research had been done in other countries—mainly Sweden but also Finland and Britain. The report emphasized that the purpose of perfusion studies on aborted fetuses was solely to obtain knowledge about normal fetal physiology for the benefit of other fetuses and infants.[116] And it went on to outline five ethical principles to which all types of fetal research must adhere, including that the woman must give her informed consent. Finally, the commission recommended an end to the moratorium on fetal research. These recommendations, approved in 1975, became the first federal regulations governing fetal research in the United States as well as research supported by US funding abroad.[117]

The liberalization of abortion in the United Kingdom and the United States was a central backdrop for the media coverage and debates that led to national

115 Dubow, *Ourselves Unborn*, 67–69, 75.

116 National Commission for the Protection of Human Subjects of Biomedical and Behavioral Research, *Research on the Fetus: Report and Recommendations*, 12–15. Reports and papers submitted to the committee were published separately as *Research on the Fetus: Appendix*, and Swedish research is described on pp. 24–25 (footnotes 111, 115–16).

117 The five ethical principles developed by the commission were: 1. Investigations on animal models and nonpregnant humans must come before research on the human fetus. 2. The knowledge must be important and not possible to obtain in any other way. 3. The risks and benefits to the mother and the fetus must have been described and thoroughly evaluated. 4. Informed consent from the mother must have been granted. 5. Subjects must be selected so that 'risks and benefits will not fall inequitably among economic, racial, ethnic and social classes.' See *Research on the Fetus: Report and Recommendations*, 63–64. The lifting of the moratorium is discussed on p. 76. For a discussion of the commission, see Dubow, *Ourselves Unborn*, 78–79.

regulations for fetal research in these countries. The reports of the Peel Advisory Group and the National Commission for the Protection of Human Subjects of Biomedical and Behavioral Research also fed directly into and mobilized opposition to abortion in the 1970s and 1980s.[118] Even if Swedish fetal research had been criticized after the coverage in the *Washington Post*, anti-abortion activists, especially in the United States, increasingly (and sometimes unknowingly) used Lennart Nilsson's pictures of aborted fetuses as evidence for fetal personhood.[119]

As discussed in Elisabet Björklund's chapter in this volume, the situation in Sweden was different. Anti-abortion movements existed and used Nilsson's images as well, but never gained momentum. Drawing on television programs from the late 1960s to the 1980s, Björklund shows that, with one spectacular exception, mainstream Swedish media avoided addressing fetal research and rarely displayed explicitly aborted fetuses. Moreover, when US anti-abortion images and films, such as *The Silent Scream* from 1984, were debated in the media, they were dismissed as propaganda. Björklund suggests that a line was thus drawn between Sweden and its 'good,' beautified fetuses, portrayed by Lennart Nilsson and symbolizing universal life, and the United States, where 'bad' pictures of often gory-looking fetuses were disseminated by anti-abortion activists. Again, it was the notion of Sweden as a rational, modern country that the mainstream media wished to evoke.

7 Regulating Fetal Research in Sweden

For most of the twentieth century, Swedish legislation on abortion, population registration, and transplantation promoted rather than hindered access to fetuses for medical research. The media and political debates in the 1960s as well as the circulation of Lennart Nilsson's images contributed to portrayals of the fetus as vulnerable and in need of protection but had no direct effects on the formal framework for conducting research. All the same, the international controversies, committees, and regulations of the 1970s put pressure on the Swedish medical community and alerted parliamentary politicians. The strategy chosen was to prefer ethical review of fetal research over regulation by law, a tendency earlier referred to as bioethicalization.

Ethical guidelines and regulations were slow to develop. Despite international attempts to establish ethical standards for medical experimentation

118 Schoen, *Abortion after* Roe, 74–75, 88–89.
119 Jülich, 'Fetal Photography,' 134–37.

following World War II, initiatives varied across national and local contexts for a considerable time.[120] As discussed by Tinnerholm Ljungberg, both in this volume and elsewhere, US measures to establish informed consent as an ethical principle for medical research were of particular importance to Sweden. As in other countries, research ethics committees were formed in response to demands from the NIH, which sponsored research at the Swedish university hospitals. The first formalized committee was created at the Karolinska Hospital (linked to the KI) in 1966 and consisted solely of medical experts, although they represented various fields, including pediatrics and gynecology. The task of the committee was to evaluate research projects involving human subjects and to make sure that the researcher asked for informed consent before conducting medical research. Tinnerholm Ljungberg shows that fetal research provoked internal debate. In practice, however, it was subjected to few restrictions.[121]

The 1974 Parliamentary Committee on Education highlighted the role of the research ethics committees. Throughout its investigation, medical representatives argued that legislation in the field would severely hinder free research and progress. Parliamentary politicians, on the other hand, pointed to the Peel Advisory Group and asked for corresponding guidelines to regulate Swedish research. Finally, the Committee on Education published a report recommending that all research on humans, including fetuses, be assessed by a local research ethics committee. It also proposed that the medical community should include lay persons in these committees to increase transparency. This new demand for the ethical review of fetal research was then confirmed by the Medical Research Council.[122] It was hardly a coincidence that medical research ethics became a central topic during the same period that Swedish fetal research appeared in the headlines of the *Washington Post* and was discussed by a US federal commission.

As in other liberal democracies, many questions concerning medical research and therapeutics involving human embryos and fetuses were increasingly handled by an expert bioethical committee.[123] The Swedish National Council on Medical Ethics was founded in 1985 as an advisory board to the Government on ethical issues in health care and biomedicine. Characteristic of the Swedish council was—and still is—that it consisted not only of ethical, legal,

120 Jacobs and Tinnerholm Ljungberg, 'How Ethics Travels.'

121 In addition to her chapter in this volume, see Tinnerholm Ljungberg, 'Regulating Research.'

122 Tinnerholm Ljungberg in this volume.

123 Littoz-Monnet, *Governing through Expertise.*

medical, and other experts, but also of representatives of political parties, who formally took the decisions of the council. This absence of lay persons is unique in an international context. Another distinctive feature is that opinions aired in the internal discussions are to be kept within the group, while the only public output is supposed to be the final consensual viewpoint. This process is seen as a guarantee of democratic legitimacy.[124]

The regulation of prenatal diagnosis was one of the issues that political and public debates brought to the forefront. Apart from the 1974 Abortion Act, which prescribed the conditions for having an abortion if a woman decided to terminate a pregnancy, there was no legislation that regulated the practice of prenatal diagnosis in Sweden. Anna Tunlid (in this volume) focuses on the 1984 Governmental Commission of the Unborn Child in order to examine various arguments for and against regulation. By using the metaphor of the 'moral landscape,' she explores how a broad set of actors, including physicians, disability organizations, and women's organizations, negotiated sometimes conflicting values and interests related to novel technologies such as obstetric ultrasound and amniocentesis. According to the commission, the fetus's right to legal protection increased during its development. Still, in the end the Government defended women's reproductive rights. Ten years after the appointment of the commission, in 1994, the Parliament decided that no special legislation on prenatal diagnosis was needed.

Around this time the Parliament also took a stance concerning fetal research. As discussed by Jülich and Tinnerholm Ljungberg elsewhere, the 1995 Transplant Act regulated the use of aborted fetuses for scientific research for the first time, and from that point, the consent of the woman is required by law. Other conditions were the lack of better means to acquire the same results and approval from an ethical committee and the National Board of Health and Welfare (from 2019 the Swedish Ethical Review Authority). New recommendations for the handling of abortion material were also introduced: fetuses older than twelve weeks should be cremated and the ash spread anonymously if the woman seeking an abortion had no other request. Material from earlier abortions should continue to be treated as biological waste.[125]

Yet controversies emerged around early embryos. In the spring of 1998, the media revealed that a hospital in the north of Sweden routinely cremated and buried the ashes from early aborted 'fetuses'; that is, those from abortions before the end of the twelfth week of pregnancy. According to the head

124 Hedlund, 'Democratic Expert Influence.'

125 Jülich and Tinnerholm Ljungberg, 'Från medicinskt avfall,' 47.

of the clinic, the increased use of medical abortion and improved ultrasound technology made it possible to distinguish human features of 'fetuses' even in very early abortions. He was supported by the Liberal People's Party parliament member Barbro Westerholm, also former director general of the National Board of Health and Welfare, who said that it was offensive to regard early aborted fetuses as medical waste. Even so, women's organizations in Norway, where a similar debate was held, criticized the fact that this approach implied blame toward women who, for various reasons, had to undergo abortion.[126]

The practice established by the National Board of Health and Welfare's guidelines and general advice in 1990, whereby older fetuses would be cremated, while embryos from early abortions would continue to be treated as 'risk waste,' remained in use for almost twenty years. In 2008 the responsibility for deciding what information would be given to abortion-seeking women was placed on the care provider. Today, in the case of early abortions that terminate in hospitals, local practice is applied. Concerning early medical abortions that end in the home environment, there are still no overall guidelines for dealing with the abortion material.[127] In a way, this situation is reminiscent of early modern times, when women privately handled and disposed of their products of miscarriage and abortion.

Although we only touch briefly upon late twentieth- and twenty-first century reproductive research and technologies such as embryonic stem cell research, cloning, and human gene editing, it is tempting to try to discern a Swedish route through this complex moral landscape. As we know, while the United States periodically has banned federal fetal research and embryonic stem cell research, such activities have continued in Sweden, and with fewer restrictions.[128] What seems to have been a recurrent theme (or path dependence) in Swedish medical and policy discussions is the view that research has to be free and unhindered. As has been noted above, the many pressing democratic issues concerning the uses of embryos and fetuses for scientific research as well as the development of prenatal diagnosis have largely been assigned to consensual-seeking bioethical expert committees.

126 Jülich and Tinnerholm Ljungberg, 48.

127 Jülich and Tinnerholm Ljungberg, 48–49.

128 On the United States, see Banchoff, *Embryo Politics*, 169–170. The Swedish case is discussed by Tydén, 'Staten och våra gener,' 73–76, and Hedlund, 'Democratic Expert Influence.'

8 Conclusion

By exploring the *longue durée* of reproduction in Sweden, we show that controversies and value conflicts surrounding fetal knowledge production are not exclusive to the 1970s and onward. As discussed, the chapters highlight, among other things, how early modern discourse on abortions and extraordinary births defined humanness and the relationship of humans to other species, as well as nineteenth-century scientists' endorsement of evolutionary theory and the interlinking of sex and race. The twentieth century saw the expansion of human fetal research, legitimated as a means to help save the nation from polio epidemics and solve the global population crisis. Through this historical lens we also see that the connection between the personified and individualized fetus on the one hand and abortion on the other began to be establish in the mid-twentieth century.

Our approach to this rich history goes far beyond narratives of research scandals and bioethics. Many historiographies have pointed to bioethics as key to the emergence of ethical contestation around embryo and fetal research in democracies on both sides of the Atlantic. Yet, bio/ethical standards came late to this history. As mentioned above, religious views on the boundaries of human fetal life were prevalent and sometimes coexisted with medical and legal criteria in early modern Sweden. For most of the twentieth century scientific definitions of dead embryos and fetuses as valuable research material dominated. But other categories of actors, such as women's movements and disability organizations, manifested their own set of standards.

In sum, we learn several things from the Swedish case. First is the striking historical continuity in the politics of population and reproduction over the centuries. Biopolitical knowledge production about human life was dependent on access to the dead bodies of women and fetuses. Early on, anatomists' and obstetricians' uses of the corpses of adults were governed by legislation, but it was not until 1995 that a new law regulated scientific research on aborted fetuses. Only then did it become mandatory by law to obtain the woman's consent before fetal research began. Women's rights in regard to their own bodies had been strengthened, especially through the introduction of abortion on demand in 1975. But their right to decide what happens to an aborted fetus came much later.

Second, Sweden's relatively liberal abortion law created a unique situation for fetal and reproductive research. Fetal research was conducted in other countries in the mid-twentieth century, but nowhere were the conditions as favorable. No regulations restricted access to aborted fetuses, and moreover the fetuses obtained were well preserved. The potential for using this human material for studies in various fields attracted foreign funders and researchers alike, but also others, such as the commercial photographer Lennart Nilsson. At the same time, it created opposition among primarily religious groups in Sweden, where abortion battles were fought decades before those in the United States. Even so, in the 1960s and 1970s anti-abortion movements became increasingly marginalized.

Third, the production of knowledge, ignorance, and secrecy in Sweden were closely intertwined. On the one hand, research in the field of human reproduction has improved the lives and health of many individuals. For instance, the 'Swedish abortion pill' contributed to the development of medical abortion, which has made abortion safer and more accessible for women. Pioneering work on obstetric ultrasound at Lund University led to a less risky procedure for diagnosing fetal conditions and anomalies than existing X-ray technology. But the risks, uncertainties, and doubts associated with reproductive knowledge, innovations, and products were not always publicly debated. Quite the contrary, as demonstrated by the National Board of Medicine's attempt to restrict reports about the dangerous side effects of thalidomide. In addition, endocrinological studies that involved living aborted fetuses were secretive or largely ignored until controversies made them public. Even after disclosure, medical actors were reluctant to share confidential information.

Fourth, ethical regulation was slow to develop but then gave way to bioethicalization. Notwithstanding the establishment of an international infrastructure for research ethics after World War II, it was mainly through pressure from US funding agencies that Swedish university hospitals accepted the ethical review of research in the mid-1960s. Moreover, another decade passed before the medical community agreed to include lay people in these research committees, and this was after Sweden had become linked to controversies associated with fetal studies internationally. Increasingly, ethical review boards and bioethical committees consisting of experts and politicians came to influence decision-making on medical-ethical questions. For several commentators today this organization signals a democratic deficit, since it tends to support medical solutions rather than involving citizens in decisions that have major impacts on their lives and health. A more pluralistic approach has been suggested that would open up the debate on complex biomedical issues, an 'ethos of controversies.'[129]

Above all, the Swedish case demonstrates the interplay of national, transnational, and global histories of fetal medicine and research. From early modern

129 Hedlund, 'Democratic Expert Influence'; Poort, Holmberg, and Ideland, 'Bringing in the Controversy.'

times until today, conditions specific to Sweden have been entangled with wider contexts in terms of both scientific knowledge production and religious and legal conceptions, as well as reproductive and population policies. In the contemporary world, a largely unregulated global bioeconomy around reproductive material is expanding, in which powerful companies, media, and funding mechanisms affect the conditions for research but also public views of the 'fetus.'

Bibliography

Åhrén, Eva. *Death, Modernity and the Body: Sweden 1870–1940*. Rochester, NY: University of Rochester Press, 2009.

Al-Gailani, Salim, and Angela Davis. 'Introduction to "Transforming Pregnancy Since 1900."' *Studies in History and Philosophy of Biological and Biomedical Sciences* 47, Pt. B (September 2014): 229–32.

Andersson, Jenny, and Mary Hilson. 'Images of Sweden and the Nordic Countries.' *Scandinavian Journal of History* 34, no. 3 (2009): 219–28.

Ankele, Monika, and Benoît Majerus, eds. *Material Cultures of Psychiatry*. Bielefeld: Transkript, 2020.

Arnberg, Klara, Pia Laskar, and Fia Sundevall, eds. *Sexualpolitiska nyckeltexter*. Stockholm: Leopard, 2015.

Arnberg, Klara, Fia Sundevall, and David Tjeder, eds. *Könspolitiska nyckeltexter: Från* Det går an *till #metoo*. 2nd ed. Göteborg: Makadam, 2019.

Asklund, Lis, and Willy Maria Lundberg. *Havandeskap, samhällets hjälp, abort: Folkskrift i abortfrågan*. Stockholm: Medicinalstyrelsen, 1947.

Banchoff, Thomas. *Embryo Politics: Ethics and Policy in Atlantic Democracies*. Ithaca, NY: Cornell University Press, 2011.

Bartholdy, Nils G. 'De danske kongers skjoldholdere.' *Heraldisk tidsskrift* 10, no. 98 (2008): 345–57.

Bauer, Susanne, and Ayo Wahlberg, eds. *Contested Categories: Life Sciences in Society*. Ashgate: Farnham, 2009.

Berg, Annika. 'Rays of Death and Visions of Life: Ultrasound Narratives, Risk Evaluations, and Prenatal Imaging.' *Technology and Culture* 65, no. 3 (2024): 933–65.

Bergenlöv, Eva. *Skuld och oskuld: Barnamord och barnkvävning i rättslig diskurs och praxis omkring 1680–1800*. Lund: Lund University, 2004.

Bidloo, Govard. *Anatomia Humani Corporis, Centum et Quinque Tabulis Illustrata*. Amsterdam: Sumptibus Viduæ Joannis à Someren, Hæredum Joannis à Dyk, Henrici & Viduæ Theodori Boom, 1685.

Björklund, Elisabet. 'Contested Pictures of Persuasion: American Images of Foetuses in Swedish Antiabortion Campaigns of the 1970s and 1980s.' In *Nordic Media Histories of Propaganda and Persuasion*, edited by Fredrik Norén, Emil Stjernholm, and C. Claire Thomson, 97–116. Cham: Palgrave Macmillan, 2023.

Björklund, Elisabet. *The Most Delicate Subject: A History of Sex Education Films in Sweden*. Lund: Lund University, 2013.

Björklund, Elisabet, and Solveig Jülich. 'Rethinking the Public Fetus: An Introduction.' In Björklund and Jülich, *Rethinking the Public Fetus*, 1–21.

Björklund, Elisabet, and Solveig Jülich, eds. *Rethinking the Public Fetus: Historical Perspectives on the Visual Culture of Pregnancy*. Rochester, NY: University of Rochester Press, 2024.

Björkman, Maria. 'The Cost of Normalization: The Thalidomide Affected and the Welfare State.' *Scandinavian Journal of History* 48, no. 3 (2023): 341–58.

Björkman, Maria, and Sven Widmalm. 'Selling Eugenics: The Case of Sweden.' *Notes and Records of the Royal Society of London* 64, no. 4 (2010): 379–400.

Blizzard, Deborah. *Looking Within: A Sociocultural Examination of Fetoscopy*. Cambridge, MA: MIT Press, 2007.

Bock von Wülfingen, Bettina, Christina Brandt, Susanne Lettow, and Florence Vienne, eds. 'Temporalities of Reproduction: Practices and Concepts from the Eighteenth to the Early Twenty-First Century.' Special issue, *History and Philosophy of the Life Sciences* 37, no. 1 (2015).

Broman, Ivar. *Människans utveckling före födelsen: En kortfattad handledning i människans embryologi*. Lund: Gleerup, 1927.

Buklijas, Tatjana, and Salim Al-Gailani. 'A Fetus in the World: Physiology, Epidemiology, and the Making of Fetal Origins of Adult Disease.' *History and Philosophy of the Life Sciences* 45, no. 44 (2023): 1–34.

Buklijas, Tatjana, and Nick Hopwood. *Making Visible Embryos* (online exhibition). 2008–10. Accessed May 6, 2023. http://www.hps.cam.ac.uk/visibleembryos/.

Busch, D. W. H. *Atlas geburtshülflicher Abbildungen, mit Bezugnahme auf das Lehrbuch der Geburtskunde*. Berlin: Hirschwald, 1841.

Carlhed, Carina. 'The Rise of the Professional Field of Medicine in Sweden.' *Professions and Professionalism* 3, no. 2 (2013): 1–15.

Carlson, H. I. *Afbildningar till förlossningsläran: Jemte inledande text*. Göteborg, 1859.

Casper, Monica J. *The Making of the Unborn Patient: A Social Anatomy of Fetal Surgery*. New Brunswick, NJ: Rutgers University Press, 1998.

Churchill, Fleetwood. *On the Theory and Practice of Midwifery*. London: Henry Renshaw; Dublin: Fannin, 1842.

Clarke, Adele E. *Disciplining Reproduction: Modernity, American Life Sciences, and 'the Problems of Sex.'* Berkeley: University of California Press, 1998.

Clarke, Adele E. 'Research Materials and Reproductive Sciences in the United States, 1910–1940.' In *Physiology in the American Context 1850–1940*, edited by Gerald L. Geison, 323–50. Bethesda: American Physiological Society, 1987.

Cohn, Victor. 'Live-Fetus Research Debate.' *Washington Post*, April 10, 1973.

Cohn, Victor. 'NIH Vows Not to Fund Fetus Work.' *Washington Post*, April 13, 1973.

Cohn, Victor. 'Scientists and Fetus Research.' *Washington Post*, April 15, 1973.

Collijn, Isak. Postscript to *Biblia: Thet är then helgha scrift på swensko: Tryckt i Uppsala 1540–1541; Gustav Vasas bibel.* Facsimile ed., 3–18. Uppsala: Almqvist & Wiksell, 1938.

Creager, Angela N. H., and Hannah Landecker. 'Technical Matters: Method, Knowledge, and Infrastructure in Twentieth-Century Life Science.' *Nature Methods* 6, no. 10 (2009): 701–5.

Czarnowski, Gabriele, and Sabine Hildebrandt. 'Research on the Boundary between Life and Death: Coercive Experiments on Pregnant Women and their Fetuses during National Socialism.' In *From Clinic to Concentration Camp: Reassessing Nazi Medical and Racial Research, 1933–1945*, edited by Paul Weindling, 73–99. London: Routledge, 2017.

de Chadarevian, Soraya. *Heredity under the Microscope: Chromosomes and the Study of the Human Genome*. Chicago: University of Chicago Press, 2020.

Dittmar, Jenna M., and Mitchell Piers. 'From Cradle to Grave via the Dissection Room: The Role of Foetal and Infant Bodies in Anatomical Education from the Late 1700s to Early 1900s.' *Journal of Anatomy* 229 (2016): 713–22.

Dolan, Brian. 'Malthus's Political Economy of Health: The Critique of Scandinavia in the *Essay on Population*.' In *Malthus, Medicine and Morality: 'Malthusianism' after 1798*, edited by Brian Dolan, 9–32. Amsterdam: Rodopi, 2000.

Donaghy, Paige. 'The Secrets of the Placenta in European Anatomy and Midwifery, 1560–1700.' *Isis* 114, no. 2 (2023): 249–71.

Dron, Heather A. *Teratology Transformed: Uncertainty, Knowledge, and Conflict over Environmental Etiologies of Birth Defects in Midcentury America*. Diss. San Francisco: University of California, 2016.

Dubow, Sara. *Ourselves Unborn: A History of the Fetus in Modern America*. New York: Oxford University Press, 2011.

Dussauge, Isabelle, Claes-Fredrik Helgesson, Francis Lee, and Steve Woolgar. 'On the Omnipresence, Diversity, and Elusiveness of Values in the Life Sciences and Medicine.' In *Value Practices in the Life Sciences and Medicine*, edited by Isabelle Dussauge, Claes-Fredrik Helgesson, and Francis Lee, 1–28. Oxford: Oxford University Press, 2015.

Elvbakken, Kari Tove. *Abortspørsmålets politiske historie 1900–2020*. Oslo: Universitetsforlaget, 2021.

Ericsson, Martin. 'What Happened to "Race" in Race Biology? The Swedish State Institute for Race Biology, 1936–1960.' *Scandinavian Journal of History* 46, no. 1 (2021): 125–48.

Fissell, Mary E. 'Man-Midwifery Revisited.' In Hopwood, Flemming, and Kassell, *Reproduction*, 319–32.

Franzén, Helena. 'Att lära sig se embryologiskt: Samlingsobjekt i forskning och pedagogiska kontexter 1870–1920.' *Scandia* 89, no. 2 (2023): 201–29.

Franzén, Helena. 'From Patient to Specimen and Back Again: Radical Surgeries and Pelvic Pathologies in the Museum Obstetricum.' *Lychnos* (2020): 33–57.

Gottweis, Herbert, Brian Salter, and Catherine Waldby. *The Global Politics of Human Embryonic Stem Cell Science: Regenerative Medicine in Transition*. Basingstoke: Palgrave Macmillan, 2009.

Guerrini, Anita. 'The Material Turn in the History of Life Science.' *Literature Compass* 13, no. 7 (2016): 469–80.

Håkansson, Håkan. 'Den lärda världen.' In *Signums svenska kulturhistoria: Renässansen*, edited by Jakob Christensson, 101–49. Lund: Signum, 2005.

Hammar, Johan August. *Några huvuddrag av fosterutvecklingen med hänsyn till förhållandena hos människan*. Vol. 2. 3rd ed. Stockholm: Bonnier, 1919.

Han, Sallie, Tracy K. Betsinger, and Amy B. Scott, eds. *The Anthropology of the Fetus: Biology, Culture, and Society*. New York: Berghahn Books, 2018.

Hedenborg, Susanna. 'En alltför stor befolkning leder till fattigdom.' In Arnberg, Sundevall, and Tjeder, *Könspolitiska nyckeltexter*, 72–76.

Hedlund, Maria. 'Democratic Expert Influence through Bioethical Advisory Commissions? The Case of PGD Legislation in Sweden.' In *Quality Issues in Clinical Genetic Services*, edited by Ulf Kristoffersson, J. J. Cassiman, and Jörg Schmidtke, 233–42. Dordrecht: Springer, 2010.

Hedlund, Maria. 'Ethicisation and Reliance on Ethics Expertise.' *Res Publica* (2023), https://doi.org/10.1007/s11158-023-09592-5

Hendriksen, Marieke. 'The Fate of the Beaded Babies: Forgotten Early Colonial Anatomy.' In *The Fate of Anatomical Collections*, edited by Rina Knoeff and Robert Zwijnenberg, 179–94. Farnham: Ashgate, 2015.

Hillgren, Karl E., and Lennart Nilsson. 'Varför måste fostret dödas?' *Se*, no. 28, July 10–16, 1952, 13–17.

Hoorn, Johan von. *Anatomes Publicae Anno MDCCV. Stockholmiae habitae Lectio Tertia. Sive Omnipotentis Mirabilia Circa Generationem Humanum*. Uppsala: Werner, 1709.

Hopwood, Nick. *Haeckel's Embryos: Images, Evolution, and Fraud*. Chicago: University of Chicago Press, 2015.

Hopwood, Nick. 'The Keywords "Generation" and "Reproduction."' In Hopwood, Flemming, and Kassell, *Reproduction*, 287–304.

Hopwood, Nick. 'Producing Development: The Anatomy of Human Embryos and the Norms of Wilhelm His.' *Bulletin of the History of Medicine* 74, no. 1 (2000): 29–79.

Hopwood, Nick, Rebecca Flemming, and Lauren Kassell, eds. *Reproduction: Antiquity to the Present Day*. Cambridge: Cambridge University Press, 2018.

Hopwood, Nick, Rebecca Flemming, and Lauren Kassell. 'Reproduction in History.' In Hopwood, Flemming, and Kassell, *Reproduction*, 3–17.

Hopwood, Nick, Peter Murray Jones, Lauren Kassell, and Jim Secord, eds. 'Communicating Reproduction.' Special issue, *Bulletin of the History of Medicine* 89, no. 3 (2015).

Hornuff, Daniel, and Heiner Fangerau, eds. *Visualisierung des Ungeborenen: Interdisziplinäre Perspektiven*. Paderborn: Brill/Fink, 2020.

Hult, Olof T. 'Benedictus Olai.' *Svenskt biografiskt lexikon*. Accessed July 8, 2023. https://sok.riksarkivet.se/sbl/Presentation.aspx?id=18477.

Hurlbut, Benjamin. *Experiments in Democracy: Human Embryo Research and the Politics of Bioethics*. New York: Columbia University Press, 2017.

Jacobs, Noortje. *Ethics by Committee: A History of Reasoning Together about Medicine, Science, Society, and the State*. Chicago: Chicago University Press, 2022.

Jacobs, Noortje, and Helena Tinnerholm Ljungberg, eds. 'How Ethics Travels: The International Development of Research Ethics Committees in the Late Twentieth Century.' Special issue, *European Journal for the History of Medicine and Health* 78, no. 2 (2021).

Johannisson, Karin. 'The People's Health: Public Health Policies in Sweden.' In *The History of Public Health and the Modern State*, edited by Dorothy Porter, 165–82. Amsterdam: Rodopi, 1994.

Jonsen, Albert R. *The Birth of Bioethics*. New York: Oxford University Press, 1998.

Jülich, Solveig. 'The Drama of the Fetoplacental Unit: Reimagining the Public Fetus of Lennart Nilsson.' In Björklund and Jülich, *Rethinking the Public Fetus*, 143–70.

Jülich, Solveig. 'Fetal Photography in the Age of Cool Media.' In *History of Participatory Media: Politics and Publics, 1750–2000*, edited by Anders Ekström, Solveig Jülich, Frans Lundgren, and Per Wisselgren, 125–41. New York: Routledge, 2011.

Jülich, Solveig. 'Fosterexperimentens produktiva hemlighet: Medicinsk forskning och vita lögner i 1960- och 1970-talets Sverige.' *Lychnos* (2018): 10–49.

Jülich, Solveig. 'The Making of a Best-Selling Book on Reproduction: Lennart Nilsson's *A Child Is Born*.' *Bulletin of the History of Medicine* 89, no. 3 (2015): 491–525.

Jülich, Solveig. 'Picturing Abortion Opposition in Sweden: Lennart Nilsson's Early Photographs of Embryos and Fetuses.' *Social History of Medicine* 31, no. 2 (2018): 278–307.

Jülich, Solveig, and Elisabet Björklund. 'The Public Fetus: A Traveling Concept.' In Björklund and Jülich, *Rethinking the Public Fetus*, 289–309.

Jülich, Solveig, and Helena Tinnerholm Ljungberg. 'Från medicinskt avfall till rättighetsinnehavare: Framväxten av värdekonflikter kring aborterade foster i Sverige.' *Tidskrift för genusvetenskap* 40, no. 3–4 (2019): 33–54.

Kent, Julie. *Regenerating Bodies: Tissue and Cell Therapies in the Twenty-First Century*. London and New York: Taylor and Francis, 2012.

Kent, Neil. *A Concise History of Sweden*. Cambridge: Cambridge University Press, 2008.

Kosmin, Jennifer F. *Authority, Gender, and Midwifery in Early Modern Italy: Contested Deliveries*. London: Routledge, 2020.

Kumlien, Mats. *Finns det ett kristet synsätt på abort?* Uppsala Faculty of Law, Working Paper 2012:2. Uppsala: Uppsala universitet, 2012.

Landecker, Hannah. *Culturing Life: How Cells Became Technologies*. Cambridge, MA: Harvard University Press, 2007.

Lee, Francis, Solveig Jülich, and Isa Dussauge. 'The Politics of Valuation: Value Disjunctures in Bioethics and Fetal Research During the Twentieth Century.' *Nordic Journal of Science and Technology Studies* 12, no. 2 (2024): 5–17.

Lemke, Thomas. *Biopolitics: An Advanced Introduction*. New York: New York University Press, 2011.

Lennerhed, Lena. 'No Backlash for Swedish Women? The Right to Abortion on Demand, 1975–2000.' *Journal of Modern European History* 17, no. 3 (2019): 326–36.

Lennerhed, Lena. 'Taking the Middle Way: Sex Education Debates in Sweden in the Early Twentieth Century.' In *Shaping Sexual Knowledge: A Cultural History of Sex Education in Twentieth Century Europe*, edited by Lutz Sauerteig and Roger Davidson, 55–70. London: Routledge, 2009.

Linnér, Birgitta. *Sex and Society in Sweden*. New York: Pantheon Books, 1967.

Littoz-Monnet, Annabelle. *Governing through Expertise: The Politics of Bioethics*. Cambridge: Cambridge University Press, 2020.

Löwy, Ilana. 'Historiography of Biomedicine: "Bio," "Medicine," and In Between.' *Isis* 102, no. 1 (2011): 116–22.

Löwy, Ilana. *Imperfect Pregnancies: A History of Birth Defects and Prenatal Diagnosis*. Baltimore: Johns Hopkins University Press, 2017.

Lundin, Per, and Niklas Stenlås. 'Technology, State Initiative, and National Myths in Cold War Sweden: An Introduction.' In *Science for Welfare and Warfare: Technology and State Initiative in Cold War Sweden*, edited by Per Lundin, Niklas Stenlås, and Johan Gribbe, 1–34. Sagamore Beach, MA: Science History Publications, 2010.

Lupton, Deborah. *The Social Worlds of the Unborn*. Basingstoke: Palgrave Macmillan, 2013.

Maehle, Andreas-Holger. *Contesting Medical Confidentiality: Origins of the Debate in the United States, Britain, and Germany*. Chicago: University of Chicago Press, 2016.

Matthews, Kirstin R. W., and Daniel Moralí. 'National Human Embryo and Embryoid Research Policies: A Survey of 22 Top Research-Intensive Countries.' *Regenerative Medicine* 15, no. 7 (2020): 1905–17.

Maynard-Moody, Steven. *The Dilemma of the Fetus: Fetal Research, Medical Progress and Moral Politics*. New York: St. Martin's Press, 1995.

Morgan, Lynn M. *Icons of Life: A Cultural History of Human Embryos*. Berkeley: University of California Press, 2009.

Morgan, Lynn M. '"Properly Disposed of": A History of Embryo Disposal and the Changing Claims on Fetal Remains.' *Medical Anthropology* 21, no. 3–4 (2002): 247–74.

Morgan, Lynn M. 'When Does Life Begin? A Cross-Cultural Perspective on the Personhood of Fetuses and Young Children.' In *Talking about People: Readings in Contemporary Cultural Anthropology*, edited by William A. Haviland, Robert J. Gordon, and Luis A. Vivanco, 35–46. Boston, MA: McGraw-Hill, 2002.

National Commission for the Protection of Human Subjects of Biomedical and Behavioral Research. *Research on the Fetus: Report and Recommendations*. US Department of Health, Education and Welfare, Publication No. (OS) 76-127. Washington, DC: Government Printing Office, 1975.

National Commission for the Protection of Human Subjects of Biomedical and Behavioral Research. *Research on the Fetus: Appendix*. US Department of Health, Education and Welfare, Publication No. (OS) 76-128. Washington, DC: Government Printing Office, 1976.

Nexø, Sniff Andersen. *Det rette valg: Dansk abortpolitik i 1930'erne og 1970'erne*. Copenhagen: Copenhagen University 2005.

Nicolson, Malcolm, and John E. E. Fleming. *Imaging and Imagining the Fetus: The Development of Obstetric Ultrasound*. Baltimore: Johns Hopkins University Press, 2013.

Nordlund, Christer. *Hormones of Life: Endocrinology, the Pharmaceutical Industry, and the Dream of a Remedy for Sterility, 1930–1970*. Sagamore Beach, MA: Science History Publications, 2011.

Nott, John, and Anna Harris, eds. *Making Sense of Medicine: Material Culture and the Reproduction of Medical Knowledge*. Bristol: Intellect Books, 2022.

Olai, Benedictus. *Een Nyttigh Läkere Book ther uthinnen man finner rådh / hielp och Läkedom til allehanda menniskiornes siwkdomar bådhe inwertes och uthwertes* [...]. Stockholm, 1578.

Olszynko-Gryn, Jesse, Patrick Ellis, and Caithan Gainty, eds. 'Reproduction on Film.' Special issue, *British Journal for the History of Science* 50, no. 3 (September 2017).

Olszynko-Gryn, Jesse, and Caroline Rusterholz. 'Reproductive Politics in Twentieth-Century France and Britain.' *Medical History* 63, no. 2 (2019): 117–33.

Park, Katharine. *Secrets of Women: Gender, Generation, and the Origins of Human Dissection*. New York: Zone Books, 2006.

Paulsson Holmberg, Tove. *Onaturlig födelse: Johan von Hoorn och det obstetriska dilemmat 1680–1730*. Lund: Lund University, 2017.

Pfeffer, Naomi, and Julie Kent. 'Framing Women, Framing Fetuses: How Britain Regulates Arrangements for the Collection and Use of Aborted Fetuses in Stem Cell Research and Therapies.' *BioSocieties* 2, no. 4 (2007): 429–47.

Poort, Looneke, Tora Holmberg, and Malin Ideland. 'Bringing in the Controversy: Re-politicizing the De-politicized Strategy of Ethics Committees.' *Life Sciences, Society and Policy* 9, no. 11 (2013): https://doi.org/10.1186/2195-7819-9-11.

Portal, Paul. *La pratique des accouchemens soutenue d'un grand nombre d'observations.* Paris: Gabriel Martin, 1685.

Quirke, Viviane, and Jean-Paul Gaudillière. 'The Era of Biomedicine: Science, Medicine, and Public Health in Britain and France after the Second World War.' *Medical History* 52, no. 4 (2008): 441–52.

Ramsey, Morag. *The Swedish Abortion Pill: Co-producing Medical Abortion and Values, ca. 1965–1992.* Uppsala: Uppsala University, 2021.

Ramsey, Paul. *The Ethics of Fetal Research.* New Haven and London: Yale University Press, 1975.

Ray, Sara. 'The Monsters of Peter and Wolff: Anatomical Preparations and Embryology in Eighteenth Century St. Petersburg.' In Björklund and Jülich, *Rethinking the Public Fetus*, 22–44.

Rothman, David J. *Strangers at the Bedside: A History of How Law and Bioethics Transformed Medical Decision Making.* 1991. New Brunswick, NJ: AldineTransaction, 2003.

Schoen, Johanna. *Abortion after* Roe. Chapel Hill: University of North Carolina Press, 2015.

'Sexualprofet på nöjesfältet.' *Se*, no. 26, June 28-July 4, 1945, 5–6.

Siegemund, Justine. *Die Chur-Brandenburgische Hoff-Wehe-Mutter.* Cölln an der Spree: Liebpert, 1690.

Sköld, Peter. 'The Birth of Population Statistics in Sweden.' *History of the Family* 9, no. 1 (2004): 5–21.

Svärd, Per-Anders, and Helena Tinnerholm Ljungberg. 'Fetal and Animal Research in Sweden: The Construction of Viable Lives in Regulatory Policy Debates, 1970–1980.' *Studies in History and Philosophy of Science, Part A* 89 (2021): 248–56.

Svendsen, Mette N., and Lene Koch. 'Unpacking the "Spare Embryo": Facilitating Stem Cell Research in a Moral Landscape.' *Social Studies of Science* 38, no. 1 (2008): 93–110.

Svenska akademiens ordbok (website). Accessed July 29, 2024. https://saob.se/.

Swedish Ministry of Health and Social Affairs. *Aborterade foster, m.m.: Betänkande.* SOU 1991:42. Stockholm: Allmänna förlaget, 1991.

Swedish Ministry of Justice. *Public Access to Information and Secrecy: The Legislation in Brief.* Stockholm: Ministry of Justice, 2020.

Takala, Tuija, and Matti Häyry. 'Physicians Controlling Women's Reproductive Choices: The Slow Liberalization of Abortion Laws in Finland.' *Cambridge Quarterly of Healthcare Ethics* 32, no. 3 (2023): 391–96.

Thornstedt, Hans. 'The Beginning and the End of Life from the Perspective of Swedish Criminal Law.' *Scandinavian Studies of Law* 14 (1970): 225–49.

Thorsén, David. 'Karolina Widerström och skolans dissektionsundervisning 1900–1920.' *Nordic Journal of Educational History* 8, no. 1 (2021): 3–30.

Tinnerholm Ljungberg, Helena. 'Regulating Research: The Origins and Institutionalization of Research Ethics Committees in Sweden.' *European Journal for the History of Medicine and Health* 78, no. 2 (2021): 267–86.

Tjeder, David. 'Mellan utlevelse och kyskhet: 1880-talets sedlighetsdebatt.' In Arnberg, Sundevall, and Tjeder, *Könspolitiska nyckeltexter*, 85–89.

Topçu, Sezin, and Irène Maffi. 'Rethinking Ignorance Production in the Field of Reproductive Biomedicine: An Introduction.' *Reproductive Biomedicine & Society Online* 14 (2022): 216–21.

Tydén, Mattias. 'The Scandinavian States: Reformed Eugenics Applied.' *The Oxford Handbook of the History of Eugenics*, edited by Alison Bashford and Philippa Levine, 363–76. New York: Oxford University Press, 2010.

Tydén, Mattias. 'Staten och våra gener.' In *Den kreativa staten: Framtidspolitiska tendenser*, edited by Torbjörn Lundqvist, 73–101. Stockholm: Institutet för framtidsstudier, 2006.

Waldby, Catherine. 'Production and Reproduction in the Bioeconomy.' Keynote for the conference 'Critical Sociology: Current Issues and Future Challenges.' Frankfurt am Main, 2014. Accessed August 14, 2022. https://anu-au.academia.edu/Catherine Waldby.

Waldby, Catherine, and Robert Mitchell. *Tissue Economies: Blood, Organs, and Cell Lines in Late Capitalism*. Durham, NC: Duke University Press, 2006.

Whiteley, Rebecca. *Birth Figures: Early Modern Prints and the Pregnant Body*. Chicago: University of Chicago Press, 2023.

Whiteley, Rebecca. 'The Limits of Seeing and Knowing: Early Modern Anatomy and the Uterine Membranes.' *Object: Graduate Research and Reviews in the History of Art and Visual Culture* 19 (2017): 95–119. Accessed July 8, 2023. https://doi .org/10.14324/111.2396-9008.026.

Widerström, Karolina, and Alma Sundquist. *Anatomiska väggtavlor*, 2nd ed. Stockholm: P. A. Norstedt & Söner, 1928.

Wilson, Duncan. *Tissue Culture in Science and Society: The Public Life of a Biological Technique in Twentieth Century Britain*. Basingstoke: Palgrave Macmillan, 2011.

Wilson, Emily K. 'Ex Utero: Live Human Fetal Research and the Films of Davenport Hooker.' *Bulletin of the History of Medicine* 88, no. 1 (2014): 132–60.

CHAPTER 1

Caring for the Liminal Dead: Lutheran Emergency Baptism and Stillbirth, ca. 1530–1720

Tove Paulsson Holmberg

> Little woman I want to comfort you with these words / although your child ended up dead / either it emerged dead from the womb or it was born with faint life / so that it could not receive baptism in the font or at home / no one should doubt the salvation of that child / and it must not be buried in mounds or in unconsecrated [pagan] ground / but in the churchyard / though without the presence of the minister / tolling of the bells / singing / and such things / so that baptism will not be degraded / and it should be buried with other baptized children / in good hope that our Heavenly Father has gracefully received it. For He is powerful enough to save a child in the womb of the mother / and to let it be baptized in its own blood / if he wants to.[1]

Birth and death are passages, openings, gateways, beginnings, and endings. For some individuals, birth is simultaneously an entrance and an exit. Emerging dead from the womb or failing to survive the first critical hours or days, they never enter the world of the living. They disappear suddenly and quietly, leaving behind ambiguous memories and feelings of emptiness, bereavement, failure, and sometimes, relief.

The history of early modern European fetal and infant health care remains marked by the manifest presence of casualties and loss. The deep impact of fetal and infant mortality on early modern families, populations, and societies has thus long been observed and analyzed by scholars in cultural history and demography.[2] Representations of fetuses and infants were fundamentally

1 Huberinus, *Tuende merckelige Tractater*, [38–39].

2 Ariès, *Centuries of Childhood*; Imhof, *Lost Worlds*; Gélis, *Les enfants des limbes*; Woods, *Children Remembered*; Woods, *Death before Birth*.

 | DOI:10.1163/9789004703759_003

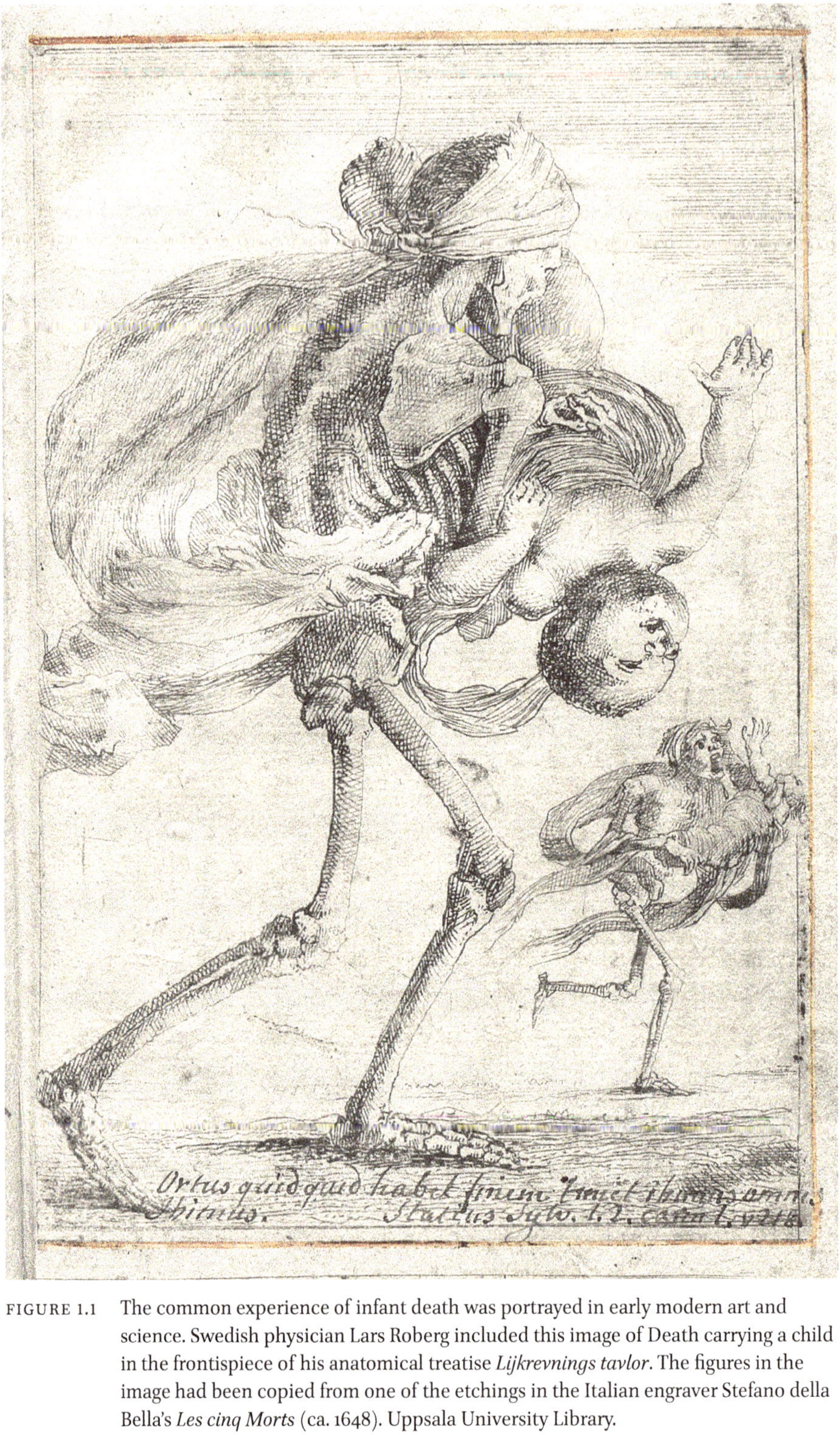

FIGURE 1.1 The common experience of infant death was portrayed in early modern art and science. Swedish physician Lars Roberg included this image of Death carrying a child in the frontispiece of his anatomical treatise *Lijkrevnings tavlor*. The figures in the image had been copied from one of the etchings in the Italian engraver Stefano della Bella's *Les cinq Morts* (ca. 1648). Uppsala University Library.

shaped by the pressure of these dark prospects. From a historical perspective, the category of 'unborn' is fundamentally fluid, and unborn entities are 'constantly changing configurations' produced by the interaction between discourses and practices in specific contexts.[3] This chapter explores the unborn and the birth transition in early modern Lutheran Sweden from the perspectives of salvation and loss. In stressing the significance of transition rites and the afterlife to notions of the unborn, it builds on previous historical and cross-cultural research that has demonstrated how concepts and depictions of the fetus and infant are inscribed in dominant religious frameworks that shape childbirth practices, family ideology, and death rites.[4]

Obstetric intervention in medieval and early modern Europe was characterized by a diversity of strategies shaped by religious, medical, and legal concerns.[5] Strategies related to the preservation of fetal and infant life and health in historical contexts are, to some degree, the result of valuations that are articulated and enacted through practices.[6] This chapter focuses on intervention strategies in sixteenth- and seventeenth-century Sweden that resulted from the influence of a Lutheran baptismal framework over religious and medical approaches to childbirth. The time period studied, ca. 1530–1720, covers two major transformations in birth intervention: the religious context of the introduction and consolidation of the Lutheran Reformation and the gradual emergence of the mechanistic paradigm in late seventeenth and early eighteenth century obstetrics. The aim is to trace how the simultaneous presence of conflicting values related to prospects of physical and spiritual survival for fetuses and infants, in combination with concern for the life of the mother, shaped the contours of a specific configuration of the unborn: the fully grown child in the liminal, 'perinatal' period before, during, and after birth.[7]

The term 'perinatal,' though not present in the early modern period, will here be used to highlight that birth is a protracted and gradual process that

---

3 Duden, 'Zwischen "wahrem Wissen" und Prophetien,' 46–47; Lupton, *Social Worlds of the Unborn*, introduction.

4 Cressy, *Birth, Marriage and Death*; Duden, Schlumbohm, and Veit, *Geschichte des Ungeborenen*; Gélis, *Les enfants des limbes*; Law and Sasson, *Imagining the Fetus*; Crowther, *Adam and Eve*; Park, 'Birth and Death'; Løkke, 'Responsibility and Emotion.'

5 See, e.g., Foscati, '"Nonnatus Dictus,"' 466; Van der Lugt, 'Formed Fetuses and Healthy Children,' 167.

6 Dussauge et al., 'On the Omnipresence,' 1–2.

7 All definitions of the term are shaped by factors influencing fetal and infant survival prospects and development in various contexts. According to the *International Statistical Classification of Diseases and Related Health Problems*, the time period begins at twenty-two completed weeks of gestation and ends seven days after birth.

is not limited to the moment of separation between mother and child, or the hours or days of labor and delivery. During this liminal phase, the fetus, and later the infant, could be described as 'hovering between life and death.' In the context of sixteenth- and seventeenth-century Sweden, 'perinatal' refers to, roughly, the time period between the seventh month of gestation, when the fetus might survive if delivered, and the first month of life, after which the infant had recovered from the ordeal of birth and stabilized itself in the world. This perinatal entity was alternatively called 'fetus,' 'fruit,' 'infant,' or 'child.' Positioned at the threshold of life, it demonstrated 'vitality' through the display of strength, activity, and movement. It was also, in many ways, looked upon as a person, a human being in possession of a soul. In her analysis of early modern birth figures, Rebecca Whiteley has identified a moment of transition, after which the fetus was 'personified' and endowed with humanity and individuality. This moment, believed to occur in mid-pregnancy, was associated with complete bodily formation, ensoulment, and quickening.[8] The fully grown fetus, at the end of pregnancy, had supposedly long since passed this moment. Surviving the perilous birth transition—achieving baptism—was necessary to the spiritual survival of the soul that resided in this liminal being.

Managing perinatal loss means coping with emergences and partings, transitions between worlds. In the following, close reading of selected birth manuals, devotional literature, and religious and legal tracts will be used to examine how narratives, concepts, and imagery related to late fetal and infant life, health, and salvation were linked to practices that produced and defended attachment and vitality, or the reverse. First, the problem of baptism and perinatal loss in Lutheran Sweden is introduced. Second, oscillations between inclusion and distance in representations of perinatal children are described, stressing the implicit imperative to secure (at least) a temporary live birth, yet accepting the conditional status of unborn entities as well as the limits of human and medical art and endeavor. Finally, some tentative conclusions are presented, framing the strategies of birth intervention in Lutheran Sweden as a compromise between Catholic and Calvinist readings of the sacrament of baptism: a process encouraging essentially utilitarian solutions and arguments.

8 Whiteley, *Birth Figures*, 62.

1 Baptismal Practices and Perinatal Loss

> The Book of Wisdom says: The righteous / though he dies early / yet is he in peace. Now when unbaptized children / through prayer and the virtue of Christ are commended to God / they are justified by Christ / and the righteousness of Christ will by grace be attributed to them. Therefore are they / regardless if they die early / in the hand of God / and no torment of death shall touch them.[9]

> The first Concern of Parents is this: as soon as possible help their new-born Child to [baptism], if they do not want to assume a firm responsibility and place themselves in grave danger.[10]

Early modern Swedish birth discourses testify of the constant pressure exercised by the presence of stillbirth, when death and birth coincide. In this context, religious practices, and baptismal practices in particular, exerted a dominant influence over the difficult processes of preventing, making sense of, and coping with perinatal loss.

During the period under consideration here, the Swedish nation-state was founded, the church was nationalized, and the Protestant (Lutheran) reformation was introduced and consolidated. Recurring wars from 1560 onward gradually transformed Sweden into a dominant power in northern Europe: a position it finally lost after the Great Northern War (1700–21). The practice of midwifery in urban and rural contexts remained relatively constant, and was to a large degree characterized as a manual trade dominated by female practitioners, surgeons and physicians generally being called upon to intervene only in desperate emergencies.[11] In the 1690s, the public training of midwives was instituted in Stockholm, to be formalized in an official set of regulations for the profession in 1711.[12] At this time, however, birth practitioners had long been surveilled by the church, with regard to the specific matter of birth-related survival and baptism.[13]

Baptism is a central sacrament in Christianity. Essentially, it removes original sin and establishes a crucial union between human individuals and God.

9 Wagner, *HWSBIBLIA*, 155.

10 Collinder, *Nödig Tröst och Underwisning*, 98.

11 Lundqvist, *Svenska barnmorskor*, 14–15.

12 Djurberg, *Läkaren Johan von Hoorn*, 58; Paulsson Holmberg, *Onaturlig födelse*, 95–96.

13 Lundqvist, *Svenska barnmorskor*, 25. For the European development, see Park, 'Birth and Death,' 21–22.

Baptism alters the status of the person completely, and that the doctrine of baptism is based on notions of death and rebirth is consistent with the understanding of the ritual as vital to personhood, humanness, and afterlife.[14] To acknowledge the transformative nature of baptism is to defend the necessity of the sacrament—and the consequent exclusion and alienation of unbaptized individuals.

To early modern Europeans, the baptism of infants functioned as a transition rite. The ceremony of baptism effected social birth, which granted the child a name and a Christian identity. If baptized infants died, they had access to the next dimension, where they were supposedly reunited with their family at the end of time. But the unfortunate individuals who died before they had received the sacrament remained lost forever, hovering in the darkness between worlds, among outsiders, pagans and non-Christians.[15]

Traditional solutions to the urgent problem of saving the souls of endangered fetuses and infants focused on emergency interventions securing the ritual: postmortem cesarean section, baptism *in utero*, and baptism of stillborn infants who seemingly displayed temporary 'life signs.'[16] Among these practices, postmortem cesarean section was the most problematic. The use of mutilating surgery on supposedly deceased mothers to secure the baptism of their living unborn children had important legal motives and consequences, since if the child survived the operation, however temporarily, the father inherited the property of his wife through the child. The operation was increasingly advocated and performed in Catholic Europe from the late medieval period onward, despite the difficult inherent ethical considerations.[17] The two latter practices, having the benefit of not affecting maternal survival, still remained questionable because of the potential violation of the sacrament that resulted from baptizing nonhuman or dead entities. The Reformation changed practices related to baptism and birth intervention. The essential Protestant response to the problem of birth-related death was to urge parents to place their unborn in the hands of God and appeal to his mercy. Since God was omnipotent, he could save whomever he wanted, and since he was loving and merciful, he would most likely respond to the prayers of pious parents. The destiny of stillborn and unbaptized children was thus to some degree placed outside the realm of

14 Davies, *Death, Ritual and Belief*, 182.

15 Imhof, *Lost Worlds*, 132–33; Gélis, *Les enfants des limbes*, 39–42.

16 For strategies related to perinatal survival and baptism in early modern Catholic contexts, see Gélis, *Les enfants des limbes*. See also Van der Lugt, 'Formed Fetuses and Healthy Children,' 171–72.

17 Keupper Valle, 'Cesarean Operation'; Park, 'Death of Isabella Della Volpe'; Foscati, '"Nonnatus Dictus."'

human control. But where Lutherans followed Luther's explicit demand that the sacrament of baptism—and infant baptism per se—still be defended and honored, Calvinists, being strong proponents of the idea that faith requires a conscious stance, tended toward a reading of the sacrament as 'symbolic' or 'external.'[18] A shared concern was the desire to remove parts of the ritual that 'devalued and compromised' the sacrament, and the performance of all baptismal practices became more closely surveilled.[19]

Stressing the fact that scripture made no reference to many aspects of the traditional baptismal ceremony, Protestant theologians warned parents not to depend on them to 'secure' the child's salvation. Instead of relying on these pointless manipulations, parents should concentrate on their relationship to God. Not trusting in divine grace was nothing less than blasphemy, and a manipulated sacrament, a simulacrum of the sacrament, was completely worthless.[20]

This inclination to entrust doubtful cases to the judgement and mercy of God conformed to the general Protestant strategy in questions where scripture remained ambiguous or silent.[21] To the parents of stillborn, the crucial change was that unbaptized children were allowed burial in the churchyard—an important sign that these unfortunate family members were no longer categorically excluded and abandoned.[22] But since they were buried with separate, and muted, rituals, the desire to pursue baptism did not abate. In popular belief, unbaptized children were described as lost souls, since they had met with a bad death and had been deprived of proper death rites. They belonged to the errant, or placeless, dead, whose ultimate destiny remained an open question. This lingering uncertainty regarding the status and dwelling place of the unbaptized dead, conforming to Catholic tradition, is reflected in Scandinavian folk belief that persisted for centuries.[23] Protecting and appeasing these entities by aiding their spiritual transformation remained a necessary priority, not only to individual families but to society at large, hence the need to continuously accept and cultivate emergency solutions.

18 Rodhe, *Doppritualet*, 37.

19 Grell, 'Protestant Imperative,' 53; Cressy, *Birth, Marriage and Death*, 123; Gélis, *Les enfants des limbes*, 216–21.

20 Gélis, *Les enfants des limbes*, 220.

21 Ferngren, *Medicine and Religion*, 156.

22 Duden, 'Zwischen "wahrem Wissen" und Prophetien,' 35.

23 Pentikäinen, *Nordic Dead-Child Tradition*, 356–57; Gélis, *Les enfants des limbes*, 42.

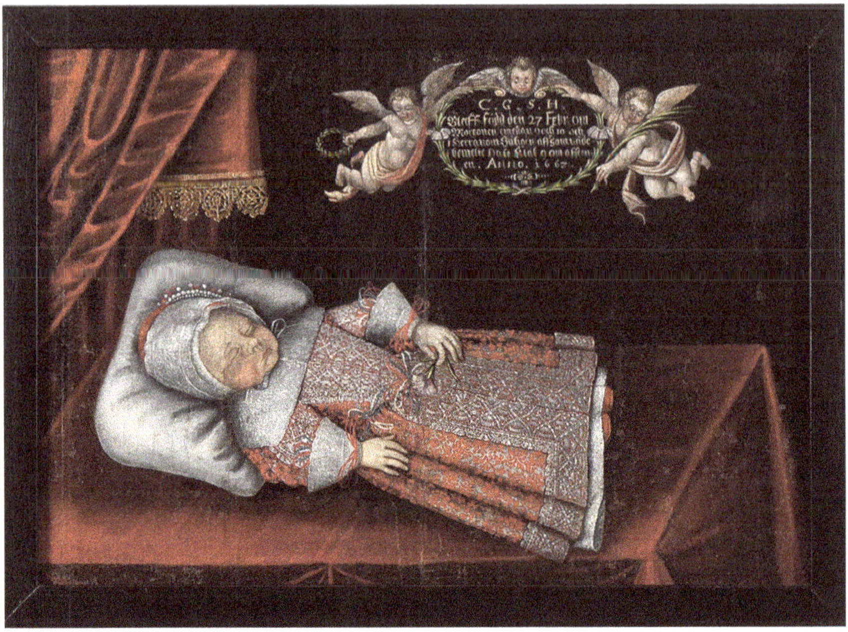

FIGURE 1.2 Memorial portrait of Carl Gustavsson Horn, by Joachim Neimann. Horn lived for less than twelve hours, yet long enough to be baptized. 'C.G.S.H. was born on the 27th Febr. in the morning between 9 and 10 and fell blissfully asleep in the Lord the same Date at 9 in the evening. Anno 1662.' He was buried in Åbo/Turku Cathedral (in Swedish Finland) wearing a gown in exclusive fabrics to show that he was a member of the high nobility. Object 68825, Nordic Museum, Stockholm.

The practice of using a reduced 'emergency' ritual to baptize weak infants in immediate connection to birth had been present since infant baptism was instituted, and it was regularly performed in medieval Sweden.[24]

Emergency baptism is a performative act that involves liquid (preferably water) and a Christian person uttering the words, 'I baptize thee [name] in the name of the Father, the Son and the Holy Ghost.' The haste and desperation inherent in the situations where it was performed, in combination with the absence of religious representatives, gave rise to the dangerous possibility that it might be invalid. Defending the status of the sacrament, Protestant theologians banned the Catholic usage of baptism 'on condition' ('If you are alive,

24 Faehn, 'Dåp,' 414.

I baptize you [...]'), and ministers were instructed to investigate whether all baptismal rituals had been performed correctly.[25]

Though the reformation process had begun in Sweden in 1527, it was the Church Council of Uppsala that ratified the first reformed Swedish Church Order (1572). This document stated that emergency baptism must be conducted at home when children are 'too weak and cannot suffer the delay to take them to church.' No child must be baptized until it was 'completely born' and distinctly alive, not even in cases of extreme need. All present shall instead 'with earnest prayers commend both mother and child in the gentle hands of God.' 'For one shall have good hope that God will embrace such prayer and service as a complete baptism. For He cares less for external deeds, which may by many means be hindered, than for the will and the heart.' Finally, emergency baptism must be strictly limited to cases of 'perfect reason'; that is, when the life of the child was in imminent danger.[26]

The security of baptism was, however, demanded by parents, who also pursued the social advantages of publicly celebrating their new family member. When the new Church Law (1686) stated that all children must be baptized in church within eight days after birth, it was a response to a growing custom favored by the elite: instant emergency baptism followed by 'christening' in connection with lavish baptismal feasts weeks or months later.[27] Underlining the importance of restricting emergency baptism to evade 'abuse, security and carelessness,' all postponement of baptism in church would henceforth lead to punishment for negligence.[28]

The Lutheran position evidently rested on a difficult dilemma: defending the status of the sacrament of baptism made statements about the effects of prenatal intercession prayers less convincing, yet such statements were necessary for both theological and practical reasons. And since baptism in any form demanded that the child survive birth, the importance of ensuring at least temporary survival continued to frame practices related to late fetal health, obstetric emergencies, and infant care. As demonstrated by Anne Løkke, parents in eighteenth-century Lutheran Denmark, who were able to accept stillbirth with equanimity, remained profoundly disturbed by their failure to secure the baptism of live-born infants.[29]

---

25 Wiesner, 'Midwives of South Germany,' 83.
26 *Laurentius Petris kyrkoordning av år 1571*, 58.
27 Sjölin, *Dopsed i förändring*, 56–60.
28 *Kyrkio-Lag och Ordning*, Chap. III, §2.
29 Løkke, 'Responsibility and Emotion,' 198–99.

The Protestant transformations of the ritual of baptism visibly transformed the ways in which fetuses and infants were conceptualized and represented. Barbara Duden has argued that the Lutheran practice of prenatal prayers strengthened the presence and childlike qualities of the unborn, resulting in a new antenatal regime directing focus toward the well-being and survival of the child.[30] Yet it is also evident that this framework created a mental opening toward the pragmatic termination of ill-timed, defective, and high-risk pregnancies, if the life of the mother was in peril. Sacrificing the child in obstructed labor is fundamentally eased if it remains conceivable that the afterlife of the unborn is not categorically compromised by failing to survive the birth transition.[31]

These changes in the configuration of the perinatal child, informed by new baptismal practices, were influenced by the introduction of new medical birth practices and technologies in the last decades of the seventeenth century. This was caused by the gradual abandonment of humoral ideas in favor of a mechanical framework in obstetrics, producing contradictory and complex concepts and imagery related to fetal and infant activity, vitality, and decay. In the following, some strategies in this process that either reached out and strengthened the bonds with the unborn, or created distance and detachment, will be identified and described in some detail.

2 Reaching Out

> Since she helps them Alive to the World, she also promotes them to the holy Baptism, so that these little ones, begotten in Sin, are washed clean from original Sin in the precious Blood of the Savior. Which is such a great Benefaction that it cannot be described by the Pen.[32]

Representations of the fully grown fetus in sixteenth- and seventeenth-century Swedish religious and medical discourses were inseparable from the assumed precedence of spiritual survival and human potentiality. The weight of the demands that this entity directed toward parents and birth practitioners granted a distinct presence to the unborn, demarcating it as a person, a member of the family and of the community of Christians.

30 Duden, 'Zwischen "wahrem Wissen" und Prophetien,' 36.
31 LaFleur, *Liquid Life*, chap. 12.
32 Hoorn, *Den Swenska Wälöfwade Jordgumman*, 5.

Residing in uterine obscurity and facing potential annihilation, the unborn were by definition exposed and vulnerable. Swedish devotional literature from the sixteenth and seventeenth centuries reflects the anxiety, concern, and attachment directed toward these liminal beings. Lutheran books of meditation repeatedly addressed the subjects of parenthood and family bonds, of coping with grief and loss and preparing for death.[33] The genre targeted women as potential mothers.[34] Johann Wagner offers in *HWSBIBLIA* (1623), chapter XII, '[a] comfort for women who miscarry, and whose children die either in the womb or in relation to birth, before they are baptized.'[35] The reader afflicted by this 'cross' was invited to contemplate seven arguments from scripture that reveal the generous compassion of Christ and the Father toward these small and innocent persons, and promise that prenatal intercessions of parents—'When Christian parents carry their unborn children to Christ upon their arms of faith and prayer'—may fully substitute for baptism. Pious parents might safely rely on the spiritual rule that if circumstances prevent access to a sacrament, the person deprived of it was not condemned for negligence. And since the unborn were inaccessible, concealed inside the womb by God himself, he would treat them with forbearance and mercy.[36]

Devotional tracts often included specific prayers to be recited during pregnancy and delivery, and regular prayers for the unborn were described as part of the antenatal care practiced by responsible parents. The prayers typically stress the courage, vulnerability, and subjectivity of the mother, and place her in a parent-child relation toward God. The unborn entity is described in emotionally charged terms as 'my little child,' 'my dear child/fruit,' 'my poor fruit.'[37]

As indicated by recurring narratives, fear of eternal loss fueled a sense of danger, urgency, and vulnerability that added emotional weight to the unborn, alternately denominated 'child,' 'fruit,' or 'fetus.' But the child itself is principally absent: eclipsed by the mother and her self-absorbed discourse with her Maker and Guardian. The physical conditions that determined and sustained the precarious liminality of unborn entities remained, if not entirely invisible, at least opaque and indistinctly conveyed.

By contrast, contemporary medical manuals reveal the complex interplay between spiritual and physical concerns that informed the management of

33 Estborn, *Evangeliska svenska bönböcker*; Lindquist, *Studier i den svenska andaktslitteraturen*, 384; Gleixner, 'Todesangst und Gottergebenheit,' 76; Veit, '"Ich bin sehr schwach."'

34 Gleixner, 'Todesangst und Gottergebenheit'; Veit, '"Ich bin sehr schwach"'; Lindgärde, 'Hon dog en Rakels död,' 178–79.

35 Wagner, *HWSBIBLIA*, 155.

36 Wagner, *HWSBIBLIA*, 154.

37 Collinder, *Nödig Tröst och Underwisning*, 42–43.

birth in a world where many mothers and children died in the process of separation. In this context, midwives were spiritual supervisors as well as medical practitioners. Physician Henrik Smid described the delivery in *Fierde Urtegaard* (Fourth garden of herbs; 1577):

> The Midwife shall comfort / ease / pray / and admonish the sickly Woman / and the other present Goodwives / so they together with her fall to their Knees / call upon God and recite the Lord's Prayer / and plead him sincerely from the bottom of the Heart / that he will be present with his holy Spirit and Grace / and extend help and succor / so that there will be blissful prosperity in the actual events. And when this has passed / the Midwife shall place the sickly Woman on the chair [...][38]

Before the second half of the seventeenth century, the process of birth was explained within a humoral framework, and complications were primarily treated with medication and spiritual and emotional support. Focusing on regulating the internal flux and supporting the 'forces,' birth practitioners preferably abstained from manipulations *in utero*. Separation in obstetric emergencies was usually restricted to the expelling of fetal remains with drugs and remedies or, in rare cases, performing postmortem cesarean section. The first method saved the life of the mother; the purpose of the second was to save living children in case of maternal demise. By waiting until one of the participants was clearly dead, birth practitioners avoided accusations of 'rashness,' cruelty, and murder. Henrik Smid advocated attentive inspection of the mother before any intervention took place. If she displayed 'signs of death' she must be left in peace, 'commended in the hands of God'; if not, the midwife might expel the (supposedly) dead fetus with purging remedies. Smid hinted that it might also be possible to extract dead children 'with Hooks and Pinchers that are convenient.' But since he anticipated censure from 'irrational women,' he prudently omitted descriptions of such dangerous practices, and closed the chapter with the less provocative method of performing postmortem cesarean section in cases of 'living Fetuses.'[39]

In *Een nyttigh Läkare Book* (A useful book for physicians; 1578), Benedictus Olai described how to detect fetal weakness and death through exterior signs of maternal ill-health. Stating that 'abortus' is critical between the fourth and the seventh month of gestation, after which 'the child is strong in the womb,' Olai used an analogy with trees that bear fruit: 'When [the fruit] is ripened, she

38 Smid, *Fierde Urtegaard*, 36–37.

39 Smid, *Fierde Urtegaard*, 23–24.

gives birth easily.'[40] Fetal death manifests itself by means of pain in the eyes and the neck, a feeling of weight in the womb, a diminished belly, and cold. A 'certain sign' was when external examinations of the belly did not provoke a response, usually resulting, some days later, in the discharge of 'nauseous matter.'[41] Olai used the term 'child' to describe the unborn entity and stated that in cases of severe maternal ill-health, it is 'not a minor question how one could help [such a] child.'[42] He also ascribed agency to this entity: it leaves the womb if it starves.[43]

Some sixty years later, physician Andreas Sparrman described birth intervention to some degree in *Sundhetenz Spegel* (A mirror for health; 1642). If the child ('fetus') does not emerge headfirst, the midwife must force back the limbs and guide the head to the exit. Sparrman also made the specific claim that dead children are to be delivered feet first: 'pulled to the Earth [grave] feet first [...] so as to separate the Entrance and Exit of this Life.'[44] Yet how these manipulations were to be effected was not explained in his brief outline.

The comparative absence of hands-on descriptions of internal manipulations of unborn bodies in late sixteenth- and early seventeenth-century manuals distinguishes them from the specialized birth manuals of the last decades of the seventeenth century, in which such manipulations are prominent. The increasing circulation of the interventionist practices described in these manuals was connected to a mechanistic conceptualization of birth, which favored the use of surgical methods, podalic version in particular. By turning the child and pulling it out by traction, birth practitioners interacted directly with unborn bodies. In the first Swedish birth manual describing podalic version, *Den Swenska Wälöfwade Jordgumman* (The well-trained Swedish midwife; 1697), a major part of the text is devoted to detailed descriptions of manipulations of fetal bodies, fully grown and ready to be born.

These new intervention practices reached out to the unborn in several ways. First, by closing in on and manipulating the unborn *in utero*, birth practitioners observed and described numerous details and phenomena related to fetal health and decay. Second, by attributing the agency exerted during birth to uterine contractions, the child was reconceptualized as passive and vulnerable, in need of assistance. If the unborn in the humoral paradigm seems obscure because its positions, limbs, and body parts remained undescribed, it

40 Olai, *Een Nyttigh Läkere Book*, [343–44].
41 Olai, *Een Nyttigh Läkere Book*, [346–47].
42 Olai, *Een Nyttigh Läkere Book*, [340].
43 Olai, *Een Nyttigh Läkere Book*, [345].
44 Sparrman, *Sundhetzens Speghel*, 361.

was still an entity that possessed independence and 'liberated itself from its prison' by force. The passive child conjured up in the mechanistic paradigm seems, by comparison, detached and reserved: a victim of forces and circumstances. Its silence and immobility carry strokes of death. Both configurations were, however, conditioned by the liminal state in which they were inscribed; as beings whose ultimate destiny depended on their successful separation from the maternal body. Contemplating this precarious and vulnerable situation, how could the fully grown, childlike, 'personified' unborn not be invested with feelings of pity, responsibility, and guardianship? And how could the determined hands of birth practitioners reaching out toward this entity in late seventeenth-century illustrations not be a mark of attachment and emotion?

The manifestations of compassion and attachment emanating from obstetric discourses and practices were not limited to fetuses that were alive. Living or dead, unborn needed help to complete their transition. But since available

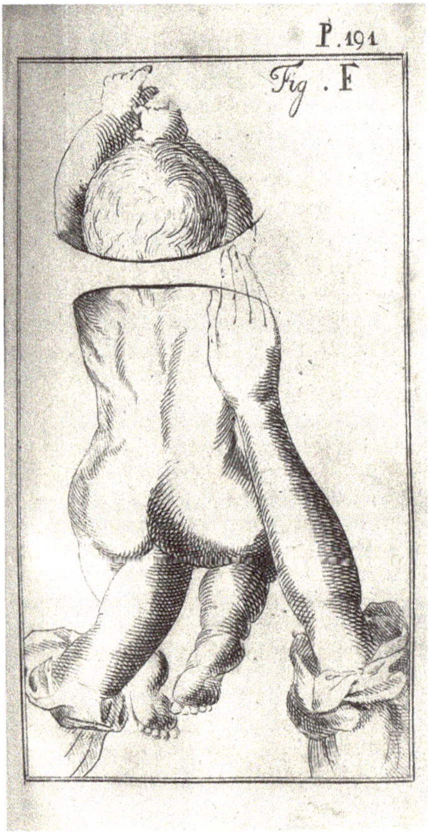

FIGURE 1.3
Loosening the arms in podalic version. This was a critical moment for the fetus. The circulation in the umbilical cord must be preserved, and the head had to follow correctly. Visualizations of this new way of intervening in the pregnant body's processes were key how to practice midwifery. From the first midwifery book in Swedish; von Hoorn's, *Den Swenska Wälöfvade Jordgumman*, 191, fig. F. Unknown artist. Hagströmer Library, Karolinska Institute.

methods of surgical separation in obstructed labor harmed the bodily integrity of the child, they were generally avoided. If birth practitioners mutilated the unborn and it emerged dead, they risked being accused of killing the child. In Lutheran contexts, surgeons and midwives had to treat the unborn as alive if not palpably dead, lacking the Catholic option described by Jacques Gélis 'to mentally treat the child as a corpse' after performing baptism *in utero*, or relying on implied permissive attitudes toward emergency baptism of lifeless and stillborn infants.[45] However, all birth practitioners desperately pursued unambiguous symptoms of fetal death, allowing them to intervene at the earliest possible moment. Declaring the unborn dead in complicated labor remained very difficult, since the cramped position of the child prevented it from moving, and once separated from the mother, it was often lifeless and extinguished, suffering from asphyxia. The demand that infants display 'distinct signs of life' before baptism moreover concealed an enduring problem: the blurred boundary between living and dead. How this dilemma was met in the event of obstructed birth, and how notions of distance and decay were attributed to unborn entities in this process, will be addressed in the next part of the chapter.

3 Distancing

> Out of a dead Fetus is nothing but evil to expect for the Mother.[46]

Death is a process, and dead bodies often show vague symptoms of life in the hours and days after the circulation of the blood and the motion of the heart have stopped. Similarly, living bodies may appear like corpses, deprived of all vital signs. These, and other phenomena in the borderland between life and death, are characteristic features of the liminal state in which perinatal children reside before and after they complete the transition of birth.[47]

Cross-cultural and historical scholarship has shown that a kind of 'ontological thickening' occurs as pregnancy progresses: the child is growing more tangible, conceivable, and present. In medieval and early modern Europe, the defining moment in the social recognition of the unborn was in mid-pregnancy

45 Gélis, *La sage-femme ou le médécin*, 358–59.
46 Hoorn, *Den Swenska Wälöfwade Jordgumman*, 238.
47 Gélis, *Les enfants des limbes*, 17; Woods, *Death before Birth*, 14–27.

when 'quickening' occurred. At this point, the distinct movements of the child displayed that it was fully formed and ensouled, after which moment terminating the pregnancy would qualify as a murder.[48] As demonstrated by Runesson in this volume, the most important factor in the valuation of a miscarried fetus was whether it had developed human form, and could be identified as a human, in which case it qualified for a 'proper' burial.[49]

Early modern obstetric discourses tend to mediate a cautious, muted, conditioned view, exuding reservation and premonition of loss. The reason for this bias lay partly in the fact that birth manuals focused on complicated, obstructed, and deviant cases. But descriptions of pregnancy care contributed as well by underlining narratives of procreation as a struggle toward fulfilment and completion, where the unborn gradually emerges from a dark multitude of chaotic alternatives and failed prospects: 'false conceptions'; mola or moon-calves; tumors; windy and watery illusions; shapeless, unfinished, and deformed drafts; remnants and leftovers; and, intensifying the fear and abjection, horrible and destructive dreams of monstra and the ever-presence of creative and intrusive evil forces.[50]

Being a ritual of transformation and inclusion, the baptismal ceremony by definition accentuated the alienation of outsiders. The first reformed Swedish ritual of baptism (1529) contained recurrent elements of exorcism: statements that marked out the newborn as a person who must dissociate him or herself from darkness and evil.

> Look upon this your servant [name] that you have called to faith, purge him [her] from all the blindness of his heart, and tear apart the ropes with which the Devil has tied him, open your door of benefaction to him, so that he may be marked with the sign of your wisdom; all dark desires vanish in him, and he may follow your holy commands and joyfully serve you in holy Christianity, transformed to the best, and be ready to come to your holy baptism and there receive true healing in Jesus Christ our Lord. AMEN.[51]

48 Park, 'Birth and Death,' 19; Van der Lugt, 'Formed Fetuses and Healthy Children,' 170–71. For legal discussions on miscarriages and abortion in early modern Sweden, see Runesson's chapter in this volume.

49 Runesson, chap. 2 in this volume.

50 See Bondestam's chapter, on early modern Swedish legal and medical discourses on fetal monstrosity, in this volume.

51 Petri, *Een handbock påå swensko*, 318.

The manifest presence of exorcism in the ritual of baptism was much debated in the late sixteenth and early seventeenth centuries, essentially regarded as problematic because of the explicit linking of infants, darkness, and sin.[52] Still, the liminal condition of the unborn invited speculations of this nature. Huberinus's devotional tract from 1577 states that the Devil pursues pregnant women relentlessly, tormenting them with 'fright, terror, eeriness, distress, fear, illness and hopelessness.' Being a sworn enemy to the children of man, he intensifies his efforts during this vulnerable period, since he knows that once they are born and baptized, they are beyond his reach: 'The holy Angels of Heaven form a circle around the baptized, and the children of the pious.'[53] In narratives like this, dark forces mercilessly haunt the innocent souls of the unborn, hoping to harvest them before their inclusion in the Kingdom of Grace. Scandinavian folklore testifies to an enduring belief in the determination, and capacity, of evil spirits to molest, steal, or harm newborn children.[54] Delivering children alive and securing their spiritual transformation and protection by the means of baptism appear in this context as an act of resistance toward chaos, evil, and annihilation.

Success in this quest was conditional on deciphering and analyzing signs of life, strength, weakness, and decay in hidden, inaccessible, and mute entities. All close investigation of unborn bodies was impeded by the general aversion toward internal examinations, except in extreme emergency.[55] In this process, religious narratives investing motherhood with heroism, resolution, and self-sacrifice tended to delay the moment when obstetric intervention was attempted, to the detriment of the health and survival of both mother and child.[56]

Early modern birth intervention evolved around the difficult problem of how to save both mother and child in complicated and obstructed birth. The status of the unborn in this process was living, dead, or 'unknown.' Whenever it was possible to declare the unborn dead, because of explicit fetal corruption, there was no delay in helping the mother to relieve herself of 'this useless and harmful burden.'[57] When in doubt, birth practitioners, family, and friends hesitated to use methods of intervention that harmed, mutilated, or destroyed the unborn body, particularly if the mother was severely weakened. In this

52 Rodhe, *Doppritualet*, 82–85.

53 Huberinus, *Tuende merckelige Tractater*, 2.

54 Burjam, *Den skandinaviska folktron*, chap. 1.

55 Siegemund, *Court Midwife*, 84; Paulsson Holmberg, *Onaturlig födelse*, 170–79.

56 Schwartz, *Milton and Maternal Mortality*, chap. 3.

57 Hoorn, *Den Swenska Wälöfwade Jordgumman*, 90.

situation, the most acceptable solution could be to support and comfort the mother in her parting, and eventually bury her undelivered. Painfully aware of their limited ability to save both mother and child in obstetric emergencies, medical authors tended to cultivate selective silence on the subject of birth-related death, and carefully avoided describing potentially dangerous methods of separation, leaving the question of survival 'in the hands of God.'[58]

As long as it was believed that the child contributed actively to birth, fetal death was deeply feared, since being unable to release themselves from fetal remains, pregnant mothers had to be purged of the matter of failed pregnancies. The very notion of 'purging,' by definition, evokes images of purifying, and discarding of nonhuman, shapeless, and unsolidified growths. Medical authors before around 1650 included numerous remedies to expel 'dead fetuses' in their manuals, which in combination with their silence on the subject of how to detect signs of fetal life and intervene manually, produced discourses that evoke images and notions of distance, detachment, failure, and decay.[59]

Mechanistically informed manuals, by contrast, generated detailed observations of fetal corporality: a focus that grants a powerful presence to the unborn. The birth manuals of obstetric surgeon Johan von Hoorn (1697, 1715, 1719) devote several chapters to the examination of signs of fetal vitality and decay. The author recommended mutilating surgery in case of fetal demise and defended the priority of the mother. Yet being a supporter of podalic version, his genuine concern was advancing early intervention, thus saving both mother and child. In his publications the promotion of manual intervention techniques is combined with methods to revive and resuscitate weak infants.[60]

Preparing for intervention in obstetric emergencies meant anticipating the need for emergency baptism. Von Hoorn initially observed that slow and obstructed delivery often results in weak and lifeless infants. To escape censure the midwife was obligated to state this to the attendant family. She would then prepare necessary objects and remedies and a bowl of clean water, proceed with the delivery, and if the child was not manifestly dead, she would put it in her lap and examine it closely. If there 'seem[ed] to be some hope of life,' she helped it to start breathing. If she then noticed 'distinct signs of life,' she immediately proceeded to baptize it. But if in doubt, she had to revive the child further by irritating and provoking it with substances and manipulations until it demonstrated explicit vitality. The decision needed to be approved of by other

58 Smid, *Fierde Urtegaard*, 14.

59 Olai, *Een Nyttigh Läkere Book*, [347].

60 Paulsson Holmberg, *Onaturlig födelse*, 229–31.

persons present: 'So that she can be free from censure, like she had abused the holy [sacrament of] Baptism and baptized a dead child.'[61]

Given that available intervention practices were hazardous and difficult to master, obstetric narratives in mechanistic birth manuals radiate distance, danger, and death. In fact, they clearly testify to the conditional state in which unborn entities resided, even as fully grown children, and regardless of the importance of their physical survival to the performance of religious transition rites. They also reveal the extent to which considerations and valuations were affected by the desperate imperative to save the mother. Once it became evident that she was in mortal danger, the child was viewed in a new light. Perhaps it was not viable at all. And if so, had not this passing traveler, failing to cross the final border, been promised a safe path to the next world through intercession prayers? Was it fair that this unknown creature, immobile, noncompliant, and passive, or decomposing, faceless, and lost, was to determine the fate of its suffering mother? If the child's survival was set against the survival of the mother, the child must be sacrificed. And sacrificing the child, of course, was facilitated if it was visibly dead. The loss was made acceptable by discourse that repressed notions of personhood and attachment and conjured up distance, decay, and defeat.

4 Conclusion

Religious and medical discourses, concepts, and images of unborn entities are the result of intervention practices that enact, articulate, and negotiate values. This chapter has explored strategies that attributed or denied attachment and vitality to perinatal children in early modern Lutheran Sweden, and tentatively outlined some possible consequences of the complex interplay between religious and medical priorities for the configuration of the unborn in this context.

The urgent problem of stillbirth and baptism displays, as argued above, constant adjustment not only to changing religious doctrine, but also to negotiations between theological priorities and obstetric emergency practices and technologies. This supports the view that the development of early modern Swedish birth intervention was intimately connected with religious responses to fetal and infant loss, and with shifting arguments about how to equally secure physical survival and salvation of mother and child in obstructed and complicated deliveries.

61 Hoorn, *Den Swenska Wälöfwade Jordgumman*, 271–72.

Caring for the spiritual survival of the unborn was an act of social and parental responsibility that testifies to the importance of the afterlife to early modern notions of personhood and humanness. This brief survey supports the idea that intervention practices informed by the Lutheran doctrine of baptism, however contradictory, strengthened notions of attachment by reaching out to and including the perinatal child before birth (through intercession prayers), and after birth (by burial in the churchyard). The results also indicate that substantial fetal and infant mortality, caused by both late-pregnancy fetal and maternal ill-health and perilous obstetric intervention technologies, counterbalanced these impulses, supporting a cautious, conditional attitude toward unborn entities, only gradually allowing them to step forward from shapelessness, obscurity, and darkness, and take their place in the world of the living.

It may be suggested that the particular strategies governing Swedish baptismal practices from late sixteenth century onward—insisting on and securing infant survival before baptism, yet accepting the prospect of salvation for the unbaptized stillborn through divine intervention—influenced representations of the perinatal child in two specific ways. First, by demanding that infants survive birth and demonstrate explicit signs of life before baptism took place, the Lutheran framework strengthened narratives that attributed individuality and potentiality to the fully grown unborn, as well as fostering birth practices that led to the improvement of birth-related survival. Since distinct signs of life were a sine qua non, birth practitioners were forced to perfect examination and resuscitation techniques, and gradually succeeded in persuading mothers to allow earlier intervention, employing utilitarian arguments to further their cause. This pragmatic position becomes further visible in more generous attitudes toward death rites for the stillborn, as well as in arguments about the priority of securing maternal survival. Second, and paradoxically, loosening the link between baptism and salvation opens up the possibility of a less condemnatory attitude toward the deliberate termination of dangerous and unsafe pregnancies—that is, the practice of induced abortion. The liminal child might be rejected in this world since it is not being denied a continued existence in the next. This solution to the enduring problem of obstetric loss did not result in articulated changes in attitudes toward abortion or infanticide—but it provided birth practitioners with room to maneuver in desperate cases, when the life of the mother could only be saved by using mutilating surgery on the obstructed child. Yet in obstetric discourses the forwarding of the pragmatic solution of sacrificing such children continuously rested on the concealment of the dubious nature of signs of fetal life and decay. Ultimately, securing survival and managing loss in the birth transition meant intervening at some time, regardless of the conditions and the outcome. All the abovementioned intervention practices participated in, and were the result of, the complex negotiation and production of conflicting values of attachment, distance, vitality, and decay which were ascribed to the perinatal child in this context, and concern for its ultimate survival.

Acknowledgments

This work was supported by Erik Philip-Sörensen Foundation and Åke Wiberg Foundation.

Bibliography

Ariès, Philippe. *Centuries of Childhood*. London: Pimlico, 1996.

Burjam, Friedrich. *Den skandinaviska folktron om barnet under dess ömtålighetstillstånd i synnerhet före dopet*. Helsingfors: Alexandersuniv., 1917.

Collinder, Johann. *Nödig Tröst och Underwisning för Äckta hafwande Qwinnor och Barnaföderskor* [...]. Stockholm, 1698.

Cressy, David. *Birth, Marriage and Death: Ritual, Religion, and the Life-Cycle in Tudor and Stuart England*. Oxford: Oxford University Press, 1997.

Crowther, Kathleen M. *Adam and Eve in the Protestant Reformation*. Cambridge: Cambridge University Press, 2010.

Davies, Douglas J. *Death, Ritual and Belief: The Rhetoric of Funerary Rites*. London and Washington, DC: Cassell, 1997.

Djurberg, Vilhelm. *Läkaren Johan von Hoorn: Förlossningskonstens grundläggare i Sverige*. Lychnosbibliotek 4. Uppsala, 1942.

Duden, Barbara, Jürgen Schlumbohm, and Patrice Veit, eds. *Geschichte des Ungeborenen: Zur Erfahrungs- und Wissenschaftgeschichte der Schwangerschaft, 17.–20. Jahrhundert*, Göttingen: Vandenhoeck and Ruprecht, 2002.

Duden, Barbara. 'Zwischen "wahrem Wissen" und Prophetie: Konzeptionen des Ungeborenen.' In *Geschichte des Ungeborenen: Zur Erfahrungs- und Wissenschaftgeschichte der Schwangerschaft, 17,–20. Jahrhundert*, edited by Barbara Duden, Jürgen Schlumbohm, and Patrice Veit, 11–48. Göttingen: Vandenhoeck and Ruprecht, 2002.

Dussauge, Isabelle, Claes-Fredrik Helgesson, Francis Lee, and Steve Woolgar. 'On the Omnipresence, Diversity, and Elusiveness of Values in the Life Sciences and Medicine.' In *Value Practices in the Life Sciences and Medicine*, edited by Isabelle Dussauge, Claes-Fredrik Helgesson, and Francis Lee, 1–28. Oxford: Oxford University Press, 2015.

Estborn, Sigfrid. *Evangeliska svenska bönböcker under reformationstidevarvet.* Lund: Lunds universitet, 1929.

Faehn, Helge. 'Dåp.' In *Kulturhistoriskt lexikon för nordisk medeltid: Från vikingatid till reformationstid 3*, edited by Ingvar Andersson and John Granlund, 413–18. Köpenhamn: Rosenkilde og Bagger, 1980.

Ferngren, Gary B. *Medicine and Religion: A Historical Introduction.* Baltimore: Johns Hopkins University Press, 2014.

Foscati, Alessandra. '"Nonnatus Dictus Quod Caeso Defunctae Matris Utero Prodiit": Postmortem Caesarean Section in the Late Middle Ages and Early Modern Period.' *Social History of Medicine* 32, no. 3 (2019): 465–80.

Gélis, Jacques. *Les enfants des limbes: Mort-néz et parents dans l'Europe chrétienne.* Paris: Louis Audibert, 2006.

Gélis, Jacques. *La sage-femme ou le médécin: Une nouvelle conception de la vie.* Paris: Fayard, 1988.

Gleixner, Ulrike. 'Todesangst und Gottergebenheit: Die Spiritualisierung von Schwangerschaft und Geburt im luterischen Pietismus.' In *Geschichte des Ungeborenen: Zur Erfahrungs- und Wissenschaftgeschichte der Schwangerschaft, 17.–20. Jahrhundert*, edited by Barbara Duden, Jürgen Schlumbohm, and Patrice Veit, 75–98. Göttingen: Vandenhoeck and Ruprecht, 2002.

Grell, Ole Peter. 'The Protestant Imperative of Christian Care and Neighborly Love.' In *Health Care and Poor Relief in Protestant Europe 1500–1700*, edited by Andrew Cunningham and Ole Peter Grell, 43–65. London: Routledge, 1997.

Hoorn, Johan von. *Den Swenska Wälöfwade Jordgumman Hwilken Grundeligen underwijser huru med en Hafwande handlas, en Wåndande hielpas, en Barna-Qwinna handteras, och det nyfödda Barnet skiötas skal* [...]. Stockholm, 1697.

Huberinus, Caspar. *Tuende merckelige Tractater, den ene om den hellige Ecteskabs Stat, den anden om fructsommelige Quinder, meget trostelige / screffne udaff Huberino: oc udsatte paa danske aff Doct. Pet. Palla.* Københaffn: [Hans Vingaard], 1556.

Imhof, Arthur E. *Lost Worlds: How Our European Ancestors Coped with Everyday Life and Why Life Is So Hard Today.* Translated by Thomas Robisheaux. Charlottesville and London: University Press of Virginia, 1996.

International Statistical Classification of Diseases and Related Health Problems. 10th revision. Geneva: WHO, 2016.

Keupper Valle, Rosemary. 'The Cesarean Operation in Alta California during the Franciscan Mission Period (1769–1833).' *Bulletin of the History of Medicine* 48, no. 2 (1974): 265–75.

Kyrkio-Lag och Ordning / som then Stormächtigste Konung och Herre/ Herr CARL then Elofte / Sweriges / Göthes och Wändes Konung / &c. Åhr 1686. hafwer låtit författa / och Åhr 1687 af Trycket utgå och publicera. Jemte ther til hörige Stadgar. Stockholm, 1687.

LaFleur, William. *Liquid Life: Abortion and Buddhism in Japan*. Princeton, NJ: Princeton University Press, 1992.

Laurentius Petris kyrkoordning av år 1571: Utgiven av Samfundet Pro Fide et Christianismo. Edited by Emil Färnström. Stockholm: Diakonistyrelsen, 1932.

Law, Jane Marie, and Vanessa R. Sasson, eds. *Imagining the Fetus: The Unborn in Myth, Religion and Culture*. Oxford: Oxford University Press, 2008.

Lindgärde, Valborg. 'Hon dog en Rakels död: Om havandeskap och barnafödande i äldre svensk andaktslitteratur.' In *Sydsvenska medicinhistoriska sällskapets årsskrift: Tema förlossningskonst*, edited by David Dunér and Tove Paulsson Holmberg, 93–124. Lund, 2009.

Lindquist, David. *Studier i den svenska andaktslitteraturen under stormaktstidevarvet*. Stockholm: SKD, 1939.

Løkke, Anne. 'Responsibility and Emotion: Parental, Governmental and Almighty Responses to Infant Death in Denmark in the Mid-eighteenth to the Mid-nineteenth Century.' In *Death, Emotion and Childhood in Premodern Europe*, edited by Katie Barclay, Kimberley Reynolds, and Ciara Rawnsley, 191–208. London: Palgrave Macmillan, 2016.

Lugt, Maaike van der. 'Formed Fetuses and Healthy Children in Scholastic Theology, Medicine and Law.' In *Reproduction: Antiquity to Present Day*, edited by Nick Hopwood, Rebecca Flemming, and Lauren Kassel, 167–80. Cambridge: Cambridge University Press, 2018.

Lundqvist, Birger. *Svenska barnmorskor*. Stockholm: Svenska barnmorskeförbundet, 1940.

Lupton, Deborah. *The Social Worlds of the Unborn*. Basingstoke: Palgrave MacMillan, 2013.

Olai, Benedictus. *Een Nyttigh Läkere Book ther uthinnen man finner rådh / hielp och Läkedom til allehanda menniskiornes siwkdomar bådhe inwertes och uthwertes* [...]. Stockholm, 1578.

Park, Katherine. 'Birth and Death.' In *A Cultural History of the Human Body in the Medieval Age*, edited by Linda Kalof, 17–37. London: Bloomsbury Academic, 2010.

Park, Katherine. 'The Death of Isabella Della Volpe: Four Eyewitness Accounts of a Postmortem Caesarean Section in 1545.' *Bulletin of the History of Medicine* 82, no. 1 (2008): 169–87.

Paulsson Holmberg, Tove. *Onaturlig födelse: Johan von Hoorn och det obstetriska dilemmat 1680–1730*. Lund: Lunds universitet, 2017.

Pentikäinen, Juha. *The Nordic Dead-Child Tradition: Nordic Dead-Child Beings; A Study in Comparative Religion*. FF Communications 202. Helsingfors: Suomalainen Tiedeakatemia, 1968.

Petri, Olaus. *Een handbock påå swensko / Ther doopet och annat mera uthi står* [1529]. In *Samlade skrifter af Olavus Petri*, edited by Bengt Hesselman, 4 vols., 2: 311–367. Uppsala: Sveriges Kristliga Studentrörelses förlag, 1915.

Roberg, Lars. *Lijkrevnings tavlor, déd ær tydelig utreedning o'm een människje-cropp til dés förnæmre fasta deelars kjænningar, om-égor och vérkan*. Uppsala: Werner, 1718.

Rodhe, Edvard. *Dopritualet i svenska kyrkan efter reformationen*. Lunds universitets årsskrift N.F. Part 1, vol. 7, no. 1. Lund, 1910.

Schwartz, Louis. *Milton and Maternal Mortality*. Cambridge: Cambridge University Press, 2009.

Siegemund, Justine. *The Court Midwife* [1690]. Edited and translated by Lynne Tatlock. Chicago and London: University of Chicago Press, 2005.

Sjölin, Ingegerd. *Dopsed i förändring: Studier av* Örebro *pastorat 1710–1910*. Lund: Lund University Press, 1999.

Smid, Henrik. *Henrick Smids fierde Urtegaard, fliteligen tilsamman læst aff lærde Lægers Bøger, saav Quindfocks oc unge Spædbørns Siugdomme*. Köpenhamn, 1577.

Sparrman, Andreas. *Sundhetzens Speghel: Uthi hwilken man beskodar Sundhetzens Natur, förnämste orsakerne til alla Siukdomar, som Sundheten förstöra plägha, såsom ock the Medels rätta Bruk, hwarigenom hon för them befrijat, til thet bestemda Målet kan underhållen warda* [...]. Stockholm, 1642.

Veit, Patrice. '"Ich bin sehr schwach, doch drückst du nach ..." Evangelisches Kirchenlied und seelsorgerische Begleitung von Schwangeren im 17. und 18. Jahrhundert.' In *Geschichte des Ungeborenen: Zur Erfahrungs- und Wissenschaftgeschichte der Schwangerschaft, 17,–20. Jahrhundert*, edited by Barbara Duden, Jürgen Schlumbohm, and Patrice Veit, 49–74. Göttingen: Vandenhoeck and Ruprecht, 2002.

Wagner, Johann. *HWSBIBLIA: Ther uthi Alle nådhehungrighe / torstighe och bekymradhe hierta/ såsom j itt Panacea Spirituali / Eller Andhelighit skadhefördreff / thet retta himmels brödh / och then liufligha Gudz barns miölk haffue til at finna / ther medh the bådhe sina och andre bedröffuadhe siälar / spijsa och wederquekia kunna* [...]. Translated by Samuel Olai. Västerås, 1623.

Whiteley, Rebecca. *Birth Figures: Early Modern Prints and the Pregnant Body*. Chicago: University of Chicago Press, 2023.

Wiesner, Merry E. 'The Midwives of South Germany and the Public/Private Dichotomy.' In *The Art of Midwifery: Early Modern Midwives in Europe*, edited by Hilary Marland, 77–94. London and New York: Routledge, 1993.

Woods, Robert. *Children Remembered: Responses to Untimely Death in the Past*. Liverpool: Liverpool University Press, 2006.

Woods, Robert. *Death before Birth: Fetal Health and Mortality in Historical Perspective*. Oxford: Oxford University Press, 2009.

CHAPTER 2

Between Blood Clots and Corpses: Valuations of Fetal Remains in Early Modern Courts

Anton Runesson

In 1715 Ingrid Guttormsdotter gave birth to what in her view was a human child, albeit premature and stillborn.[1] The infant had not been baptized, yet she sought to have it buried in consecrated ground. Since Ingrid had shortly before been accused of stealing another woman's child in order to use it for magical purposes, representatives of the church were suspicious of her request. They demanded to see what she wanted to have buried. After the small coffin was opened, a conflict of interpretations unfolded over what her product of conception was, and how it should be properly handled. According to the vicar, for example, the alleged child showed no signs of being a stillborn human. Since it lacked bones and other body parts, to him it was merely 'some coagulated blood,' a 'so-called corpse,' and therefore did not merit a churchyard burial. Similarly, a woman who had been present during Ingrid's delivery, Ella Andersdotter, testified to the form of what she had given birth to, or rather its absence thereof. She, too, asserted that it lacked any human shape and merely consisted of 'two bundles of blood, the size of a fist.' Consequently, there was nothing to bury.[2]

Whereas the previous chapter by Tove Paulsson Holmberg explored early modern attempts at securing the salvation of unborn humans in perilous situations, the abovementioned case highlights an attempt to secure salvation through burial. In detailing the ways in which the unborn was handled, it offers insights into how the life of this uncertain entity was understood. At stake here was the issue of how to distinguish between those bodies to whom life was ascribed, which in turn made them worthy of a Christian burial, and those ineligible for such treatment. In effect, the account thus raises the question

1 Throughout the chapter, I follow the accepted practice of referring by name, instead of surname, to people without family names.

2 Larsen and Rauø, *Jukkasjärvi og Enontekis tinglag*, 22–23. For a similar case, see Richardsson, *Revsunds tingslags domboksprotokoll*, 75, 87. For a study of secret burials of stillborn children, and specifically of the three coffins depicted and described on next page, see Kättström Höök, 'Från foster till dop.'

 | DOI:10.1163/9789004703759_004

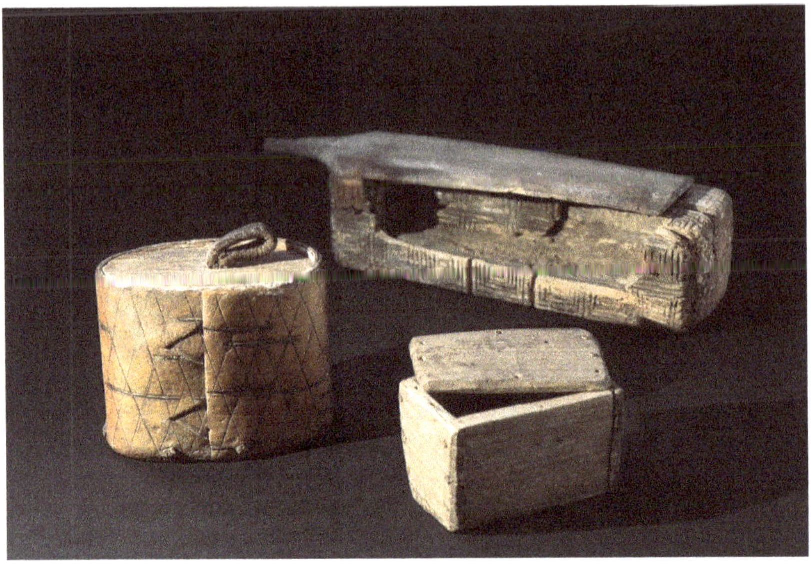

FIGURE 2.1 Three small coffins for burial of fetal remains, found within a cavity in the wall surrounding the church in Odensjö, Småland (a province in the southern part of Sweden), measuring between 15.1 and 5.5 centimeters. Radiocarbon dating proves the content of the largest coffin to be from 1675, plus or minus thirty-five years. Objects 0285615, 0285614, 0285616, Nordic Museum, Stockholm.

of how unborn entities were perceived and valued in seventeenth- and eighteenth-century Sweden. By examining cases similar to Ingrid Guttormsdotter's, this chapter investigates the handling of unborn entities in order to understand how they were defined and valued in a nonmedical context.

To address these questions, I focus on the different ways in which women accused of terminating pregnancies, as well as witnesses and representatives of the court, described products of conception and how they dealt with them, so as to see how they attributed notions of humanness and personhood to them. Adopting a valuography approach, I analyze the conflicting criteria of valuation that underpinned various definitions of and ways of handling fetal bodies as described in Swedish court cases between 1600 and 1750.[3] In order to do so, I apply the concepts of humanness and personhood, as developed by anthropologist Lynn Morgan. As Morgan has argued, a fetus or newborn must first of all be categorized as a member of the human species and be ascribed humanness. Following this, the newborn can then be elevated to the status of

3 Dussauge, Helgesson, Lee, and Woolgar, 'On the Omnipresence,' 1–2.

a person—invested with personhood—and as such, it becomes charged with legal and moral rights, among them the right to live.[4]

This approach differs somewhat from previous scholarship. Anthropologists and sociologists have contributed important insights into the social lives of the unborn. However, they have at times taken (modern) embryologists' descriptions of embryological material as 'waste' for granted.[5] In so doing, they have bypassed the various and nuanced ways in which people in history have made sense of fetal remains. For instance, Deborah Lupton has stated that in past eras 'dead embryos and fetuses from miscarriage and abortions were routinely disposed of as garbage [...] with little concern for a respectful burial or disposal, regardless of their stage of development.' As I will show, this does not hold true for the early modern practices of designating, categorizing, and disposing of the remains of a pregnancy loss or a stillbirth under consideration here.

My study contributes fresh perspectives on the history of the early modern unborn, which has primarily been addressed from the point of view of histories of science, medicine, and theology. In these studies, attention has been given to the legacies of epigenetic theories, the rise of preformationism, and the confessionalization of the fetus. According to the epigenetic stance, which was part of Galenic physiology, fetal development unfolded in three stages, from unformed matter into an ensouled being. During the first stage, the fetus had only a nutritive soul and was similar to a plant, but in the second stage—as its heart began to pulsate—the fetus started to function as a lowly animal. Finally, as it approached delivery, the fetus was endowed with a rational soul.[6] However, with the gradual development of mechanical embryology in the seventeenth century, the fetus was no longer understood to be organized out of unformed matter; rather, it represented the growth of a preformed embryo.[7] From the moment of conception onward it had only to mature within the womb, a process that was likened to fermentation in Swedish medicine.[8]

4 The moments of attribution of humanness and personhood may or may not coincide. See Morgan, 'When Does Life Begin?,' 35–46. For a historical discussion of notions of personhood, see Kosmin, 'When the Fetus Becomes a Child.'

5 Lupton, *Social Worlds of the Unborn*, 29. Cf. Casper, 'At the Margins of Humanity.' However, see Morgan, *Icons of Life*, and Jülich's chapter in this volume, for more in-depth analysis of how early twentieth-century embryologists classified dead embryos and fetuses as waste with no other value than as material for their own scientific research. This conception only gradually became contested, as dead specimens were fraught with political meanings.

6 Flemming, 'Galen's Generations of Seeds,' 102–3.

7 Keller, 'Embryonic Individuals.' See also Bondestam's chapter in this volume.

8 Dunér, *Tankemaskinen*, 223.

Studies on the confessionalization of the fetus instead highlight how its animation was imagined in terms of its relation to the Christian soul. These studies have proved that the fetus was envisioned and valued differently across the confessional divide, with the Protestant fetus being conceived of as alive, in terms of being eligible for salvation, at an earlier stage than the Catholic one. Within Catholicism the unborn had to be born and baptized in order to be saved, whereas within Protestantism it might be saved through intercession prayers.[9] For example, the Swedish clergy was influenced by the theological doctrine of traducianism, held that a fetus was alive and ensouled at the moment of conception.[10] Most recently Rebecca Whiteley has studied early modern visualizations of the unborn in prints. Specifically, with regard to what she terms 'the personification of the fetus,' she states that the dominant stance among religious authors was that it required both complete bodily formation and ensoulment, and that the latter could take place at any time during pregnancy, but most probably after four months of pregnancy.[11]

Notwithstanding the importance of these conceptual frameworks, we do not know much about how they corresponded with the practical handling of unborn or stillborn entities. Applying the concepts of humanness and personhood with regard to how these entities were categorized and valued at a more mundane level offers a new perspective, while at the same time illuminating how notions of human life were interconnected with cultural notions of personhood and possible salvation grounded in a particular context. Thus, rather than emphasizing ensoulment as the beginning of life, I argue that human shape and awareness outside the womb were the essential criteria for ascribing humanness and personhood, which in turn were prerequisites for baptism and burial. A similar investigation has been conducted by Maaike van der Lugt, who examined medieval ideas on abortion, baptism, and burial, and how they related to notions of embryonal ensoulment, humanness, (legal) personhood, and salvation.[12] Following her lead, I look into similar causalities, but from practices described in court records rather than legal stipulations, as the practices recounted in testimony seem more closely related to the lived realities of ordinary people.

---

9 Kosmin, 'When the Fetus Becomes a Child.' See also Veit, '"Ich bin sehr schwach,"'; Gélis, 'Lebenzeichen—Todeszeichen.'

10 Bergenlöv, *Skuld och oskuld*, chap. 6. Traducianism was favored by Luther and is the belief that the soul, the immaterial aspect of a human being, is transmitted through natural generation along with the body, the material aspect. Creationism, on the other hand, holds that God directly creates all souls.

11 Whiteley, *Birth Figures*, 62–63.

12 Lugt, 'Formed Fetuses and Healthy Children.'

The empirical material consists of a sample of roughly two hundred court cases from various parts of Sweden.[13] I focus on cases of suspected infanticide in which accused women maintained that they had miscarried, or flat out denied ever having been pregnant. These suspected infanticides are also complemented with cases of other crimes related to pregnancy and childbirth.[14] The majority of the cases were brought before courts in rural areas where there were no trained midwives or physicians serving as expert witnesses, but instead honorable women with experiences of pregnancy, childbirth, and in some cases, miscarriages.[15] Using these sources thus offers insights into how a broader stratum of society in everyday contexts solved the medico-legal problem of defining fetal life.

To the extent that studies on early modern infanticide have engaged with the accused women's accounts of pregnancy loss, they have not highlighted what these enunciations reveal with regard to how products of pregnancy loss were made sense of and valued.[16] Recently, however, Paige Donaghy has drawn attention to the wide range of physical events—from fetal to potentially fetal or nonfetal pregnancies—that in early modern England were experienced as pregnancy losses. In passing, she touches upon the fact that the products of these pregnancy losses were handled in various ways, but she does not elaborate.[17] And since her study is based on medical casebooks and letters—that is, sources filtered by medical frameworks—we still lack a history of the early modern unborn from the more everyday perspectives of women with firsthand experience of miscarriage and dealing with fetal remains.

---

13 The cases have been located by scrutinizing printed and digitized protocols of lower courts for the period between 1600 and 1750. Additionally, the online database Gender and Work (GaW), hosted by the Department of History at Uppsala University and comprising 2,866 Swedish court cases concerning various crimes, has been searched for cases of interest. In the following, cases collected from GaW are referred to by their case number in the database. For a fuller discussion of the selection of the sources, as well as a list of all of the cases, see Runesson, *Blod, kött och tårar*, 38–39, 43–48, 226–34.

14 For a discussion of combining criminal sources regulating illicit sexuality this way, see Sjöberg, *Kvinnors jord, manlig rätt*, 69–74.

15 As Sofia Ling has shown in her study of conflicts between trained physicians and those whom they considered "quacks" in Sweden between 1770 and 1870, the medically trained were few in number, and concentrated in the urban areas. See Ling, 'Kärringmedicin och vetenskap.'

16 See, e.g., Fischer-Homberger, *Medizin vor Gericht*, 222–92; Jackson, 'Suspicious Infant Deaths.' For a recent study of 'the openness of the miscarrying female body,' which overlooks the products of miscarriage, see Evans and Read, '"Before Midnight She Had Miscarried,"' 2–32.

17 Donaghy, 'Miscarriage, False Conceptions.' For her brief discussion of how unborn entities were buried, see 1143–44.

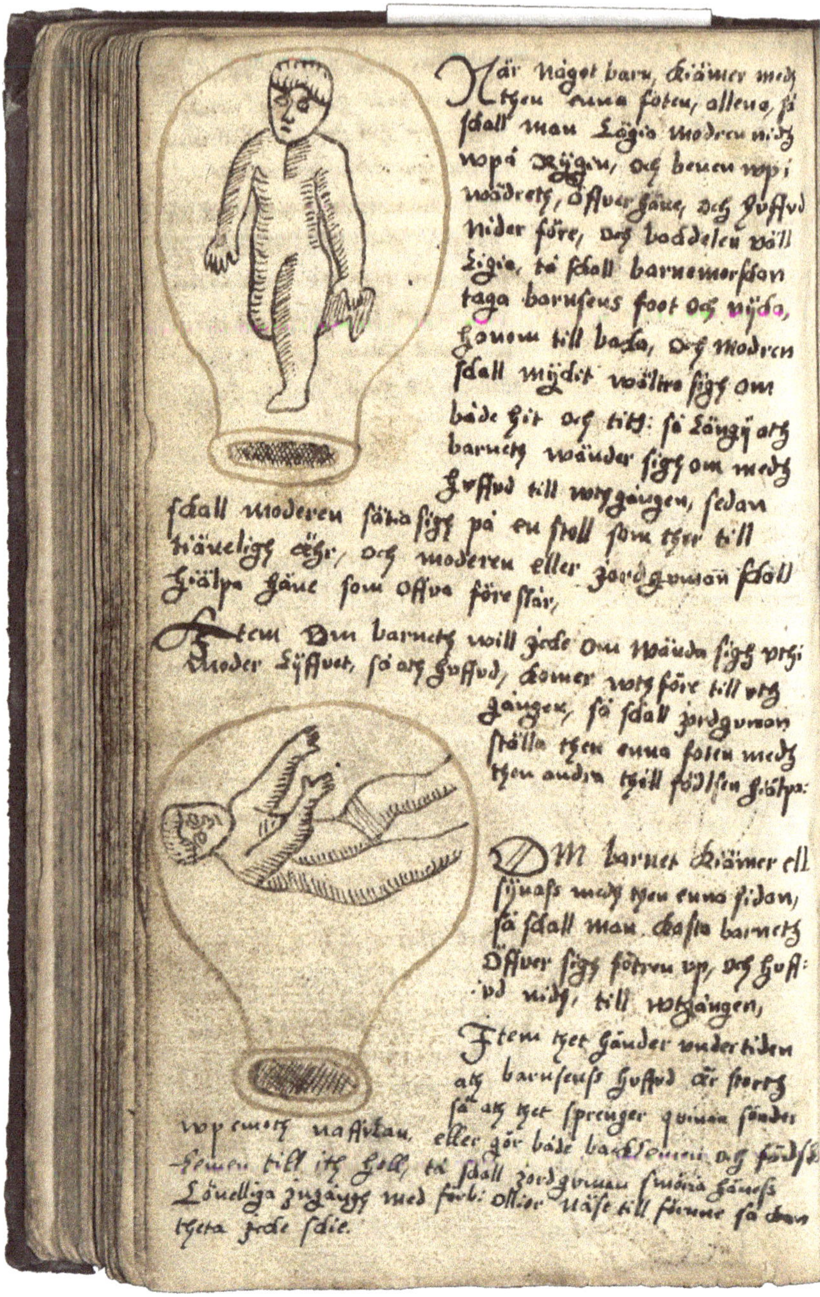

FIGURE 2.2 There are very few visual testimonies of how pregnancy and fetal activity were envisioned in Swedish early modern culture. These drawings of the fetus *in utero* on an unpublished manuscript were most likely adopted from the birth figures pictured in Rösslin's German midwifery manual *Der Swangern Frawen und Hebammen Roszengarten* from the beginning of the sixteenth century. The manuscript was bound together with (and probably created by the same author) Månsson's medicine book *Practica* published in 1654. Hagströmer Library, Karolinska Institute.

Om Något barn kommer medh axlorna fram, så skall man taga in medh handen och om wända thet öffver sigh, med föterna till uth gången, män thet war bäst, om möijeligh ähr att huffud komme för uth, eller hon må skiuta axlorna sin koss, och ställa huffud till uthgången.

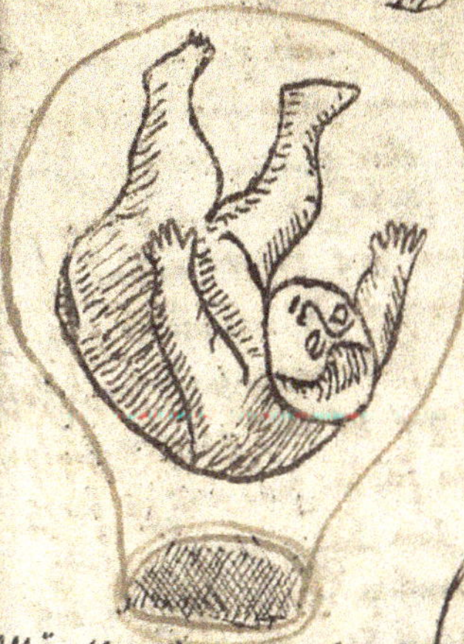

Män thet gör qwinnan swårliga ondt så att många måste döö ther igenom som swaga ähr till naturen.

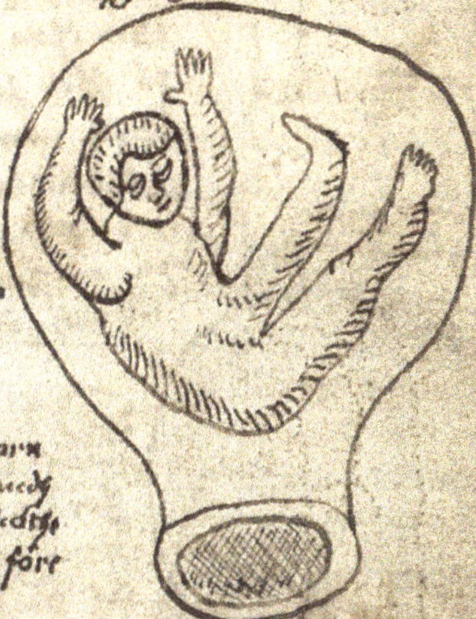

Item När något barn kära sigh för inna medh händerna, och med ansichtet så skall hon göra som före sagdt ähr,

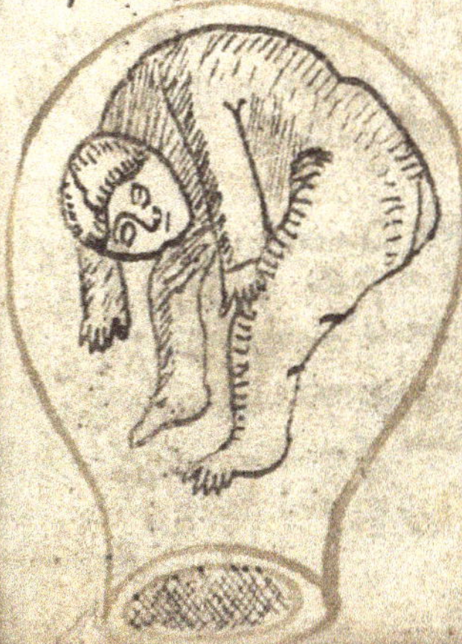

Om barnet kära sigh för inna medh både föterna och medh en eller medh både händerna, och med huffud, så skall dass Hebam, grijpa wthi huffud, och wända barnsens föter öffver huffud, och uth hiälpa barnet till födelsen.

As statements made in court occurred within a legal frame of reference, a rudimentary explanation of the modern statutes against infanticide is needed. In 1608 excerpts from the Old Testament—the Mosaic Law—were added to criminal law, an indication of the conjoining of nation-state and church commonly understood as confessionalization.[18] All sexual activity outside marriage was punishable by law; thus it was mostly unmarried women employed as maids who were accused of infanticide.[19] The crime of infanticide included premeditated killings of newborns as well as concealed miscarriages. Accordingly, it did not matter whether the accused women had willingly terminated pregnancies or miscarried accidentally. But it was crucial whether these events had taken place in secret or not. The specific statutes against infanticide that were proclaimed in 1655, 1669, and 1684 all stressed that women claiming accidental miscarriage or stillbirths were not to be treated lightly. In order to counter such claims, the statute of 1655 stated that fetuses were to be inspected to determine how advanced in maturity they were. However, as of 1684 an accused woman could be found guilty if she had concealed a pregnancy, given birth in secret, and disposed of the remains. Nevertheless, women could forestall accusations of infanticide by presenting the stillborn child or the miscarried fetus to witnesses who could then testify on their behalf. For women suspected of terminating pregnancies, the evidentiary burden was clearly reversed, as they had to prove their innocence to avoid being convicted on circumstantial evidence.[20]

In what follows, I demonstrate that cases of alleged infanticide in which miscarriage was presented as a defense are a fruitful way of grasping historical processes of valuation via cultural attributions of humanness and personhood, since miscarriage brings cultural definitions of life to the fore.[21] First, however, I will briefly discuss how experiences of pregnancy and miscarriage were described in court, as these accounts in turn highlight the importance of studying the practical handling of products of pregnancy loss.

1 Sensing Fetal Life and Death

In her study of correspondence between female patients and an eighteenth-century German physician, Barbara Duden has shown that the initial

18 Sundin, *För Gud, staten och folket*, 135–39, 447–56.

19 Thunander, *Hovrätt i funktion*, 134–35.

20 Bergenlöv, 'Barnamord.'

21 See Morgan, 'When Does Life Begin?,' on the problems of applying the term 'infanticide' to killings of neonates prior to their having been recognized as persons.

movements of the unborn—its 'quickening' inside the womb—constituted the beginning of a pregnancy. After having sensed this initial movement, women conceived of themselves as pregnant.[22] The court cases under scrutiny confirm this. Generally, when accused women in court described how they came to know that they were pregnant, they referred to feeling fetuses or children quicken inside the womb. This was noticed roughly four months after conception.[23] Asked if she had any knowledge at all about conception and the coming into being of a fetus, Ingrid Guttormsdotter flatly stated that she knew that a fetus was to be carried *in utero* for four months dead and then five months alive.[24] In other words: before quickening there was merely dead matter inside the womb, which became alive when it began to move. But this live matter was not necessarily animated in the sense of being ensouled, as previous scholarship has argued.[25] On the contrary, no case in my sample explicitly suggests that this movement was simultaneous with the fetus's being endowed with a soul. Instead, they indicate that this happened at a later stage, which I will discuss below.

Along the same lines, women who had noticed the life-announcing signal of their fetuses' quickening could also sense them ceasing to move, which they interpreted as a sign of that life ceasing.[26] Absence of fetal movements meant that the woman in question was no longer pregnant with a living child, and that a miscarriage had occurred or would occur. And miscarriages, in turn, were described as accidents that befell the pregnant body. In such descriptions, terms for intended abortion were used, but formulated in the passive voice. In several cases, the court records simply state that miscarried children or fetuses departed in different ways from the pregnant body.[27] Pain was then rarely, if ever, mentioned.

In these statements, the verb indicating how the fetus was expelled from the maternal body signaled whether it was alive or not. But the same word did

---

22 Duden, 'Quick with Child,' 335–44. See also Bergenlöv, *Skuld och oskuld*, 391–96. For a more nuanced account highlighting that quickening was not necessarily understood as a guarantee of a true pregnancy, see McClive, 'Hidden Truths of the Belly.'

23 See, e.g., Norberg, *Ångermanlands domsagas dombok och tingsprotokoll*, 15:47, 152.

24 Larsen and Rauø, *Jukkasjärvi og Enontekis tinglag*, 21.

25 Ensoulment coinciding with the first fetal movements is discussed in Bergenlöv, *Skuld och oskuld*, 391–96.

26 For an example, see Norberg, *Avskrift av Ångermanlands domsagas dombok*, 18:81–82.

27 See, e.g., Norberg, *Laga ting i Ångermanland*, 14:92–93, 114; GaW, case 141; Uppsala universitet, *Akademiska konsistoriets protokoll*, 15:231; GaW, case 6142. Cf. Paulsson Holmberg's chapter in this volume, for early modern instructional material emphasizing the uterine forces as agents.

not necessarily indicate whether this entity had human traits nor whether it should be valued as a person. Moreover, as a consequence of 'child' and 'fetus' being interchangeable in descriptions of miscarriage, we need to examine the practical handling of these entities to determine how they were valued.

2 Absence of Human Shape and Form

When Brita Axelsdotter was accused of infanticide in 1638, she denied having killed a child by three times asserting that what had come out of her body did not have human life. She insisted that it 'neither had life, nor was it mature, nor did it have any [human] shape.'[28] Humanness depended on both human form and the degree of maturity this form had reached, two criteria that Brita's product of conception did not meet. Asked what she had done with what she had miscarried, Brita retorted that she had thrown it into the fire.[29] This way of disposing of products of miscarriage was not unusual, as it emerges in other cases as well.[30] In one sense it was, of course, a way of destroying evidence. Yet the motivations for getting rid of the products of pregnancy loss are interesting in their own right: what had been miscarried and disposed of in the fire had lacked resemblance to a human body—the first yardstick of humanness and a prerequisite for being valued as a person. Accordingly, these unformed entities were disposed of in a way corresponding to their value, or lack thereof.

Another example adduces a more elaborate and explicit motivation for disposing of fetal remains in the fire. The case is unusual, as a married woman with experience of eight births was accused of terminating her pregnancy. Märitha Pedersdotter defended herself against the allegation of infanticide by explaining that she had miscarried by accident, adding that the fetus she had lost was nothing but a 'blood-liver the size of a hand.'[31] She did refer to it as a fetus, since it was the result of conception, which she as a married woman did not need to conceal. But this did not mean that it was to be valued as a human coming into being. She maintained that it had no resemblance to a human body, which was why it was of no use or worth. Explaining why she had thrown it into the fire, she explicitly stated that 'it was of no value.'[32]

28 Norberg, *Ångermanlands domsagas dombok och tingsprotokoll*, 16:95.

29 Norberg, *Ångermanlands domsagas dombok och tingsprotokoll*, 16:95.

30 Norberg, *Ångermanlands domsagas dombok och tingsprotokoll*, 15:5–6, 36, 102–3; GaW, case 1242; GaW, case 681.

31 Hellbom, *Tingsprotokoll för Njurunda*, 2:303.

32 Hellbom, *Tingsprotokoll för Njurunda*, 2:305.

Again, humanness was defined on the basis of the form or formlessness of the product of conception. What is more, in this case the relation between an evaluation based on form and a valuation with practical implications was spelled out. If it did not resemble a human body, the product of conception was not a developing human body and consequently could not be valued as such. It was disposed of accordingly.

A similar line of argument appears in yet another case, in which the fetal remains were partly burned and partly buried. Gunilla Larsdotter recounted how she once had been swollen as if she was pregnant, but what had then emanated out of her body was merely blood and a 'lump.'[33] She had burned and washed away the liquid parts, and despite the lump's showing no signs of being a child-to-be she had buried it, although not in the churchyard's consecrated ground, as Ingrid Guttormsdotter had attempted to do. The lump, with both its solid form and its lack of human shape, could have been something human coming into being, which was why it should be buried rather than burned. Gunilla Larsdotter's handling of the lump thus testifies to an absence of clear-cut divisions between persons and nonpersons; what she buried perhaps can be conceived of as a 'quasi-person.'[34] Mimicking a proper burial by burying it in unconsecrated ground became the fitting ritual for its disposal.

The denials that clots and lumps of blood were developing humans resonate with the early modern notion of false conception. In the end, bodies could swell up, look pregnant, and expel coagulated blood without this being the result of conception, even if sexual intercourse had preceded it.[35] The case of the young widow Karin Ivarsdotter, who was accused of infanticide, illustrates this. The charges against Karin were based on the fact that the people she lived with and worked for had noticed her body undergoing a transformation for some months. As she had been observed to have been swollen 'as if she was pregnant,' she was reproached for having given birth to a child which she then had killed.[36] Or so read the charge against her.

Denying these accusations, Karin maintained that she had not been pregnant, but had instead suffered from severe constipation as the result of her monthly period coinciding with the onset of the full moon. She designated this state of being as both 'moon-illness' and 'mother-passion.'[37] In her defense,

33 Larsen and Rauø, *Kautokeino, Aviovara, Teno, Utsjok Tingsteder*, 200.

34 For this terminology, see Lupton, *Social Worlds of the Unborn*, 19.

35 For an excellent discussion of different types of 'false pregnancies,' see Donaghy, 'Miscarriage, False Conceptions.'

36 Larsen and Rauø, *Kautokeino, Aviovara, Teno, Utsjok Tingsteder*, 166.

37 Larsen and Rauø, *Kautokeino, Aviovara, Teno, Utsjok Tingsteder*, 201.

people with experiences of a wide variety of constipations witnessed and corroborated her story. They all made the point that even if the coagulated blood was the result of conception, it was not an unborn human unless it looked like one. The former county sheriff, for example, recounted how his late wife once had been constipated for a month, her stomach swelling so that she appeared to be pregnant. They had both assumed that she was expecting a child, but the swelling had passed when her blood started to flow normally again, whereupon coagulated blood had poured out of her, yet without any traces of anything with a human form. Widow Margetta Amunsdotter testified to having been swollen for four months, and that she too had seemed to be pregnant, but what finally emanated from her body as the constipation passed had no resemblance to a child. In fact, she did not know how to classify it. Yet another corroborating witness put it similarly, as she explained that something unknown had emitted from her body after a year of constipation that had made her look pregnant; it was thickened blood without any traces of bodily shape.[38]

Clearly, coagulated blood emanating from a maternal body—even when assumed to be the result of conception—was not necessarily a pregnancy loss, at least when it had no recognizable human form. Thus far, the cases investigated have remained rather silent on what a product of conception should look like in order to be valued as a developing human. Cases of fetal inspection shed light on the matter.

3 Shape and Form of a Human

Reproductive and fetal knowledge in early modern Europe was a sphere for married women who themselves had experience of childbirth.[39] This explains why married women considered to be honorable in the local community at times were summoned to inspect fetal remains or stillborn children when these were at hand as material evidence in court. As there were no trained midwives or physicians serving as experts in the Swedish cases under scrutiny, the depositions of these women were rarely questioned for their want of medical training.[40] After performing an inspection of reportedly killed, miscarried, or stillborn children, it was the duty of these women to establish how advanced

38 Larsen and Rauø, *Kautokeino, Aviovara, Teno, Utsjok Tingsteder*, 194–201.

39 Gowing, *Common Bodies*, 40–51.

40 By contrast, Cathy McClive has shown that in early modern France, where there was 'tighter medical regulation,' women serving as expert witnesses in court were often distrusted by professional physicians. See McClive, 'Blood and Expertise,' 105–7, quotation on 106.

in pregnancy the woman claiming miscarriage or stillbirth had been, and then to testify to this in court.[41] They might not have experienced miscarriage themselves, but if they had, by virtue of their being married women they would not have had to conceal it.

It is evident that the inspecting women had certain knowledge of how the unborn took on human shape in the womb. For instance, after inspecting a product of conception, three women testifying in court as expert witnesses stated that it would have been a complete human child after another eight weeks or so of gestation.[42] Unfortunately they did not explain how they came to this conclusion: whether, for instance, they drew on medical texts or—which is probably more plausible owing to the scarcity of medically trained persons in Sweden in this period—from personal experience.[43] Testimonies of fetal inspections are often rather sparse. This could be due to the fact that what they held to be signs of humanness were obvious and taken for granted, and did not need to be laid out in detail.[44]

However, when conflicting interpretations of the form of the products of conception emerge, the accounts are more substantial and give glimpses into what constituted the shape of human persons coming into being. Generally, in such cases the accused woman claimed to have been pregnant for only a short time, whereas the material evidence contradicted this and became proof of an advanced pregnancy.

For instance, in a case in which the inspecting women found that a supposedly miscarried child had both a 'head-skull and a complete skeleton,' they classified it as a complete and mature human being.[45] The accused woman's assertion that she had been pregnant for merely five months could thus be disregarded, as the form of the stillborn indicated a fairly extended pregnancy. In inspections such as this one, heads were surely important signs of

41 Here, I discuss only cases in which signs of life are debated on the basis of shape, form, and traits. For an inspection searching for signs of trauma, see, e.g., Norberg, *Ångermanlands domsagas dombok och tingsprotokoll*, 15:30, 41, 77–78.

42 Norberg, *Ångermanlands domsagas dombok och tingsprotokoll*, 15:50.

43 For a discussion of how knowledge traveled between the fields of medicine and law from the nineteenth century onward, see Ruberg, 'Travelling Knowledge and Forensic Medicine.'

44 Records of a case from Stockholm in 1618, for example, simply read that the stillborn had been dead inside the womb for quite some time ('aff the tekn och mercken the hade seett, hade barnet vthi moder lijffuedh lenge warit dödt'), but the inspecting women did not indicate how they came to this conclusion. See Wikström, *Stockholm tänkeböcker från 1592*, 369.

45 GaW, case 541. For a similar case, cf. *Jämtlands domböcker och landstingsprotokoll*, 51, 72, 77.

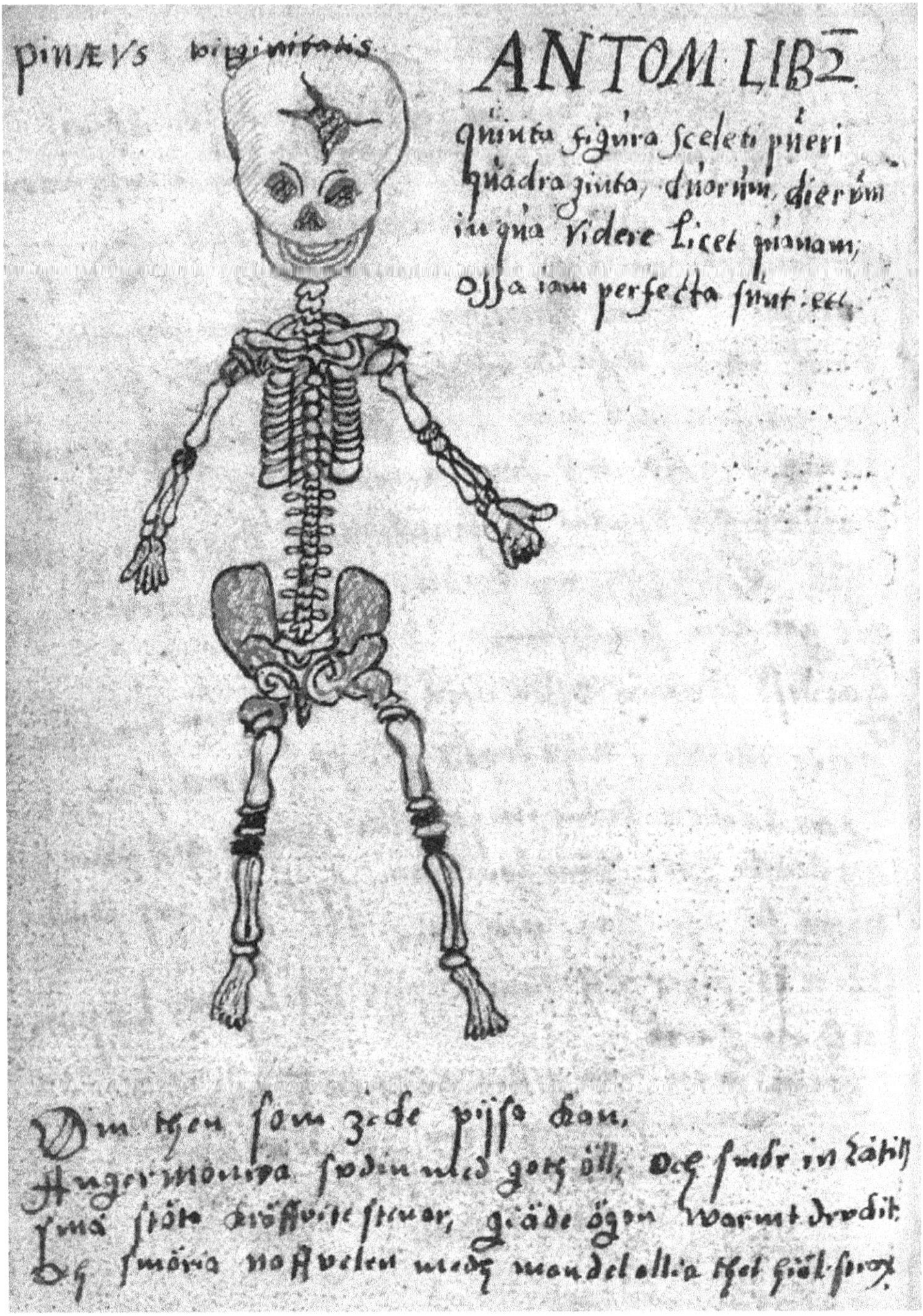

FIGURE 2.3 A drawing of a fetal skeleton from an unpublished manuscript bound together with Månsson's *Practica*. The original image was published in Pineau's *De integritatis et corruptionis virginum notis*, 102. Hagströmer Library, Karolinska Institute.

humanness, but they did not yet stand out as the primary mark of a human body.[46] Instead, the overall impression is that in order to be defined as a human, the inspected assemblage needed to demonstrate as many human body parts and attributes as possible.

The case of Brita Andersdotter illustrates this tendency. Her product of conception was found in a coffin by her brother, who then laid information against her in court. She rejected all claims that it was a dead infant, and asserted that she had not sensed any fetal movements before some coagulated blood had poured out of her.[47] Brita claimed that her pregnancy was no further along than four months. Against her denial that the fetus had been alive, based on the absence of quickening, the material remains of her pregnancy loss indicated otherwise, according to the women summoned to inspect it. They found it to have 'all bones, an umbilical cord, a skull as well as two hands with fingers.'[48] The material evidence thus proved it to be a human body, which was why the court dismissed Brita's claim as to the length of her pregnancy.

Rather than stressing certain parts of the products of conception as more indicative of humanness than others, inspecting women seem to have found the assemblage of human body parts decisive. A rare case of a malformed stillbirth exemplifies this. Its feet were attached to its head and the arms to its back, yet it was nevertheless classified as a human child that had been born into the world.[49] Although it was malformed to the extent that one might expect it to be defined as a monster, this was not the case. The malformed child was not taken to reveal any rules of nature or transgressions of nature's boundaries, as would become the case in the nineteenth century.[50] Instead, the court's investigation circled around the question of whether the extraordinary body was alive and aware at birth, indicating that this might well have been the case notwithstanding its unusual composition. Again, no specific body parts were emblematic of a real human being, but rather it was the assemblage of human traits that indicated a body's status as a human person, even if the ordering of the parts was deviant.

Moreover, in the cases under discussion, there is never talk of performing lung tests on stillborn children—that is, of submerging them in water to determine whether they had been able to breath *ex utero*, as was a common practice in eighteenth-century Europe.[51] No case makes reference to the lung as a

46 See Bondestam's chapter in this volume.

47 Bark, *Undersåkers tingslags domboksprotokoll*, 48.

48 Bark, *Undersåkers tingslags domboksprotokoll*, 48.

49 Larsen and Rauø, *Jukkasjärvi og Enontekis tinglag*, 159.

50 See Bondestam's chapter in this volume.

51 For this practice, see Jackson, 'Suspicious Infant Deaths,' 75–81; Ruberg, 'Travelling Knowledge and Forensic Medicine,' 369.

privileged sign of a living human. Instead, the ultimate criterion for a human person was having been awake, and thus aware, outside the womb.

Two such inspections, although not concerning concealed pregnancies, speak to questions of determining personhood by virtue of human shape, as well as practical handling as an enactment of values. Both put early modern notions of spiritual personhood at the fore. By moving beyond cases revolving around miscarriages to one related to a stillbirth and another involving an emergency baptism, we can better understand how human persons were valued.

In the first case, a woman who inspected the stillbirth of Märit Andersdotter testified in favor of the accused, stating that Märit's child unfortunately had not been born alive.[52] Being a stillborn child, it was thus a liminal figure, since it was not breathing and living when it entered the world. Consequently, the child was buried in unconsecrated ground and without ceremony. After all, although the child was clearly human, it had not been baptized, which was a prerequisite for a Christian burial.[53] Its handling thus corresponded with its liminal status as stillborn.

In the second case, the court investigated Brita Johansdotter to determine whether her child had been stillborn or if she had killed it intentionally after delivery. The women who had attended her childbirth were asked whether the child in question had been 'born into the world'; that is, if it had been born alive.[54] One of them testified that it had been 'wide awake' but had only been alive for a day and a night.[55] Another woman substantiated that it had looked like other 'mature and waking children,' yet had been weak and frail.[56] The fact that the child had been aware was a sure sign of humanness and elevated it to a person, which was why an emergency baptism had been performed. This in turn enabled the child to be buried in consecrated ground and to be eligible for salvation. By having been alive in the world—even if very briefly—the child was to be included in the Christian community of the dead and potentially saved.

'Awake' in this context referred to awareness outside the womb and indicated having been 'born alive.'[57] Thus defined as a human person, the child was handled and valued as an ensouled being in need of the cleansing effects

52 Hansen, *Hammerdals tingslags domboksprotokoll*, 93.

53 Cf. Paulsson Holmberg's chapter in this volume, on burials of unbaptized children.

54 Uppsala universitet, *Akademiska konsistoriets protokoll*, 54.

55 Uppsala universitet, *Akademiska konsistoriets protokoll*, 54.

56 Uppsala universitet, *Akademiska konsistoriets protokoll*, 54.

57 *Svenska akademiens ordbok*, s.v. 'vacker,' 'vaken.' According to the historical dictionary, 'vacker' refers to 'vaken,' which in turn is defined as being alive, being in a conscious state of mind and susceptible to sensory impressions.

of baptism.[58] In this case humanness and personhood were ascribed to the child not only by virtue of its shape, but above all, by its having been awake and aware *ex utero*, which meant that it had been ensouled and was susceptible to salvation. Human shape and awareness in tandem had elevated it to an ensouled person, and enabled its baptism and proper burial.

In conclusion, instead of focusing on the initial movements inside the womb as the moment of animation or ensoulment of the early modern unborn, the empirical evidence suggests a necessary accord between body and soul depending on the shape and form of the product of conception. Only an ensouled human body was eligible for the burial rites proper to what in this context could be called a Protestant person—which in turn made salvation possible—and only the products of conception that looked human enough qualified for this treatment.

4 Conclusions

Ways of designating, categorizing, and disposing of the remains of a pregnancy loss or a stillbirth differ across times and cultures according to how these unborn entities are perceived. Underpinning such processes are culturally specific notions of life. Yet scholars investigating the social lives of the unborn have tended to overlook historical practices that preceded the establishment of modern embryology, emphasizing that dead embryos and fetuses from miscarriages and abortions were considered to be garbage, not worthy of burial. We can conclude that this assertion is somewhat misguided: in the early modern period the handling of a product of pregnancy loss corresponded to the extent to which it had assumed human form.

Drawing on early modern Swedish court cases, this chapter has studied the practical handling of unborn entities as a means of understanding how people attributed life to them, and how they valued that life. In contrast to previous historical scholarship that stresses quickening as the moment at which the fetus became animated and ensouled, the empirical evidence presented here suggests that these characteristics were instead attributed to unborn assemblages at a later stage of gestation, depending on their shape and form. In more general terms, although the concept of the soul was never explicitly invoked, this study indicates that there was a necessary accord between body and soul based on form and appearance: regardless of the sex of the unborn, it needed to look like a human to be or to have been an ensouled person.

58 For emergency baptism, see Paulsson Holmberg's chapter in this volume.

I have shown that there were three main ways of handling products of conceptions, which in turn reflect the cultural criteria for defining humanness and personhood in early modern Sweden. These three approaches corresponded to vaguely defined, yet in the sources clearly discernible, yardsticks for attribution of humanness and personhood. First, products of miscarriages were disposed of in the fire when they lacked any human form and were thus ascribed no value. Second, they were buried in unconsecrated ground when humanness was perceptible, but not to the extent that they could be classified as fully human and, by extension, ensouled. Finally, they were properly buried in consecrated ground when they appeared human to the extent that they could be conceived of as human persons, not least by virtue of their having been awake outside the womb. Personhood corresponded with form and shape in the sense that only the products of conception that presented several human traits, and thus looked like a human, could be conceived of as a true human person. Having reached this state, the entity was included in the confessional community and accordingly buried as one, with the expectation of an afterlife and hopes for salvation.

Bibliography

Bark, Karin, ed. *Undersåkers tingslags domboksprotokoll 1649–1690*. Östersund: Landsarkivet i Östersund and Jämtlands läns fornskriftssällskap, 2011.

Bergenlöv, Eva. 'Barnamord: Från fördömelse till förståelse.' In *Offer för brott: Våldtäkt, incest och barnamord i Sveriges historia från reformationen till nutid*, edited by Eva Bergenlöv, Marie Lindstedt Cronberg, and Eva Österberg, 237–89. Lund: Nordic Academic Press, 2002.

Bergenlöv, Eva. *Skuld och oskuld: Barnamord och barnkvävning i rättslig diskurs och praxis omkring 1680–1800*. Lund: Lunds universitet, 2004.

Casper, Monica J. 'At the Margins of Humanity: Fetal Positions in Science and Medicine.' *Science, Technology & Human Values* 19, no. 3 (1994): 307–23.

Donaghy, Paige. 'Miscarriage, False Conceptions, and Other Lumps: Women's Pregnancy Loss in Seventeenth- and Eighteenth-Century England.' *Social History of Medicine* 34, no. 4 (2021): 1138–60.

Duden, Barbara. 'Quick with Child: An Experience That Has Lost Its Status.' *Technology in Society* 14, no. 3 (1994): 335–44.

Dunér, David. *Tankemaskinen: Polhems huvudvärk och andra studier i tänkandets historia*. Nora: Nya Doxa, 2012.

Dussauge, Isabelle, Claes-Fredrik Helgesson, Francis Lee, and Steve Woolgar. 'On the Omnipresence, Diversity, and Elusiveness of Values in the Life Sciences and

Medicine.' In *Value Practices in the Life Sciences and Medicine*, edited by Isabelle Dussauge, Claes-Fredrik Helgesson, and Francis Lee, 1–28. Oxford: Oxford University Press, 2015.

Evans, Jennifer, and Sara Read. '"Before Midnight She Had Miscarried": Women, Men, and Miscarriage in Early Modern England.' *Journal of Family History* 40, no. 1 (2015): 3–23.

Fischer-Homberger, Esther. *Medizin vor Gericht: Gerichtsmedizin von der Renaissance bis zur Aufklärung*. Bern: Huber, 1983.

Flemming, Rebecca. 'Galen's Generations of Seeds.' In *Reproduction: Antiquity to Present Day*, edited by Nick Hopwood, Rebecca Flemming, and Lauren Kassel, 95–108. Cambridge: Cambridge University Press, 2018.

Gélis, Jacques. 'Lebenzeichen—Todeszeichen: Die Wundertaufe totgeborener Kinder in Deutschland der Aufklärung.' In *Rituale der Geburt: Eine Kulturgeschichte*, edited by Barbara Duden, Jürgen Schlumbohm, and Patrice Veit, 269–88. München: Beck, 1998.

Gender and Work (website). Uppsala University. Accessed July 4, 2023. https://gaw.hist.uu.se/.

Gowing, Laura. *Common Bodies: Women, Touch and Power in Seventeenth-Century England*. New Haven, CT: Yale University Press, 2003.

Hansen, Georg, ed. *Hammerdals tingslags domboksprotokoll 1649–1690*. Östersund: Landsarkivet i Östersund and Jämtlands läns fornskriftssällskap, 2011.

Hellbom, Algot, ed. *Tingsprotokoll för Njurunda*. Vol. 2, *Ur Medelpads domböcker 1673–1699*. Sundsvall: Medelpads fornminnesförening, 1983.

Jackson, Mark. 'Suspicious Infant Deaths: The Statute of 1624 and Medical Evidence at Coroners' Inquests.' In *Legal Medicine in History*, edited by Michael Clark and Catherine Crawford, 64–86. Cambridge: Cambridge University Press, 1994.

Jämtlands domböcker och landstingsprotokoll: Jämtlands domböcker 1621–1628. Östersund: Jämtlands läns fornskriftsällskap, 1933.

Kättström Höök, Lena. 'Från foster till dop: Hur man skyddar en hedning.' *Fataburen: Kulturhistorisk tidskrift* (2015): 12–37.

Keller, Eve. 'Embryonic Individuals: The Rhetoric of Seventeenth-Century Embryology and the Construction of Early-Modern Identity.' *Eighteenth-Century Studies* 33, no. 3 (2000): 321–48.

Kosmin, Jennifer. 'When the Fetus Becomes a Child: Some Reflections from the Long Eighteenth Century.' In *Rethinking Medical Humanities: Perspectives From the Arts and the Social Sciences, edited by* Rinaldo F. Canalis, Massimo Ciavolella, and Valeria Finucci, 51–70. Berlin: De Gruyter, 2023.

Larsen, Dag A., and Kåre Rauø. *Dombok Torneå Lappmark: Jukkasjärvi og Enontekis tinglag 1715–1726*. Finnsnes: Lenvik bygdemuseum, 1994.

Larsen, Dag A., and Kåre Rauø. *Dombok Torneå Lappmark: Kautokeino, Aviovara, Teno, Utsjok Tingsteder 1726–1735*. Finnsnes: Lenvik bygdemuseum, 1999.

Ling, Sofia. *Kärringmedicin och vetenskap: Läkare och kvacksalverianklagade i Sverige omkring 1770–1870*. Uppsala: Uppsala universitet, 2004.

Lugt, Maaike van der. 'Formed Fetuses and Healthy Children in Scholastic Theology, Medicine and Law.' In *Reproduction: Antiquity to Present Day*, edited by Nick Hopwood, Rebecca Flemming, and Lauren Kassel, 167–80. Cambridge: Cambridge University Press, 2018.

Lupton, Deborah. *The Social Worlds of the Unborn*. Basingstoke: Palgrave Macmillan, 2013.

Månsson, Arvid. *Practica, eller een liten doch nyttigh vnderwijszning, om åderlåtande, hwilka ådrer man för åtskillige siukdomar vplåta kan, begynnandes på hufwudet, och sedan nedher til fötterna*... Stockholm: [Ignatus Meurer] 1654.

McClive, Cathy. 'Blood and Expertise: The Trials of the Female Medical Expert in the Ancien-Régime Courtroom.' *Bulletin of the History of Medicine* 82, no. 1 (2008): 86–108.

McClive, Cathy. 'The Hidden Truths of the Belly: The Uncertainties of Pregnancy in Early Modern Europe.' *Social History of Medicine* 15, no. 2 (2002): 209–27.

Morgan, Lynn M. *Icons of Life: A Cultural History of Human Embryos*. Berkeley: University of California Press, 2009.

Morgan, Lynn M. 'When Does Life Begin? A Cross-Cultural Perspective on the Personhood of Fetuses and Young Children.' In *Talking about People: Readings in Contemporary Cultural Anthropology*, edited by William A. Haviland, Robert J. Gordon, and Luis A. Vivanco, 35–46. Boston, MA: McGraw-Hill, 2002.

Norberg, Sture, ed. *Ångermanlands domsagas dombok och tingsprotokoll*. Vol. 15, *1628–1633*. Huddinge: Sture Norberg, 2000.

Norberg, Sture, ed. *Ångermanlands domsagas dombok och tingsprotokoll*. Vol. 16, *1634–1638*. Huddinge: Sture Norberg, 2000.

Norberg, Sture, ed. *Avskrift av Ångermanlands domsagas dombok och tingsprotokoll*. Vol. 18, *1643–1644*. Huddinge: Sture Norberg, 2003.

Norberg, Sture, ed. *Laga ting i Ångermanland*. Vol. 14, *1612–1624*. Huddinge: Sture Norberg, 2000.

Pineau, Severin. *De integritatis et corruptionis virginum notis: graviditate item & partu naturali mulierum, opuscula*. Lugduni-Batavorum, apud Franciscum Hegerum, 1641.

Richardsson, Ingegerd, ed. *Revsunds tingslags domboksprotokoll 1649–1700*. Östersund: Landsarkivet i Östersund and Jämtlands läns fornskriftssällskap, 2011.

Rösslin, Eucharius. *Der Swangern Frawen und Hebammen Roszengarten*. Strasbourg and Hagenau, 1513.

Ruberg, Willemijn. 'Travelling Knowledge and Forensic Medicine: Infanticide, Body and Mind in the Netherlands, 1811–1911.' *Medical History* 57, no. 3 (2013): 359–76.

Runesson, Anton. *Blod, kött och tårar: Kroppslig erfarenhet i Sverige ca 1600–1750*. Stockholm: Stockholms universitet, 2021.

Sjöberg, Maria. *Kvinnors jord, manlig rätt: Äktenskap, egendom och makt i äldre tid.* Hedemora: Gidlund, 2001.

Sundin, Jan. *För Gud, staten och folket: Brott och rättskipning i Sverige 1600–1840.* Stockholm: Institutet för rättshistorisk forskning, 1992.

Svenska akademiens ordbok (website). Accessed July 4, 2023. https://saob.se/.

Thunander, Rudolf. *Hovrätt i funktion: Göta hovrätt och brottmålen 1635–1699.* Stockholm: Institutet för rättshistorisk forskning, 1993.

Uppsala universitet. *Akademiska konsistoriets protokoll*, edited by Hans Sallander. Vol. 15. Uppsala: Uppsala universitet, 1968.

Veit, Patrice. '"Ich bin sehr schwach, doch drückst du nach …" Evangelisches Kirchenlied und seelsorgerische Begleitung von Schwangeren im 17. und 18. Jahrhundert.' In *Geschichte des Ungeborenen: Zur Erfahrungs- und Wissenschaftsgeschichte der Schwangerschaft 17.–20. Jahrhundert*, edited by Barbara Duden, Jürgen Schlumbohm, and Patrice Veit, 49–74. Göttingen: Vandenhoeck & Ruprecht, 2002.

Whiteley, Rebecca. *Birth Figures: Early Modern Prints and the Pregnant Body.* Chicago: University of Chicago Press, 2023.

Wikström, Lars, ed. *Stockholm tänkeböcker från 1592*. Vol. 10. Stockholm: Stockholms stadsarkiv, 1973.

CHAPTER 3

Beyond the Human Fetus: Monstrous Births and Emerging Biopolitics around 1800

Maja Bondestam

Not all fetuses delivered from women have been recognized as humans in Western law and medicine. By following the category of so-called monstrous births and medico-legal discussions about the presence of souls, it is possible to trace important hierarchies and power relations at the borders of life. In early modern Sweden, monstrous births could remind people of the offspring's subhuman dimensions but also of an original state, a playful and wondrous nature, free to deviate from expected habits. Their natural, legal, and spiritual status was still debated in late eighteenth-century medicine and law, whereas by the early nineteenth century, the monster was no longer a category of interest in these domains. How can one explain this shift, and what were the consequences for human fetuses, definitions of personhood, and legal hierarchies?

Earlier research has discussed the disappearance of monsters from nature and medicine in terms of normalization. Lorraine Daston and Katharine Park have emphasized the emergence of absolute regularity, both of nature's customs and God's rules, in European elite culture in the late seventeenth century. Monsters now submitted, not to secular powers, but to strict norms, and this process is traceable for many decades. Daston and Park end their investigation in 1750, when monsters were no longer prestigious and rare but reduced to an incomplete part of nature, which in itself had become uniform over time and place.[1]

In turning to the Swedish case and a specific discussion about human and nonhuman fetuses, I attempt to place earlier research on the disappearance of monsters in relation to a little-studied local context.

The research field describes a well-known pathologization of extraordinary bodies, which is relevant in the search for new power relations in modernity. Before 1800, physically irregular persons sometimes had a prominent place in society, offering reminders of God's presence and a playful nature. They were displayed, displayed themselves, traveled, and aroused wonder and

1 Daston and Park, *Wonders and the Order of Nature*, 10, 14, 18, 176, 187, 189, 202, 205–8, 214.

 | DOI:10.1163/9789004703759_005

excitement. During the eighteenth century, however, people with unusual bodies transformed into mute deformations. In an anatomical framework, conjoined twins and fetuses with too many or too few limbs, or other unexpected features, were approached as organisms that had failed to achieve their perfect final form. The value of extraordinary fetuses depended, not on their rarity or singularity, but on the body's capacity to reveal rigid rules of nature.[2] How did new questions about the procreative capacity of the population relate to this shift? In what ways did viability, the capacity to live on independently of the mother and to develop and reach maturity, start to operate as a placeholder for the recognition of personhood at the beginnings of life?[3]

The history of monstrous births is connected with changing valuations and meanings of the fetus and in a broader sense with the ordering of differences, bodies, identities, rights, and power relations in modern democracies from the late eighteenth century onward. Who should enjoy legal and economic privileges? How did monstrous births relate to this heated debate? Did they become objects of curative operations, of comparison on a universal scale, and of examination in relation to some average body in the statistical middle?[4] As Lennard J. Davis has noted, the concept of the norm invited the majority of the population to be part of, or to relate itself to, the norm, conforming to the common type or average standard.[5] In addition to these aspects of normalization, I also pay attention to the emerging notion of nature as regular and universally homogenous, as described by Daston and Park.

By analyzing the legacy of Carl Linnaeus's classification of the human species, I discuss how the distinctions between humans, monsters, and animals changed around 1800. My claim is that from the early nineteenth century the old distinction between human newborns and offspring beyond human identity, such as animalistic monsters and mixed categories, disappeared and was replaced by malformed, dead, or dying children. The focus of interest changed from transgressed boundaries between species to gradual differences among humans and the indicated viability of the human fetus. As far as I know this shift has never been discussed in the historiography of extraordinary births. Jennifer Kosmin shows how medico-legal definitions of fetal life increasingly shaped decision-making over rights and inheritance in eighteenth-century Europe and how the viable fetus came to exist as a conceptual and legal

2 Hagner, 'Enlightened Monsters,' 178; Foucault, *Abnormal*, 50.

3 On viability as an organizing principle in the management of birth today, see Christoffersen-Deb, 'Viability,' 65–66.

4 Bondestam, 'Introduction,' 11–19; Ray, 'From Monsters to Malformations.'

5 Davis, *Enforcing Normalcy*, 24.

entity during the century. According to her, monstrous births, the limits of humanity, and the importance of souls continued to trouble religious and legal categories of life in this period.[6] I can confirm her results while also studying the early nineteenth century and analyzing shifts in relationships between the species, a diminishing interest in the human soul, and a normalization of monstrosities as important in the medico-legal definitions of the fetus and the emerging focus on its supposed capacity for future independent life.

Inspired by Michel Foucault's writing on monsters, I examine sources not only in medicine and natural history but also in forensic medicine and civil law. As Foucault claims, the breach of natural laws in the seventeenth and eighteenth centuries was not enough to constitute monstrosity. Only when a body also created disorder in social life, when it overturned or disturbed civil or canon laws, was it seen as a monster.[7] For a closer examination of this phenomenon, I have studied Swedish handbooks in forensic medicine and civil law, published between 1776 and 1851, in which the terse paragraphs of the law were expanded and explained for professionals such as physicians, priests, midwives, obstetricians, lawyers, and judges. The handbooks needed continual revision in accordance with shifting legislation, which makes it possible to follow legal categories such as 'humans' and 'monsters' over time.

On the following pages, I also discuss these disappearing monsters in relation to a certain type of modern power, which took as its object the management of life. In the 1970s, Foucault identified a distribution of so-called biopower or biopolitics, which in Western societies from the second half of the eighteenth century combined with an intensified production of the *knowledge of life*. Biopolitics framed the body as an organism with certain abilities, as utilizable, amenable to profitable investment, with prospects of survival, and capacities for being trained.[8] This 'biopower' became manifest in the use of statistics on the life of human population to encourage reproduction or, as it was called in less abstract and more active terms in the eighteenth century, generation.[9] As I will show, in Sweden, with its early population censuses, these tendencies formed a political technology of life that had to do with analyzing, disciplining,

6 Kosmin, 'When the Fetus,' 50–52.

7 Foucault, *Abnormal*, 63, 64. About stillbirths as transboundary in a similar way to monsters, see Paulsson Holmberg, 'Ambiguous and Transitional Bodies.'

8 Foucault, *History of Sexuality*, 1:139–48; Foucault, Senellart, and Davidson, *Security, Territory, Population*, 1–8, 55–59, 63; Foucault, 'Politics of Health,' 93–96; Foucault, *'Society Must Be Defended,'* 242–46; Lemke, *Biopolitics*, 5, 35, 39, 47.

9 Rusnock, 'Biopolitics and the Invention of Population,' 334. On the words 'generation' and 'reproduction,' see Hopwood, 'Keywords,' 287–304.

and regulating bodies and populations. This process eventually included monstrous births.

First, I describe the signs of humans and monsters in eighteenth-century forensic medicine and the subsequent homogenization of humankind around 1800, which made monstrous births less strange, frightening, erroneous, transgressive, and wondrous. Then I turn to civil law and its definitions of the person, the human, and the citizen, before discussing the disappearance of the monster and the intensified production of knowledge about the population. Finally, I examine the specificity of monstrous births and emerging biopolitics in late eighteenth- and early nineteenth-century Sweden.

1 Classification of the Human Kind

The early modern vision of nature was a coherent, hierarchical continuum with no sudden breaches or gaps, and the human species was always placed above the animals. The two groups shared a number of significant traits but, as emphasized in the physico-theological literature of the eighteenth century, it was easy to distinguish humans from the rest of creation, since they used their reason daily. The natural order reached from the lowest lifeless matter, through plants, animals, and humans, to the angels and the highest spiritual substances. Humans were of heavenly origin and had an elevated nature, which created a boundary between them and animals. As stated in a zoological handbook in 1750, the human head is the home of reason, the soul, and morality, and accordingly must be the most important feature of the species. Humans' exceptional quality lay in thinking, behavior, virtue, and the capacity for mastery and judgement—traits emanating from the heart and the soul or perhaps from the head and the brain.[10]

In the early editions of *Systema naturae*, in the dissertation *Antropomorpha*, and in the text *Menniskans cousiner*, Carl Linnaeus discussed the vague distinctions between humans and apes. He divided the animal kingdom into six classes, and in the first one (quadrupeds), the manlike animals, *Homo* and *Simia*, constituted the first order.[11] Later on, Linnaeus gave humans the name *Homo sapiens* and replaced the order Antropomorpha with Primates, in which he continued to place both humans and apes since no physical traits distinguished them from each other. Nature was supposed to move slowly

10 Orrelius, *Historia animalium*, L § 200.

11 Linné, *Systema naturae*; Linné, *Menniskans cousiner*, 4–5; Linné, *Dissertatio academica, in qua Antropomorpha*.

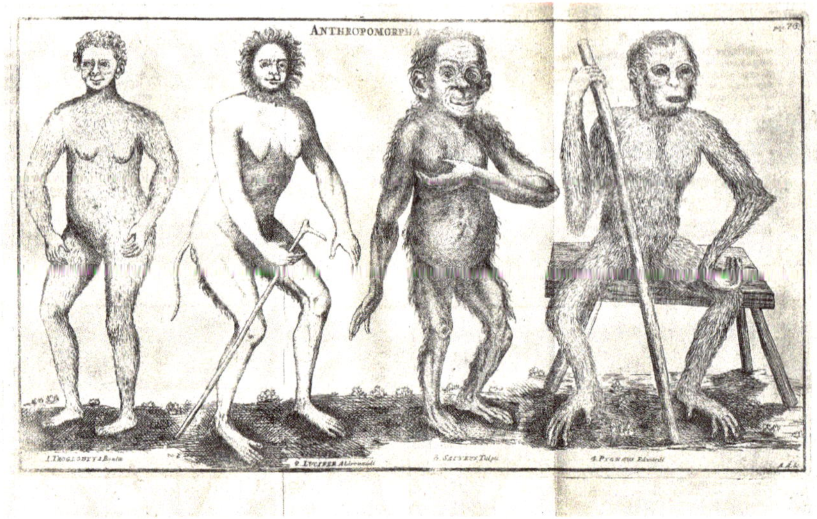

FIGURE 3.1 *Antropomorpha* was a dissertation published in 1760, defended by Christian Emmanuel Hoppius but written by his professor Carl Linnaeus. It describes the Antropomorpha (humanlike beings), who, according to Linnaeus, stood between *Homo sapiens* and the lower apes in the class 'Quadrupedia,' later 'Mammalia,' and even later 'Primates.' The famous engraving by Andreas Åkerman shows, from the left, the troglodyte, the tail man, the satyr, and the pygmy. Uppsala University Library.

from one thing to another, and Linnaeus saw night humans or 'Ourang Outan' (*Homo nocturnus*) as a middling link between the humanlike species in the first order.[12] According to Linnaeus the human genus (*Homo*) contained four species. Besides *Homo sapiens* and *Homo troglodytes*, there were also *Homo lar* and *Homo caudatus*. *Homo lar* was described as tailless, with erect posture and of human height, whereas *Homo caudatus* was also called 'Lucifer' or the 'tail human.'[13]

Certain attributes, not least zoomorphic ones, could cast doubt on whether a newborn offspring was human or not, and thorough discussions on the subject were held in forensic medicine in the last decades of the eighteenth century. This field of knowledge itself transcended disciplines, as it connected law with medicine and helped legal scholars resolve court cases that had to do with rape, induced abortion, and infanticide. As Anton Runesson states in this volume, medical experts were seldom consulted in the seventeenth-century courts. In the eighteenth century, however, physicians and surgeons participated more

12 Linné, *Menniskans cousiner*, 16; Broberg, *Homo sapiens L*, 192–95.
13 Broberg, *Homo sapiens L*, 190, 205–12, 237.

frequently in court proceedings, and forensic medicine became a subject in medical journals around Europe.[14]

When it came to the subject of extraordinary births in the late eighteenth century, authors of forensic handbooks focused on the presence of the human soul. So-called monsters were at the center of attention, and they seemed to occupy a space between species. It was possible that they had no souls and accordingly could not be ascribed human status. In 1776, Jonas Kiernander, physician and district medical officer, emphasized that the human head harbors the soul and, consequently, distinguished a human from an animal offspring. Kiernander wrote for people who decided the lives, rights, and futures of newborns, such as midwives, obstetricians, and judges. He stated that some observers spoke of *monsters* (*Monstrum*) while others saw *animals* or *prodigies* in deformed bodies, which in shape and build differed from their genus. A number of subcategories were identified, such as people with double limbs or two heads connected to one body, those without required body parts, or those who had body parts that were unusual or even created against the order of nature. Deviations in size were less significant, but giants and dwarfs belonged to the monster category, as did newborn babies that looked like animals, such as frogs, apes, and puppies. Kiernander referred to the famous sixteenth-century surgeon Ambroise Paré, who claimed that a human offspring could have the head of an ox, a calf, an elephant, or a dog, while the rest of the body was humanlike. However, many learned authorities doubted the capacity of soulless animals to give birth to humans, and vice versa, and Kiernander was far from convinced of the existence of such mixed beings. At the same time, he found it hard to explain the existence of newborn babies covered with hair, displaying broken limbs or animalistic traits. Was the origin of such monsters in the egg, or did the extraordinary shape appear later in the life of the fetus, owing to a moldable material or body, a so-called *Materia Plastica*?[15]

This was a major question in eighteenth-century medicine. Epigenetic theories described how the embryo takes shape in the uterus and how complex organic structures emerge from simple, undifferentiated ones.[16] According to the competing theory of preformation, the fetus was a fully formed miniature human being, shaped by God from the beginning. All essential organs and complex structures were in place in the seed or the egg, and no profound

14 Gustafsson, 'Läkaren, döden och brottet,' 17–20, 24–25, 45–105; Crawford, 'Legalizing Medicine.' An important seventeenth-century contribution to the field is Zacchia, *Quaestiones medico-legales*.

15 Kiernander, *Utkast til Medicinal-lagfarenheten*, 697–99, 705–10.

16 Hagner, 'Enlightened Monsters,' 196–99.

development or change was associated with the fetus, whose body parts only grew in size from the moment of conception to birth. The epigenesists argued, with a different starting point, that nature itself acts in relation to new life and that every embryo develops gradually, out of unorganized matter. They considered the living body to have a creative, formative, and organizing potential—the embryo not only unfolded preformed parts, as preformationists thought, but also built itself up from the inside. For the epigenesists, this made the act of procreation a dynamic and unpredictable course of events, full of hindrances and invisible processes.[17]

Kiernander only commented briefly on these tensions in European medicine in his efforts to understand the appearance of monstrous births. A more widespread theory explaining why infants sometimes deviated from their parents' physical shape proposed a fundamental communication between pregnant women and their fetuses, mediated by nerves and fantasy. As the theory stated, women sometimes processed outer images and imprinted them on the fetuses through a shaping power, which mainly produced minor deviances in the children's bodies.[18] In Kiernander's words, 'There is almost daily evidence of children who are tainted either by the imagination or the fright of the mother, such as the hare-lipped.'[19] An offspring with too many or unusually placed inner organs could not, however, be the result of even the strongest impression on the mother's soul. Some monstrous formations were simply against the order of nature, such as a fetus born with a lump of flesh in place of the head, or with no head at all. Such births made up a class of their own called creatures (*kreatur*) and, like children resembling soulless animals, had no right to be baptized. A physician's difficult decision to kill a monstrous birth was indicated only if it, or its father, was definitely a soulless animal, such as when a woman delivered an offspring with a dog's, or some other animal's, head.[20]

One might expect that the body's perfections or deviances guided Kiernander in this discussion, but of greater importance was the soul, or the absence thereof. The essence of a human being lay in her spiritual dimensions, and Kiernander stated that a well-shaped head was the distinguishing mark of human identity. Children with two heads attached to one body should accordingly be baptized with two different names but would perhaps not inherit as two individuals or write separate wills.[21]

---

17 Roe, *Matter, Life, and Generation*, 1; Hagner, 'Enlightened Monsters,' 194–99.

18 Huet, *Monstrous Imagination*, 1.

19 Kiernander, *Utkast til Medicinal-lagfarenheten*, 701.

20 Kiernander, *Utkast til Medicinal-lagfarenheten*, 702–8, 712. On fears of the headless body, see Cressy, 'Lamentable, Strange, and Wonderful,' 41, 63.

21 Kiernander, *Utkast til Medicinal-lagfarenheten*, 712.

Relevant for Kiernander was the ecclesiastical law of 1686, which prevailed as the principal moral and legal code for church practices, such as baptisms and burials, into the early twentieth century. It reserved baptisms and funerals for living beings with a human appearance, according to a distinction between humans and monsters: 'Monsters (*Monstra*), without human shape, although delivered by a woman, should neither have the right to be baptized or buried.'[22] Unbaptized infants were left without names or godparents and excluded from burial in consecrated ground. They did not qualify for eternal life.[23] The harsh statement of the ecclesiastical law echoes the Aristotelian notion of a necessary congruence between the body and the soul, implying that bodies that did not look human had no souls. It differs from Augustine's inclusive vision of humanity, in which an immortal soul was limited neither to bodies with certain physical attributes nor to people with full rational capacities, and in which all infants were welcomed as God's creatures. In medieval theology, canon law, and manuals for priests, the discussion about monsters did not address whether they should be baptized, but how to do so, whereas from the fourteenth century, a well-formed head became a sufficient criterion for human status.[24]

In 1783, the Swedish physician and surgeon Roland Martin specified that the soul had its home in the brain. He also stated that a child was ideally the image of its parents, that the amount of spirituality corresponded to the shape of the head, and that a well-shaped head was a sign of a perfect procreative process. To deny newborn children human rights simply because they suffered from ascites, had a swollen head, no brain, or an inclined forehead appeared to Martin, however, as unnecessarily harsh. The terminology was important here. A child without a brain should be called deformed (*wanskapad*), not a freak nor a monster (*missfoster*), since the soul in such creatures pervaded the whole body. To call a child with civil and spiritual rights a freak violated all principles, since the word indicated that the offspring definitely had no soul and that its ability to live and move came only from the body. Such offspring got their nourishment from the mother's blood, through the umbilical cord, and deviated from human nature in their whole existence. An unusually shaped head or a missing brain was no certain sign of soulless monstrosity. When the whole being deviated from the expected shape, one could doubt whether a human had birthed it and whether the egg in the uterus had acquired life with a soul.[25]

---

22 *Sveriges kyrkolag af år 1686*, 210.

23 Paulsson Holmberg's chapter in this volume.

24 Lugt, 'Formed Fetuses and Healthy Children,' 174, 176.

25 Martin, *Läkare-Grunder*, 563.

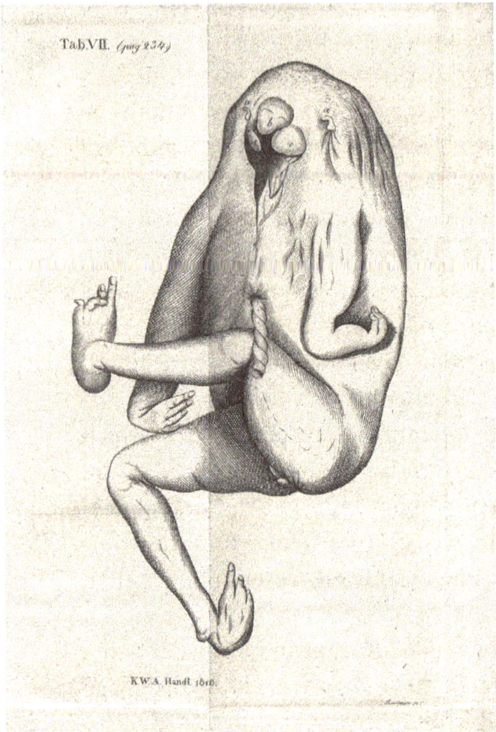

FIGURE 3.2
An engraving of a 'freak' that had been delivered in 1785 from a woman by the physician Eric Odehelius. Reporting in the transactions of the Royal Swedish Academy on this event and the following anatomical dissection, he held it likely to be one of the strangest 'freaks' ever observed. Yet, he still thought of it as a human offspring, not an animalistic creature or soulless monster. From Odhelius, 'Beskrifning på et Missfoster,' 175, Tab. VII. Unknown artist. Uppsala University Library.

Both Kiernander and Martin saw the presence of a soul, or at least signs of such presence, as the essence of humanity in a fetus and doubted that humans actually could deliver soulless creatures, so-called freaks or monsters. For Kiernander, the absence of humanity manifested itself in a number of physical features, such as a missing head or an animal's head, whereas for Martin absent humanity was less obvious to detect. All this changed, as we will see, in the nineteenth century, as the focus moved from mixed beings, animalistic monsters, and signs, to malformed, dead, or dying children.

2 From Soulless Creature to Nonviable Fetus

In the 1770s, the anatomist and physical anthropologist Johann Friedrich Blumenbach challenged Linnaeus's classification of humankind when he claimed that there was only one human species. Comparisons of pregnancy, life span, and sensitivity to diseases demonstrated obvious differences between humans and apes. Blumenbach constantly came back to the idea of humanity as a

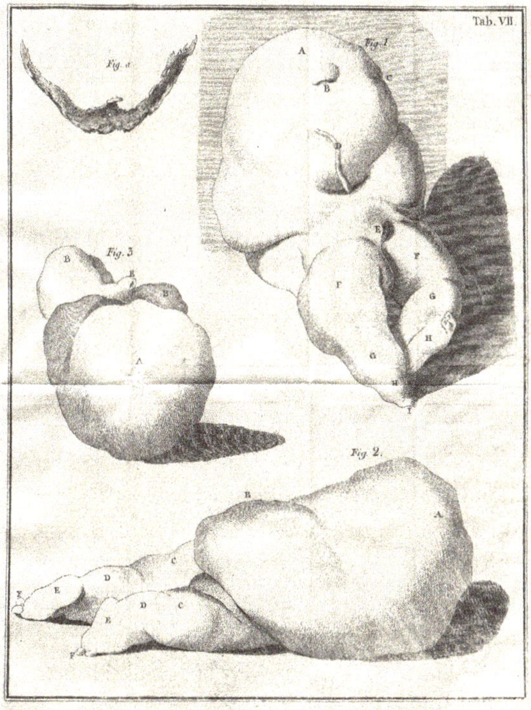

FIGURE 3.3
This miscarriage was delivered in 1816 by a 28-year-old woman in her fourth month of pregnancy. The provincial physician Carl Nordblad provided a brief description of the 'deformed fetus' in the transactions of the Royal Swedish Academy. Although the sex was unclear he did not question its human identity. From Nordblad, 'Beskrifning På ett Foster,' 234, Tab. VII. Engraving by Johan Gustaf Ruckman. Uppsala University Library.

single, united category and stated that the brain, soul, and consciousness were the same among groups of humans. He also emphasized that human beings' upright posture, two-handedness, developed speech, and reason distinguished them from apes.[26]

Around 1800, there was intense discussion on this subject, and in 1809, Carl Iser, a Swedish physician and author of popular works on anthropology, claimed that 'the sharp minded LINNAEUS' was mistaken on how many species there were in the human genus.[27] Iser stated, with references to Blumenbach, that there was no more than one kind of human, that *Homo troglodytus* was a variety of the human species, and that *Homo lar* was an ape.[28] In this way, an assortment of human types gathered in one single species, and a considerable gap appeared between humans and the rest of the four-limbed animals.

This reduction from four human species to one occurred at the same time as human offspring were redefined according to new patterns in Swedish

26 Hannaford, *Race*, 206; Stepan, *Idea of Race in Science*, 10.
27 Funke and Lippold, *Naturalhistoria*, 40.
28 Funke and Lippold, *Naturalhistoria*, vii.

medico-legal literature. Eric Gadelius, physician and professor of medicine at the Karolinska Institute, was teaching pathology, anatomy, physiology, and forensic medicine in the early nineteenth century. In 1804, he defined the difference between misshapen persons (*vanlytta*) and freaks (*missfoster*) as gradual. Following Martin, and in contrast to Kiernander, Gadelius made no specific distinction between body and soul, human and animal, or fetuses with and without well-shaped heads. He stated that all offspring of human parents were human, but viable to different degrees, and discussed errors in their organic structure.[29] Humans were supposed to have a natural shape, sometimes so abrogated that the infant died immediately after birth and consequently failed to fulfil its constitution. In such cases, it was appropriate for the physician to use the term freak (*missfoster*) and to examine and present a medical opinion on the offspring to the judge.[30]

For Gadelius, human identity was defined in relation, not to soulless monsters, but in a gradual sense to infants who lacked the ability to live—who were nonviable. Transboundary fetuses with animalistic traits, who during the previous century symbolized a crucial absence of thinking, reason, and morality, were not beyond human identity. For Gadelius it was rather the malformed, dying, or stillborn fetuses who lacked full human status.[31]

In 1838, the physician August Timoleon Wistrand, who specialized in the medico-legal sphere, wrote a handbook on forensic medicine in which he claimed that the freak (*missfostret*) appeared as an ontological noncategory. The classifying principle so far had been that an offspring was human if 'the formation of the head indicates a human soul.'[32] Wistrand preferred another definition and believed that a fetus should be an object of forensic examination only if it deviated from 'the normal human formation' to such an extent that its human rights were called into doubt.[33] Attention was paid to both the presence of the head and the viability of the fetus: '*Freaks*, monstra, are such human fetuses, by whom the brain or some other essential organ is missing or is so abnormally formed, that they cannot live an autonomous life. Therefore, they usually die soon after the delivery.'[34]

---

29 The Swedish words closest to viability are probably *livsduglig* and *livskraftig*, which mean 'capable,' 'strong,' and 'healthy enough to live on.' They became used in a broader sense from the second half of the nineteenth century.

30 Gadelius, *Handbok*, 141–43.

31 Gadelius, *Handbok*, 141–43.

32 Wistrand, *Handbok*, 40.

33 Wistrand, *Handbok*, 39.

34 Wistrand, *Handbok*, 40.

Both Gadelius and Wistrand argued that proper humans were capable of autonomous life, whereas monsters were either stillbirths or about to die, and consequently did not constitute a relevant category. No monsters were moving around among humans, producing disorder in social life, taxonomy, or the legal system. Instead, there were stillbirths or fetuses about to die because of some missing or underdeveloped essential organ.

At the same time as monsters disappeared from forensic medicine, a growing gap between humans and animals appeared. This was partly thanks to Blumenbach's critique of Linnaeus's classification of the quadrupeds and to the consolidation of four human species into one. In the new century, there were only humans and animals, nothing in between. No mixed bodies and no subcategories narrowed the gap between humans and apes.

For centuries, the soul and its physical mark, the well-shaped head, separated humans from animals, but suddenly, beginning with Gadelius, viability and the supposed capacity for future independent life distinguished human newborns from offspring beyond human identity. A presumed capacity of the infant to live, develop, and reach maturity replaced the old focus on a certain feature, essence, or shape of the infant's head. At the same time, the category of the monster disappeared from forensic medicine. Can this shift also be seen in other parts of early nineteenth-century culture? To deepen our understanding of the human fetus and its conceptual limits I will now examine, first, definitions of *the person* and its legal status in early nineteenth-century civil law and, second, the intensified production of statistical knowledge about *the population* from the middle of the eighteenth century onward.

3 Who Is a Person?

In the early nineteenth century, three handbooks explaining Swedish legislation for civilians pointed out that a person is a being of the human kind and that the words 'person,' 'human,' and 'monster' overlap to some extent.

The author of one of these was Ebbe Samuel Bring, professor of history and philosophy, and with formal qualifications and practical experience in jurisprudence. In 1817, he emphasized that a *person* is an intelligent being with full rights and a subject of legal relationships with the ability to undertake free activities prescribed by the law. He clarified that a person according to the civil law was a Swedish man, over twenty-one years old, who was not ill, insane, or deformed. In relation to this standard, there were also children; women; disabled, insane, or ill persons; foreigners; Jews; and so-called Tartars and Gypsies. They could also enter into legal relationships, but not in the full sense, owing to a perceived difference in human nature. To include them in the general set of rules, civil law used the category *physical person*, and Bring claimed that all human individuals were counted as such, from birth to death.[35]

At the center of the judicial concept of the person was the healthy adult male Swede, whereas all others inhabited the periphery of legal relationships and rights. In the margins of the judicial concept of the person, we find beings hardly acknowledged as humans at all. Bring stated that certain defects of the body influenced civil law, such as 'hideous errors and infirmities, for example deformity.'[36] As monsters were their own category, they were not considered deformed. Now, a monster (*monstrum*) was a creature delivered by a woman, but without a human head. Someone who was procreated and delivered by humans, should be supported, taken care of, and have human rights. If a newborn *partus acephalus*, a fetus with no skull and no brain, showed signs of life, it should have the right to inherit. This was especially the case if the defects had other causes than ones associated with the parents.[37]

The interesting thing about Bring is that he discussed not only persons, humans, and physical persons but also headless monsters as subjects of the law. In this way, he is similar to Kiernander, although he had fewer problems with the monster category. There was no need to kill or exclude monsters from eternal life, the Christian community, human rights, care, or support. For Bring, the monster did not create disorder in social life, or overturn or disturb civil or canon laws. It was a human, so it seems, especially if we read him in relation to Foucault's definition of monsters as disturbing not only the laws of nature but also civil or religious laws.

A clearer separation of humans from monsters is present in Fredrik Schrevelius's handbook of Swedish civil law from 1844: 'Only humans are, as earlier said, physical persons. From this follows, that a monster (*monstrum*), also when it is delivered by a human mother, is not a person.'[38] Schrevelius clung to the old distinction between humans and monsters and stated that someone with a human head was a human, no matter how deformed he or she was in other aspects, whereas someone without a head was beyond human identity.[39] Here Schrevelius agreed with medico-legal authors from the eighteenth century, such as Kiernander and Martin, but in a later edition of his book from

35 Bring, *Grunderna till swenska civil-lagfarenheten*, 66–67, 117–31.

36 Bring, *Grunderna till swenska civil-lagfarenheten*, 129.

37 Bring, *Grunderna till swenska civil-lagfarenheten*, 130.

38 Schrevelius, *Lärobok*, 39.

39 Schrevelius, *Lärobok*, 39–40.

1851, he moved closer to Wistrand and Bring when he questioned whether a freak or a monster (*missfoster* or *monstrum*) could exist at all.[40]

Schrevelius now defined monsters as fetuses whose malformations prevented them from continuing to live, such as stillbirths, dying newborns, or fetuses without heads. This resulted in a situation where lawyers and judges no longer had to engage with the monster category, and its definition appeared in Swedish civil law for what was likely the last time. Now only humans remained in the legislation, as in forensic medicine, but as clearly indicated by Bring, there were also significant differences between humans. An important hierarchy, stretching from the intellectually and physically healthy adult Swedish man to a number of other persons, was established in the first decades of the new century. From the middle of the eighteenth century onward, all fetuses delivered by human mothers counted as humans in Swedish civil law, and all *physical persons* had rights, although not in the full sense. This is a central paradox in the history of bodies and eighteenth-century democracy. A number of new groups achieved human identity but, simultaneously, were denied full legal rights.

4 Valuing Viability

Swedish authorities have a long history in the field of population registration, and in the early days, they embraced not only bodies and aspects of the population that were easy to quantify but also extraordinary births. In 1668 the ecclesiastical law stated that priests must write yearly reports, not only on births, marriages, and deaths in the parishes, but also on '[r]are occurrences, people's especially good or bad achievements, or such things displaying themselves, which are beyond the order of nature, in the elements, or living or dead, and are worth recording.'[41]

This formulation was still common in 1749, when the public statistical authority, the Office for Tabulation, was founded in Stockholm. The Office for Tabulation was to systematically examine and take stock of national resources, including humans, but also of rare events in nature. In 1757, one such report described a child born in the parish of Källa, on the island of Öland, who had no skull or proper skin on the back of the head. There was only a thin membrane over the brain, through which the blood vessels clearly appeared. Among a number of other physical irregularities, the child had no eyes, no

40 Schrevelius, *Lärobok*, 59.

41 Sidenbladh, *Sällsamma händelser*, 3.

nose, and no upper jawbone. According to the reporting priest, the child died within twenty-four hours of its birth.[42]

The registration of this case was part of the larger production of knowledge about the size, health, and quality of the population. In the middle of the eighteenth century, inadequate care for small children was seen as the cause of depopulation and infant mortality. On the basis of the first collected numbers of births and deaths in the Swedish parishes, the Office for Tabulation claimed that 20–30 percent of all children died during their first year.[43]

The initiative to create a public administrative authority that collected and processed statistics about the population came from the Royal Swedish Academy of Sciences, founded in 1739 to promote studies in natural history and to use the results of such studies. The Office for Tabulation and the academy worked together and published a number of essays on demography and small children. The essays discussed the utility of yearly charts of the number of births in the nation. Diseases of infants, misshapen births (*vanskapligt födda*), and the number of twins being born every year were analyzed, as well as the distribution of boys and girls. When during the year were children most frequently born in Sweden? Which were the most common diseases among them? How many women died during childbirth? How many children were born without legitimate fathers, and with different faults (*lyten*)?[44]

Statistical reports represented information about the population in tables showing numbers about births, deaths, marriages, and diseases. Complex realities gave way to overviews, which in turn enabled comparisons and were supposed to clarify ongoing discussions about the nation's health, strength, and wealth. In political arithmetic, new techniques of inquiry were used to observe, count, analyze, classify, and order the population—the normative core to which every singularity, more or less deviant, was now compared. Quantitative information enabled the exact treatment of any subject, and local observations contributed to discussions about subjects of national debate. The origin of biopolitics lay in similar studies of the population and can be seen in a growing interest in human bodies as objects of surveillance, intervention, and modification.[45]

Biopolitics was not concerned with individuals, but with physical signs, measured and aggregated at the level of the population. Statistics on the lives,

42 Sidenbladh, *Sällsamma händelser*, 30.

43 Wannerdt, *Den svenska folkbokföringens historia*, 21; Nyström, 'Nils Rosén von Rosenstein,' 425.

44 Ståhl, *Register*, 217–18, 496.

45 Rusnock, 'Biopolitics: Political Arithmetic,' 50–51, 56–67; Rusnock, *Vital Accounts*, 16–19.

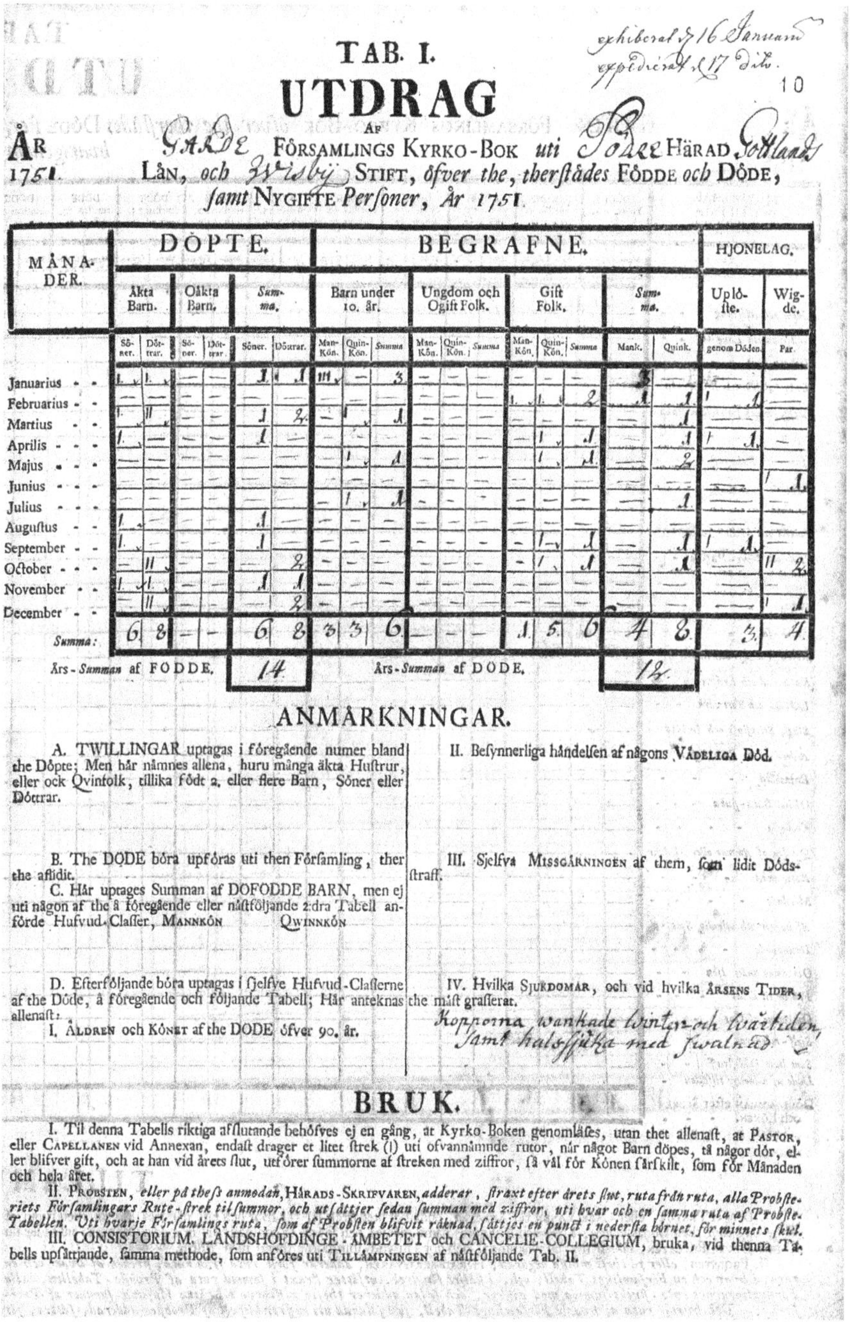

exhiberat d. 16 Januarii
expedierat d. 17 dito.

10

TAB. I.

UTDRAG

AF

ÅR 1751. Garde FÖRSAMLINGS KYRKO-BOK *uti* [illegible] HÄRAD Gottlands LÄN, *och* Wisby STIFT, *öfver the, therſtädes* FÖDDE *och* DÖDE, *ſamt* NYGIFTE *Perſoner, År* 1751.

MÅNADER.	DÖPTE. Åkta Barn. Söner.	Döttrar.	Oäkta Barn. Söner.	Döttrar.	Summa. Söner.	Döttrar.	BEGRAFNE. Barn under 10. år. Mankön.	Quinkön.	Summa	Ungdom och Ogift Folk. Mankön.	Quinkön.	Summa	Gift Folk. Mankön.	Quinkön.	Summa	Summa. Mank.	Quink.	HJONELAG. Uplöſte genom Döden.	Wigde. Par.
Januarius	1	1	–	–	1	1	111	–	3	–	–	–	–	–	–	3	–	–	–
Februarius	–	–	–	–	–	–	–	–	–	–	–	–	1	1	2	1	1	1	–
Martius	1	11	–	–	1	2	–	1	1	–	–	–	–	–	–	–	1	–	–
Aprilis	1	–	–	–	1	–	–	–	–	–	–	–	–	1	1	–	1	1	–
Majus	–	–	–	–	–	–	–	1	1	–	–	–	–	1	1	–	2	–	–
Junius	–	–	–	–	–	–	–	–	–	–	–	–	–	–	–	–	–	–	1
Julius	–	–	–	–	–	–	–	1	1	–	–	–	–	–	–	–	1	–	–
Auguſtus	1	–	–	–	1	–	–	–	–	–	–	–	–	–	–	–	–	–	–
September	1	–	–	–	1	–	–	–	–	–	–	–	–	1	1	–	1	1	–
October	–	11	–	–	–	2	–	–	–	–	–	–	–	1	1	–	1	–	2
November	1	1	–	–	1	1	–	–	–	–	–	–	–	–	–	–	–	–	–
December	–	11	–	–	–	2	–	–	–	–	–	–	–	–	–	–	–	–	1
Summa:	6	8	–	–	6	8	3	3	6	–	–	–	1	5	6	4	8	3	4

Års-*Summan* af FÖDDE. 14 Års-*Summan* af DÖDE. 12

ANMÅRKNINGAR.

A. TWILLINGAR uptagas i föregående numer bland the Döpte; Men här nämnes allena, huru många äkta Huſtrur, eller ock Qvinfolk, tillika födt 2. eller flere Barn, Söner eller Döttrar.

B. The DÖDE böra upföras uti then Förſamling, ther the aflidit.

C. Här uptages Summan af DÖFÖDDE BARN, men ej uti någon af the å föregående eller näſtföljande 2:dra Tabell anförde Hufvud-Claſſer, MANNKÖN QWINNKÖN

D. Efterföljande böra uptagas i ſjelfve Hufvud-Claſſerne af the Döde, å föregående och följande Tabell; Här anteknas allenaſt:

I. ÅLDREN och KÖNET af the DÖDE öfver 90. år.

II. Beſynnerliga händelſen af någons VÅDELIGA Död.

III. Sjelfva MISSGÄRNINGEN af them, ſom lidit Döds-ſtraff.

IV. Hvilka SJUKDOMAR, och vid hvilka ÅRSENS TIDER, the mäſt graſſerat.

Kopporna wankade wintern och wårtiden, samt halssjuka med swulnad.

BRUK.

I. Til denna Tabells riktiga afſlutande behöfves ej en gång, at Kyrko-Boken genomläſes, utan thet allenaſt, at PASTOR, eller CAPELLANEN vid Annexan, endaſt drager et litet ſtrek (|) uti ofvannämnde rutor, när något Barn döpes, tå någor dör, eller blifver gift, och at han vid årets ſlut, utförer ſummorne af ſtreken med ziffror, ſå väl för Könen ſärſkilt, ſom för Månaden och hela året.

II. PROBSTEN, *eller på theſs anmodan,* HÄRADS-SKRIFVAREN, *adderar, ſtraxt efter årets ſlut, ruta från ruta, alla Probſteriets Förſamlingars Rute-ſtrek til ſummor, och utſättjer ſedan ſumman med ziffror, uti hvar och en ſamma ruta af Probſte-Tabellen. Uti hvarje Förſamlings ruta, ſom af Probſten blifvit räknad, ſättjes en punct i nederſta hörnet, för minnets ſkul.*

III. CONSISTORIUM, LANDSHÖFDINGE-ÄMBETET och CANCELIE-COLLEGIUM, bruka, vid thenna Tabells upſättjande, ſamma methode, ſom anföres uti TILLÄMPNINGEN af näſtföljande Tab. II.

FIGURE 3.4 Annual table completed by a parish priest, summarizing monthly births, deaths, and marriages, according to age and sex. This example, dated 1751, is from the parish of Garde on the island of Gotland. Priests were required to report whether children were born out of wedlock or not, any births of twins, common diseases, and peculiar events that led to someone's death. National Archives of Sweden.

longevity, births, deaths, health, sexuality, procreation, and disability of many people enabled the governing of individuals and collectives. This specific knowledge and power also made particular bodies and experiences disappear. Life became a collective reality and a generalizable, independent, measurable, and objective factor as, in the interests of fixed norms, standards, and average numbers, it was separated from actual, living beings and experiences.[46]

Extraordinary births, however, had a history of their own in relation to biopolitics and population censuses. Whereas information about births, deaths, and marriages was listed in tables and abstracted as numbers and names, the written reports on rare deviances in nature consisted of whole narratives with details, specificity, and descriptions of actual beings. The very essence of an extraordinary birth was that it was worth reporting. It was singular and beyond the expected order of nature. Even until the 1800s, the cases, reported and sometimes published in the proceedings of the Academy of Sciences, were often illustrated and exhaustively described (see figures 3.2, 3.3). It seems the national census, at least in the first century of systematically recorded rarities, did not lead particular bodies and experiences to disappear into abstracted numbers and charts. Instead, they displayed and drew attention to unexpected and unusual bodies. By the end of the seventeenth century, extraordinary births were reported systematically to the authorities, but they were not represented in tables and charts before the early twentieth century.[47]

Despite their absence from statistical charts during the 1800s, extraordinary births were part of a biopolitical project as they were objects of surveillance, analysis, classification, and measurement of life, health, and quality. In medico-legal definitions of humans and monsters, the concept of *viability* or capacity for future independent life became important around 1800 and established during the first part of the century. In 1825 a German professor of law and jurisprudence at Heidelberg had, according to a Swedish dissertation, claimed that 'the life of an unfit fetus is a life of pretense, without value and impossible to compare and measure with real human life.'[48] Health, strength, and the fetus's ability to live on independently came into focus across nineteenth-century European medicine and law, and now it seemed as if the urge to measure, compare, and value specific lives in relation to some kind of standard included extraordinary births. The Swedish case shows that biopolitics was part of this development and, in a wider sense, of the modernization

46 Lemke, *Biopolitics*, 5.

47 Sidenbladh, *Sällsamma händelser*, 7. Since 1964 congenital malformations have been recorded in the Swedish Register of Congenital Malformations and the Medical Birth Registry. See Lee's chapter in this volume.

48 Bergstrand, 'Till frågan,' 65–66.

of the human fetus. It was a new way to approach life—not by looking for the defining traits of the human body, which in earlier centuries had revealed nature's purposive order and helped to determine what a human was, but by grading corporeal capacities.

5 The Disappearing Monster

Swedish forensic medicine and civil law confirm earlier research on the normalization and pathologization of monstrosity and extraordinary births around 1800, but also bring new knowledge to the fore. By focusing on the number of human species in natural history, the widening gap between humans and animals, the changing definitions of *monsters*, *persons*, and *humans* in forensic medicine and civil law, and finally on the governing of physical deviances in emerging population censuses, this chapter contributes to the history of the human fetus, extraordinary birth, and the disappearing monster.

Before the nineteenth century, Swedish monsters appear far from normalized. Until the second half of the eighteenth century, they blurred the limits of the human body, mixed categories and species, and created disorder in delivery rooms and in the law. This occurred to the extent that it seemed justifiable to kill some of them. Inspired by Foucault's observation that the early modern monster disturbed not only natural but also civil and canon law and created disorder in social life, I have followed the changing definitions of extraordinary births in forensic medicine and civil law and in the prevailing ecclesiastical law of 1686. I conclude that around 1800, physically unusual fetuses not only brought definitions of human identity and human rights to the fore but also were incorporated into biopolitical knowledge of life, although with remaining elements of display, originality, and the specificity of actual bodies.

Why did the discussion of extraordinary births shift from transgressed boundaries between the species and the offspring's resemblance with animals, to the child's capacity for life? I have mentioned new classifications of the human species, the growing gap between humans and animals, and the homogenization of all human offspring after Blumenbach. Another aspect worth discussing is the new medical interest in life, living organisms, the strength of the species, and the health and quality of populations and persons that arose around 1800. In relation to this, I want to make two major points.

First, to focus on *animalistic features* or on *emblematic body parts*, as the authors of handbooks in forensic medicine did in the eighteenth century, was to examine signs of truth and order pertaining to a higher and often invisible level of reality. The presence of a certain organ or feature, such as the human head, could indicate that the body possessed a human soul and reason, and therefore belonged in a specific place in the hierarchy of nature, wherein everything alive, from the simplest stone to God himself, was connected. Emblematic signs determined what a particular offspring was, they revealed nature's purposive order and the categories through which it operated or, accidentally, violations of this order. The last alternative was brought to the fore when a woman delivered a monster, an animalistic creature, an offspring without head, or a fetus with an animal's head. To kill such a being immediately after birth, as Kiernander suggested, meant that there was no violation of the natural hierarchy and no mixing of categories.

Second, to focus on a body's *capacity for life* and to define a human being as someone dying or incapable of autonomous life, as medico-legal and judicial authors did from the early nineteenth century, was to aim at the body itself, to analyze what promoted life and strengthened the species. Extraordinary births had by that time been recorded systematically for more than a century, in line with the ecclesiastical law of 1668, although they were notoriously difficult to abstract from experiences, lives, and contexts; reduce to numbers; and insert in tables. Every case demanded its own narrative, and the routine of recording extraordinary births did not immediately incorporate them into a political technology that compared, valued, and measured life in relation to utility.

In the early nineteenth century, however, the distinctions between humans, animals, and monsters gave way to valuations and comparisons between different fetuses' capacity for life and to questions of the health and quality of the population as a whole. Records of conjoined twins and classifications of fetuses with too many, too few, or unusually composed body parts were now part of a larger effort to observe the population, to measure, quantify, compare, value, and relate bodies to a normal standard. The number of human species was at the same time reduced from four to one in European natural history, while the gap between apes and humans widened, and the demarcation of human identity shifted from an offspring's animalistic features to its capacity for life. Unruly monsters disappeared from both medicine and law, and the focus of interest shifted to viable infants and to national health and strength.

Bibliography

Bergstrand, Hilding. *Till frågan om vad som bör innefattas i begreppet mänskligt liv i rättslig mening*. Stockholm: Karolinska Institutet, 1916.

Bondestam, Maja. 'Introduction.' In *Exceptional Bodies in Early Modern Culture: Concepts of Monstrosity before the Advent of the Normal*, edited by Maja Bondestam, 11–36. Amsterdam: Amsterdam University Press, 2020.

Bring, Ebbe Samuel. *Grunderna till swenska civil-lagfarenheten, uti systematisk ordning*. Lund, 1817.

Broberg, Gunnar. *Homo sapiens L: Studier i Carl von Linnés naturuppfattning och människolära*. Stockholm: Almqvist & Wiksell, 1975.

Christoffersen-Deb, Astrid. 'Viability: A Cultural Calculus of Personhood at the Beginnings of Life.' *Medical Anthropology Quarterly* 26, no. 4 (2012): 575–94.

Crawford, Catherine. 'Legalizing Medicine: Early Modern Legal Systems and the Growth of Medico-Legal Knowledge.' In *Legal Medicine in History*, edited by Michael Clark and Catherine Crawford, 89–116. Cambridge: Cambridge University Press, 1994.

Cressy, David. 'Lamentable, Strange, and Wonderful: Headless Monsters in the English Revolution.' In *Monstrous Bodies/Political Monstrosities in Early Modern Europe*, edited by Laura Lunger Knoppers and Joan B. Landes, 40–63. Ithaca, NY: Cornell University Press, 2004.

Daston, Lorraine, and Katharine Park. *Wonders and the Order of Nature, 1150–1750*. New York: Zone Books, 1998.

Davis, Lennard J. *Enforcing Normalcy: Disability, Deafness, and the Body*. London: Verso, 1995.

Foucault, Michel. *Abnormal: Lectures at the Collège de France, 1974–1975*. Edited by Valerio Marchetti and Antonella Salomoni. Translated by Graham Burchell. London: Verso, 2003.

Foucault, Michel. *The History of Sexuality. Vol. 1, The Will to Knowledge*. Translated by Robert Hurley. Harmondsworth: Penguin, 1990.

Foucault, Michel. 'The Politics of Health in the Eighteenth Century.' In *The Essential Foucault: Selections from Essential Works of Foucault, 1954–1984*, edited by Paul Rabinow and Nikolas Rose, 90–105. New York: New Press, 2003.

Foucault, Michel. *'Society Must Be Defended': Lectures at the Collège de France, 1975–76*. Edited by Mauro Bertani. Translated by David Macey. London: Penguin, 2004.

Foucault, Michel, Michel Senellart, and Arnold Ira Davidson. *Security, Territory, Population: Lectures at the Collège de France, 1977–1978*. Basingstoke: Palgrave Macmillan, 2007.

Funke, Carl Philipp and Georg Heinrich Christian Lippold. *Naturalhistoria, hämtad ur Funkes och Lippolds skrifter*. Vol. 1, no. 3. Örebro, 1809.

Gadelius, Eric. *Handbok i medicinal-lagfarenheten*. Stockholm, 1804.

Gustafsson, Tony. *Läkaren, döden och brottet: Studier i den svenska rättsmedicinens etablering*. Uppsala: Uppsala universitet, 2007.

Hagner, Michael. 'Enlightened Monsters.' In *The Sciences in Enlightened Europe*, edited by William Clark, Jan Golinski, and Simon Schaffer, 175–217. Chicago: University of Chicago Press, 1999.

Hannaford, Ivan. *Race: The History of an Idea in the West*. Washington, DC: Woodrow Wilson Center Press, 1996.

Hopwood, Nick. 'The Keywords "Generation" and "Reproduction."' In *Reproduction: Antiquity to the Present Day*, edited by Nick Hopwood, Rebecca Flemming, and Lauren Kassell, 287–304. Cambridge: Cambridge University Press, 2018.

Huet, Marie-Hélène. *Monstrous Imagination*. Cambridge, MA: Harvard University Press, 1993.

Kiernander, Jonas. *Utkast til Medicinal-lagfarenheten, domare til uplysning, läkare til hjelpreda och barnmorskor til underwisning i ämnen, som röra människo-kroppen*. Stockholm, 1776.

Kosmin, Jennifer. 'When the Fetus Becomes a Child: Some Reflections from the Long Eighteenth Century.' In *Medical Humanities: Perspectives from the Arts and the Social Sciences*, edited by Rinaldo F. Canalis, Massimo Ciavolella, and Valeria Finucci, 51–70. Berlin: De Gruyter, 2023.

Lemke, Thomas. *Biopolitics: An Advanced Introduction*. New York: New York University Press, 2011.

Linné, Carl von. *Dissertatio academica, in qua Antropomorpha, consens. experient. Facult. Medic. in Reg. Academ. Upsaliensi, præside … Dn. Doct. Carolo Linnæo … publico examini submittit Christianus Emmanuel Hoppius, Petropolitanus. In audit. Carol. Maj. die VI. Septemb. anno MDCCLX. H. A. M. S.* Uppsala: Evald Ziervogel, 1760.

Linné, Carl von. *Menniskans cousiner: Antropomorpha, efterskrift och noter av Telemak Fredbärj*. Uppsala: Svenska Linnésällskapet, 1955.

Linné, Carl von. *Systema naturae, sive regna tria naturæ systematice proposita per classes, ordines, genera & species*. Lugduni Batavorum, 1735.

Lugt, Maaike van der. 'Formed Fetuses and Healthy Children in Scholastic Theology, Medicine and Law.' In *Reproduction: Antiquity to the Present Day*, edited by Nick Hopwood, Rebecca Flemming, and Lauren Kassell, 167–80. Cambridge: Cambridge University Press, 2018.

Martin, Roland. *Läkare-Grunder: Til biträde för Styresmän och Domare, Ifrån Kunskapen om Människans kropp och allmänna Naturläran, efter D. J. Ern. Hebenstreits Anthropologia Forensis*. Stockholm, 1783.

National Archives of Sweden (website). 'Statistiska tabeller.' Accessed July 14, 2023. https://riksarkivet.se/statistiska-tabeller.

Nordblad, Carl. 'Beskrifning På ett Foster, af en märkvärdig missbildning.' *Kongl. Vetenskaps Akademiens Handlingar* 2 (1818): 234–36.

Nyström, Eva. 'Nils Rosén von Rosenstein.' In *Svenskt biografiskt lexikon*. Vol. 30, 425. Stockholm: Svenskt biografiskt lexikon, 1999.

Odhelius, Erik. 'Beskrifning på et Missfoster.' *Kungl. Vetenskaps Akademiens nya handlingar* 3 (1785): 175–80.

Orrelius, Magnus. *Historia animalium, eller Beskrifning öfwer diur riket*. Stockholm, 1750.

Paulsson Holmberg, Tove. 'Ambiguous and Transitional Bodies: Stillbirth in Stockholm, 1691–1724.' In *Exceptional Bodies in Early Modern Culture: Concepts of Monstrosity before the Advent of the Normal*, edited by Maja Bondestam, 163–84. Amsterdam: Amsterdam University Press, 2020.

Ray, Sara. 'From Monsters to Malformations: Anatomical Preparations as Objects of Evidence for a Developmental Paradigm of Embryology, 1770–1850.' *Journal of the History of Biology* 55, no. 1 (2022): 35–57.

Roe, Shirley A. *Matter, Life, and Generation: 18th-Century Embryology and the Haller-Wolff Debate*. Cambridge: Cambridge University Press, 1981.

Rusnock, Andrea A. 'Biopolitics: Political Arithmetic in the Enlightenment.' In *The Sciences in Enlightened Europe*, edited by William Clark, Jan Golinski, and Simon Schaffer, 49–68. Chicago: University of Chicago Press, 1999.

Rusnock, Andrea A. 'Biopolitics and the Invention of Population.' In *Reproduction: Antiquity to the Present Day*, edited by Nick Hopwood, Rebecca Flemming, and Lauren Kassell, 333–45. Cambridge: Cambridge University Press, 2019.

Rusnock, Andrea A. *Vital Accounts: Quantifying Health and Population in Eighteenth-Century England and France*. New York: Cambridge University Press, 2002.

Schrevelius, Fredrik. *Lärobok i Sveriges allmänna nu gällande Civil-rätt*. Vol. 1. Lund: Berling, 1844.

Schrevelius, Fredrik. *Lärobok i Sveriges allmänna nu gällande Civil-rätt*. Vol. 1. 2nd ed. Lund: Berling, 1851.

Sidenbladh, Elis. *Sällsamma händelser i Sverige med Finland åren 1749–1801 och i Sverige 1821–1859: Ur Uppgifter af prästerskapet antecknade*. Stockholm, 1908.

Ståhl, Anders Johan. *Register öfver Kongl. Vetenskaps-Academiens Handlingar ifrån deras början år 1739 till och med år 1825*. Stockholm: Norstedt & söner, 1831.

Stepan, Nancy. *The Idea of Race in Science: Great Britain 1800–1960*. London: Macmillan in association with St Antony's College, 1982.

Sveriges kyrkolag af år 1686: Jemte stadganden, hvarigenom den blifvit i vissa fall upphäfven, ändrad och tillökt, utgifven af A. J. Rydén. Jönköping, 1844–45.

Wannerdt, Arvid. *Den svenska folkbokföringens historia under tre sekler*. Solna: Riksskatteverket, 1982.

Wistrand, August Timoleon. *Handbok i forensiska medicinen*. Stockholm: Zacharias Hæggström, 1838.

Zacchia, Paolo. *Quaestiones medico-legales: In quibus omnes eae materiae medicae, quae ad legales facultates videntur pertinere, proponuntur, pertractantur, resolvuntur* [...] Vols. 1–4. Leipzig: F. Lanckisch for E. Rehefeld, 1630.

CHAPTER 4

Visualizing the Early Stages of Life: Embryology and Fetal Anatomy at the Karolinska Institute, 1820s–1920s

Eva Åhrén

It was 1910 and department chair Emil Holmgren was pleased: the Karolinska Institute's Department of Histology had inaugurated new, state-of-the-art premises, with enlarged spaces for teaching and research. The new laboratories all had sinks with running water, ventilation, and cabinets for chemicals and optical instruments, thermometers, microtomes, and other necessary equipment. New microscopes were installed for students and scientists, and separate labs set up for the teaching assistant, the specimen preparator, and the department chair. There was a library, a room for wall charts, photomicrography equipment, and a good many cabinets for microscopy specimens mounted on glass slides. The embryological teaching collection contained slide series of fish, amphibian, bird, and mammal embryos in different stages of development. Complete series also existed of human embryos from the third, fourth, and fifth weeks, as well as series from later stages of development.[1] The new facilities and their equipment displayed a commitment to an empirical research tradition that had a long history at the Karolinska Institute (KI).

Embryology was a vital field of medical scientific research and teaching at the time, in Sweden as well as internationally. The field included studies of human and animal gametes, fertilization, and embryonal and fetal development (normal as well as pathological). Like other branches of biological science, it depended on developing technologies and methods of observation and circulation. This chapter will explore and discuss material and visual aspects of research on the early stages of life, covering human as well as animal embryology and fetal anatomy. It will investigate the work of a few scientists at the KI. First, prominent rector and anatomy chair Anders Retzius, who ushered in a new era in Swedish anatomical study (including comparative, microscopic, and pathological anatomy), based on empirical observation. Second, his son Gustaf Retzius, a leading figure in histology, neuroanatomy, and physical

1 Holmgren, 'Histologiska institutionen,' 476–80.

DOI:10.1163/9789004703759_006

anthropology, committed to studying and visualizing large series of materials. And last, Emil Holmgren and his contemporary colleague, anatomy professor Erik Müller, both working in a time when embryology was well established as a subject of research and teaching in anatomy and histology. My aim is to add to the understanding of historical practices of embryonic and fetal knowledge production by focusing on this local history. I will show that, although research questions as well as methods and observational technologies changed over time, there was significant continuity in the research practices at the KI from the 1820s to the 1920s. Embryological knowledge production was a visual and material way of knowing throughout the period of study, with researchers using a multitude of methods to analyze, compare, describe, and communicate.[2]

The KI was founded in 1810, ostensibly as a school for field surgeons. But its leading men aimed at building an institution for combined medical and surgical education, founded on the principles of scientific research—a novelty within higher education at the time.[3] Throughout the nineteenth century, KI professors were striving for a position as Sweden's leading medical school and research institute, in constant competition with the medical faculties of the old universities at Lund and Uppsala. While the medical faculty at Uppsala long adhered to an idealist tradition, KI professors promoted medicine founded on empirical science and clinical practice. KI scientists thus created a productive milieu that became a driving force in the renewal of Swedish medical training and a dynamic node in the transnational circulation of knowledge. They learned from, applied, and developed approaches from the Paris school of anatomy, with its focus on hands-on experience, pathology, and morphological comparison across species. But, beginning in the 1820s, attention shifted to the German lands, where the most interesting research in microscopic anatomy was happening.[4] The Nordic networks of scientific exchange were already strong, but were further strengthened during the nineteenth century, with the start of regular conferences in 1839.[5] KI scientists participated in and contributed to the transnational scientific exchange through publishing internationally (mostly in German, but also in French and English); presenting

2 Cf. Hopwood, 'Embryology'; Hopwood et al., 'Introduction'; Nyhart, *Biology Takes Form*, part 3.

3 Nilsson, 'Vetenskapen'; *Karolinska institutets historia*, vol. 3; Rocca, *Forging a Medical University*.

4 On anatomy at KI, see Åhrén, 'Museerna'; Gustafson, 'Anatomi.' On nineteenth-century German life science, see Nyhart, *Biology Takes Form*; Schickore, *Microscope*.

5 The Scandinavian Association of Naturalists was inspired by the Society of German Natural Scientists and Physicians, which held its first meeting in 1822, and the British Association for the Advancement of Science, which started in 1831. See Eriksson, '*I andans kraft*.'

their research findings at conferences on the European continent and the British Isles; and exchanging letters, publications, drawings, and specimens with their peers. Over time, they developed a particular way of knowing the early stages of life, sharing and maintaining an emphasis on materializing and visualizing their objects of research.[6] Practices of collecting, preparing, observing, drawing, photographing, exhibiting, and printing were central to their work.[7]

Research on embryos and fetuses was a process of visualization and materialization; observation, analysis, and communication depended on creating objects to study by applying a multitude of techniques, instruments, and chemicals. Embryonic specimens—once received in the anatomy museum or histology lab—had to be stabilized, cut, colored, mounted on glass slides, suitably lit, and enlarged in order to be studied and depicted. Drawings and, from around 1900, photomicrographs were integral to the research process, and producing images a primary concern for the scientists. Plaster casts, wax models, and stereoscopic photography gave stable three-dimensional form to fragile embryonic and fetal bodies. Therefore, studying visualizations is key to understanding anatomical (including embryological) knowledge production in history. Published images were not just complementary to written accounts of research findings: making images was an integral part of the research process, and the resulting visuals could be as valuable as textual descriptions and arguments (if not more). For this reason, I prefer to call them visualizations rather than 'illustrations,' which would indicate that the images were secondary to the words. Visualizations were stand-ins for specimens, and were necessary to communicate research findings, facilitating circulation and remote witnessing of the museum specimens. Specimen collections, in turn, functioned as libraries of existing research at the same time as they offered material for new studies.[8] A well-functioning university department needed a high-quality and up-to-date infrastructure of equipment for research and teaching. Published research articles, monographs, and textbooks included detailed discussions of methods and technologies used, and reflections on the epistemic merits of their use—what Jutta Schickore has called 'second-order,' or reflexive, research concerns.[9] I will analyze visual and material aspects of the research process by focusing on such reflections on methods and technologies,

6 Pickstone, *Ways of Knowing*.

7 See Nick Hopwood's work, most notably 'Producing Development' and *Haeckel's Embryos*. See also Morgan, *Icons of Life*.

8 Åhrén, 'Figuring Things Out'; Åhrén, 'Museerna.' See also Hallam, *Anatomy Museum*; McLeary, *Science in a Bottle*. On visualization, see Fiorentini, 'Induction of Visibility.'

9 Schickore, *Microscope*, 3.

including microscope apertures and light sources, fixation chemicals, and coloring agents.

1 Mammalian Eggs, Embryonal Gills, and Fetal Malformations

Embryology appeared as a focused scientific pursuit around the turn of the nineteenth century, when comparative anatomists, physiologists, and zoologists began a systematic analysis of developing embryos, reaching for an understanding of the earliest stages of life.[10] Whereas nineteenth-century zoologists mainly focused on invertebrates, vertebrate embryology was studied in the departments of anatomy, histology, and physiology at medical faculties and institutes. But even though embryology became an essential part of anatomy and zoology curricula, and a central field of biological research, it did not become a unified discipline, with its own departments, chairs, and journals.[11] At the KI, human embryos and fetuses were studied at the anatomy department, in comparison with other mammals. But embryos and fetuses also showed up in research and curricula in histology (microscopic anatomy), pathological anatomy, gynecology and obstetrics, physiology, and forensic medicine.[12]

Anders Retzius established embryonic and fetal anatomy as part of the medical students' anatomy curriculum in the 1820s. During his time as professor of anatomy at the KI (from 1824 until his death in 1860), he also researched normal and pathological embryology, introduced new findings and literature in the field to the readers of the proceedings of the Swedish Society of Medicine, and prepared a multitude of fetal specimens for the KI's anatomy museum.[13] And the topic of embryology became an important part of the effort to make medicine more scientific, as did microscopic anatomy in general.

On his first trip abroad in 1828, Anders Retzius traveled to Berlin, to attend the meeting of the Society of German Natural Scientists and Physicians, convened by the Humboldt brothers at Berlin University. The European continent was opening up after the Napoleonic Wars: traveling, correspondence, and the circulation of print material became easier, which made it possible for scientists to expand their networks and communicate in new ways. In Berlin, Retzius connected with a cohort of young men who were reshaping the life sciences at

10 Hopwood, 'Producing Development'; Buklijas and Hopwood, 'Making Visible Embryos.'
11 Nyhart, *Biology Takes Form*, chap. 3; Hopwood, 'Embryology,' 294.
12 *Karolinska institutets historia*, vol. 3.
13 Nilsson, 'Vetenskapen.'

this time, most notably Johannes Müller, who became a close friend. Comparative embryology was at the very heart of these scientists' pursuits, and Anders Retzius witnessed firsthand demonstrations of some spectacular new findings that were about to fundamentally change the understanding of the development of humans and other mammals: Karl Ernst von Baer demonstrated his own discovery of the mammalian ovum in the ovary of a dog, and Martin Rathke showed gill slits in mammalian embryos.[14] Upon returning to Stockholm, Retzius started studying some of the anatomical structures he learned about in Berlin, and introducing his colleagues to these novelties. For example, he presented embryonal gill slits in a lecture at the Swedish Society of Medicine in 1829, where he also demonstrated specimens and drawings. The talk was summarized in print, giving Swedish doctors around the country a glimpse into cutting-edge research in embryology. Retzius took Rathke's finding to be an astonishing confirmation of the recapitulation theory. In Retzius's words, it was proof that 'the fetus of higher animals, during its development, undergoes organizational changes that correspond to the lower degrees of development of the entire lower chain of the animal kingdom.'[15] This early form of the recapitulation theory was first formulated by Carl Friedrich Kielmeyer in 1793, and adopted by German Romantic scientists like Lorenz Oken and the influential anatomist Friedrich Tiedemann. But it was highly contested in Anders Retzius's time. The most pointed criticism was formulated by von Baer in *Über Entwicklungsgeschichte der Thiere* (1828), where he argued that embryonic development instead progressed from a common simple germ into successively more complex forms according to four basic schemata.[16] It is unclear whether Retzius had read von Baer's ideas of development, but he seemed to hold on to the recapitulation theory, which was, perhaps, easier to grasp.

Just like Johannes Müller and other post-Romantic German colleagues, Retzius was committed to careful empirical study, and skeptical of speculation. The new achromatic microscopy lenses of the 1820s and 1830s made it possible to study tissues at greater resolutions than before, down to the cellular level. And the new embryology depended on these instruments of observation.[17] The excitement about embryology went hand in hand with this development of new technologies. But the focus of study was not just human

14 Hopwood, *Haeckel's Embryos*, 19–21. On the emerging science of biology, and embryology's place in it, see Lenoir, *Strategy of Life*; Nyhart, *Biology Takes Form*, pt. 1; Otis, *Müller's Lab*; Schickore, *Microscope*, chap. 6.

15 *Anders Retzius bref*, 65–66, 76–77; Swedish Society of Medicine, *Årsberättelse*, 14–15.

16 Baer, *Über Entwicklungsgeschichte*; Hopwood, *Haeckel's Embryos*, 18–19.

17 Hopwood, *Haeckel's Embryos*, chap. 2; Schickore, *Microscope*, 139.

embryonal development—it was a comparative effort, where animal embryos of all species were collected, studied, visualized, and compared. It was a gigantic collective project to advance the understanding of the development of organisms over the course of history, as well as the development of individuals from the moment of fertilization to full-grown creature.

One central goal of embryological studies at this time was to distinguish abnormal forms of development by studying structural abnormalities, stillbirths, and other unusual manifestations of generation and fetal development. Case reports of unusual births were common in journals and meetings throughout the nineteenth century, although their character changed over time. In the first half of the century, many accounts of malformed fetuses were based on the maternal impression theory, which connected malformations to events during pregnancy. As detailed studies on embryonal and fetal development accumulated over the years, the collective body of knowledge increased, and the questions regarding malformations became more precise. What, exactly, was it that went wrong in the developmental process, when a baby was born with a specific malformation? Explanations began to be sought more often in the process of fetal development than in the mother's experiences during gestation.[18]

Anders Retzius took an interest in both normal and abnormal fetal development, and reported on the development of genitalia as early as 1828.[19] Retzius prepared specimens of normal and abnormal embryos and fetuses for the KI's anatomy museum, and put them on display alongside wet and dry normal and pathological specimens of adult humans, a growing series of racial crania, and a large number of animal skeletons and preparations. The KI's professors and affiliated physicians collected fetal specimens in their practices and clinics. But specimens could also be sent to the KI by provincial physicians hoping to make a name for themselves and strengthen their position within contemporary medical networks. The museum thus became a network hub, with Anders Retzius at its center. The trade in specimens helped establish and uphold relationships and hierarchies within the community of medical doctors. Published case accounts and catalogue entries mentioned donors' names and gave them a recognized place in the scientific network (although the KI's museum catalogues were lost in a fire in 1892).[20] When Retzius received embryonic and fetal

18 Bondestam, *Tvåkönad*; Bondestam [Larsson], 'From Frightening Beast'; Hopwood, 'Embryology,' 288.

19 Swedish Society of Medicine, *Årsberättelse*, 16–18.

20 Åhrén, 'Museerna'; Åhrén, 'Making Space'; Müller, 'Anatomiska institutionen'; see also Franzén's chapter in this volume. On museums in nineteenth-century medical education

specimens, he was especially interested in finding abnormal genital shapes. He 'gave several of these specimens such a position and preparation so as to well demonstrate the parts in question' in the museum, showed them at the Swedish Society of Medicine, and included printed drawings of normal genital development in an 1854 article on a case of 'hypospadia' and 'mistaken gender.' On the fold-out lithographic plate, eight schematic drawings visualize the progressive fetal development of genitals, four male and four female.[21]

Retzius's museum-based, comparative research method was an analytical and visual way of knowing. The visualizing work started at the dissection table and went on to materialize specimens for research and display. For early nineteenth-century embryology, this method was perfect. Creating series of specimens helped scientists understand what was normal development and what was not. Comparative analysis was necessary and depended

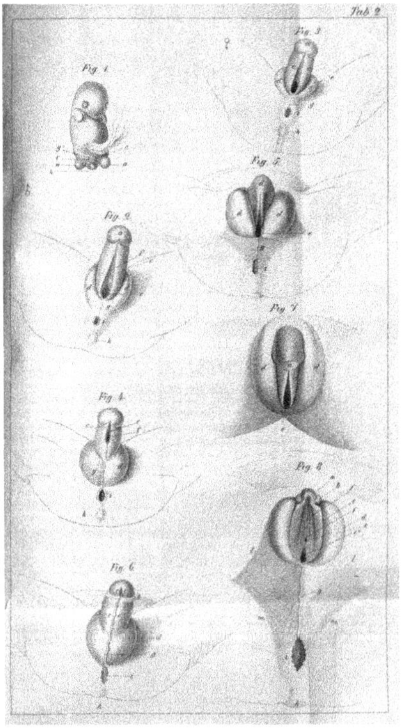

FIGURE 4.1
Schematic drawings of genital development in human embryos of both sexes, from specimens in the KI's Anatomy Museum. Lithographic prints in Anders Retzius, 'Händelse af Hypospadi,' 9, Tab. 2. Hagströmer Library, KI.

and research, see Alberti, *Morbid Curiosities*; Hallam, *Anatomy Museum*; McLeary, *Science in a Bottle*; Reinarz, 'Museum Medicine.'

21 A. Retzius, 'Händelse af Hypospadi.' Invented in 1798, lithography is a printing method which uses a polished stone surface to transfer images onto paper. Gascoigne, *How to Identify Prints*, 19a.

on accumulation of specimens over time, but also on published visualizations. Other scientists could then use the printed images for comparison with their own museum specimens or drawings. And since human embryos could be hard to come by, the collective effort of scientists slowly created a virtual reference collection.[22] Embryos were also difficult to study: they were tiny, delicate, fragile, and perishable. Stabilizing embryos in the form of specimens and visualizations made it possible to study and compare them, and facilitated circulation in time and space.[23]

2 Comparative Studies of Fetal Development: Brains and Proportions

Although Anders Retzius was a very productive researcher and author of research papers, he very rarely theorized or made statements of scientific principles. And he never published comprehensive monographs or atlases, preferring active research work to writing. In a rare exception to his usual empirical focus, however, Retzius ventured a theoretical approach to brain development in an 1844 lecture at the Royal Swedish Academy of Sciences. Referring again to the recapitulation theory, he claimed that human fetal brain development goes through the shapes of the 'lower classes of animals.' This was a 'natural law' described by Friedrich Tiedemann, who had also shown that the brain hemispheres developed from front to back in his 'classical' work on the fetal development of the human brain from 1816. How to understand and locate the higher functions of the brain was, according to Retzius, 'one of the greatest problems of our time.' Retzius connected the theoretical perspective to his own embryo specimens in the KI museum, and showed drawings of these to the audience. The printed lecture is instead accompanied by four diagrammatic representations of human brain development, which visualize the theory rather than actual brain specimens.[24]

While Anders Retzius dominated Swedish anatomy from around 1830 until 1860, his son Gustaf Retzius was the most prolific Swedish researcher in the anatomical sciences from 1876 to the mid-1910s. Continuing in his father's footsteps, Gustaf studied a wide range of subjects in comparative anatomy,

22 Hopwood, Schaffer, and Secord, 'Seriality'; Pickstone, *Ways of Knowing*, chap. 5; Rudwick, 'Paper Museum.'

23 Latour, 'Drawing Things Together.'

24 Retzius, 'Om bildningen,' 194, 196–97; cf. Tiedemann, *Anatomie*. Other publications by Retzius are less clear on the subject of recapitulation and seem to support von Baer's general laws of embryonal development from a simple form to more complex ones, which diverged within four types rather than developing in parallel.

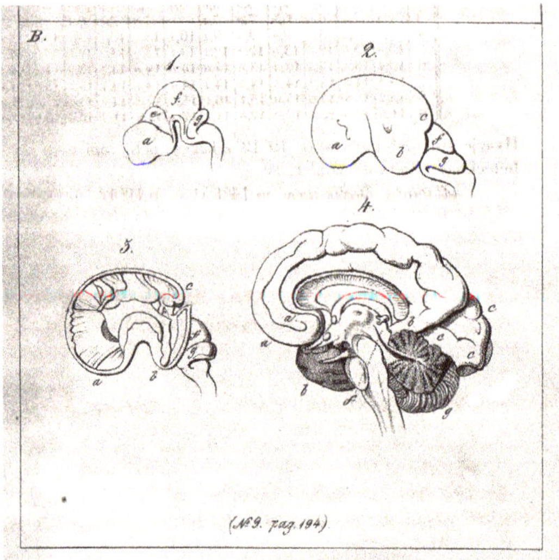

FIGURE 4.2
Diagrammatic representation of fetal brains. Lithographic prints in Anders Retzius, 'Om bildningen,' Tab. B. Hagströmer Library, KI.

histology, neuroanatomy, and physical anthropology. He famously published lavish books and his own oversized periodical, *Biologische Untersuchungen*, including expertly printed plates, often based on his own drawings.[25] And, just like his father, Gustaf was an active and highly respected member of international networks of scientists. He held professorships in histology and anatomy at the KI from 1878 until 1890, when he chose to continue his work as an independent scientist, a career move made possible by his marriage to wealthy philanthropist Anna Hierta in 1877.[26] Retzius's oeuvre stood out in his time (and still does) because of his meticulous dissections, often comparing a large number of specimens, which added detail to detailed analysis, plus the many thousands of beautifully crafted and printed images in his publications.

One of Gustaf Retzius's main research interests was comparative brain anatomy: morphological and macroscopic, as well as microscopic. Methods of preparation were crucial to this study, and Retzius's publications always reflect on methodology and 'second-order' research questions in great detail. One lecture, presented to the Swedish Society of Biology in 1889, is particularly noteworthy in this regard. It is entirely devoted to brain preparation and accompanied by demonstrations of specimens and drawings. 'A badly preserved brain is of little value,' Retzius asserts in the opening sentence of the printed talk. And he devotes a section to fetal specimens, comparing various techniques and fluids for fixation and preservation of this delicate organ. For

25 Åhrén 'Figuring Things Out.'
26 On Gustaf Retzius's life, see Uddenberg, *Skallmätaren*.

fresh specimens, he favors soaking the brains before removing them from the cranium, using a solution of chrome, osmium, and acetic acid. Although it turns the specimen a grayish green, this method preserves volume and shape better than solutions of ethanol, which shrink the brains. Fetal brains preserved in this chrome solution make excellent museum pieces and are well-suited models for depictions. Along with a number of brain specimens, Retzius demonstrated some drawings made using 'Lucae's orthoscope,' a 'mathematical' drawing device designed to reduce perspectival distortions.[27]

In 1896, Retzius published a book on the macroscopic anatomy of the human brain, *Das Menschenhirn*, which contained case studies of adult and fetal brains in two oversize tomes. The text in the first volume is mostly descriptive, containing few and modest conclusions: women's brains did not differ from men's brains in any significant way, even if they were generally smaller, less complex, and displayed a tendency to be lighter, which could possibly influence creativity and intellectual processing. Retzius came to a similar conclusion regarding fetal brain development—he had not been able to see any differences between male and female brain development. And in a typically cautious manner, he deferred to the need for more comparative studies, which should also take into account possible racial differences.[28] Gustaf Retzius seemed to believe that future studies would, or could, reveal such differences in the structure of brains, but, on the basis of his own meticulously empirical research, he could not agree with those scientists who had made strong claims that placed white men in an exceptional category of neurological refinement.[29]

Many of the plates in *Das Menschenhirn* are full-size photographs of adult brains, hand printed in collotype on expensive paper by printer G. Tholander. Retzius only worked with greatly skilled collaborators, demanding the highest quality every step of the way: from his own preparations to the photographs by Christian Westphal and the drawings by medical artists Sigrid Andersson-Rissler, Hilma Bundsen, Ebba Flodman, and Gustaf Wennman.[30] Whereas adult brain morphology is represented in full-size photographic reproduction,

27 Retzius, 'Om metoderna,' 123–24. The 'orthoscope' was invented by D. M. Soemmering and further developed by his Frankfurt colleague J. C. G. Lucae. Lucae, *Zur organischen Formenlehre*, 30.

28 Retzius, *Das Menschenhirn*. Cf. Chorell, 'Neurovetenskap,' 250–52; Uddenberg, *Skallmätaren*, 213–15.

29 On Gustaf Retzius, physical anthropology, and race, see Ljungström, *Oscariansk antropologi*, chaps. 3–5; Uddenberg, *Skallmätaren*, 356–411.

30 Retzius, *Das Menschenhirn*, vol. 2; Lindblad, *Gustaf Retzius*, 121–22. The collotype process was invented in 1855 and became the first commercially viable method of printing photographs. It entailed transferring photographs to light-sensitized gelatin-coated glass

the many fetal brains in the book are visualized in a variety of techniques: drawings emphasizing three-dimensionality, simple line drawings, photographs, or hybrids of these. The specimens of fetal brains and spines in figure 4.3 float isolated from each other on the plate, with explanations printed on the opposite page. One of the photographed specimens (nos. 6 and 7) shows a face in profile, making it less abstract and detached than the others. The ensemble of techniques used on the plates indicate that each was carefully chosen for its ability to convey particular aspects of the anatomical structures. Retzius had collected the brains for this study from bodies autopsied at Stockholm hospitals while he worked at the KI, which gave him the opportunity to claim material for the museum and for his own research. He could now present examinations of 'fetal brains in the highest possible number of stages' of development.[31]

Eight years later, Retzius published a study on the proportions of human fetuses, with a particular focus on extremities. He again collaborated with artist Gustaf Wennman and photographer Christian Westphal, who this time

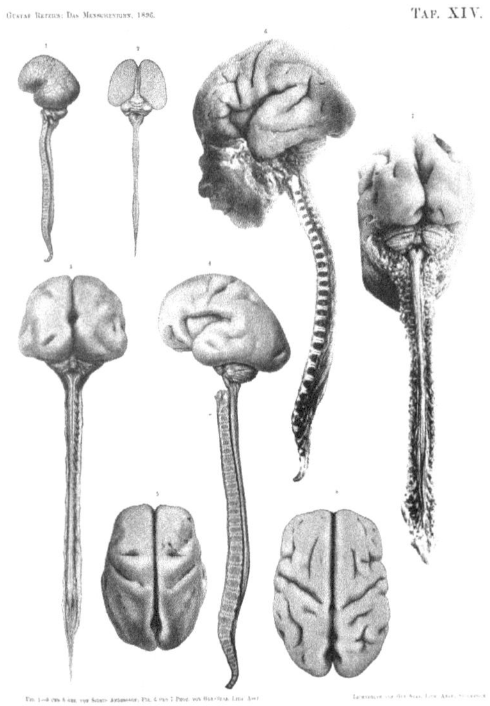

FIGURE 4.3
Fetal brains and spinal cords produced by photographer Christian Westphal, together with artists and technicians. Collotype plate in Gustaf Retzius, *Das Menschenhirn*, Taf. XIV. Hagströmer Library, KI.

surfaces for printing, which enabled their exact reproduction. Gascoigne, *How to Identify Prints*, 40.

31 Retzius, *Biografiska anteckningar*, 2:162.

also acted as printer of the many collotype reproductions. Retzius defers to the embryological publications of Albert von Kölliker, Wilhelm His, Oscar Hertwig, and others regarding the first two months of development.[32] He was an active member of the primarily German-speaking network of leading anatomists, attending conferences and engaging in dialogue with many of them. Kölliker, especially, was a dear friend and mentor of Retzius's, but he also corresponded with other leading embryologists, such as His.[33] While he had originally planned to include the earliest embryonic development in the study, Retzius had found that it was impossible to acquire enough 'fresh, normal material,' even though physicians in his network had supplied him with a 'considerable amount' of fetuses from spontaneous abortions. He thus chose to focus on fetal proportions in the third and fourth months of development.[34] Wennman's pencil drawings of disembodied hands and feet have an uncanny three-dimensional quality, even on the lithographed plate, where they are interspersed with simple outlines of the specimens.

The topic of fetal proportions needs further study, Retzius claims, and goes on to describe in detail the relative size and length of fetuses and their arms and legs, from the second to the third month of gestation. The text is complemented by tables of measurements, taken from skeletonized fetuses, wet specimens, and some fresh, unprepared specimens. When this study was published, Retzius was no longer officially affiliated with the KI, but the text makes clear that he was still very well connected with its faculty. One series of fetuses in the study consists of thirty-nine skeletons, which had been preserved in a mixture of water, glycerin, and alcohol by a preparator credited as Mr. Roth, when Retzius was chair of the anatomy department and director of the museum of anatomy, in 1888–89. Another series had whole, undissected fetuses, which were conserved in various fluids. He had received most of these fetuses after 1890, from his colleagues at the KI, including the current museum director, anatomy chair Erik Müller. Some of the specimens belonged to the Anatomy Museum, but most of them were in Retzius's own possession.[35]

Gustaf Retzius's meticulous care in procuring, dissecting, preparing, studying, and visualizing the specimens was a method in and of itself. The goal of his comparative anatomical research was often to study large series of particular

32 Retzius, 'Zur Kenntnis der Entwicklung,' 33–76, 53.

33 Letters to Gustaf Retzius and Gustaf Retzius's correspondence, bound series, Hierta–Retzius collection.

34 Retzius, 'Zur Kenntnis der Entwicklung,' 53.

35 KI colleagues who supplied Retzius with fetuses include professors M. Sondén and Westermark, and doctors Alin, C. G. Jonsson, and Reuterskiöld. Retzius, 'Zur Kenntnis der Entwicklung,' 41, 53.

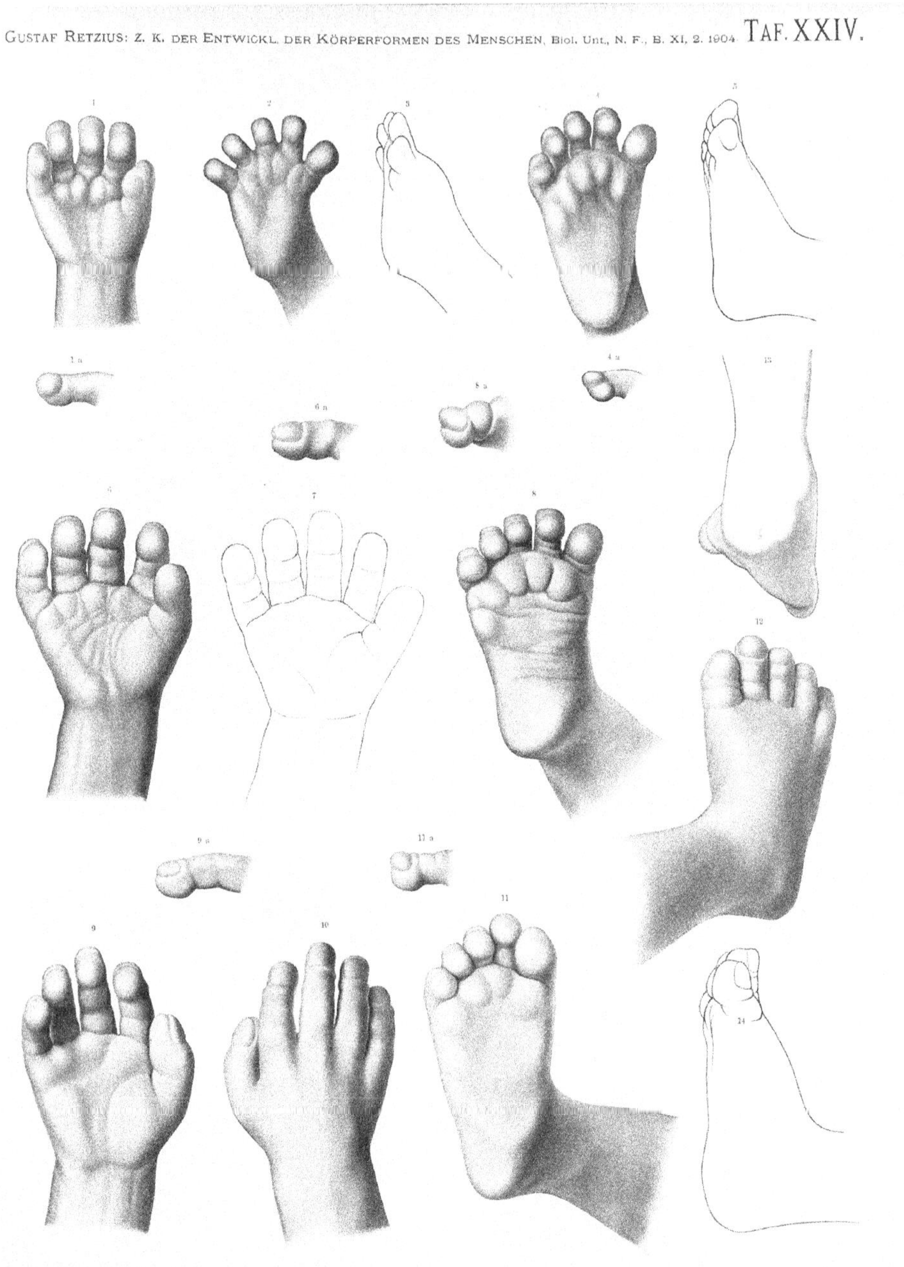

FIGURE 4.4 Pencil drawings of fetal hands and feet by Gustaf Wennman. Lithographic print in Gustaf Retzius, *Biologische Untersuchungen*, Taf. XXIV. Hagströmer Library, KI.

species or structures in order to clarify, develop, or expand research that had been published by others. His research was focused on the visual, structural, and morphological, and the presented results were always visual as well. His texts explain and support the images, and discuss the methods he used to make them, rather than the text being 'illustrated' and supported by the images.

3 Variations on a Theme: Sperm, Ova, and Chromosomes

Around the same time as the study of fetal proportions, Retzius began collecting, visualizing, and analyzing sperm and egg cells from humans and animals. Detailed investigations of gametes were, he believed, necessary in order to understand the process of fertilization. In 1902, he published a couple of articles on the subject of sperm morphology, following up on an earlier paper from 1881. These were followed by another fifty papers on the subject in his own publication series, *Biologische Untersuchungen*, the last of which was published posthumously in 1921.[36] All of them contained lithographic prints from his own drawings, more than three thousand figures in all. Retzius made these precise drawings at his apochromatic Zeiss microscope, observing the specimens, which were usually fixed with osmium tetroxide or Zenker's fixative, preferably with sunlight as his light source. As always, he carefully described the methods and materials he used. Judging from oversized wall charts preserved in the archive of the Royal Swedish Academy of Sciences, Retzius also gave lectures on the subject of sperm morphology. In a plate from 1912, human sperm cells are lined up next to sperm of other primates to facilitate visual comparison.

Gustaf Retzius managed to obtain specimens from more than four hundred different species from all over the world, covering sperm of every type of organism, from primitive marine gastropods to apes and humans. He purchased fresh or prepared specimens (testicles or whole animals) from dealers and hunters or received gifts and donations from scientists, curators, and collectors within his immense international scientific network. Some of the animals came from zoos or museums; others were killed in the wild. Some were rare, such as the Australian echidna and Japanese giant salamander. Others—such as mussels, clams, sea worms, starfish, and jellyfish—Retzius fished out of the waters near

36 E.g., Retzius, 'Zur Kenntniss der Spermatozoen'; 'Weitere Beiträge'; 'Ueber einen Spiralfaserapparat'; 'Noch einige Beiträge,' *Biologische Untersuchungen*.

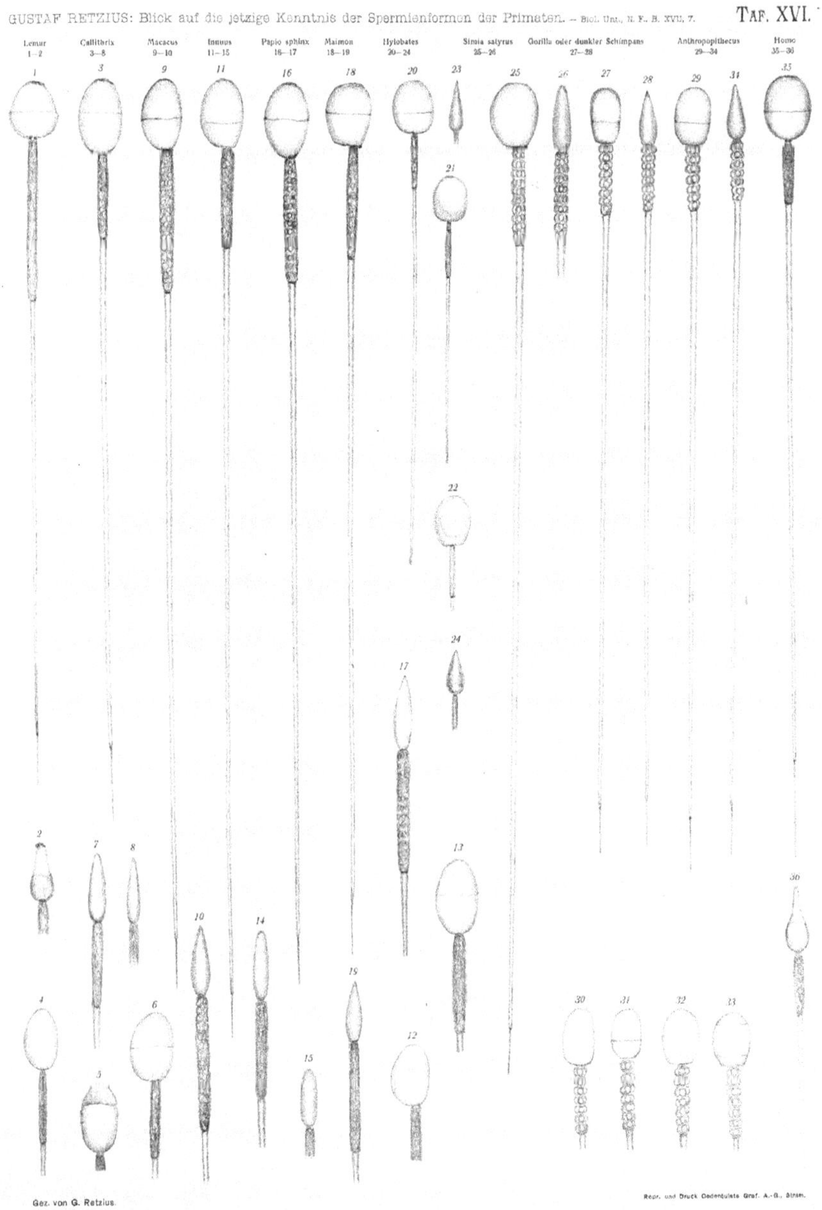

FIGURE 4.5 Gustaf Retzius's own drawings of primate sperm cells. Lithographic plate in Retzius, *Biologische Untersuchungen*, Taf. XVI. Hagströmer Library, KI.

the Kristineberg marine zoology research station on the Swedish west coast, where he and his wife used to spend time in the summer.[37]

Retzius also devoted time to studying ova, as well as the first phases of cell division after fertilization. Volumes 16, 17, and 18 of *Biologische Untersuchungen* contain a number of papers on the subject, based on careful preparation, staining, and analysis. In the introduction to three papers published in 1911, Retzius writes that the investigations are the results of his efforts to find a method that would stain the chromosomes of egg cells and sperm cells in different colors, so that he would be able to study the process of development immediately following fertilization. In Echinoderms (starfish, sea urchins, and the like), he had found that a particular staining method made the chromosomes in the nucleus of sperm cells retain a green color after entering the egg cell, whereas the ovum's chromosomes stood out in red. This method could not easily be used in mammals, however, and this paper is devoted entirely to discussing methods of fixating, staining, and studying these minuscule parts of the cell nuclei of invertebrates. Hoping to solve some of the problems of fertilization, Retzius turned to studying fertilized eggs of the nematode *Ascaris megalocephala*, an intestinal parasite of horses and an 'old, well-known ideal object for chromosome research.' He found the quality of the images in his 'esteemed colleagues" published research on the subject unsatisfactory and set out to produce something superior. The *Ascaris* was a popular research subject because it had only two chromosomes in its cells and was easy to study. It was not easy to acquire the necessary specimens, though. Retzius failed to find worms at horse slaughterhouses in Stockholm and then turned to his colleagues Theodor Boveri and Friedrich Meves—leading researchers on the subject—to ask for specimens, which they willingly sent. He found these unusable because of the effect of injected dyes, and so was back to square one. Finally, he received some fresh specimens from a colleague at the KI, Emil Holmström, and could start the research.[38] In the foreword as well as in his autobiography, Retzius acknowledges technician Anna Edman, who masterfully 'performed the difficult and time-consuming work of embedding, microtomizing [slicing], coloring, and mounting [the ova specimens] in Canada turpentine.'[39]

37 Afzelius, 'Gustaf Retzius,' lists the four hundred species Retzius examined. See also Uddenberg, *Skallmätaren*, 219–23; Retzius, *Biografiska anteckningar*, 2:165–67, 241–58. On the history of research on sperm and its role in fertilization, see Vienne, 'Eggs and Sperm.'

38 Retzius, 'Einleitung,' 1–6, quotation on 1.

39 Retzius, *Biografiska anteckningar*, 2:166.

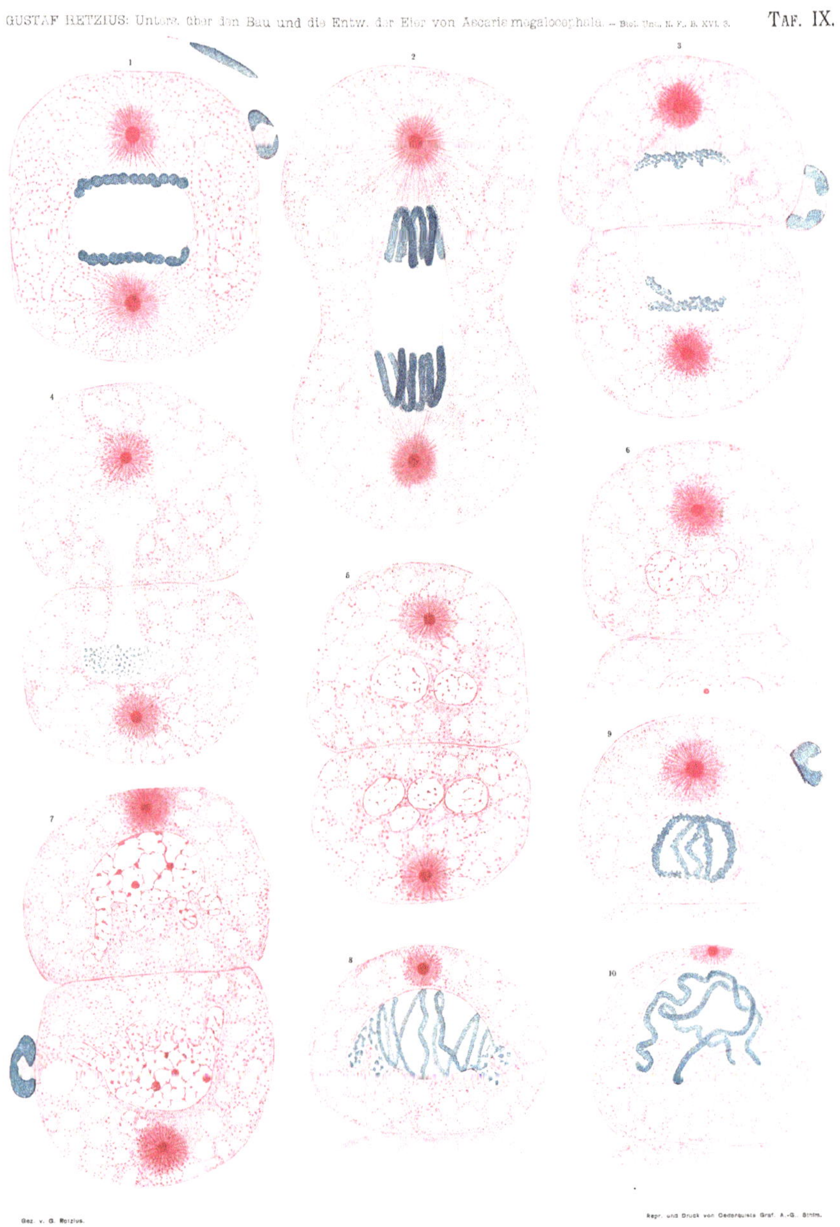

FIGURE 4.6 Gustaf Retzius' own drawings of colored specimens visualizing the first stages of cell division in fertilized ova of *Ascaris megalocephala*. Chromolithographic plate in Retzius, *Biologische Untersuchungen*, Taf. IX. Hagströmer Library, KI.

Germ cells and cell division had become the focus of much research in physiology, anatomy, and zoology, after German anatomist Oscar Hertwig first described the process of how the sperm cell enters the ovum in 1876, based on studies of sea urchins. Soon thereafter, Walther Flemming described 'chromatin,' structures in the cell nucleus that stood out after staining, and then Wilhelm Waldeyer coined the term 'chromosomes' in 1888.[40] The term derived from the Greek words *chroma*, 'color,' and *soma*, 'body,' thus naming the structure after the visualization process. Although decades had passed since Theodor Boveri's famous study of fertilization and cell division of the *Ascaris megalocephala*, and many scientists since had published on the topic, Retzius still felt that the existing images were not good enough to demonstrate the *structure* of the stages of cell division. His own chromolithographic plates are indeed superior, both artistically and scientifically, displaying large, detailed visualizations of the microscopic specimens, colored to also show the effect of dyes on the cell nucleus, not just the structure.[41] Retzius was not, however, concerned with the questions of heredity, which Boveri, Roux, and others addressed. This is typical of Retzius's work: he homes in on a question, often a structural detail, that needs to be resolved, and then sets out to perfect the methods of observation and representation. As the process of cell division after fertilization was a central problem in morphological embryology, studying the *Ascaris* fitted into Retzius's wider concerns of refining the understanding of shape and structure through visualization. And he continued this line of work—the incredibly detailed visualizations of cell division in the *Ascaris megalocephala* were followed by other studies, where Retzius continued to add pieces to the puzzle. But although his specified aim was to understand fertilization, Retzius did not formulate any synthesizing conclusions from his studies of sperm, ova, and cell division. Instead, his work is, again, distinctly empirical and *serial*, displaying a method of collecting massive amounts of material to analyze and compare.[42]

Gustaf Retzius learned, and further developed, the latest methods of fixating and coloring microscopic specimens, which he also discussed in detail in his publications. He used the best available microscopes and printing technology.[43] The outcome of his studies has the character of 'museum science': a collecting

40 Uddenberg, *Skallmätaren*, 219; Nyhart, *Biology Takes Form*, chap. 7, 302–3. On the history of chromosomes and early biological research on heredity, see Churchill, 'From Heredity Theory.'

41 'Chromolithography' signified all kinds of lithographic color printing during the second half of the nineteenth century, the 'heyday of reproductive color lithography.' Gascoigne, *How to Identify Prints*, 28b.

42 Hopwood, Schaffer, and Secord, 'Seriality.'

43 Åhrén 'Figuring Things Out'; cf. Schickore, *Microscope*.

and comparative practice, an analytical way of knowing. A style of working that could seem out of step with his time, when the experimental way of knowing became increasingly dominant in biology, including embryology. But, in fact, museum-based research practices overlapped with laboratory science, and were still very productive, at least up to the First World War.[44] Retzius's publications, taken together, make up a 'paper museum,' where his collections, preparations, and analyses of embryos, fetuses, germ cells, and chromosomes were documented, visualized. The studies circulated widely, thus facilitating comparison and further study by other scientists.[45]

When Erik Müller gave his inaugural lecture as chair of histology at the KI in 1896, he also dealt with chromosomes, but in the setting of a discussion of scientific studies and theories of generation, from the eighteenth century on. Müller, who had studied with Oscar Hertwig and Wilhelm His, stressed the importance of microscopic technology, and favored 'the most exact of all methods of research, […] experiment.' While his arguments regarding evolutionists and epigeneticists in his own era are obscure, his opinion on the importance of chromosomes is clear: 'the most important substance in all living organisms is the so-called chromatin.' Fertilization is a process through which nuclear parts of the sperm cell are introduced into the egg cell, Müller continues, connecting the chromatin from the father and the mother. Chromatin is what makes up the chromosomes, and it carries the inherited characteristics from the parents and start the ontogenetic development of the individual. Supporting Oscar Hertwig and Wilhelm Roux, and criticizing Ernst Haeckel and his biogenetic law ('ontogeny recapitulates phylogeny'), Müller sees cellular science as the foundation of modern biology. He ends his talk by hailing recent research findings in histology and embryology, and their influence on medical practice. Although a new approach to development and heredity was underway, Müller still emphasized the foundational character of microscopic anatomy, for both the scientist and the practicing physician.[46]

4 Microscopic Slides and Plaster Casts: New Approaches to Embryology

Much as the conditions of science and society had changed between the 1820s of Anders Retzius and the early 1900s of Erik Müller and Emil Holmgren, one theme connects their work at the KI: the collection, preparation, study, and

44 Pickstone, *Ways of Knowing*, chap. 6; Reinarz, 'Museum Medicine.'
45 Cf. Rudwick, 'Paper Museum.'
46 Müller, 'Några nyare åskådningar,' 498–516.

visualization of specimens. In Anders Retzius's time, the use of achromatic microscopes was beginning to make it possible to study the tiniest structures of life. But the main focus of work in the anatomy museum was still on procuring and studying gross anatomy specimens. By the first decades of the twentieth century, the technological possibilities had proliferated, to say the least, and macroscopic anatomy specimens were losing their attraction as objects of investigation and as symbols of scientific knowledge. Instead, special cabinets were filled with series of microscopic slides of tissues and organs harvested from humans and animals. Thousands of slides could fit into one cabinet. And in the Department of Histology, many of these cabinets had thin slices of embryos arranged in series upon series.[47] Gross anatomical specimens and models were, however, still on display in the KI's first-class anatomy museum in the early twentieth century, and they were actively used in medical instruction together with visualizations in other media: models in wax, plaster, or wood; prints and wall charts; drawings on the blackboard; projected photographs and slides. The KI had bought wax models from the Ziegler workshop to be used in embryology class, but unlike at Uppsala University, there was no local production of wax models.[48]

Dominant as it was in embryology, microscopic study was not suitable for all research topics. The method of observation and visualization had to be adapted to the research question. In a monograph from 1896, Erik Müller studied fetal development of abdominal organs, particularly the small intestine. Müller spent the spring and summer researching this topic, first in Stockholm, and then in Leipzig, at Wilhelm His's anatomical department. He acknowledges His in the introduction, along with the sculptor Franz Josef Steger, who had taught him to make plaster casts. Steger and His had collaborated to make durable plaster models for anatomical instruction, and plaster was used in many scientific and cultural settings at the time, including anatomy: to produce molds for wax moulages and models, and to make death and life masks, anthropological casts, and copies of sculptures, portrait busts, architectural details, and archaeological objects.[49] The method Müller used to study the fetuses was unusual, however. After injecting fetuses with a formalin solution through thc carotid artery, and then hardening them suspended in formalin, Müller dissected the fetuses using a method developed by His, removing tissues and organs layer by

47 Åhrén, 'Museerna,' 152–54. See also Franzén, 'Att lära sig se'; Tybjerg, 'From Bottled Babies,' 263–78.

48 Åhrén, 'Making Space,' 110–11. On Ziegler's collaboration with His and others, see Hopwood, *Embryos in Wax*; Hopwood, 'Plastic Publishing.' On wax models in Uppsala, see Franzén, 'Att lära sig se,' 9–12.

49 Cf. Franzén's chapter in this volume; Hallam, *Anatomy Museum*, 127–29, 193–94.

layer. After each layer, he made a plaster cast of the specimen, creating a series of casts for each fetus, which made it possible to study the shape and relative position of the organs at particular stages of fetal development.[50]

The ten image plates of the article show a combination of lithographed drawings and photographs of the plaster casts, thus visualizing a series of progressively larger fetal specimens, from five centimeters long up to fifty-five centimeters. Plate IV (figure 4.7) also shows the gradual dissection of two fetuses, by laying out a series of plaster casts next to each other. By applying this method, Müller claims to have been able to better examine and visualize the topography of abdominal organs of the fetus 'in situ,' compared to studies that, for example, used sections made from frozen specimens. Müller's conclusion ends up comparing his own results with publications of his peers, and the methodological discussion is as crucial here as it ever was for Anders and Gustaf Retzius.[51]

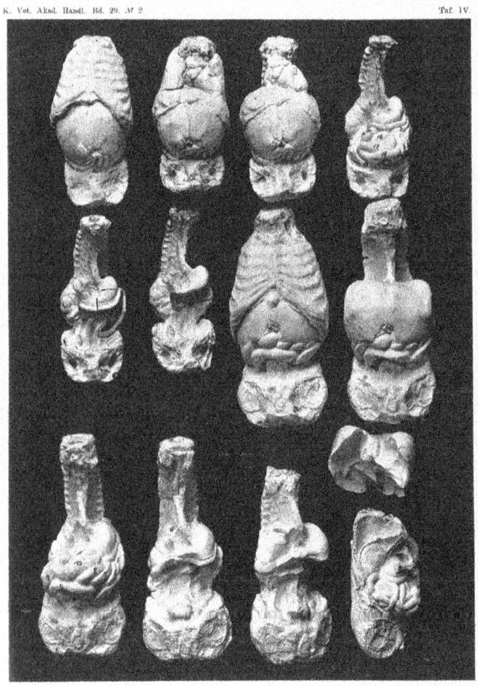

FIGURE 4.7
Photograph of a series of plaster casts displaying progressive dissections of the intestines of two fetuses, seventeen and twenty centimeters long. Photo-lithographic plate in Müller, 'Beiträge zur Anatomie,' Taf. IV. Hagströmer Library, KI.

50 Müller, 'Beiträge zur Anatomie.' William Hunter used a similar method in the 1770s—plaster casts of pregnant women and fetuses are preserved in the Hunterian Museum, Glasgow. Hallam, *Anatomy Museum*, 126–29. On Steger and His, see Cornwall and Smith, 'Anatomical Models.'

51 Müller, 'Beiträge zur Anatomie,' 70–73. On frozen sections in topographical anatomy, see Al-Gailani, '"Ice Age."'

As microscopic tissue studies became more and more the norm in embryology, Erik Müller also primarily used an ensemble of different technologies of visualization. In the 1912 volume of *Kongl. Vetenskaps-Akademiens handlingar* (Proceedings of the Royal Swedish Academy of Sciences), for example, he published a study of connective tissue in dogfish shark embryos, accompanied by lithographs of microscopic specimens. The entire volume was dedicated to Gustaf Retzius on the occasion of his seventieth birthday, and the articles were all written by some of Retzius's closest friends and students. Emil Holmgren, Müller's successor as chair of histology at the KI, was one of the contributors, as were embryologists Ivar Broman of Lund University, and J. August Hammar from Uppsala University.[52]

Emil Holmgren, who proudly described the modern equipment of the histology department of the KI in 1910, made use of the laboratory equipment for teaching and research, but also used its photographic studio for publishing a textbook in histology in 1920.[53] This volume contained 742 reproduced photographs of microscopic specimens in the department's collections. Photographic micrography (not to be confused with micro-photography; i.e., minute photographs), was a technique to take images of specimens through the lens of a microscope. It had by this time become the preferred, and most modern, form for visualizing, reproducing, and circulating histological knowledge.

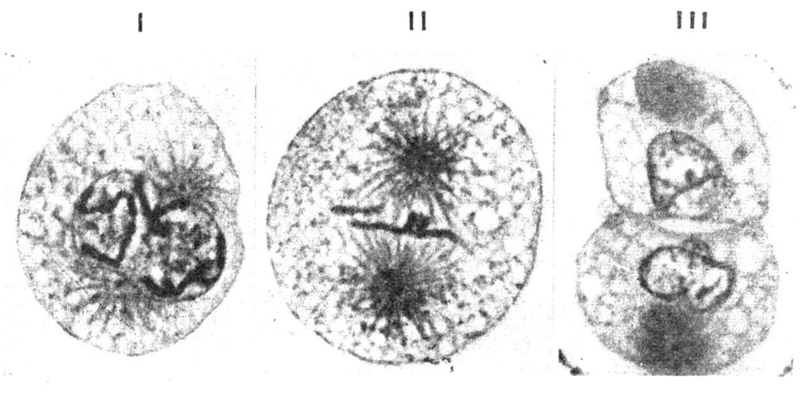

FIGURE 4.8 Photomicrographs of the first stages of cell division in a fertilized ovum of *Ascaris megalocephala*, produced at the Department of Histology at the KI. Halftone print in Holmgren, *Lärobok i histologi*, 91, fig. 34. Hagströmer Library, KI.

52 Müller, 'Untersuchungen'; Retzius, *Biografiska anteckningar*, 2:156, and on the merits of Müller, Holmgren, Broman, Hammar, and others, 234.

53 Holmgren, *Lärobok*.

Although the published images are modest, small halftone prints, and less visually striking than Gustaf Retzius's large-scale color lithographs, they had other qualities speaking for them. The photograph had acquired an aura of objectivity, a valued quality in scientific contexts favored by Holmström precisely for this reason.[54] And it signaled epistemic authority as well as access to (institutional) resources. Holmgren's images of the ovular cell division of the *Ascaris megalocephala* are thus just as authoritative as Gustaf Retzius's, but with other means.

5 Conclusion: the Embryo as Model of Development

Between Anders Retzius's first dissections of sheep embryos to study their gill slits and Emil Holmgren's handbook in histology lies a dramatic century of societal transformation. Sweden went from a poor and war-ridden country to a modern industrial state. Science and technology were at the heart of this nation-building, modernizing effort. The KI established itself as a modern research institution and medical school with high standards, dedicated to the empirical study of medicine and life science. During the nineteenth century, research in anatomy—medicine's foundational science—became increasingly based on comparative methods and microscopic investigations. Embryology as a subject for research and teaching was at the center of this development.[55] The KI's professors of anatomy and histology were enthusiastically teaching the latest in embryology, as well as pursuing research and participating in international networks of scientific exchange.

Scientific knowledge about generation and embryonal development increased tremendously during the nineteenth century, following von Baer's description of the mammalian ova, Rathke's demonstration of fetal gill slits, and the establishment of the cell theory in the 1830s. Life scientists found the embryological field of inquiry central to their pursuit of knowledge. This had deeper connotations than mere delight in novel research findings or individual contributions that expanded the general body of knowledge. Embryonal development had taken on a symbolic meaning. Whether or not an individual scientist supported the recapitulation theory—as formulated by Ernst Haeckel or earlier by Johann Friedrich Meckel and his contemporaries—embryology described a development from the simple to the complex, from the general

54 Cf. Daston and Galison, 'Image of Objectivity'; Daston and Galison, *Objectivity*.
55 Hopwood, 'Embryology,' 285–94.

to the differentiated.[56] This developmental model fitted nicely together with nineteenth-century idealism, which was remarkably persistent well into the twentieth century. The development of human and animal anatomy through history could, then, be seen in analogy with embryonal development. Culture and society, too, were generally understood to develop from the primitive to the advanced, in a progressive pattern, toward perfection. This developmental, perhaps evolutionary, view of natural and cultural history was shared by most Swedish scientists at the time, including the main actors of this article, Anders and Gustaf Retzius, Erik Müller, and Emil Holmgren.[57]

What I have focused on here, however, is not the grand theories of life and evolution, but practices of embryonic and fetal knowledge production at the KI, the work that scientists performed in their laboratories and transferred to the pages of their publications. This work was inherently visual and material. Studying, analyzing, and comparing gametes, fertilization, or embryonic and fetal development in different species required a chain of practices of collection and preparation. They involved technologies of staining, cutting, slicing, and magnifying. Artists, hunters, doctors, janitors, photographers, instrument makers, chemists, technicians, and printers were necessary collaborators in this pursuit. Specimens, which grounded the scientific value of the study, remained in the collections of the anatomy and histology departments. As I have shown, the end results were not just scientific texts, but, more importantly, *visualizations* based on observations of specimens, thus reflecting the process of knowledge production—a visual and material way of knowing.

Acknowledgements

I wish to thank Michael Sappol, Carrie Greenwood, and Anna Lantz for their expertise and support.

Bibliography

Afzelius, Björn A. 'Gustaf Retzius and Spermatology.' *International Journal of Developmental Biology* 39, no. 5 (1995): 675–85.

56 Hopwood, 'Embryology,' 290; Hopwood, 'Producing Development.'

57 Cf. Lenoir, *Strategy of Life*; Gustafsson, 'En harmonisk och hierarkisk ordning.'

Åhrén, Eva. 'Figuring Things Out: Visualizations in the Work of Anders and Gustaf Retzius, 1829–1921.' *Nuncius: Journal of the Material and Visual History of Science* 32, no. 1 (2017): 166–211.

Åhrén, Eva. 'Making Space for Specimens: The Museums of the Karolinska Institute, Stockholm.' In *Medical Museums: Past, Present, Future*, edited by Samuel J. M. M. Alberti and Elizabeth Hallam, 102–15. London: Royal College of Surgeons of England, 2013.

Åhrén, Eva. 'Museerna: Vetenskap i tre dimensioner.' In Johannisson, Nilsson, and Qvarsell, *Medicinen blir till vetenskap*, 126–69.

Alberti, Samuel J. M. M. *Morbid Curiosities: Medical Museums in Nineteenth-Century Britain.* Oxford: Oxford University Press, 2011.

Al-Gailani, Salim. 'The "Ice Age" in Anatomy and Obstetrics: Hand and Eye in the Promotion of Frozen Sections around 1900.' *Bulletin of the History of Medicine* 90 (2016): 611–42.

Anders Retzius bref till A. H. Florman: Ett bidrag till medicinens historia i Sverige. Edited by Carl M. Fürst. Lund: Gleerups, 1896.

Baer, Karl Ernst von. *Über Entwicklungsgeschichte der Thiere: Beobachtung und Reflexion.* Vol. 1. Königsberg: Bornträger, 1828.

Bondestam, Maja. *Tvåkönad: Studier i den svenska hermafroditens historia.* Nora: Nya Doxa, 2010.

Bondestam, Maja. *See also* Larsson, Maja.

Buklijas, Tatjana, and Nick Hopwood. *Making Visible Embryos* (online exhibition). 2008–10. Accessed December 4, 2020. http://www.hps.cam.ac.uk/visibleembryos/.

Chorell, Torbjörn Gustafsson. 'Neurovetenskap: Hjärna och psyke.' In Johannisson, Nilsson, and Qvarsell, *Medicinen blir till vetenskap*, 238–26.

Churchill, Frederick B. *August Weismann: Development, Heredity, and Evolution.* Cambridge, MA: Harvard University Press, 2015.

Churchill, Frederick B. 'From Heredity Theory to *Vererbung*: The Transmission Problem, 1850–1915.' *Isis* 78 (1987): 337–64.

Cornwall, Jon, and Chris Smith. 'Anatomical Models by F. J. Steger (1845–1938): The University of Otago Collection.' *European Journal of Anatomy* 18, no. 3 (2014): 209–11.

Daston, Lorraine, and Peter Galison. 'The Image of Objectivity.' *Representations* 40 (Fall 1992): 81–128.

Daston, Lorraine, and Peter Galison. *Objectivity*. New York: Zone Books, 2007.

Eriksson, Nils. *'I andans kraft, på sannings stråt…': De skandinaviska naturforskarmötena 1839–1936.* Göteborg: Göteborgs universitet, 1991.

Fiorentini, Erna. 'Induction of Visibility: Reflections on Histological Slides, Drawing Visual Hypotheses and Aesthetic-Epistemic Actions.' *History and Philosophy of the Life Sciences* 35 (2013): 379–94.

Fleck, Ludwik. *Genesis and Development of a Scientific Fact*. Translated by F. Bradley and T. J. Trenn. Chicago: University of Chicago Press, 1979.

Franzén, Helena. 'Att lära sig se embryologiskt: Samlingsobjekt i forskning och pedagogiska kontexter 1870–1920.' *Scandia* 89, no. 2 (2023): 201–229.

Gascoigne, Bamber. *How to Identify Prints: A Complete Guide to Manual and Mechanical Processes from Woodcut to Inkjet*, 2nd ed. London: Thames & Hudson, 2004.

Gustafson, Tony. 'Anatomi: Praktik och pedagogik.' In Johannisson, Nilsson, and Qvarsell, *Medicinen blir till vetenskap*, 170–99.

Gustafsson, Torbjörn. 'En harmonisk och hierarkisk ordning: Synen på utveckling i 1800-talets svenska biologi.' *Lychnos* (1994): 87–113.

Hallam, Elizabeth. *Anatomy Museum: Death and the Body Displayed*. London: Reaktion Books, 2016.

Holmgren, Emil. 'Histologiska institutionen.' In *Karolinska mediko-kirurgiska institutets historia*, 3:462–82. Stockholm: Karolinska mediko-kirurgiska institutet, 1910.

Holmgren, Emil. *Lärobok i histologi*. Stockholm: Norstedts, 1920.

Hopwood, Nick. 'Embryology.' In *The Cambridge History of Science*, vol. 2, edited by Peter J. Bowler and John V. Pickstone, 285–315. Cambridge: Cambridge University Press, 2009.

Hopwood, Nick. *Embryos in Wax: Models from the Ziegler Studio*. Cambridge: Whipple Museum of the History of Science, 2002.

Hopwood, Nick. *Haeckel's Embryos: Images, Evolution, and Fraud*. Chicago: University of Chicago Press, 2015.

Hopwood, Nick. 'Plastic Publishing in Embryology.' In *Models: The Third Dimension of Science*, edited by Soraya de Chadarevian and Nick Hopwood, 170–206. Stanford, CA: Stanford University Press, 2004.

Hopwood, Nick. 'Producing Development: The Anatomy of Human Embryos and the Norms of Wilhelm His.' *Bulletin of the History of Medicine* 74, no. 1 (2000): 29–79.

Hopwood, Nick, Rebecca Flemming, and Lauren Kassel, eds. *Reproduction: Antiquity to the Present Day*. Cambridge: Cambridge University Press, 2018.

Hopwood, Nick, Peter Murray Jones, Lauren Kassel, and James Secord. 'Introduction: Communicating Reproduction.' *Bulletin of the History of Medicine* 89, no. 3 (Fall 2015): 379–404.

Hopwood, Nick, Simon Schaffer, and Jim Secord. 'Seriality and Scientific Objects in the Nineteenth Century.' *History of Science* 48, no. 3–4 (2010): 251–85.

Johannisson, Karin, Ingemar Nilsson, and Roger Qvarsell, eds. *Medicinen blir till vetenskap: Karolinska Institutet under två århundraden*. Solna: Karolinska University Press, 2010.

Karolinska mediko-kirurgiska institutets historia. Vols. 1–3. Stockholm: Karolinska mediko-kirurgiska institutet, 1910.

Kungl. Svenska vetenskapsakademiens handlingar 49 (1912).

Larsson, Maja. 'From Frightening Beast to Primitive Stage: On the Normalization of the Monstrous Body in Swedish Medicine.' In *Body Claims*, edited by Janne Bromseth, Lisa Folkmarson Käll, and Katarina Mattsson, 26–57. Uppsala: Uppsala University, 2009.

Larsson, Maja. *See also* Bondestam, Maja.

Latour, Bruno. 'Drawing Things Together.' In *Representation in Scientific Practice*, edited by Michael Lynch and Steve Woolgar, 19–68. Cambridge, MA: MIT Press, 1990.

Lenoir, Timothy. *The Strategy of Life: Teleology and Mechanics in Nineteenth-Century German Biology*. Dordrecht: Reidel, 1982.

Lindblad, Tomas. *Gustaf Retzius: A Biography*. Stockholm: Hagströmerbiblioteket, 2007.

Ljungström, Olof. *Oscariansk antropologi: Etnografi, förhistoria och rasforskning under sent 1800-tal*. Hedemora: Gidlunds, 2004.

Lucae, Johann Christian Gustav. *Zur organischen Formenlehre*. Frankfurt am Main: Varrentrapp, 1844.

McLeary, Erin Hunter. 'Science in a Bottle: The Medical Museum in North America, 1860–1940.' PhD diss., University of Pennsylvania, 2001.

Morgan, Lynn M. *Icons of Life: A Cultural History of Human Embryos*. Berkeley: University of California Press, 2009.

Müller, Erik. 'Anatomiska institutionen.' In *Karolinska mediko-kirurgiska institutets historia*, 3:69–138. Stockholm: Karolinska mediko-kirurgiska institutet, 1910.

Müller, Erik 'Beiträge zur Anatomie des menschlichen Foetus.' *Kongl. Svenska Vetenskaps-akademiens handlingar* 29, no. 2 (1897): 1–74, plus ten image plates.

Müller, Erik. 'Några nyare åskådningar inom utvecklingsläran.' *Hygiea* 58 (1896): 498–516.

Müller, Erik. 'Untersuchungen über ein faseriges Stützgewebe bei den Embryonen von Acanthias vulgaris.' *Kungl. Svenska vetenskapsakademiens handlingar* 49 (1912): 5–18, plus four image plates.

Nilsson, Ingemar. 'Vetenskapen: Medicinens teori.' In Johannisson, Nilsson, and Qvarsell, *Medicinen blir till vetenskap*, 12–41.

Nyhart, Lynn K. *Biology Takes Form: Animal Morphology and the German Universities, 1800–1900*. Chicago: University of Chicago Press, 1995.

Otis, Laura. *Müller's Lab*. Oxford: Oxford University Press, 2007.

Pickstone, John V. *Ways of Knowing: A New History of Science, Technology and Medicine*. Chicago: University of Chicago Press, 2001.

Reinarz, Jonathan. 'The Age of Museum Medicine: The Rise and Fall of the Medical Museum at Birmingham's School of Medicine.' *Social History of Medicine* 18, no. 3 (2005): 419–37.

Retzius, Anders. 'Händelse af Hypospadi, som gifvit anledning till misstag om kön, iakttagen af Hr Stadsläkaren Doctor C. W. Engelbrecht i Söderköping och beskrifven, jemte tillägg om de yttre genitaliernas utvecklingsformer.' *Hygiea* 16 (1854): 549–53, plus two image plates.

Retzius, Anders. 'Om bildningen af hjernans hemisphaerer och hvalf.' *Öfversikt af Kongl. Vetenskaps-akademiens förhandlingar*, no. 9 (1844): 194–98.

Retzius, Gustaf. *Biografiska anteckningar och minnen*. Vol. 2. Edited by Otto Walde. Uppsala, 1948.

Retzius, Gustaf. *Das Menschenhirn: Studien in der makroskopischen Morphologie*. Vols. 1–2. Stockholm, 1896.

Retzius, Gustaf. 'Einleitung zu den zunächst folgenden Mitteilungen über das Verhalten des chromatins in der verschiedenen physiologischen Zuständen.' *Biologische Untersuchungen, Neue Folge* 16 (1911): 1–6.

Retzius, Gustaf. 'Noch einige Beiträge zur Kenntnis der Spermien bei den Affen.' *Biologische Untersuchungen, Neue Folge* 19 (1921): 57–61.

Retzius, Gustaf. 'Om metoderna att konservera hjärnor.' *Biologiska föreningens förhandlingar* 1 (1888–89): 118–30.

Retzius, Gustaf. 'Ueber einen Spiralfaserapparat am Kopfe der Spermien der Selachier.' *Biologische Untersuchungen, Neue Folge* 10 (1902): 61–64.

Retzius, Gustaf. 'Weitere Beiträge zut Kenntnis der Spermien des Menschen und eineger Säugethiere.' *Biologische Untersuchungen, Neue Folge* 10 (1902): 45–60.

Retzius, Gustaf. 'Zur Kenntnis der Entwicklung der Körperformen des Menschen während der fötalen Lebensstufen.' *Biologische Untersuchungen, Neue Folge* 11 (1904): 33–76.

Retzius, Gustaf. 'Zur Kenntnis der Spermatozoen.' *Biologische Untersuchungen* 1 (1881): 77–88.

Rocca, Julius. *Forging a Medical University: The Establishment of Sweden's Karolinska Institutet*. Stockholm: Karolinska Institutet University Press, 2006.

Rudwick, Martin. 'George Cuvier's Paper Museum of Fossil Bones.' *Archives of Natural History* 27, no. 1 (2000): 51–68.

Schickore, Jutta. *The Microscope and the Eye: A History of Reflections, 1740–1870*. Chicago: University of Chicago Press, 2007.

Swedish Society of Medicine. *Årsberättelse om svenska läkare-sällskapets arbete*. Stockholm: Svenska läkaresällskapet, 1829.

Tiedemann, Friedrich. *Anatomie und Bildungsgeschichte des Gehirns im Foetus des Menschen nebst einer vergleichenden Darstellung des Hirnbaues in den Thieren*. Nürnberg: Steinischen Buchhandlung, 1816.

Tybjerg, Karin. 'From Bottled Babies to Biobanks: Medical Collections in the Twenty-First Century.' In *The Fate of Anatomical Collections*, edited by Rina Knoeff and Robert Zweinenberg, 263–78. Farnham: Ashgate, 2015.

Uddenberg, Nils. *Skallmätaren: Gustaf Retzius—hyllad och hatad*. Stockholm: Fri tanke, 2019.

Vienne, Florence. 'Eggs and Sperm as Germ Cells.' In *Reproduction: Antiquity to the Present Day*, edited by Nick Hopwood, Rebecca Flemming, and Lauren Kassel, 413–26. Cambridge: Cambridge University Press, 2018.

Archival Sources

Retzius, Gustaf. Correspondence, bound series. Hierta–Retzius collection. CHS.
Retzius, Gustaf. Letters from various persons. Hierta–Retzius collection. CHS.

CHAPTER 5

'Pelves of Various Nations': Race and Sex in a Mid-nineteenth-Century Obstetric Collection

Helena Franzén

In the eighteenth century, physicians claimed the management of difficult labors, in which the fetus got stuck in the pelvic canal, as a field of expertise. They had an array of tools, such as forceps, at their disposal to facilitate delivery.[1] Into the following century, questions regarding whether and how racial differences manifested physically were debated by scholars conducting anatomical studies of reproduction.[2] Collections of instruments and preserved bodies were a vital resource for the production of knowledge and authority in the nineteenth century.[3]

In 1867, Alfred Higgins, a member of the newly founded Anthropological Society of London, traveled to Stockholm to meet the physician and anatomist Gustaf Retzius at the Karolinska Institute, at the time known as the Caroline Medico-Surgical Institute, which was a combined medical and research institute.[4] The purpose was to discuss plans for an English translation of the 'anthropological works' of Gustaf's renowned father, Anders Retzius.[5] Higgins had set out with the intention of visiting several Scandinavian museums, but was unable to fulfil this aim. He saw the anatomical museum at the Karolinska Institute, where a collection of human skulls assembled by Anders Retzius was on display; the Swedish History Museum; and the Natural History Museum, all

1 Martin, *Woman in the Body*, 54.

2 Hendriksen, 'Fate of the Beaded Babies.'

3 Pickstone, *Ways of Knowing*; Reinarz, 'Age of Museum Medicine,' 419–37.

4 Higgins, 'Note,' 14. In the historiography this society is described as promoting scientific racism, in the sense that several of the leading members, such as James Hunt, stated that there was an inherent hierarchy between peoples. Qureshi, 'Robert Gordon Latham,' 160–63.

5 A collection of Anders Retzius's texts regarding human diversity had been published posthumously in Swedish and German a few years earlier. Retzius, *Anders Retzii samlade skrifter*; Retzius, *Ethnologische schriften*.

 | DOI:10.1163/9789004703759_007

situated in Stockholm.[6] Later, he complained that he had not had the opportunity to visit Uppsala University:

> The time at my disposal did not admit of my visiting the anatomical museum at Upsala [sic], which contains some few race-skulls and has, moreover, been recently enriched by the extensive collection of pelves of various nations, collected by the brother of Professor Anders Retzius, Dr. Magnus Retzius, Professor of Obstetrics at his [Anders Retzius's] Caroline Institute in Stockholm.[7]

Magnus Retzius had sold the collection to the medical faculty at Uppsala University in 1862, but he had assembled it in Stockholm over the previous decades. In the inventory accompanying the sales contract, the pelves mentioned by Higgins were listed under the heading 'race pelves.'[8] The collection also contained osteological preparations of pelves—that is, preserved body parts—labeled with conditions such as rickets. Fetal crania, casts of pelves in plaster and papier mâché, models of the pregnant body, and obstetrical instruments were also part of the collection. All the pelves were remnants of women's bodies which had been skeletonized, mounted, written on, and labeled: practices which made them into collection objects.

After the sale, the Uppsala collection was housed in the museum at the Department of Anatomy for many years. In 1903 the pelves, along with the obstetrical instruments, were moved to the Uppsala University Hospital, and over time items were added, removed, and destroyed. In the mid-1990s and in 2006 the pelves and instruments were moved to the Museum of Medical History in Uppsala, where they remain today.[9]

This chapter explores this hitherto unexamined obstetric collection in the context of Swedish nationalism in the first half of the nineteenth century. By investigating the remaining pelvis preparations in relation to archival sources and scientific publications, the aim is to uncover how Magnus Retzius's collection was used as evidence in the Swedish nation-building project. In particular, I will demonstrate that tension between interpretations of the pelvis and the skull had a bearing on ideas about national identity in Sweden. Moreover, I will

6 Ljungström, 'Swedish Golgotha.'

7 Higgins, 'Note,' 17.

8 'Professor C M Retzius salubrev.'

9 Sixty-seven pelves still remain, of which about twenty are casts, as well as two unlabeled fetal crania of unknown origin.

highlight that ideas about sex and race, along with antiquarian artifacts, were intertwined and involved in the making of 'the Swedish people.'

The formation of skull collections internationally and in Sweden has been the subject of historically oriented studies, with a focus on the 1860s onward, whereas the existence and uses of racialized pelvis collections have barely been addressed.[10] Previous scholarship, most dating from the 1980s and 1990s, has shed light on only a few collections containing pelves categorized according to racial groupings, largely in passing, with the focus on how women's genitals were described and how hierarchies were thereby produced. It has been shown that women of African descent were subjected to particularly close scrutiny.[11] More recently, it has been demonstrated that preparations of women's pelves have been used as means of constructing national identity and 'the indigenous.'[12] This strain of research has outlined the potential of racialized pelvis collections as sources in the investigation of identity formation, and this study takes a similar approach.

In the first section of this chapter, the collectors, their scientific context, and the interplay between their collections are analyzed. The second section demonstrates that these collections were deeply intertwined with inquiries into prehistory within the spheres of Scandinavianism and antiquarianism, which in turn were linked to nationalism. The conclusion emphasizes that race and sex were constituted through Magnus Retzius's collection in the context of the Swedish nation-building project of the first half of the nineteenth century, as a means to define the 'Swedish people.'

1 The Collectors of Pelves and Skulls

Magnus and Anders Retzius were born in Lund, where their father, Anders Jahan Retzius, a student of Linnaeus, was professor of natural history. After completing his medical studies, Magnus started a career as a military physician in 1815. In 1819 he assumed the position of assistant physician at the Pro Patria

10 On Sweden, see Ljungström, 'Oscariansk antropologi'; Svanberg, 'World as Collected,' 398–404; Svanberg, *Människosamlarna*, 124–35. Internationally, see, e.g., MacDonald, *Human Remains*; Fabian, *Skull Collectors*; Conklin, *In the Museum of Man*; Sysling, *Racial Science*.

11 Schiebinger, *The Mind Has No Sex?*, 211–13; Schiebinger, *Nature's Body*, 156–60; Fausto-Sterling, 'Gender, Race, and Nation'; Qureshi, 'Displaying Sara Baartman.'

12 This study focused on Mexico around 1900, but it illustrates that this phenomenon occurred in a country during a time of identity crisis. Cházaro, 'From Anatomical Collection.'

Lying-In Hospital in Stockholm, where he was appointed chief physician in 1830. After working in obstetrics for thirty years, he was appointed to the chair of obstetrics at the Karolinska Institute in 1849.[13]

When Magnus started working at the Pro Patria Lying-In Hospital, there were small-scale teaching and research collections of anatomical and zoological preparations, as well as surgical instruments, at the universities in Lund and Uppsala, and at the Karolinska Institute.[14] It was not uncommon for physicians to possess collections of their own. In the first half of the nineteenth century, naturalists, who were also often physicians, collected, described, and classified the world through its contents.[15] Dead animals, plants, and rocks from all over the globe found their way into the naturalists' private collections, acquired on their own travels or by their associates.[16] In line with the tradition of natural history, Magnus's collection was privately owned, but as I will show, it was also a product of his ties to the Karolinska Institute.

During the nineteenth century, as medicine became more specialized, existing collections were reorganized and extended to serve emerging fields of research and education.[17] At the Karolinska Institute this process was headed by Anders Retzius, who became an increasingly influential professor and expanded his employer's collections from the 1830s onward. He is particularly known for assembling the collection of human skulls, but the museum also contained many dry and wet preparations of human and animal remains.[18] Anders also established an index to categorize human variation, in terms of cranial form, in the early 1840s.[19] The Retzius brothers represented different models of ownership relative to these collections, yet their collecting activities and scholarly works were closely enmeshed.

Anders considered the brain as key in giving form to the cranium—for men in particular—and argued that those forms were distinct for people of different races.[20] He was, however, not a phrenologist and distanced himself from those teachings because he considered them to lack an empirical foundation for the claim that personality traits, morals, and intelligence correlated to the

13 'Biografi'; Qvarsell, 'Patriotism, paternalism och offentlig vård,' 88.

14 Svanberg, *Människosamlarna*, 49–50, 167; Åhrén, 'Museerna,' 127–29.

15 Curry et al., *Worlds of Natural History*.

16 MacGregor, *Naturalists in the Field*.

17 Alberti, *Nature and Culture*.

18 Åhrén, 'Making Space for Specimens.'

19 Anders Retzius introduced this index in Retzius, 'Om formen af Nordboarnes kranier'; Gould, *Mismeasure of Man*.

20 Retzius, 'Om formen af Nordboarnes kranier,' 2, 4–5; Retzius, 'Om formen af hufvudets benstomme,' 43–44.

form of designated regions of the cranium.[21] Anders associated skull form with degrees of 'cultural development'—that is, civilization:

> Within nations which live in the natural state, and within those which otherwise find themselves at a lesser stage of cultural development, the individual differences appear less. On the other hand, greater individual differences also emerge in the cranial form to the same extent that higher and broader education has appeared. One should therefore preferentially extract the material for the investigations from the actual people, less from the higher classes, and more from the distant countryside than in the cities.[22]

Magnus, with his interest in obstetrics, instead focused his attention on pelves, which were also thought to manifest racial differences. In his dissertation from 1848 about narrow pelves, Magnus stated that 'the form of the pelvis, like the skull, is more or less specific for each particular human race. It is most prominent in the female pelvis.'[23] He also discussed race in relation to giving birth. Some of his contemporaries had argued that the size of the fetus corresponded with pelvic form and width in different groups:

> Winterbottom affirms, that negresses, who generally have small and narrow pelves, give birth to small children, while mestizos (a mix of Europeans and colored), who live in the same areas as the negroes, have wide pelves and give birth to big, plump children.[24]

Magnus shared this notion and connected it to ideas about relations between the body and civilization, stating that the physical constitution of some groups of people was closer to that of animals, hinting that this was due to their more primitive state:

> the more a nation's particular pelvic form approaches the animalistic form, the more unrefined and crude such a pelvis appears, and the less developed are the internal pelvic planes, but yet the fetus passes more easily through them, and the less painful and drawn-out is the labor, such as for example for the women of the Bushmen and the primeval Negroes.[25]

21 Retzius, 'Frenologien bedömd från anatomisk-ethnologisk ståndpunkt,' 97–98.
22 Retzius, 'Om formen af hufvudets benstomme,' 42.
23 Retzius, *Afhandling*, 14.
24 Retzius, *Afhandling*, 6.
25 Retzius, 'Om bäckenplanerna,' 66.

Some obstetricians abroad argued that 'civilized' women had difficult and painful labors because of their refinement—an idea based in part on biblical references, in which the notion of original sin provided a model for linking increased knowledge with greater suffering.[26] In his publications, Magnus did not spell out that train of thought. Nonetheless, the Retzius brothers seem to have associated the form and the size of pelves, fetal skulls, and brains with each other, on a scale which they considered to reflect a ladder of civilization. Race and reproduction were thus thought to be intertwined.

Magnus conceptualized giving birth as a mechanical process, which he also related to race. In his dissertation he wrote about 'labor-mechanics,' describing how the obstetrician could intervene when a fetus could not pass through the pelvic channel.[27] The core of Magnus's dissertation discusses how to determine that a woman's pelvis is too narrow for the fetus to pass through and how to make suitable interventions. Problematic childbirths were thus defined relative to the woman's bodily constitution; the pathology was thought to be situated in her and, implicitly, in her race.

Like skulls, pelves were examined by taking measurements—a practice known as pelvimetry.[28] Specific instruments, craniometers and pelvimeters respectively, were used for this purpose.[29] The first pelvimeters seem to have been constructed in France in the 1770s by Jean-Louis Baudelocque and were used for determining whether a woman's pelvic channel was wide enough for a fetus to pass through.[30] There were six of these instruments in Magnus's collection.[31] As shown in previous research, pelvimeters were also used to co-construct race and pathology. By establishing the common form and width of a certain group, potential problems such as 'too-narrow pelves' could be diagnosed, which in turn could serve as a basis for decision-making about interventions when the fetus could not pass through the pelvic channel.[32] In Magnus's collection, ideas about race and pathology were also present; some pelves were described according to racial categories and others in terms of pathological conditions. Magnus and several of his international colleagues aspired to

26 Rich, 'Curse of Civilised Woman,' 60–61.

27 Retzius, *Afhandling*, 8, 193.

28 Dias, 'Visibility of Difference,' 38.

29 Grant, '"Those Parts Peculiar to Her Organization."' Magnus Retzius used the term 'pelvimensores' for instruments for measuring the pelvis and the Swedish term 'bäckenmätning,' which literally translates to 'pelvimetry.' Retzius, *Afhandling*, 54.

30 Hoyme, 'Physical Anthropology and Its Instruments.'

31 'Professor C M Retzius salubrev.'

32 Cházaro, 'Mexican Women's Pelves,' 100–115.

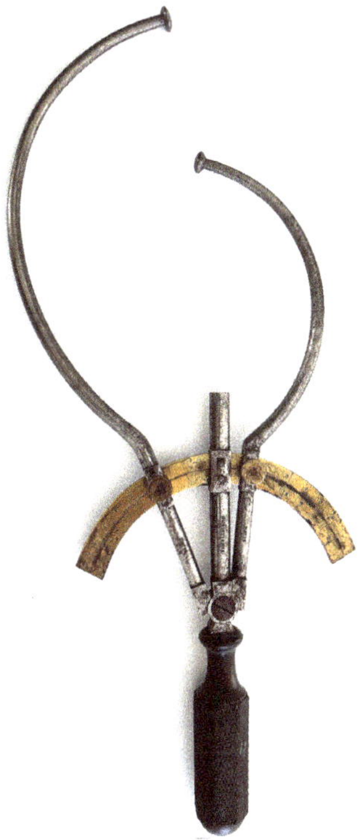

FIGURE 5.1
Wellenbergh's pelvimeter from Magnus Retzius's collection (the middle brace missing). UMM 0247, Museum of Medical History, Uppsala.

ascertain average measurements of pelves, as well as fetal skulls. Their collections and patients constituted the basis of their efforts.[33]

2 The Need for Collections

In previous centuries human bodies had been understood as directly linked to social organization, faith, and surrounding climate.[34] Throughout the first half of the nineteenth century, there were overlapping and conflicting understandings of human origins and variations, as well as what these meant for people's place in society. Monogenesis, the theory that all humans had the same origin, competed with polygenesis, which held that there were different species of humans with distinct geographical origins.[35]

33 Retzius, *Afhandling*, 35, 47–48.
34 Augstein, *Race*.
35 Stocking, *Victorian Anthropology*.

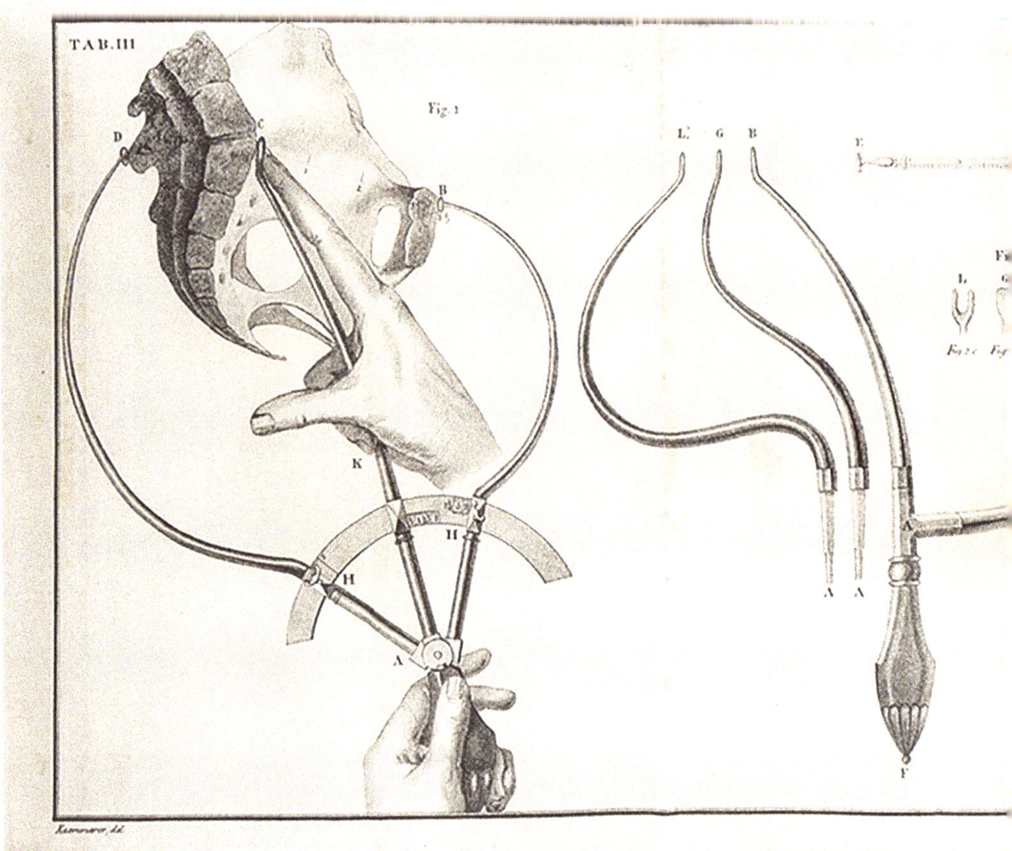

FIGURE 5.2 Pelvimeters were used to measure women's pelves internally and externally. An instructional figure from Wellenbergh, *Abhandlung über einen Pelvimeter*, Tab. III. The Internet Archive.

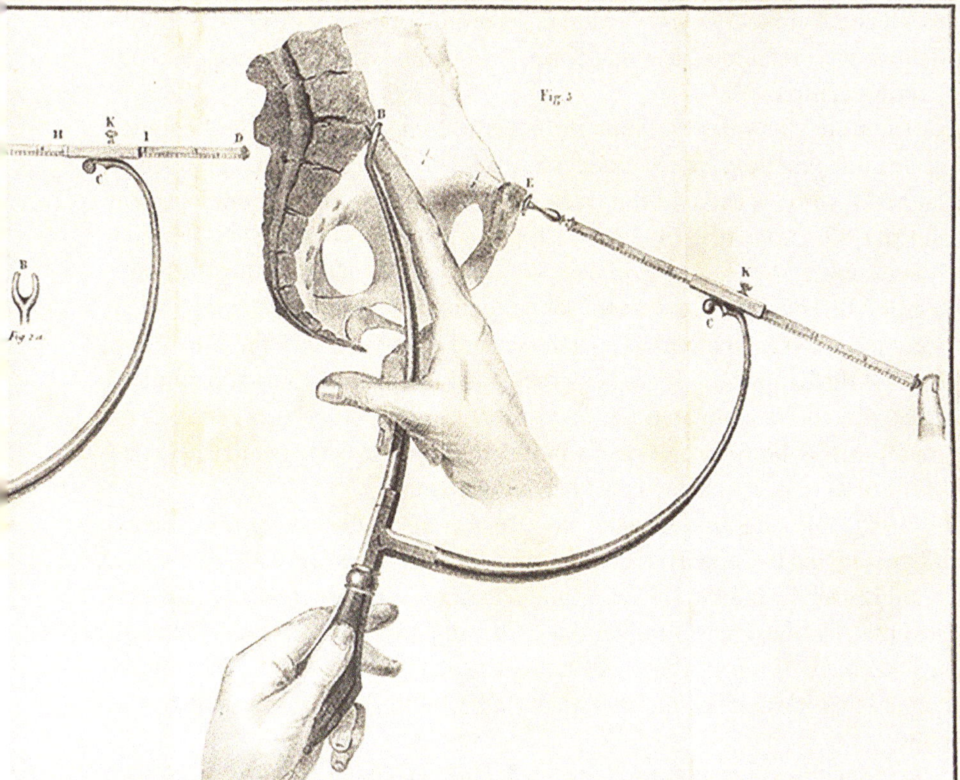
H
K
I
D
C
B
Fig 2 a
B
Fig 3
E
K
C

Comparative anatomy emerged in the second half of the eighteenth century as a way to study differences between humans and animals, as well as variations within these groups. The skull and the pelvis became established as empirical material through which comparative anatomists studied human variation. This development triggered a change in the function of collections and opened the way for new approaches to systematization, which required an increased number of specimens to analyze in relation to each other. Johann Friedrich Blumenbach was one of the first to reorganize an existing collection of skulls, to which he also added new material, according to racial categories that were defined with reference to cranial form. Collections were thus crucial for comparative anatomy.[36]

The study of human variation through the comparison of anatomical specimens was practiced by several scholars, such as Georges Cuvier, professor of natural history in Paris. In the research literature, the case of Sara Baartman illustrates this practice. In 1815, Baartman, a Khoisan woman, died. Her body was examined by Cuvier, who described her as belonging to the 'Bushmen,' a group he considered to be the closest to animals. Parts of Baartman's body were prepared as anatomical specimens and integrated into the Museum of Natural History in Paris. It has been noted that in Cuvier's report of his autopsy of Baartman, he compared her pelvis with those of other 'races' kept at the museum. It is, however, not clear whether these pelves belonged to whole skeletons or were kept as a dedicated pelvis collection.[37]

Arvid Florman introduced the practice of comparative anatomy to Sweden. After studying in Copenhagen in the 1780s, he became professor of anatomy at Lund University in 1801. He taught and remained in close contact with Anders, and this relationship was influential in shaping Anders's approach to anatomical studies.[38] It is probable that Florman also taught Magnus. In 1844, Anders argued that it was by no means established what the term 'race' entailed:

> Of all the parts of natural history, knowledge about the human family is the most uncharted. On the one hand, the differences between specific human races are so great that one is tempted to consider them as separate species of a family. On the other hand, no valid characteristics can be found that would justify such an assumption. Instead, the terms varieties of humankind or folk races have been articulated, but an assured notion

36 Dias, 'Séries de crânes,' 205–7.

37 Fausto-Sterling, 'Gender Race, and Nation,' 35–36, 38.

38 Åhrén, 'Museerna,' 135–38.

> of how the word human race should be understood has however not been determined, and it is even less determined which these races are.[39]

This uncertainty fueled the need to assemble and expand collections. In Magnus's hands, such collections also became evidence for demonstrating the origins of the 'Swedish people.'

It is possible that Magnus began collecting pelves in the 1820s—at least those that he labeled according to pathologies, which appear to have been sourced mainly from autopsies he performed on women who died at Pro Patria Lying-In Hospital. For instance, in 1846 a patient perished in the aftermath of an embryotomy, and her pelvis was made into a preparation, as an example of a type of pelvis considered pathological because of its 'narrowness.'[40]

Twenty-one pelves were listed under the heading of 'race pelves' in the inventory of 1862, and these came from other sources. They were specified as 'Eskimo,' 'Slavic,' 'Samoyed,' 'Negro,' 'Mulatto,' 'Abyssinian,' 'Mongolian,' 'Javan,' 'Arabian,' 'from the Nicobar Islands,' 'from Peru,' 'from Mexico,' 'Norwegian,' 'Finnish,' 'Greenlandic,' 'Lapp?,' and 'Botocud.'[41] The evidence of the specimens themselves, their labels, and the inventory of 1862 can be correlated to the collecting enterprise and scientific networks of Anders, whose skull-collecting activities began in the 1820s and intensified in the 1840s.[42]

Like the 'race skulls,' the 'race pelves' came from numerous contexts.[43] While Anders published several articles on his theories of race in relation to the skull collection at the Karolinska Institute, documenting where and from whom the specimens had been procured, Magnus rarely made explicit statements about the provenance of his specimens in his publications. Yet names mentioned in Anders's articles appear on labels in Magnus's collection. For example, the pelvis 'from Mexico' was probably sent by the Swedish-Norwegian consul in Montevideo, J. Tarras, who played an active role in describing peoples in South America.[44] Swedish consuls abroad were central for facilitating contact with international colleagues and for the exchange of specimens. The Swedish corvettes and frigates that embarked on trade missions also had a diplomatic role

39 Retzius, 'Om formen af hufvudets benstomme,' 40.

40 Retzius, *Afhandling*, 86.

41 'Professor C M Retzius salubrev.'

42 Ljungström, 'Swedish Golgotha,' 167–68.

43 Ninety-five names of people who supplied Anders Retzius with skulls or plaster casts thereof have been identified, the majority being active in the study of anatomy. Ljungström, 'Swedish Golgotha,' 168.

44 Pelvis preparation, object D75, text on the label: 'Pelv. Femina. Mexikana. Dedit Tarras. Nautica. Mus. Obstetr.' Tarras is mentioned in Retzius, 'Cranium af Pampasindian,' 191.

in establishing relationships with local powers. By way of this infrastructure, scholars in Sweden were supplied with observations and specimens of various kinds—geological, botanical, and ethnographic.[45]

Magnus went abroad on study trips to the German lands, France, and England four times over the years, but never ventured beyond the borders of Europe.[46] Consequently he was dependent on other means of obtaining specimens from distant lands. Collecting enterprises in general relied on available means of communication and networks for accessing and transporting objects from afar.[47] Trade and nation-building projects were features of the colonial context in which pelves and skulls were acquired.[48]

3 Prehistory, Scandinavianism, and the Nation-Building Project

The specimens in the Retzius brothers' collections related to how Sweden participated in world trade and politics in different ways, as well as being associated with the wider connections between borders and form in the sense of territory, epochs, and bones. The map of the world was being redrawn by European powers when Magnus and Anders started assembling their collections. The Napoleonic Wars reshaped alliances and borders, with major consequences for Sweden. In 1809 Sweden lost Finland to Russia. In 1814 it lost Eastern Prussia and entered a union with Norway. Finally, in 1818 it gained a new royal dynasty, headed by one of Napoleon Bonaparte's former generals.[49]

In the following decades new collective identities were forged in response to these changes, which defined who belonged together, who did not, and in what ways.[50] Many European states struggled with the formation of new identities in the political turmoil that followed the Napoleonic Wars, and in this context the construction of a shared past was central.[51] When a new Swedish constitution was ratified after a coup d'état in 1809, the nation was no longer equivalent

45 The corvette *Carlskrona* had been instructed by the king, when mooring in Buenos Aires in 1846, to sign a declaration of acknowledgement of the newly founded Argentinian Confederation. Sylvan, *Korvetten Carlskrona sista resa*, 36–38.

46 'Biografi.'

47 Sysling, *Racial Science*, 28–30.

48 This broad approach to colonialism has been put forward as fruitful. Naum and Nordin, 'Introduction'; Fur, 'Colonialism and Swedish History.'

49 Björk, 'Overlapping Histories,' 20–24.

50 Hall, 'Social Construction of Nationalism,' 94–95.

51 Jensen, 'Makten över forntiden.'

with the sovereign alone; instead 'the people' became integral and thus newly in need of definition.[52]

Professionals within the Swedish state gained influence and were involved in shaping the new identity of the nation, of which the construction and preservation of historical heritage was part.[53] In the early and mid-nineteenth century, the discipline of archaeology emerged from antiquarianism and played a key role in nationalistic discourses. In 1811 the Geatish Society was founded in Stockholm by a group of friends. Part of the state administration of antiquities and history, these individuals were influential in shaping the new Swedish nationalism by investigating, and at the same time constructing, Sweden's past. The term 'Göthisk' hinted at a group of people and emphasized a quintessential Swedishness.[54]

As the individual nations of Norway, Sweden, and Denmark were reshaped and consolidated in the early nineteenth century, a sense of a shared identity called Scandinavianism was also promoted.[55] In the previous century this academic movement had centered on professional collaborations, especially between scholars in Lund and Copenhagen. In the 1820s political tension limited contact, but when restrictions were lifted in the 1830s, several scholars on both sides romanticized the idea of a shared identity as 'Scandinavians.' This notion became politically prominent in the 1840s, when the desire to merge the Scandinavian countries into a single political entity was articulated in academic circles.[56] The Retzius brothers largely conducted their inquiries into human variation within this context.

In July 1839 meetings of the Scandinavian naturalists were inaugurated in Gothenburg, Sweden. Based on German and British models, this would become a regular event throughout the century, held in different cities in the region.[57] In this setting, the Danish professor of anatomy Ib Pedersen Ibsen became a supplier for the Retzius brothers. Several specimens found their way into the Stockholm collections through Ibsen.[58]

52 Hilson, 'Denmark, Norway, and Sweden,' 195–97.

53 Jensen, 'Makten över forntiden,' 54–55.

54 Molin, 'Den rätta tidens mått.'

55 Hilson, 'Denmark, Norway, and Sweden.'

56 Eriksson, '"I andans kraft, på sanningens stråt… ."'

57 Eriksson, '"I andans kraft, på sanningens stråt … ,"' 151.

58 Ibsen donated two unspecified anatomical preparations to the museum at the Karolinska Institute during the meeting of the Scandinavian naturalists in 1842, and these gifts were considered so valuable that he was thanked with a gold medal. Protocol for September 5, 1842, paragraph 11.

Among other things, Magnus received the 'Greenlandic' pelvis plaster cast from the Danish professor. The pelvis 'from the Nicobar Islands' was also bought from Ibsen, who likely acquired it, as well as the 'Greenlandic' original, through the Danish colonial infrastructure.[59] At the meeting of the Scandinavian naturalists in 1850, 'Professor Ibsen held a lecture about the inhabitants of the Nicobarian Islands and showed crania along with pelves of these subjects of the Danish crown.'[60] Lecturing and displaying specimens in this setting were ways of connecting near and distant geographies, as well as authenticating specimens. The meetings of the Scandinavian naturalists provided a space where nation-building projects were articulated and reinforced through the display and exchange of such objects.

The mere specimens were not sufficient in themselves. Recording and organizing information about their provenance and related observations was also considered imperative.[61] The names of the individuals who donated, exchanged, or sold a preparation to the collector were often written on the very bones of the pelves, as they were on skulls. The racial category to which the pelvis was assigned was also often inscribed on the surface and announced membership in a group, either by a racial designation or a geographical/national origin.

The colonial enterprises of European kingdoms, such as Denmark, had created opportunities for obtaining and transporting bodies and ethnographic materials from different parts of the world to collectors in Europe. Even though Sweden was not one of the major colonial powers, Swedish collectors still took part in this flow of goods. Moreover, Sweden had a long colonial history in the northern parts of the country, where the Sámi population (the so-called Lapps) in the Sápmi region ('Lapponia') was subjected to a colonial regime.[62]

It is likely that the question mark in 'Lapp pelvis?' in the inventory of 1862 indicates uncertainties about its provenance. For the Retzius brothers it was important to know whether a skull or a pelvis could be authenticated as having derived from a specific group of people. This concern was shared by other scholars interested in the reasons for human variation, such as the British skull collector Joseph Barnard Davis.[63] The question mark probably signifies that

59 'Professor C M Retzius salubrev.' The Danish colonial infrastructure is mentioned in Naum and Nordin, 'Introduction,' 6.

60 Retzius, 'Kort redogörelse,' 446.

61 Roque, 'Stories, Skulls, and Colonial Collections.'

62 Nordin and Ojala, 'Collecting, Connecting, Constructing.'

63 MacDonald, 'Corpse Stories.'

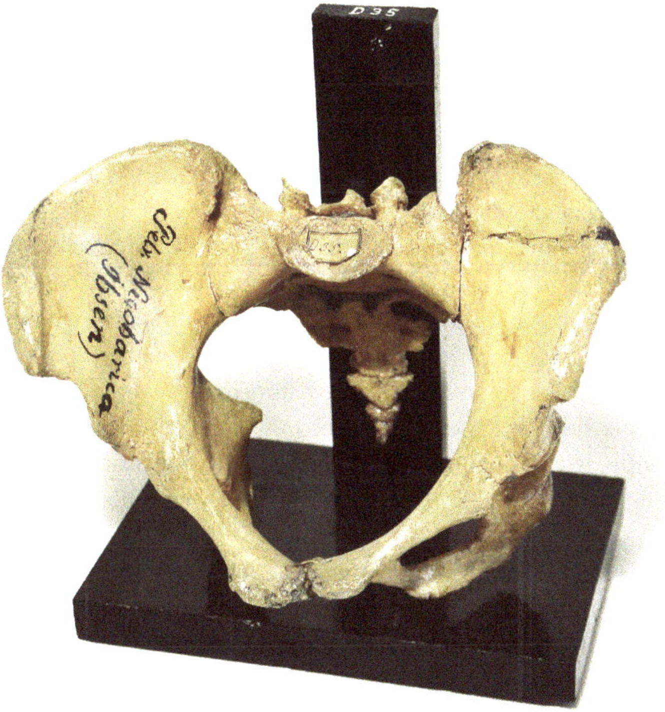

FIGURE 5.3 The pelvis preparations in the collection were often, like skulls, separated from the rest of the skeleton and a racial category, such as 'Nicobarian,' written on the bones. Through this practice, scholars produced the very same racial categories. Magnus Retzius bought this specimen from Ib Pedersen Ibsen around 1850. Object D35, UMM 408, Museum of Medical History, Uppsala. Photo: Helena Franzén.

the provenance had not been properly established, or that the specimen had been obtained from someone who was not deemed entirely trustworthy.[64]

A pelvis in Magnus's collection was labeled as 'Finnish,' and in the inventory of 1862 it was annotated as 'genuine Finnish.'[65] This is a likely indication that the pelvis was considered to be representative for Finns. This pelvis was a gift from Evert Julius Bonsdorff, a professor of anatomy in Finland who had studied with Anders in Stockholm. Anders had received several crania deemed

64 Sysling, '"Not Everything That Says Java."'

65 'Professor C M Retzius salubrev'; Pelvis preparation, object D90, described as 'Finnish' on the label.

'genuine' from Bonsdorff, and the authenticating factor was his credibility, underscored by their personal relationship.[66]

Multiple factors had to be considered in the authentication of Sámi individuals. Anders stated that since they were buried in the same churchyards as Swedish and Finnish settlers, it could not be assumed that disinterred bodies belonged to one or the other group. Nevertheless, he asserted that several reliable individuals had supplied him with crania from the Sámi, which were acquired from contexts in which their origins were certain, such as forensic autopsies when the physician knew the ethnicity of the deceased person.[67]

The issue of authenticity and representativeness was entangled with antiquarianism, which, like natural history, was associated with categorizations of territory, epochs, and form. Enquiries into prehistory and concerns that specimens have 'genuine' origins tapped into the ongoing Swedish nation-building project, along with ideas about a shared past, cultural customs, and language. Similar developments occurred in Britain, France, Germany, Finland, Norway, and Denmark.[68]

Many of Anders's inquiries into racial categorization were closely connected to questions about European prehistory. According to his presentation in 1842, 'the European nations, due to emerging culture and lively trade [have] already been in quite close contact with each other for several centuries,' a situation that called for caution: 'one has to make sure that the specimens used for examinations are of pure and unmixed stock.'[69] Anders regretted, for example, that while it would have been easy to obtain specimens from the dissections halls in Copenhagen, it would not be possible to ascertain which group they belonged to, since people were too mobile in that area.[70]

One way to access bodies that could be securely attributed to a certain group was to unearth prehistoric burials. This practice represents a key intersection between early nineteenth-century inquiries into human variation and antiquarianism. Anders and Sven Nilsson, professor of zoology at Lund University, were prominent figures in this area, and they influenced each other's works. Nilsson published *Den Skandinaviska Nordens Ur-Invånare* (1838–43), in which he presented a chronology of Sweden's prehistory sorted into 'ages,' which in turn were defined by the material properties of unearthed artifacts.[71]

66 Åhrén, 'Museerna,' 143–44.
67 Retzius, 'Om formen af Nordboarnes kranier,' 23–24.
68 Stig Sørensen, 'Fall of a Nation'; Barton, 'Scandinavianism, Fennomania'; Barton, 'Finland and Norway'; Manias, *Race, Science, and the Nation.*
69 Retzius, 'Om formen af Nordboarnes kranier,' 1.
70 Retzius, 'Om formen af Nordboarnes kranier,' 11.
71 Nicklasson, 'Sven Nilsson,' 161–78.

In this work Nilsson also equated certain artifacts and ages with certain groups of people, by examining skulls found together with objects such as tools.[72] Anders referenced this publication in 'Om formen af Nordboarnes kranier' (1842) and declared his own intentions to further investigate Nilsson's results, as Nilsson had requested.[73]

Like the Retzius brothers, Nilsson used the comparative method, for which collections of material objects—excavated artifacts and bodies—were imperative. For Nilsson, the locations of the finds were also vital, as they were thought to indicate which regions different 'peoples' had inhabited. Groups of people, territory, and epochs were thought to be interlocking. As highlighted in previous research, Nilsson was influenced by Cuvier, with whom he had studied; thus, sorting people and things into types was a given feature in his research.[74] Several specimens from prehistoric burials were incorporated into the collection at the Karolinska Institute. For example, Sven Lovén had obtained a cranium from Norway in this way; he brought it back to Sweden and gifted it to the museum.[75]

4 The 'Swedes' and the 'Others'

At the meeting of the Scandinavian naturalists in Copenhagen in 1847, Magnus presented his investigations into the form of female pelves from people inhabiting the Scandinavian peninsula, which he later published in a short article. Judging from the setting and the topic, this paper was heavily influenced by the current tides of Scandinavianism and nationalism. In his account, Magnus distinguished the following categories of pelvic forms: 'Geatish,' 'Lapp,' and 'Finnish.' This division was based on previous studies, which, he remarked, demonstrated distinctive differences between the cranial forms of these peoples.[76] This declaration most likely hinted at his brother's influential publication 'Om formen af Nordboarnes kranier.' In contrast to pelvis preparations implicitly categorized as 'Swedish,' which he could easily access via the lying-in hospital, pelves attributed to other racial categories were fewer. Magnus shed

72 Nilsson, *Skandinaviska Nordens Ur-Invånare*.
73 Retzius, 'Om formen af Nordboarnes kranier,' 1.
74 Ljungström, 'Oscariansk antropologi,' 226–38.
75 Retzius, 'Om formen af Nordboarnes kranier,' 17–18.
76 Retzius, 'Bäckenets form,' 836–39.

light on what he considered to be racial differences of the pelvis in terms of general form, as well as the shape and angles of the pelvic canal.[77]

In the same vein as the abovementioned article, Magnus also produced *Icones pelvium gentium Scandinavia*.[78] The nature of this work is not firmly established, and we do not know when, or whether, it was published. It was likely an atlas in which the forms of the 'Scandinavian pelves' were illustrated and probably produced in the late 1840s. Moreover, the overlaps between the contents of the collection, the article, and the atlas itself suggest that the illustrations were drawings based on specimens in the collection. The title accentuated that although Magnus's collection contained pelves from farther away, the 'Scandinavian forms' interested him the most, and his perceptions were entangled with those of his brother and Nilsson.

Magnus stated that Finland was not part of Scandinavia, but that many Finns lived within the northern peninsula, along with Sámi; thus it was of interest to identify them. He argued that the form of the 'Norwegian pelvis' was equivalent to 'the Geatish,' which in turn was considered to be similar to those of the 'Germanic tribes.'[79] Previous research has noted Nilsson's proposal that 'Germanic tribes' immigrated to what was to become Sweden at the beginning of the Iron Age.[80] Nilsson argued that the 'ages' corresponded to different degrees of cultural development; thus he considered the 'Germanic tribes' to be more advanced than the peninsula's previous inhabitants, of whom he considered the Sámi to be the last remnants.[81]

In his 1848 dissertation, Magnus stated that he had chosen to focus on 'the situation in our own country and the Swedish-Geatish species of the Germanic folk tribe, which inhabit the Scandinavian peninsula from Scania to the Lapponian mountains.'[82] His obstetrical practice was thus implicitly enmeshed in ideas about race. Magnus noted that even though forms could be attributed to specific groups, they did not necessarily correspond to contemporary patients. This, he thought, was due to mixing between individuals from different groups.[83] Magnus's perception of human variation involved groups that were inherently different from each other, as well as static, if there was no 'mixing.' This notion of differences between 'Scandinavian pelves' was rooted in the idea that such differences were congenital, not the consequence of external stimuli:

77 Retzius, 'Bäckenets form,' 836–39.

78 It is listed as a printed work in 'Biografi.'

79 Retzius, 'Bäckenets form.'

80 Ljungström, 'Oscariansk antropologi,' 295, 311.

81 Nilsson, *Skandinaviska Nordens Ur-Invånare*, 2, 103.

82 Retzius, *Afhandling*, 15. His use of the word 'species' is probably a slip, since he did not explicitly take the position of polygenesis.

83 Retzius, *Afhandling*, 14–15.

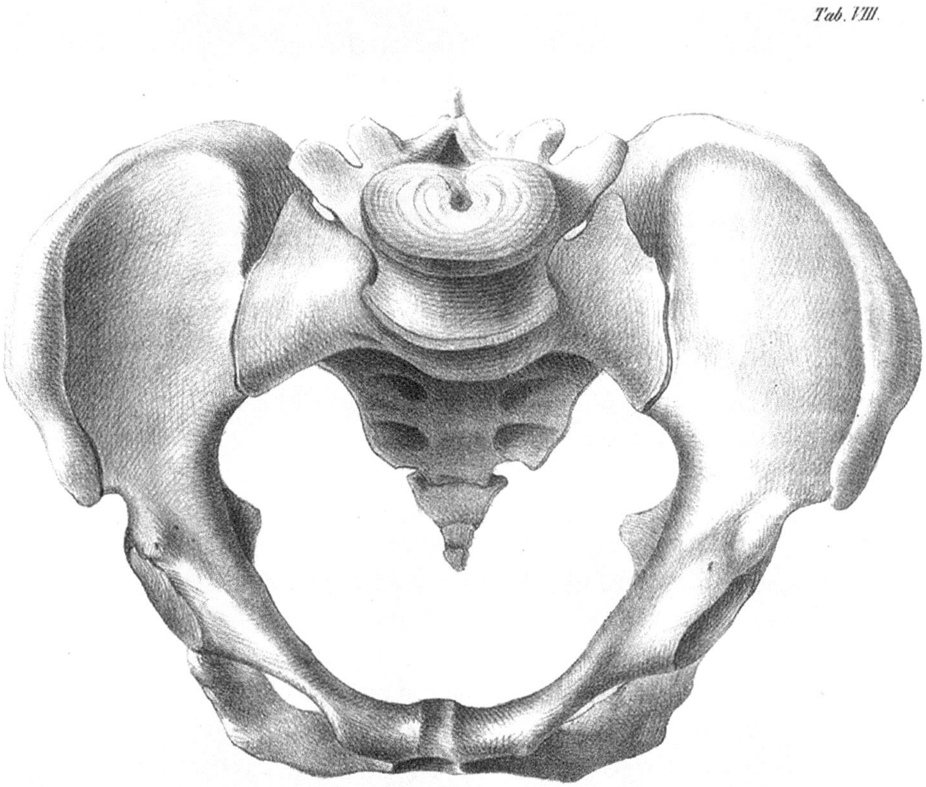

FIGURE 5.4 Lithograph of the form of a 'Swedish' pelvis in an atlas of pelvic forms. It is likely that the atlas is a copy, or a proof, of Magnus Retzius, *Icones pelvium gentium Scandinavia* (late 1840s). This particular volume was part of the library which previously belonged to the Swedish Society of Medicine. Neither originator or date is attached, but the content suggests that this is Magnus Retzius's work. Private collection of Olof Edlund.

> The differences, which this examination exposes, seem to me to have been too great to be explained only as consequences of the habits, customs, and ways of living influencing these races. Therefore, there is substantial reason to assume that they [the differences] stem from a specific destined development type, which is congenital, and which has remained as true to form as the form of their crania.[84]

While Magnus stated that the 'Finnish' and 'Lapp' pelves had their own distinct forms, he discerned no differences between the 'Geatish' and the 'Norwegian'

84 Retzius, 'Bäckenets form,' 839.

types. It is likely that this stance was influenced by the fact that Finland was no longer a part of Sweden, while Sweden and Norway had been unified. The Sámi, who for a long time had been described as other by representatives of the Swedish state, were continually articulated as different. Pelves were used as identity markers of peoples. The peoples were simultaneously described and created in determining who belonged and who did not. Political circumstances were therefore paramount in the identity formation of the Swedish nation, and women's pelves were one means to distinguish who were Swedes and who were others.

5 Conclusion

This chapter has demonstrated that the motivations for assembling and designating 'race pelves' in Magnus Retzius's collection were entangled with nationalism. The collecting and use of the pelves were connected to the formation of Swedish national identity in the first half of the nineteenth century, through the construction of a past in which antiquarianism and Scandinavianism were enmeshed. Material artifacts and the forms of bones were used as evidence in inquiries into prehistory, to attest to the presence of certain groups of people in a certain territory, at a specific point in time. Thus pelves were, along with skulls and artifacts, empirical foundations of the nation-building project and means of defining who the 'Swedish people' were.

While Anders Retzius focused on skulls, Magnus opted for pelves because of his obstetrical interests. The study of pelves enabled him to theorize about connections between women's bodies and civilization, in which ideas about sex and race intersected. The core of what constituted the connection between race and sex was the idea that women's bodies had a mechanical function, which manifested when giving birth. This tied in with ideas about race and pathology, in which the pathological was constructed in terms of function. Magnus did not explicitly state in his writings that he considered 'Swedish' pelves pathological by default, but that narrow pelves were a common problem. However, he positioned himself as an expert who had the knowledge to manage difficult labors brought on by this condition. The Retzius brothers used their collections as empirical foundations and argued that the degree of 'cultural development' dictated the form of the skull and the pelves, which in turn generated consequences in childbirth. The pathology of 'too-narrow' pelves was constructed in relation to the size of fetuses and implied to be a result of civilization.

Bibliography

Åhrén, Eva. 'Making Space for Specimens: The Museums of the Karolinska Institute, Stockholm.' In *Medical Museums: Past, Present, Future*, edited by Samuel J. M. M. Alberti and Elizabeth Hallam, 102–15. London: Royal College of Surgeons, 2013.

Åhrén, Eva. 'Museerna: Vetenskap i tre dimensioner.' In *Medicinen blir till vetenskap: Karolinska Institutet under två århundraden*, edited by Karin Johannisson, Ingemar Nilsson, and Roger Qvarsell, 126–69. Stockholm: Karolinska Institutet University Press, 2010.

Alberti, Samuel J. M. M. *Nature and Culture: Objects, Disciplines and the Manchester Museum*. Manchester: Manchester University Press, 2009.

Augstein, Hannah Franziska. *Race: The Origins of an Idea, 1760–1850*. Bristol: Thoemnes, 1996.

Barton, H. Arnold. 'Finland and Norway, 1808–1917.' *Scandinavian Journal of History* 31, no. 3–4 (2006): 221–36.

Barton, H. Arnold. 'Scandinavianism, Fennomania, and the Crimean War.' *Journal of Baltic Studies* 36, no. 2 (2005): 131–56.

Björk, Ragnar. 'The Overlapping Histories of Sweden and Norway: The Union from 1814–1905.' In *Disputed Territories and Shared Pasts: Overlapping National Histories in Modern Europe*, edited by Tibor Frank and Frank Hadler, 17–34. New York: Palgrave Macmillan, 2011.

Cházaro, Laura. 'From Anatomical Collection to National Museum, ca 1895: How Skulls and Female Pelvises Began to Speak the Language of Mexican National History.' In *Beyond Alterity: Destabilizing the Indigenous Other in Mexico*, edited by Paula López Caballero and Adriana Acevedo-Rodrigo, 173–98. Tucson: University of Arizona Press, 2018.

Cházaro, Laura. 'Mexican Women's Pelves and Obstetrical Procedures: Interventions with Forceps in Late 19th-Century Medicine.' Translated by Paul Kersey. *Feminist Review* 79, no. 1 (2005): 100–115.

Conklin, Alice L. *In the Museum of Man: Race, Anthropology, and Empire in France, 1850–1950*. Ithaca, NY: Cornell University Press, 2013.

Curry, Helen Anne, Nick Jardine, James Secord, and Emma Spary, eds. *Worlds of Natural History*. Cambridge: Cambridge University Press, 2018.

Dias, Nélia. 'Séries de crânes et armée de squelettes: Les collections anthropologiques en France dans la seconde moitié du xixe siècle.' *Bulletins et Memoires de la société d'anthropologie de Paris Nouvelle Séri* 1, no. 3–4 (1989): 203–30.

Dias, Nélia. 'The Visibility of Difference: Nineteenth-Century French Anthropological Collections.' In *The Politics of Display: Museums, Science, Culture*, edited by Sharon MacDonald, 36–52. London: Routledge, 1998.

Eriksson, Nils. *'I andans kraft, på sannings stråt ...': De skandinaviska naturforskarmötena 1839–1936*. Göteborg: Göteborgs universitet, 1991.

Fabian, Ann. *The Skull Collectors: Race, Science, and America's Unburied Dead*. Chicago: University of Chicago Press, 2010.

Fausto-Sterling, Anne. 'Gender, Race, and Nation: The Comparative Anatomy of "Hottentot" Women in Europe, 1815–1817.' In *Deviant Bodies: Critical Perspectives of Difference in Science and Popular Culture*, edited by Jennifer Terry and Jacqueline Urla, 19–48. Bloomington: Indiana University Press, 1995.

Fur, Gunlög. 'Colonialism and Swedish History: Unthinkable Connections?' In *Scandinavian Colonialism and the Rise of Modernity: Small Time Agents in a Global Arena*, edited by Magdalena Naum and Jonas M. Nordin, 17–36. New York: Springer, 2013.

Gould, Stephen Jay. *The Mismeasure of Man*. 1981. London: Penguin Books, 1997.

Grant, Joanna. '"Those Parts Peculiar to Her Organization": Some Observations on the History of Pelvimetry, a Nearly Forgotten Obstetric Sub-speciality.' In *The Female Body in Medicine and Literature*, edited by Andrew Mangham and Greta Depledge, 135–47. Liverpool: Liverpool University Press, 2011.

Hall, Patrik. *The Social Construction of Nationalism: Sweden as an Example*. Lund: Lund University, 1998.

Hendriksen, Marieke. 'The Fate of the Beaded Babies: Forgotten Early Colonial Anatomy.' In *The Fate of Anatomical Collections*, edited by Rina Knoeff and Robert Zwijnenberg, 179–94. Farnham: Ashgate, 2015.

Higgins, Alfred. 'Note on Certain Scandinavian Museums.' *Journal of the Anthropological Society of London* 5 (1867): 14–19.

Hilson, Mary. 'Denmark, Norway, and Sweden: Pan-Scandinavism and Nationalism.' In *What Is a Nation? Europe 1789–1914*, edited by Timothy Baycroft and Mark Hewitson, 192–209. Oxford: Oxford University Press, 2006.

Hoyme, Lucile E. 'Physical Anthropology and Its Instruments.' *Southwestern Journal of Anthropology* 9, no. 4 (1953): 408–30.

Jensen, Ola Wolfhechel. 'Makten över forntiden: Exempel från den svensk-finska arkeologin och minnesvården.' In *Att återupptäcka det glömda: Aktuell forskning om forntidens förflutna i Norden*, edited by Påvel Nicklasson and Bodil Peterson, 51–70. Lund: Lund University, 2012.

Ljungström, Olof. *Oscariansk antropologi: Exotism, förhistoria och rasforskning som vetenskaplig människosyn*. Uppsala: Uppsala universitet, 2002.

Ljungström, Olof. 'Swedish Golgotha: Anders Retzius' Collection of Human Crania at the Karolinska Institutet According to an 1862 Manuscript.' *Lychnos* (2014): 159–71.

MacDonald, Helen. 'Corpse Stories: Anatomy, Bodies and a Colonial World.' In *Bodies beyond Borders: Moving Anatomies, 1750–1950*, edited by Kaat Wils, Raf de Bont, and Sokhieng Au, 73–90. Leuven: Leuven University Press, 2017.

MacDonald, Helen. *Human Remains: Dissection and Its Histories*. New Haven, CT: Yale University Press, 2006.

MacGregor, Arthur, ed. *Naturalists in the Field: Collecting, Recording and Preserving the Natural World from the Fifteenth to the Twenty-First Century*. Leiden: Brill, 2018.

Manias, Chris. *Race, Science, and the Nation: Reconstructing the Ancient Past in Britain, France, and Germany*. New York: Routledge, 2013.

Martin, Emily. *The Woman in the Body: A Cultural Analysis of Reproduction*. Boston: Beacon Press, 1987.

Molin, Torkel. *Den rätta tidens mått: Göthiska förbundet, fornforskningen och det antikvariska landskapet*. Umeå: Umeå universitet, 2003.

Naum, Magdalena, and Jonas M. Nordin. 'Introduction: Situating Scandinavian Colonialism.' In *Scandinavian Colonialism and the Rise of Modernity: Small Time Agents in a Global Arena*, edited by Magdalena Naum and Jonas M. Nordin, 3–16. New York: Springer, 2013.

Nicklasson, Påvel. 'Sven Nilsson och Den skandinaviska Nordens Ur-Invånare.' *Fornvännen* 106 (2011): 161–78.

Nilsson, Sven. *Skandinaviska Nordens Ur-Invånare, ett försök i komparativa Ethnografien och ett bidrag till människoslägtets historia*, 1838–43. Stockholm: Norstedt, 1862–64.

Nordin, Jonas M., and Carl-Gösta Ojala. 'Collecting, Connecting, Constructing: Early Modern Commodification and Globalization of Sámi Material Culture.' *Journal of Material Culture* 23, no. 1 (2018): 58–82.

Pickstone, John V. *Ways of Knowing: A New History of Science, Technology, and Medicine*. Chicago: University of Chicago Press, 2001.

Qureshi, Sadiah. 'Displaying Sara Baartman, the "Hottentot Venus."' *History of Science* 42, no. 2 (2004): 233–57.

Qureshi, Sadiah. 'Robert Gordon Latham, Displayed Peoples, and the Natural History of Race, 1854–1866.' *Historical Journal* 54, no. 1 (2011): 143–66.

Qvarsell, Roger. 'Patriotism, paternalism och offentlig vård: Pro Patrias barnbördshus 1774–1951.' In *För det allmänna bästa: Ett kungligt sällskap mellan stat och marknad under 250 år: Kungl. Sällskapet Pro Patria 1766–2016*, edited by Erik Amnå, 49–115. Stockholm: Kungl. Sällskapet Pro Patria och Bokförlaget Atlantis, 2016.

Reinarz, Jonathan. 'The Age of Museum Medicine: The Rise and Fall of the Medical Museum at Birmingham's School of Medicine.' *Social History of Medicine* 18, no 3 (2005): 419–37.

Retzius, Anders. 'Cranium af Pampasindian [1855].' In *Anders Retzii samlade skrifter af ethnologiskt innehåll*, edited by Gustaf Retzius, 190–97. Stockholm: Svenska läkaresällskapet, 1864.

Retzius, Anders. 'Frenologien bedömd från anatomisk-ethnologisk ståndpunkt [1847].' In *Anders Retzii samlade skrifter af ethnologiskt innehåll*, edited by Gustaf Retzius, 95–120. Stockholm: Svenska läkaresällskapet, 1864.

Retzius, Anders. 'Kort redogörelse för Skandinaviska Naturforskare-Sällskapets 6:te möte i Stockholm år 1851.' *Hygiea* 13, no. 7 (1851): 432–48.

Retzius, Anders. 'Om formen af hufvudets benstomme hos olika folkslag [1844].' In *Anders Retzii samlade skrifter af ethnologiskt innehåll*, edited by Gustaf Retzius, 40–57. Stockholm: Svenska läkaresällskapet, 1864.

Retzius, Anders. 'Om formen af Nordboarnes kranier [1842].' In *Anders Retzii samlade skrifter af ethnologiskt innehåll*, edited by Gustaf Retzius, 1–36. Stockholm: Svenska läkaresällskapet, 1864.

Retzius, Gustaf, ed. *Etnologische Schriften: Nach dem Tode des Verfassers gesammelt*. Stockholm: Svenska läkaresällskapet, 1864.

Retzius, Magnus. *Afhandling om bäckenförträngning*. Stockholm: Norstedt, 1848.

Retzius, Magnus. 'Bäckenets form hos de folk, som bebo den skandinaviska halfön.' *Forhandlinger ved de Skandinaviske Naturforskarnes femte Møde, der holdtes i Kiøbenhavn fra den 12te till den 17te Juli 1847* 5 (1849): 836–39.

Retzius, Magnus. 'Om bäckenplanerna och deras inflytande på fosterhufudets rörelser under en kronbjudnings-förlossning.' *Hygiea* 9 (1847): 65–79.

Rich, Miriam. 'The Curse of Civilised Woman: Race, Gender and the Pain of Childbirth in Nineteenth-Century American Medicine.' *Gender and History* 28, no. 1 (2016): 57–76.

Roque, Ricardo. 'Stories, Skulls, and Colonial Collections.' *Configurations* 19 (2011): 1–23.

Schiebinger, Londa. *The Mind Has No Sex? Women in the Origins of Modern Science*. Cambridge, MA: Harvard University Press, 1989.

Schiebinger, Londa. *Nature's Body: Gender in the Making of Modern Science*. Boston: Beacon Press, 1993.

Stig Sørensen, Marie Louise. 'The Fall of a Nation, the Birth of a Subject: The National Use of Archaeology in Nineteenth-Century Denmark.' In *Nationalism and Archaeology in Europe*, edited by Margarita Díaz-Andreu and Timothy Champion, 24–47. London: UCL Press, 1995.

Stocking, George. *Victorian Anthropology*. New York: Free Press, 1987.

Svanberg, Fredrik. *Människosamlarna: Anatomiska museer och rasvetenskap i Sverige, ca 1850–1950*. Stockholm: Historiska museet, 2015.

Svanberg, Fredrik. 'The World as Collected: Or, Museum Collections as Situated Materialities.' In *Museum Theory*, edited by Andrea Wicomb and Kylie Message, 389–415. Chichester: John Wiley, 2015.

Sylvan, O. R. *Korvetten Carlskrona sista resa: Inmönstrad 5/8 1845, förlist i Floridagolfen 30/4 1846*. Stockholm: Marinlitteraturföreningen, 1996.

Sysling, Fenneke. '"Not Everything That Says Java Is from Java": Provenance and the Fate of Physical Anthropology Collections.' In *The Fate of Anatomical Collections*, edited by Rina Knoeff and Robert Zwijnenberg, 195–210. Farnham: Ashgate, 2015.

Sysling, Fenneke. *Racial Science and Human Diversity in Colonial Indonesia.* Singapore: National University of Singapore Press, 2016.

Wellenbergh, J. H. J. *Abhandlung über einen Pelvimeter; nebst Wahrnehmungen* über die *Anwendung desselben.* Haag 1831.

Archival Sources and Museum Collections

'Biografi.' Sekreterarens arkiv, k. 27c:1. CHS. [Unsigned, handwritten document about the life of Magnus Retzius, registered at the archive March 10, 1869]

Pelvis preparation, object D75, UMM 408. Museum of Medical History, Uppsala. [Many of the objects which once constituted Magnus Retzius's collection are now catalogued under the organizational unit UMM.]

Pelvis preparation, object D90, UMM 408. Museum of Medical History, Uppsala.

'Professor C M Retzius salubrev på åtskilliga instrumenter och preparater till kirurgiska institutionen 1862.' Medicinska fakulteten, FIV Övriga handlingar 1:5. Uppsala University Archive. [Sales contract between Magnus Retzius and Uppsala University with an inventory of the objects]

Protocol for September, 5, 1842. Karolinska Institutet kansliet 1828–1964, AIA Protokoll med bilagor, 4. NAS, Täby.

Retzius, Magnus. An atlas of lithographs of 'Scandinavian pelves,' probably the unpublished *Icones pelvium gentium Scandinavia* from the late 1840s. Private collection of Olof Edlund.

Wellenbergh's pelvimeter. UMM 0247. Museum of Medical History, Uppsala.

CHAPTER 6

Embryology and the Clinic: Early to Mid-twentieth-Century Stories of Pregnancy, Abortion, and Fetal Collecting

Solveig Jülich

Embryological collections at Lund University in the south of Sweden date back to the eighteenth century. As elsewhere, anatomists started to assemble dead fetuses from humans and animals, transforming them into specimens for scientific and educational purposes. Both normal fetal bodies and 'teratological monsters' were sought after. In tandem with the establishment of modern embryology and evolutionary theory, these collections expanded in number and scope, and also came to include scaled-up wax models of fetal development. In 1934 Lund University became a location for an embryological research institute: the Tornblad Institute for Comparative Embryology, modeled on the famous Department of Embryology of the Carnegie Institution of Washington in Boston as well as the Hubrecht Laboratory in Utrecht. It was made possible through a donation from the Swedish businessman Hjalmar Tornblad, and directed by the anatomist Ivar Broman.[1]

This chapter explores the expansion of the embryological collection at Lund University, first located within the Anatomy Department and then the Tornblad Institute, in the first half of the twentieth century. Focusing on the human specimens in the collection, I aim to show how a reproductive bioeconomy emerged around the collecting of embryos and fetuses from women's interrupted pregnancies. Drawing on annual reports from Lund University as well as letters in Broman's archive, I highlight how the collection relied on the establishment of an informal network of physicians and midwives—and increasingly, gynecological clinics—who eagerly saved specimens for science. In addition, I use a selection of patient records to bring to light the stories of

1 For a more extensive history of the Tornblad Institute and its embryological collection, see Thomas Nilsson and Jülich, *Embryologiska rum*. A smaller part of the specimens has been preserved and is now kept at the Biological Museum at Lund University, whereas the records and other objects are held at Lund University Archive and the Medical Faculty of Lund University, respectively. For the two other institutes, see Maienschein, Glitz, and Allen, *Centennial History*, vol. 2; Faasse, Faber, and Narraway, 'Brief History.'

 | DOI:10.1163/9789004703759_008

some of the women whose miscarriages and abortions made the collection possible. Finally, I discuss to what extent ethical principles and values guided Broman and his colleagues in their collecting enterprise.[2]

My chapter draws on international research that has highlighted the emergence of reproductive bioeconomies during the twentieth century.[3] In particular, I rely on the work of scholars who have shown how the establishment of the embryological view of development intersected with the social, cultural, and material history of embryo collecting. Nick Hopwood has detailed how, in the 1870s, the German anatomist Wilhelm His set up an exemplary 'supply network' of scientists and physicians to obtain early embryos from abortions and miscarriages for his foundational work in human embryology.[4] Lynn Morgan's account of the American anatomist Franklin P. Mall's embryo collecting in the early twentieth century describes the 'embryo economy' that had to be in place before the Carnegie Institution of Washington collection could be consolidated.[5] With a few exceptions, neither Hopwood nor Morgan was able to trace back or gain access to the patient records related to the specimen collections of His and Mall.[6] Thus, this chapter contributes an important perspective that has been largely missing in earlier historical studies on embryo and fetal collecting.[7]

1 Establishing a Reproductive Bioeconomy

Ivar Broman was born and raised in Skåne, southern Sweden. He studied medicine at Lund University and became a doctor of medicine in 1899. After spending a few years as a professor in Uppsala, he returned to Lund and was appointed professor of anatomy. In 1927 he was elected as a member of the

2 In the medical context I study, the words 'egg,' 'embryo,' and 'fetus' are used interchangeably. I largely follow the actors' practice.

3 For instance, Catherine Waldby has used the concept of 'reproductive bioeconomy' to highlight how female reproductive biology has increasingly come to function as a valuable economic asset, albeit one that is often positioned outside economic value, including surplus embryos left over from IVF. See Waldby, 'Production and Reproduction.' For an extended analysis, see Waldby and Cooper, 'Biopolitics of Reproduction.'

4 Hopwood, 'Producing Development,' 38–39.

5 Morgan, *Icons of Life*, 61, 69–90. For a discussion on how embryologists converted fetal remains into valuable scientific material see also her "'Properly Disposed of.'"

6 Morgan, *Icons of Life*, 141; Hopwood, 'Producing Development,' 41. This is also true of Franzén's work on the embryo collecting of Swedish anatomist August Hammar. See Franzén, "'Precious Material.'"

7 For an account that builds on women's private correspondence, see Withycombe, *Lost*.

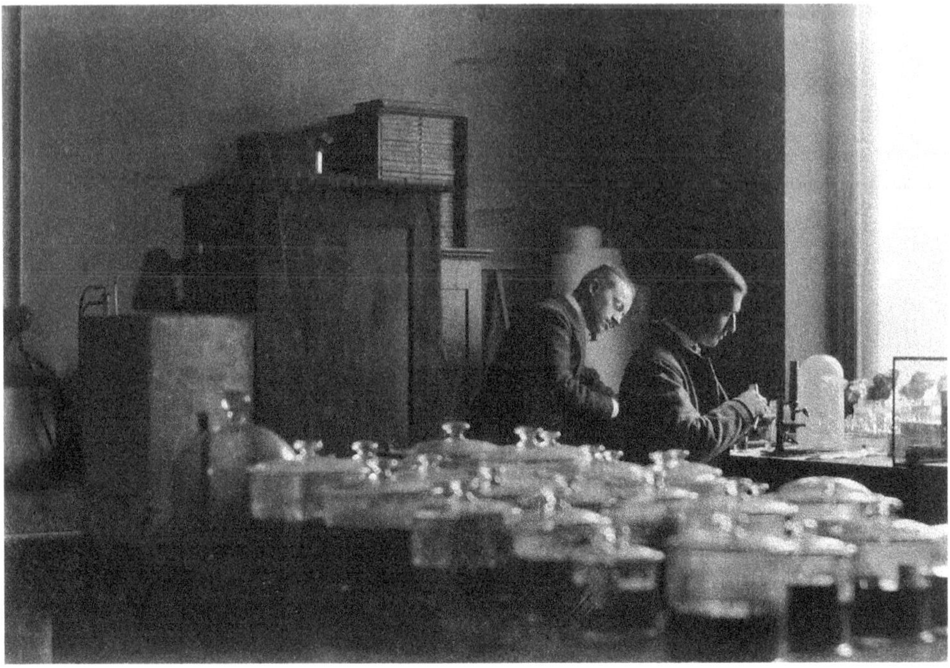

FIGURE 6.1 Two students at the histological laboratory of Lund University in 1893. Ivar Broman (*right*) drawing sections for his first reconstruction of a human embryo (three millimeters) and Elis Essen-Möller (*left*) cutting sections. Photographer: unknown. The Tornblad Institute Collection, Medical Faculty of Lund University.

Royal Swedish Academy of Sciences and joined international societies such as the Institut International d'Embryologie (today the International Society of Developmental Biologists). In 1933, around the same time as he retired from his position as professor of anatomy, he became the director of the Tornblad Institute, and continued to work until his untimely death in 1946.[8]

Throughout his career, Broman was a diligent writer and lecturer on various topics within biology and sexual science. He often presented this work as popular science to signal that the target audience was a larger public. The author's stated intention was to dissolve outdated beliefs about sexuality, reproduction, pregnancy, marriage, and family life. But from today's perspective, the reading is hard to digest, to say the least. Broman, like many others at the time, embraced a hierarchical value system with a supposed biological basis. All creatures, living and dead, were assigned a 'human value' or an 'animal value' that determined their place in a biological hierarchy. Drawing on his research

8 On Broman's biography, see Jülich, 'Historier kring Tornbladinstitutet,' 167–72.

and often using pictures of various kinds, Broman argued that the state should intervene and sterilize deficient individuals, and he was critical of 'race mixing' as well as legal abortion and women who worked outside the home, which he considered to be against their nature. These positions were decidedly eugenic and also aligned with a conservative view of women and the family. As for his opposition to abortion, Broman shared this perspective with an overwhelming majority of physicians in Sweden.[9]

Broman first came into contact with embryology when, as a young assistant at the histological laboratory, he was asked to build a model of the exterior of a three-millimeter-long human embryo (figure 6.1). During his years in Uppsala and more actively after moving back to Lund in 1905, he began to collect embryological material from humans as well as animals. Mainly on the basis of this collection, he wrote a book in German that dealt with normal development and the origin of malformations and 'monstrosities.' This special interest in comparing the development of various animal species was linked to evolutionary theory, including the biogenetic law, proposed by Ernst Haeckel in the 1860s, which stated that the development of an embryo rehearsed the evolutionary history of the species. A second area of interest, also adopted from the German embryological community, was the concept of a 'Bauplan' (body plan), a set of morphological features shared by many members of a group of animals such as vertebrates. Third, he considered some malformations of organs as a regression of development (atavism).[10] In this focus on comparative embryology, Broman relied on collaborative partners who sent him embryos and fetuses from places near and far. Through these partially informal networks, a form of reproductive bioeconomy was created, based on transactions and exchanges other than purely economic ones.

Broman had long experience of coping with the lack of dead bodies for research and education. The difficulty of obtaining dissection material is in fact a recurring problem in the history of anatomy. From the anatomists' point of view, laws and regulations were a double-edged sword: they could either limit or increase the influx of dead bodies. As the expert who led the 1922 government investigation into the procurement of corpses, Broman pushed for regulations that would facilitate medical access to both deceased adults and stillborn children. In this way, 'feebleminded' people and patients who died at publicly funded health care facilities could pay back their debt to society, he

9 Broman's views on these topics are described in Jülich, 'Historier kring Tornbladinstitutet,' 231–44.

10 Broman, *Normale und abnorme Entwicklung des Menschen*. On Broman's scientific interests, see Källén, *Tornblad Institute in Lund*, 7–8.

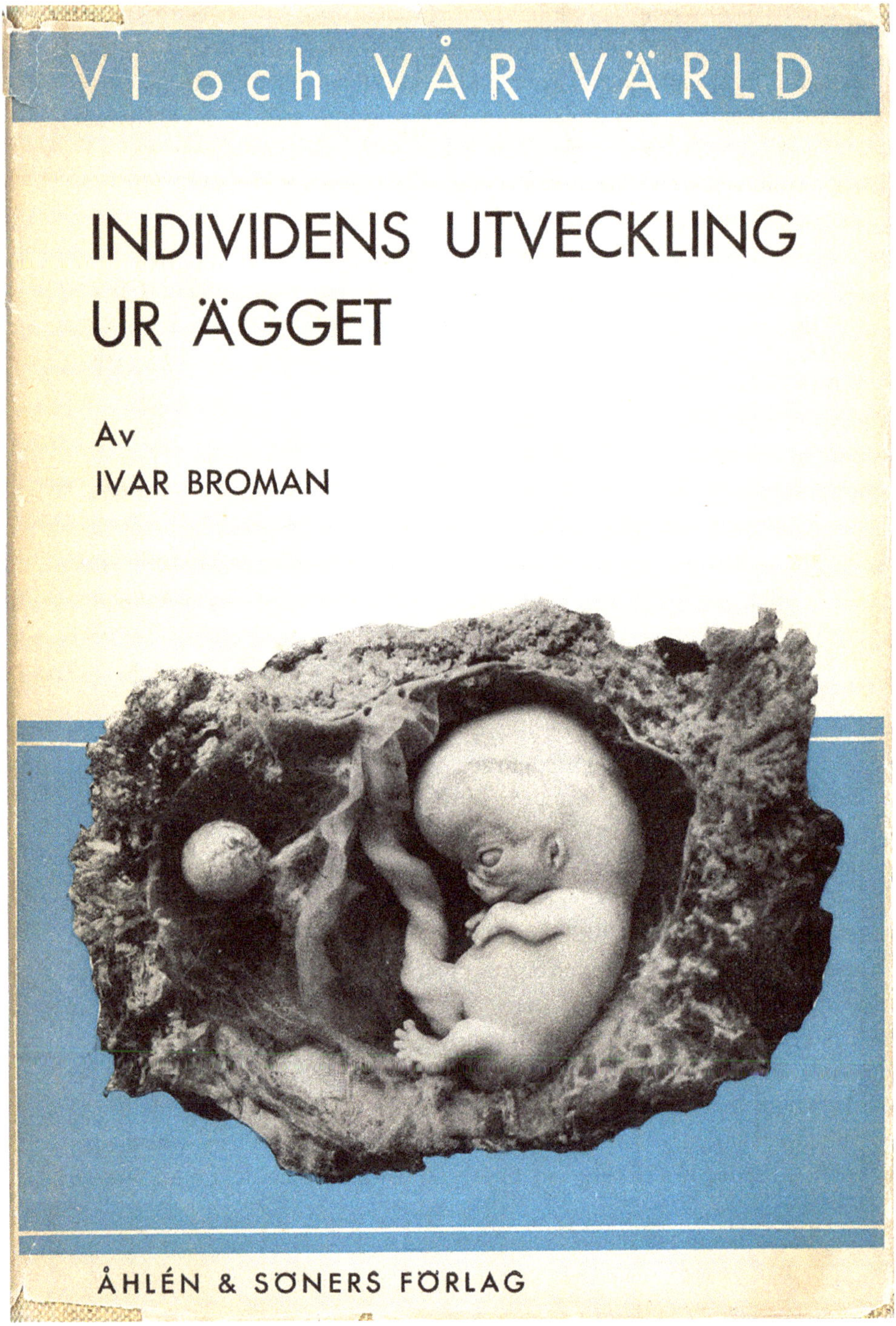

FIGURE 6.2 Pictures of human specimens from the Tornblad Institute collection were widely disseminated. From Broman, *Individens utveckling ur ägget*, front cover.

suggested. Women who sought medical services for miscarriage or abortion could similarly benefit society by leaving their embryos and fetuses to embryological research. This point is not explicitly stated by Broman but follows from his way of arguing.[11]

Yet there was no clear legislation surrounding embryos and fetuses that—through miscarriages, ectopic pregnancies, and abortions—became available for medical purposes. Until the Second World War, a fetus/child had to be born alive in order to be recorded as a child in the population register. In 1940, the definition was changed so that 'child' meant 'every new-born, who breathed after birth, as well as every stillborn of at least thirty-five centimeters in length' (later, length was replaced by age, consistent with the recommendations of the World Health Organization).[12] In practice, this indicated that spontaneously or surgically aborted embryos and fetuses did not have to be reported to the population register (unless illegal abortion was suspected). During Ivar Broman's entire career, abortion material was thus a kind of residual category that did not fall under any existing regulations.

The biggest problem for building Broman's collection was not legal but practical and logistical. The number of dead bodies that accrued to the Anatomy Department was limited, and the majority were male.[13] Material from women's interrupted pregnancies was hard to come by, especially the 'precious' tiny, millimeter-sized embryos that were hidden in blood clots and tissues. Through appeals in medical publications, several anatomists tried to persuade physicians and midwives not to discard tissues from miscarriages and abortions, but instead to preserve and send the material to anatomical institutions. In return, compensation was promised for the preservation and shipping costs.[14] Competition in this reproductive bioeconomy came from obstetricians at the maternity hospitals who advertised in the midwives' magazine *Jordemodern* with similar appeals. These clinically oriented physicians were—in a different way than anatomists and embryologists—interested in transforming the more abstract doctrine of the cause, development, and typology of malformations into concrete knowledge of how to handle complicated births when women's lives and health were at risk.[15] Moreover, Broman urged butchers and hunters

11 Broman, *Utredning och förslag*, 57.

12 Jülich, 'Fosterexperimentens produktiva hemlighet,' 19–20.

13 This is based on a review of annual reports in Lund University, *Lunds universitets årsberättelse*, for the years 1905–33.

14 See, e.g., Hammar, 'Upprop.' This advertisement is discussed in Franzén, '"Precious Material,"' 183.

15 Jülich, 'Historier kring Tornbladinstitutet,' 182. See also the discussion in Franzén, 'From Patient to Specimen.'

not to throw away malformed animal fetuses but rather to send them to a research institution for the benefit of science. What, in the eyes of the public, might be seen as waste could become valuable scientific material in the hands of embryologists.[16]

2 The Fetal Collecting Network

Through these calls and previous personal and institutional contacts, Broman managed to build up an extensive network of people who supplied him with human embryological material. Following the strategy of Wilhelm His and Franklin P. Mall, he recruited various medical actors from near and far. Alongside academics—from medical students to assistants and professors—there were physicians of many different kinds, including private practitioners and those with public posts, as well as a few midwives. One female physicians was included.[17] The majority of these individuals were located in Skåne, but some of them lived and worked in other regions of Sweden. Preserved letters to Broman provide clues that the specimens were sent through the postal service, by train, to Lund.[18]

Increasingly, the fetuses that were transported to the Anatomy Department and the Tornblad Institute came from women's clinics and lying-in hospitals in the region. But this traffic was still highly dependent on Broman's informal contacts and agreements. For instance, Elis Essen-Möller, a former fellow student, supplied fetuses to Broman for more than three decades.[19] He was a professor and chief physician at Lund Hospital's Obstetrics-Gynecology Department from 1901 to 1935 and a driving force behind the new women's clinic that was opened in 1918. Both he and Broman were active members in the Swedish Society for Racial Hygiene, and Essen-Möller carried out the first eugenic sterilizations in Sweden on a female 'idiot' and a woman suffering from epilepsy 'with regard to the offspring and thus also to society.'[20] This happened in 1906 and 1914, respectively—long before the practice was regulated by law.[21]

---

16 Broman, *Vidunder och missfoster*, 128.

17 The persons are listed in Lund University, *Lunds universitets årsberättelse*, under 'Anatomiska institutionen' (1905–1931) and 'Embryologiska institutionen' (1932/33–1934/35 to 1946/47). In the following I refer to these sections and years, unless otherwise indicated.

18 Lund University, *Lunds universitets årsberättelse*; Swedish letters, vols. 1–7, Ivar Broman's archive.

19 Lund University, *Lunds universitets årsberättelse*; Swedish letters, vols. 1–7, Ivar Broman's archive.

20 Chalfork, '"När svartrockar" blev "vitrockar."'

21 A sterilization law was pushed through in 1934. It allowed sterilization only for the 'insane' and on a voluntary basis for the mentally normal. The law was significantly expanded

One category of suppliers consisted of some of Broman's former students, who, after graduating in Lund, found employment at hospitals in various towns and cities. Following several years of work in Skåne, Yngve Plym Forshell took a job as a physician at the Central Hospital in northern Gävle's combined obstetrics and gynecology ward. In a letter in 1939, he thanks Broman for 'many moments of celebration and joy' during his time at university and also for the personal friendship he has enjoyed: 'To your charming wife and you together a warm thank you for your hospitality!'[22] In another letter, Plym Forshell informs Broman that 'a shipment of specimens'—two fetuses from the fifth month of pregnancy, a surgically removed pregnant uterus, and a two-month-old fetus with intact membranes—were prepared to be sent to Lund: 'Undeniably, it looks as if I conducted a better angel-making, when chance joined it so that many such cases lumped together. You are welcome![23]

Sebastian von Wachenfeldt was younger than Broman but trained at the same medical faculty. In 1935 he became chief physician at Helsingborg's Maternity Hospital, fairly close to Lund, and the source of many specimens that are mentioned in the annual reports. Through letters from von Wachenfeldt, it is possible to follow the routine handling and delivery of fetuses. The first letters he wrote are more formal, addressed to 'Herr Professor I. Broman' and signed 'With respectful regards S. v. Wachenfeldt,' but quite soon the tone shifted to 'Brother!' and 'Yours Affectionately.' The majority of letters begin with a statement that it has become possible to send 'another fetus,' followed by information about how it has been fixed in a jar with some liquid (so as not to be destroyed) and sometimes a few words about the surgical method used and the patient in question. Indirectly it appears that von Wachenfeldt was instructed that the fetuses should be 'fresh' and fixed as quickly as possible after the operation: 'It was probably almost alive then!'[24]

Broman is anxious that von Wachenfeldt should use 'Bouin'—a mixture of picric acid, acetic acid, and formalin—as a fluid for preserving the fetuses (it was considered more durable), and bottles of the liquid are sent from Lund to Helsingborg but soon run out: 'P.S. The bouin flasks out! D.S.'[25] He also offers von Wachenfeldt compensation for the postage costs in connection with the

in 1941 and came to include both sterilizations without consent and formally 'voluntary' sterilizations, which meant that the person in question signed a sterilization application. On this history, see Tydén, 'Scandinavian States.'

22 Plym Forshell to Broman, July 24, 1939.

23 Plym Forshell to Broman, September 25, 1941. 'Angel-making' (*änglamakeri*) was a term used to describe foster parents' deliberate killing of foster children through neglect, thereby turning them into little angels.

24 Von Wachenfeldt to Broman, January 13, 1940.

25 Von Wachenfeldt to Broman, n.d.

transport of the specimens, but the physician declines: 'Thank you for your kind concern for my cash, but the package and also previous shipments have gone as service shipments. If the accountant or other authorities argue, I can come up with a bill; until then, we'll leave it be.'[26] This shows that the trafficking of fetuses could take place in a kind of gray zone between civil service and private contacts.

During Broman's tenure, it was considered important that the exchange of fetuses be organized as a gift economy rather than a market. Scientific credibility was not to be confused with grave robbing and the commercial trade in human remains. Memories remained of events in Edinburgh a hundred years earlier, when it was discovered that a series of murders had been committed by two perpetrators (William Burke and William Hare) who sold the bodies to the medical faculty for dissection.[27] In the written report on the 1922 government investigation into the procurement of corpses, Broman distanced himself from practices involving payment. Buying corpses of newborn babies from privately practicing midwives, a 'custom' in some places in Germany, he regarded as 'in several ways questionable and therefore not desirable.'[28]

All the same, the gift economy was based on reciprocity: the 'givers' ('donor' was not yet an established term) of embryos and fetuses expected something in return. Broman regularly gave—as a gesture of gratitude—his publications to the physicians who sent him embryological material. In Lund University's annual reports, everyone who had presented such gifts was mentioned by name—their contribution thus received a kind of official recognition.[29] Broman also worked to ensure that the individuals who made major contributions—such as Hjalmar Tornblad—were named honorary doctors in the medical faculty and received other awards. Although the language was idealistic—almost religious—and celebrated the givers' selfless contribution to science, this reproductive bioeconomy was thus based on the gifts being reciprocated in some symbolic form.[30]

However, the border between 'gift' and 'commodity' was not always clear. Lund University's annual reports mention several examples of commercial transactions involved in the acquisition of human specimens for the Anatomy

26 Von Wachenfeldt to Broman, June 13, 1940.

27 Jülich, 'Historier kring Tornbladinstitutet,' 188. On the embryo exchange as gift economy, see also Morgan, *Icons of Life*, 65–66.

28 Broman, *Utredning och förslag*, 48. I am not aware of any historical evidence that supports Broman's view on the German practice.

29 Lund University, *Lunds universitets årsberättelse*. After 1949 the external givers are no longer mentioned by name.

30 See, e.g., Axelsson to Broman, November 27, 1931.

Department and the Tornblad Institute. For instance, in the early 1930s Broman managed to acquire the deceased Austrian histologist Walter Kolmer's sections of human embryos. These were 'nerve colored' and therefore completed the department's own collection. Kolmer's human specimens were not a gift but a purchase from the firm Theodor Oswald Weigel in Leipzig.[31]

The embryological collection was thus based on a network of 'givers' that created a reproductive bioeconomy where gift and counter-gift were in the foreground. But this predominantly noncommercial network was not only a prerequisite for the enterprise; it also helped to strengthen existing social relationships, as well as create new ones. Several individuals in the network had been Broman's fellow students—perhaps they had participated in the same student burlesque performances (*spex*)—or were students he himself had taught. Over the years, these friends and colleagues gathered in various local societies in Lund and the Scania region that were only open to men. Thus male friendship—I cannot resist using the word 'Bromance'—was affirmed through the sense of chosenness and community.[32]

Yet there was a key category of people who were not compensated by either symbolic or economic payments in this reproductive bioeconomy: the female patients. Medical representatives were well aware that embryological research presupposed access to reproductive bodies, but this fact was rarely acknowledged in public. Who were the women who contributed embryos and fetuses to Broman's collection? And more broadly, what were the conditions encountered by pregnant women who needed gynecological-obstetrical care in early and mid-twentieth century society?

3 The Female Patients

Getting pregnant and giving birth around the turn of the twentieth century was, for many women, associated with great risks: ectopic pregnancy, preeclampsia, and other serious illnesses were part of everyday life. Complicated births and cesarean sections could lead to death. Contraceptives were hard to come by and illegal abortions dangerous. At the same time, conditions differed significantly, depending on the circumstances. Being married or unmarried, working at home or elsewhere, living in a city or in the countryside, ethnically Swedish or not, and whether the child was born in or out of wedlock—all these factors affected the women who became pregnant and their potential children.

31 Lund University, *Lunds universitets årsberättelse*, 1932/33–1934/35, 32.

32 On this theme, see Jülich, 'Historier kring Tornbladinstitutet,' 188, 193.

The situation radically changed around the mid-twentieth century. Instead of home births where midwives had a great deal of responsibility, especially in smaller towns, the majority of births took place in hospitals with specialist physicians, nurses, and laboratory staff on site. An expansion of gynecological health care was underway, and new methods for the diagnosis and treatment of women's diseases were introduced. As the welfare state expanded, maternity and child-care centers began to be established, and through child benefit and other measures, society's support for families with children increased. In 1938 a new law came into force allowing abortion for medical, humanitarian, and eugenic reasons. At the same time, the ban on contraceptive information was abolished, pharmacies were obliged to sell contraceptives, and in 1955 sex education was made compulsory in elementary schools.[33]

In Lund, until the beginning of the twentieth century, gynecological operations were performed in the surgical ward of the hospital. Obstetrics still belonged to the maternity hospital. A new women's clinic was inaugurated in 1918 and was the first in Sweden to combine maternity care and obstetric/ gynecological surgery. The maternity hospital in Helsingborg opened in 1926 and, organizationally speaking, belonged to the adjacent infirmary. At Malmö Municipal Hospital, beginning in 1907, the patients were treated in a maternity ward, which was later expanded to include gynecology; around 1940 a new women's clinic was inaugurated, and from 1948 the hospital was a teaching hospital attached to the medical faculty in Lund.[34]

By compiling information from different sources, I have been able to trace about thirty patient records of women whose fetuses from interrupted pregnancies were sent to the Anatomy Department and the Tornblad Institute in Lund. The earliest of these records is from the maternity ward at Malmö Municipal Hospital in 1916 and the latest from Lund Hospital's women's clinic in 1951. Most of the patients were registered in the 1930s and 1940s, the majority after the decriminalization of abortion in 1938.[35] Given their limited number, it is difficult to say how representative these records are, but they do offer glimpses into life stories and hint at gender and socioeconomic patterns.

33 These developments are described in Jülich, 'Historier kring Tornbladinstitutet,' 193.

34 Jülich, 'Historier kring Tornbladinstitutet,' 194.

35 Information related to preserved specimens in the Tornblad collection, found on labels of jars as well as in catalogues and correspondence, was used to track the patient records that are now kept at Skåne Regional Council Archive. The catalogues were moved to a storehouse of the Medical Faculty in 2017. These records are not classified as confidential since they are more than seventy years old. Nevertheless, I have changed the names of the patients and other personal data to protect their identities.

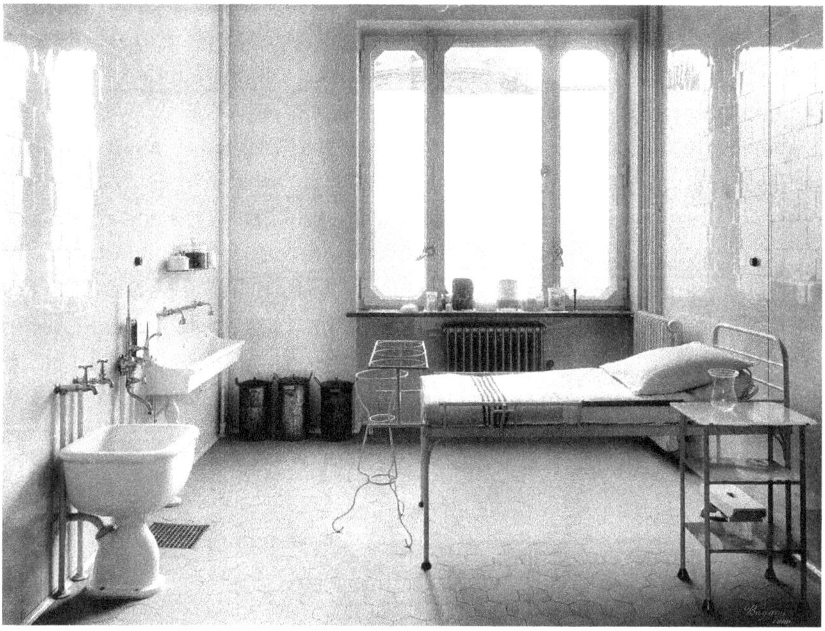

FIGURE 6.3 Examination and delivery room at the women's clinics of Lund University in the 1920s. Photographer: Per Bagge. South Swedish Society for the History of Medicine.

Several of the women who were treated for miscarriage or underwent abortion at hospitals in the region were unmarried and thus dependent on paid work. Some had probably moved from the countryside to the growing cities and taken up employment in new industries or as servants of the middle class. Under 'occupation' in the patient records, 'maid,' 'housekeeper,' 'cleaner,' and 'dishwasher' have been entered. Some earned a livelihood in business and could work alongside men but probably with lower wages; one woman is a 'clerk,' another a 'telephone operator,' a third a 'shop assistant.' But many are registered in rural areas. One is a 'daughter living at home' (*hemmadotter*), the term for a woman who stayed at home and never married. For those who did marry, an occupation is rarely given; instead, that of the husband appears. Records for unmarried women listed the father's work: 'farmer,' 'groom,' 'mill worker,' 'carpenter,' and 'fisherman.' In only a few cases, the husband is employed by the state: there is a 'civil servant' and a 'railway servant.'

Alongside aspects of gender and class, another pattern emerges when reviewing the patient records: the majority are abortion cases. Of the thirty women, twenty-one were admitted for an abortion, while eight were treated for miscarriage and one for ectopic pregnancy. The abortion cases can be sorted into different categories, depending on the reason for granting permission to terminate the pregnancy: medical or eugenic. Nine of the women had been granted an abortion on medical grounds, which included 'weakness' and being 'worn-out' from too many pregnancies. In a total of twelve cases, the abortion was performed for eugenic reasons with subsequent sterilization. Both mental illness and 'mental retardation' as well as severe physical illnesses of the woman, the male partner, or their relatives are cited as grounds for certification in the records. These abortion records often include attachments with an investigation and a decision in the form of a telegram from the National Board of Medicine. Humanitarian indication, the third type, when the abortion was justified by the woman's becoming pregnant after incest or rape, does not appear in the material. Also absent are examples of abortions on socio-medical grounds—a fourth indication introduced in the 1946 Abortion Act.

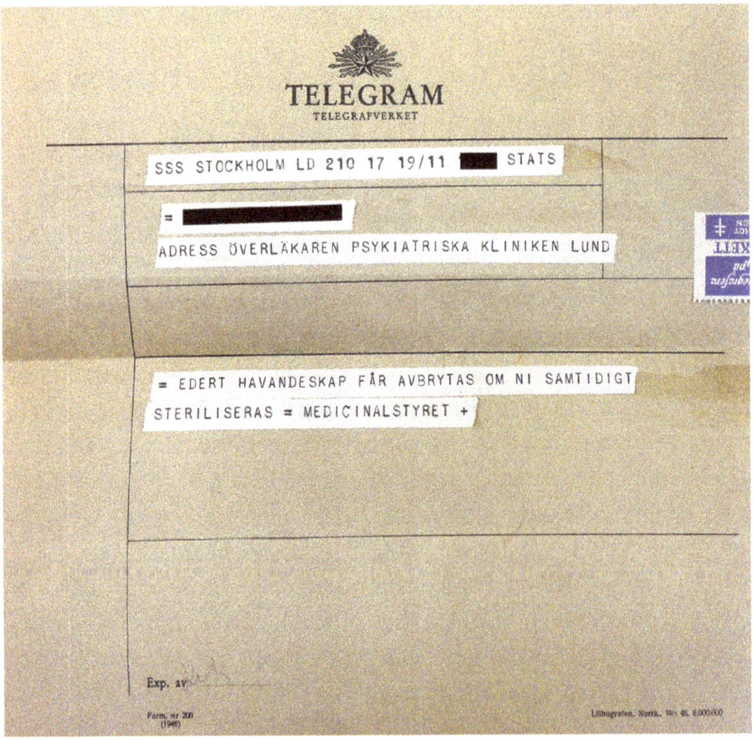
TELEGRAM
TELEGRAFVERKET
SSS STOCKHOLM LD 210 17 19/11 ▇▇ STATS
= ▇▇▇▇▇▇▇
ADRESS ÖVERLÄKAREN PSYKIATRISKA KLINIKEN LUND
= EDERT HAVANDESKAP FÅR AVBRYTAS OM NI SAMTIDIGT
STERILISERAS = MEDICINALSTYRET +
Exp. av

FIGURE 6.4 Telegram sent in 1947 from the National Board of Medicine in Stockholm to an (anonymized) patient at the psychiatric ward at Lund University Hospital indicating that her abortion application had been approved on the condition that she was sterilized. Photo: Solveig Jülich.

The procedure for applying for an abortion was complicated. A woman who wanted to terminate her pregnancy sought an appointment with a physician or one of the counselling agencies established after the Parliament had decided to legalize abortion in 1938. A first option was for an application to be sent to the National Board of Medicine, where a decision was made by the forensic psychiatric board (later the social-psychiatric board). A second alternative was for two physicians to jointly decide on an abortion and subsequently report to the National Board of Medicine. Decisions concerning abortion for eugenic reasons, however, were always made by the board, and as a condition in the majority of cases the woman would be sterilized at the same time. The woman signed the abortion application herself, but several certificates from relatives, counsellors, and physicians were also required: describing her living conditions, family relationships, physical and mental status, and stating the reason why she wanted an abortion. The relationship between the woman seeking an abortion and her physician was thus anything but equal, but we do not know much about how individual physicians treated patients in practice.

The most common method of abortion in the earliest phase of pregnancy (the first trimester) was the surgical one. After the woman was sedated, a rod

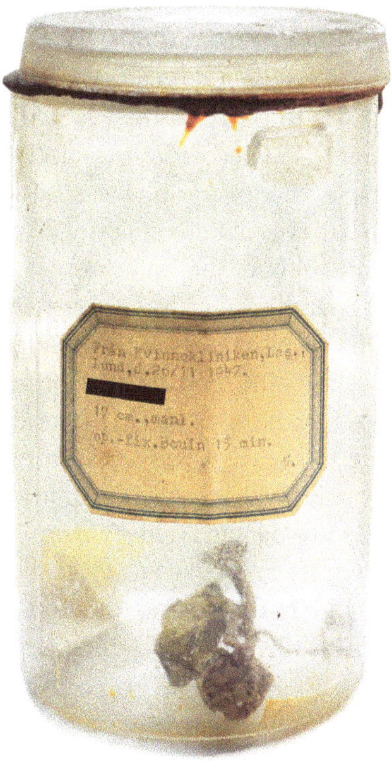

FIGURE 6.5
Preserved specimen, originating from this patient's abortion operation in 1947, photographed by Malin Thomas Nilsson at the Tornblad Institute in 2015. Courtesy of Malin Thomas Nilsson.

was inserted into the cervix to dilate and then scrape it with a blunt spoon. In the case of abortions during the second trimester (after about thirteen weeks), an operative procedure was performed from the vagina or through an incision in the abdomen. The method was called 'small cesarean section' (hysterotomy) and was used for eugenic abortions with subsequent sterilization, when a piece of the fallopian tubes was cut away. For Broman and the other embryologists, this abortion technique offered an advantage: the fetus and its surrounding amniotic membranes were removed intact, which made it possible to use the material for research. The techniques developed from the 1960s onward would make this more difficult or impossible. The saline method, injecting saline to induce miscarriage, involved destroying the fetus before it was removed. In the 1990s, abortion pills were introduced that allowed abortions to be performed at an earlier stage.[36]

One of the records, which is very brief, concerns an illegal abortion that took place during the period when abortion was still prohibited by law. The patient was a twenty-six-year-old cleaner who in April 1921 was sent to Malmö Municipal Hospital after being admitted to Trelleborg's infirmary. She was three months pregnant, bleeding profusely, and in pain. The physician in charge, Otto Gröné, one of Broman's former fellow students, diagnosed 'Abortus crim.' It is not clear from the record how she had tried to terminate the pregnancy, but there were several methods available. Stockings, probes, or other objects were inserted into the uterus by women who tried to abort themselves—sometimes resulting in their death or ruined health. Uterine syringes that could be purchased over the counter in health-care stores were filled with soap solution and injected into the uterus to induce miscarriage. There were also illegal abortionists who, without being physicians, more or less skillfully performed the operations for payment. Gröné assessed the situation for the twenty-six-year-old as urgent, and after a vaginal cesarean section, the uterus was 'evacuated.' The woman survived the operation and was discharged from the hospital ten days later. Whether she was prosecuted I do not know. The penalty for aborting a fetus was still prison, but almost all women (not the abortionists) received a suspended sentence. However, it is possible to say what happened to the aborted fetus. This is the only example of a record entry that explicitly confirms the connection to Broman's collection: the fetus was 'sent to Lund.'[37]

The language in the records is consistently terse and effective: it is not a genre that invites empathy, and some sentences hit hard. A twenty-three-year-old woman with 'Int.[elligence] age = 9 years' was registered at Helsingborg's

36 See Ramsey's chapter in this volume.

37 Patient records, D3B:87, 1921, record 407, and D3B:91, 1921, operation record 55.

Maternity Hospital in 1942 for 'sterilization operation in connection with termination of pregnancy due to imbecility.' According to the physician, the patient did not know who the father of the child was: 'stating that "they never say their name, so you can't know."' She has '4 mentally retarded siblings. The father is moderately retarded.' The operation was performed through small cesarean section followed by sterilization. The 'egg' was then picked out together with parts of the placenta. The patient record contains notes on the patient's condition after the operation. The next day she feels 'terrible' and wants to go to the toilet, but asks for permission first: 'Behaves in speech and action hardly like a 9-year-old.' Soon the woman asked to go home—she has bought a return ticket that only lasts 10 days. The physician comments ironically on her wish: 'Why, this indicates certain human characteristics!'[38]

Physicians appear to have been more empathic and also more likely to support women's abortion applications in cases of an alcoholic partner and domestic abuse. The record for Britta Johansson depicts an unsustainable situation with a husband who abused her during intoxication, hangovers, and hallucinations. The two children, aged thirteen and eleven, 'had tried to protect the appl. against his violence.' She had filed for legal separation in 1945, but after constant threats from her husband, she and the children moved back home, which she now regretted. Six years later, she was pregnant again and wanted an abortion. The physician describes her as '[n]ormally gifted' tired, anxious, and depressed. Her application was approved by the National Board of Medicine, with no requirement for sterilization. Perhaps officials did not hold Britta Johansson responsible for the situation that had arisen—unlike the women who had brought on their pregnancy through 'promiscuity.' Or the physicians might have wanted to avoid asking the husband for a certificate, and thereby giving him an opportunity to influence the outcome of the application. The operation was performed—despite no sterilization—with hysterotomy via the abdomen, and the fetus could thus be taken out intact: 'Length of the fetus 20 cm, weight 180 grams.' No justification for the choice of technique is given.[39]

These records are unreliable sources for tapping into patients' motivations. Yet, in several cases, it appears that the patients themselves wanted to be sterilized. Viola Olsson was forty-two years old when she was registered at the gynecology ward of Helsingborg's Maternity Hospital. She had undergone twelve pregnancies (her eleven children were aged two to seventeen), was pregnant again, and applied for abortion and sterilization. According to the physician's

38 Gynecological records, F2:14, 1942, record 51.

39 Patient registry, Gynecological ward, D4A:48, 1951, record 1007.

statement, there was '[h]ereditary deafness in the family,' and the patient and several of her siblings had severe hearing loss. In combination with goiter, this disability had made life increasingly difficult: 'She has always been "peculiar" as to her temper, but knew how to keep order at home until lately. In recent years, there has been a laxity in the care of the children, both in terms of feeding and clothing, apparently due to her worn-out condition.' Her husband was 'a hard-working' man but a seasonal worker and intermittently unemployed. The previous winter, when the family lived on unemployment benefits, there was 'almost poverty at home.' The physician noted that she had difficulty holding discussions because of the hearing damage and was resigned but 'clear, orderly, well oriented.' It was 'her distinct desire to be freed from yet another pregnancy, when she realizes that "now it won't work anymore."' The abortion operation and subsequent sterilization were done by von Wachenfeldt. A letter to Broman indicates that he then sent a 'larger fetus originating from the deaf woman' to the Tornblad Institute.[40]

There are also examples of physicians supporting women's desire not to be sterilized. Ella Gustavsson was a thirty-three-year-old unmarried woman who applied for an abortion at the women's clinic in Lund in 1947. She already had one small child and was now five months pregnant with another man who had withdrawn a promise of marriage. An investigation was carried out, which showed that the patient had psychotic symptoms. Mental illness ran in the family on both the father's and the mother's side. Ten years ago, she had suffered from schizophrenia: 'everything was so strange, [she] heard and saw things that weren't there, a person was singing as if otherworldly, someone else was standing behind her and wanted to take her over, the milk in the glass was drunk by somebody else.' A few years later, a probable relapse occurred, 'thought she was dead, someone was behind her, wanted to inject her with syringes.' She is 'thin, impassive, fragile' and suffers from paramimia (a psychomotor disorder that has similarities to tics). In the record it appears that the application for abortion was granted but that sterilization was not carried out: 'The patient has feared that a sterilization would not help her but instead increase her inferiority, and the certifier has been inclined to postpone the question of sterilization to a time when the patient considers herself capable of making a decision.' It is not clear who the person giving the certificate was, but apparently those responsible for the abortion application took into account Ella Gustavsson's own wish not to be sterilized, despite her 'hereditary' burden in the form of severe mental illness. Owing to the advanced pregnancy,

40 Gynecological records, F2:18, 1943, record 29; Tornblad Institute Collection catalogue, card B56; von Wachenfeldt to Broman, February 2, 1943.

the fetus, which was '19 cm long and of male sex,' could not be 'extracted whole' but was perforated first.[41]

The reproductive bioeconomy steered by male embryologists required access to raw material from women's bodies. The relationships were not symmetrical: the male 'givers' of this material (the majority were men) belonged to a social elite, and their 'gifts' were rewarded with symbolic payments in the form of honors, fraternal bonding, and scientific prestige. The patients often came from poor circumstances, had low-paying jobs, and lacked the ability to influence their situations to a greater extent. Their contribution to the bioeconomy was not recognized in the same way—female reproductive bodies were a form of a capital that was talked about quietly. Is it still possible to say something about how Broman and his colleagues reasoned about ethical principles and values?

4 Ethics and Values in Another Age

However we choose to value Broman's research practices, it is essential to understand them in their historical context. During the period he worked as a doctor and researcher, from the 1890s until his death in 1946, there existed no formal ethical rules or ethical regulations in Sweden. It was only in 1951 that the Swedish Medical Association adopted a *codex ethicus*. The background was the Nuremberg Declaration, which came about in light of the Nazis' deadly medical experiments as well as various international initiatives. Among other things, it required that researchers obtain informed consent from people participating in an experiment. The Declaration of Helsinki, adopted by the World Medical Association in 1964 and still applied in revised form today, contains several additions on biomedical research involving humans. It was not until 1995 that the use of aborted fetuses in medical experiments became the subject of legislation in Sweden. Research that includes tissues from fetuses can only be carried out today if the woman consents, and after approval by the Swedish Ethical Review Authority and the National Board of Health and Welfare.[42]

This is not to say that there were no professional regulations and moral values in Broman's time. The so-called physicians' oath (*läkareden*) had been part of the state's administrative apparatus since the sixteenth century and rested on parliamentary legislation. The rules prescribed, among other things, that physicians should not unduly worry their patients by sharing too much information

41 Patient registry, Gynecological ward, D4A:44, 1947, record 4406.

42 Jülich and Tinnerholm Ljungberg, 'Från medicinskt avfall till rättighetsinnehavare,' 49.

about an illness and that physicians were also bound by a duty of confidentiality: delicate personal conditions were not to be revealed to others, unless the patient expressed the wish to do so. Toward the end of the nineteenth century, the physicians' oath came under question, and it was abolished in 1887, along with a number of other official oaths. A decisive objection was that the duty of confidentiality could be in conflict with the public interest. In the first general medical instruction of 1890, the duty of confidentiality was subordinated to legal obligations—for example, physicians' obligation, as state officials, to report venereal diseases. In addition, there were very few requirements of an ethical nature laid out in laws, statutes, or regulations concerning the medical profession.[43]

It is therefore unsurprising that no surviving documents clearly express Broman's reasoning about ethical issues connected to the collecting and handling of embryological material. Nor did the physicians who provided him with fetuses and information about patients describe wrestling with ethical dilemmas around personal integrity or human dignity. There is no indication that the women were asked about their participation: the records contain no notes on consent or similar principles.[44]

Broman's disregard appears as an expression of a more general phenomenon. The use of women's bodies as an experimental field is a prominent feature in the history of modern medicine.[45] But there are, after all, examples suggesting that Broman considered the collecting of human fetuses from pregnant women as a sensitive—in a sense ethical—issue. A radio program recorded at the Tornblad Institute in 1939 is interesting in this context. Broman takes the reporter on a tour of the building, but when he is asked where the human material comes from, he answers evasively. He praises his collegial network and claims that the Swedish medical profession is characterized by its high-level scientific approach. Collecting material is presented as a purely technical procedure: the practiced ability to handle and preserve specimens. The female patients are not mentioned at all—but the silence is telling.[46]

43 Eklöf, *Läkarens ethos*, 193, 246; Eklöf, 'Då tystnadsplikt ersätts av informationsdelning'; Öberg, 'Varför svär inte svenska läkare ed?'

44 On the early history of patient consent in Sweden, see the introduction of this volume and Franzén, 'From Patient to Specimen,' 42. For perspectives from other national contexts, see Claes, '"By What Right"'; Maehle, *Contesting Medical Confidentiality*; Maehle, *Doctors, Honour, and the Law*, 69–94.

45 In a Swedish context, this theme has been discussed by, among others, Johannisson, *Den mörka kontinenten*, chap. 3; and Nilsson, *Kampen om kvinnan*, chap. 5.

46 'I vetenskapens verkstad.'

How should the lack of references to pregnant women be understood? Women's sexuality was bounded by strong cultural norms, and scientific fields that related to sexual and reproductive issues were particularly vulnerable to criticism and questioning from laypeople. Gynecologists involved themselves in various kinds of public activities to establish authority and trust. The connection to women's abortions made the use of embryos and fetuses for research especially sensitive. Abortions—even legal ones—were seen as shameful, and for many physicians it was a measure that could only be resorted to in cases when the woman's life was in danger. The risk of public scandal if it came to be known that specimens in the embryological collection came from sexually active, often unmarried women—in some cases abortion patients—was thus not negligible.[47]

On the other hand, the silence surrounding the patients who contributed material from their interrupted pregnancies to the Tornblad Institute collection can be interpreted as stemming from the principle of confidentiality. That Broman perceived this as an important issue is suggested by a press clipping in the archive he left behind. It concerns a court case in which a physician had been fined for refusing to testify about what he had been told in confidence by a patient; passages in the text have been underlined in red.[48] More importantly, the preserved correspondence between Broman and individuals in his informal network give the impression that the protection of the patients' identity and personal information was considered important. Von Wachenfeldt and the other physicians rarely mention the women's names in their letters to Broman. Instead, 'patient' is used, and correspondents provide depersonalized information about age, last menstrual period, and medical history. A patient record number may also be noted.

A perhaps less benevolent interpretation is that those who were considered in need of protection were not primarily the patients but the colleagues in Broman's network. That physicians' correct and considerate behavior was sometimes perceived as a central ethical or moral principle is evident, for example, in an article by Israel Holmgren published in the journal of the Swedish Medical Association in 1932: 'The physician shall think about his duties to society, he shall sacrifice his strength for the sick and behave toward them as an honorable man and a good person, he must always be a gentleman towards his colleagues.' In another article, lawyer Eric Carlquist emphasized that the medical profession must stick together vis-à-vis the public and that they should guard their 'legitimate interests,' scientific as well as economic and social. The ideal physician was

47 Jülich, 'Historier kring Tornbladinstitutet,' 204.

48 'Physicians assert their duty.'

engaged with various forms of public outreach or as a politician to establish public trust and authority.[49]

There was thus no lack of ethical considerations surrounding the reproductive bioeconomy that emerged around the collecting of embryos and fetuses in Lund during the first half of the twentieth century. The traffic in human embryological material was considered to be sensitive for several reasons—not primarily the scientific use of the fetuses, but rather the association with women's sexuality, reproduction, and abortions. The practices that Broman developed show that he took patient confidentiality seriously, but at the same time he was anxious to protect his colleagues and the medical profession against potential criticism. He dealt with this situation by using different layers of transparency and degrees of proximity in the circulation of embryonic and fetal knowledge. The academic world gained significant insight into the network's organization and its bioeconomic exchanges (for instance, through the annual reports). On the other hand, the audiences for his popular science writings and public performances—who were at a greater distance—could only form a fragmentary knowledge of the apparatus around the acquisition of human fetuses.[50]

One might wonder whether the women who applied for abortion or sought treatment for pregnancy-related complications would have denied the embryologists access to dead fetuses if they had been asked. This is a hypothetical question since I lack material that can shed light on the patients' own experiences. In contrast, Shannon Withycombe, drawing on private correspondence and other unpublished material, has shown that American women in the latter part of the nineteenth century confidently left the products of their miscarriages to physicians with a sense of participation in embryological knowledge production. For some, the miscarriage may have come as a relief, and the idea that the residue was of scientific use could be satisfying or possibly a consolation.[51] Neither can we be sure that women in general would have been critical of Broman's collecting. As we have seen, midwives and a female physician formed part of his network, and some of them actively contributed to the Tornblad Institute collection. Issues of consent and integrity are unusually complicated in this historical context.

After Broman's death, the collecting of human embryos and fetuses for the Tornblad Institute continued, but to a diminishing extent. Comparative embryology lost its scientific attraction, and interest in the collection waned. But even experimental embryology, which started to have a greater impact

49 These two articles are discussed in Eklöf, *Läkarens ethos*, 214–19.

50 On this argument, see Jülich, 'Historier kring Tornbladinstitutet,' 208.

51 Withycombe, *Lost*, 129.

in Sweden in the 1950s, depended on human material from legal abortions to produce tissue cultures where, for example, the effects of drugs and carcinogenic chemicals could be studied. In the early 1960s, in connection with the thalidomide scandal, the Tornblad Institute gained greater societal relevance, especially when it became home to the Swedish Register of Congenital Malformations.[52]

5 Conclusions

During the first part of the twentieth century, a reproductive bioeconomy was built around Ivar Broman's acquisition of embryos and fetuses from women's interrupted pregnancies for an embryological collection at Lund University. In the hands of an embryologist, this 'waste' could be converted into valuable research material. On a general level, the establishment and activities of the Anatomy Department and the Tornblad Institute presupposed various types of legislation and practical arrangements that facilitated researchers' access to miscarriages and aborted fetuses. By virtue of their positions as government officials and scientific experts, the embryologists could gain real influence, but they could not act alone. The production of embryonic and fetal knowledge required an informal network of physicians and midwives who provided Broman with human material. The collection not only relied on these social relations but also helped to strengthen existing and male friendships and to shape new ones.

Ideally, this exchange of embryos and fetuses would be organized as a gift economy rather than a commercial market. Scientific credibility demanded that these activities not be associated with grave robbing or a trade in dead human bodies. 'Gifts' from Broman's network of colleagues and former students were rewarded by mentions in academic and scientific publications as well as honorary titles. Serving science was a tribute in itself. All the same, the distinction between gift and commodity was not always easy to maintain.

Women's role in the reproductive bioeconomy has not been easy to grasp. The patients who contributed material from their interrupted pregnancies to embryological knowledge production were not asked for permission. The analysis of patient records shows that in the majority of cases these were unmarried and working people with low incomes—because they sought public care for unwanted pregnancies, they were perceived to owe a debt to society that

52 See Lee's chapter in this volume.

could be repaid by leaving their reproductive waste to the embryologists. It was hardly a coincidence that several of the specimens in the collection came from abortions with subsequent sterilization, since this method secured whole fetal bodies for research. However, it appears that some women themselves asked to be sterilized for various reasons. No one seemed to question the scientific use of human fetuses. Rather, it was the association with sexuality, reproduction, and abortion that made the traffic in fetal bodies a sensitive issue.

By today's protocols, Broman and his network acted unethically. But in their own time, their collecting practices were grounded in rules and norms that physicians and government officials were required to follow: the person who was ill should not be troubled with too much information, and the physician was bound by patient confidentiality unless the state law required otherwise. In addition, the physician must act as a gentleman in his relationships with colleagues and protect the medical profession against society's criticism. Both of these principles can be drawn from the various sources discussed in this chapter.

In our current age, egg donations, egg freezing, sperm donations, uterus transplants, and the availability of embryonic stem cells have created entirely new opportunities for reproductive medicine and biomedical research. Yet important elements of this reproductive bioeconomy can be traced back to the making of modern human embryology, including anatomists' collection of material from women's miscarriages and abortions in Sweden during the first half of the twentieth century.

Bibliography

Broman, Ivar. *Individens utveckling ur ägget*. Stockholm: Åhlén & Söner, 1937.

Broman, Ivar. *Normale und abnorme Entwicklung des Menschen: Ein Hand- und Lehrbuch der Ontogenie und Teratologie speziell für praktische Ärzte und Studierande der Medizin*. Wiesbaden: J. F. Bergmann, 1911.

Broman, Ivar. *Utredning och förslag rörande förskaffande av lik för den för läkareutbildningen nödvändiga anatomiska undervisningen*. SOU 1922:57. Stockholm: Ecklesiastikdepartementet, 1922.

Broman, Ivar. *Vidunder och missfoster i fantasi och verklighet*. Stockholm: Bonnier, 1929.

Chalfork, Fredrik. 'När "svartrockar" blev "vitrockar": Om Ivar Bromans bidrag i den rasbiologiska och rashygieniska allmänupplysningen under åren 1920–1940.' *Scandia* 72, no. 1 (2006): 72–92.

Claes, Tinne. '"By What Right Does the Scalpel Enter the Pauper's Corpse?" Dissections and Consent in Late Nineteenth-Century Belgium.' *Social History of Medicine* 31, no. 2 (2018): 258–77.

Eklöf, Motzi. 'Då tystnadsplikt ersätts av informationsdelning.' *Läkartidningen* 111, no. 43 (2014): 1912–14.

Eklöf, Motzi. *Läkarens ethos: Studier i den svenska läkarkårens identiteter, intressen och ideal 1890–1960*. Linköping: Linköpings universitet, 2000.

Faasse, Patricia, Job Faber, and Jenny Narraway. 'A Brief History of the Hubrecht Laboratory.' *International Journal of Developmental Biology* 43 (1999): 583–90.

Franzén, Helena. 'From Patient to Specimen and Back Again: Radical Surgeries and Pelvic Pathologies in the Museum Obstetricum.' *Lychnos* (2020): 33–57.

Franzén, Helena. '"The Precious Material": Obtaining Human Fetal Bodies for an Embryological Collection at Uppsala University ca. 1890–1930.' *Scandinavian Journal of History* 47, no. 2 (2022): 178–202.

Hammar, August. 'Upprop.' *Jordemodern* 14, no. 12 (1901): ad attachment.

Hopwood, Nick. 'Producing Development: The Anatomy of Human Embryos and the Norms of Wilhelm His.' *Bulletin of the History of Medicine* 74, no. 1 (2000): 29–79.

Johannisson, Karin. *Den mörka kontinenten: Kvinnan, medicinen och fin-de-siècle*. Stockholm: Norstedt, 1994.

Jülich, Solveig. 'Fosterexperimentens produktiva hemlighet: Medicinsk forskning och vita lögner i 1960- och 1970-talets Sverige.' *Lychnos* (2018): 10–49.

Jülich, Solveig. 'Historier kring Tornbladinstitutet.' In Thomas Nilsson and Jülich, 151–268. *Embryologiska rum*.

Jülich, Solveig, and Helena Tinnerholm Ljungberg. 'Från medicinskt avfall till rättighetsinnehavare: Framväxten av värdekonflikter kring aborterade foster i Sverige.' *Tidskrift för genusvetenskap* 40, no. 3–4 (2019): 33–54.

Källén, Bengt. *The Tornblad Institute in Lund: From Comparative Embryology to Reproduction Epidemiology*. Lund: Royal Physiographic Society of Lund, 2014.

Lund University. *Lunds universitets årsberättelse*. Lund: Lunds universitet, 1876–1947.

Maehle, Andreas-Holger. *Contesting Medical Confidentiality: Origins of the Debate in the United States, Britain, and Germany*. Chicago: University of Chicago Press, 2016.

Maehle, Andreas-Holger. *Doctors, Honour, and the Law: Medical Ethics in Imperial Germany*. Basingstoke: Palgrave Macmillan, 2009.

Maienschein, Jane, Marie Glitz, and Garland E. Allen, eds. *Centennial History of the Carnegie Institution of Washington*. Vol. 2, *The Department of Embryology*. Cambridge: Cambridge University Press, 2004.

Morgan, Lynn M. *Icons of Life: A Cultural History of Human Embryos*. Berkeley: University of California Press, 2009.

Morgan, Lynn M. '"Properly Disposed of": A History of Embryo Disposal and the Changing Claims on Fetal Remains.' *Medical Anthropology* 21, no. 3–4 (2002): 247–74.

Nilsson, Ulrika. *Kampen om kvinnan: Professionalisering och konstruktioner av kön i svensk gynekologi 1860–1925*. Uppsala: Uppsala universitet, 2003.

Öberg, Lisa. 'Varför svär inte svenska läkare ed?' *Läkartidningen* 98, no. 37 (2001): 3935–37.

Thomas Nilsson, Malin, and Solveig Jülich. *Embryologiska rum: Tornbladinstitutets samling av foster från människor och djur*. Göteborg: Makadam, 2022.

Tydén, Mattias. 'The Scandinavian States: Reformed Eugenics Applied.' In *The Oxford Handbook of the History of Eugenics*, edited by Alison Bashford and Philippa Levine, 363–76. New York: Oxford University Press, 2010.

Waldby, Catherine. 'Production and Reproduction in the Bioeconomy.' Keynote for the conference 'Critical Sociology: Current Issues and Future Challenges,' Frankfurt am Main, 2014. Accessed August 22, 2014. https://anu-au.academia.edu/Catherine Waldby.

Waldby, Catherine, and Melinda Cooper. 'The Biopolitics of Reproduction.' *Australian Feminist Studies* 23, no. 55 (2008): 57–73.

Withycombe, Shannon. *Lost: Miscarriage in Nineteenth-Century America*. New Brunswick, NJ: Rutgers University Press, 2019.

Audio-Visual References

'I vetenskapens verkstad: Besök på Tornbladinstitutet i Lund.' Swedish Radio, April 4, 1939.

Archival Sources and Museum Collections

Axelsson, Petter, to Ivar Broman, November 27, 1931. Swedish letters, vol. 5, Ivar Broman's archive. LUL.

Bagge, Per. Photograph of examination and delivery room at the women's clinics of Lund University in the 1920s. Image archive of SHM.

'The physicians assert their duty of confidentiality,' n.d. Biographica, vol. 16, Ivar Broman's archive. LUL.

Gynecological records, F2:14, 1942, record 51. Women's Clinic, Helsingborg Hospital. SRCA.

Gynecological records, F2:18, 1943, record 29. Women's Clinic, Helsingborg Hospital. SRCA.

Patient records, D3B:87, 1921, record 407, and D3B:91, 1921, operation record 55. Women's Clinic, Malmö University Hospital MAS. SRCA.

Patient registry, Gynecological ward, D4A:44, 1947, record 4406. Women's Clinic, Lund University Hospital. SRCA.

Patient registry, Gynecological ward, D4A:48, 1951, record 1007. Women's Clinic, Lund University Hospital. SRCA.

Photograph of Ivar Broman and Elis Essen-Möller, 1893. Tornblad Institute Collection. Medical Faculty of Lund University, storehouse at Gastelyckan, Lund.

Plym Forshell, Yngve, to Ivar Broman, July 24, 1939. Swedish letters, vol. 5, Ivar Broman's archive. LUL.

Plym Forshell, Yngve, to Ivar Broman, September 25, 1941. Swedish letters, vol. 5, Ivar Broman's archive. LUL.

Tornblad Institute Collection. Biological Museum, Lund University.

Tornblad Institute Collection catalogue, card B56. Medical Faculty of Lund University, storehouse at Gastelyckan, Lund.

von Wachenfeldt, Sebastian, to Ivar Broman, January 13, 1940. Swedish letters, vol. 7, Ivar Broman's archive. LUL.

von Wachenfeldt, Sebastian, to Ivar Broman, June 13, 1940. Swedish letters, vol. 7, Ivar Broman's archive. LUL.

von Wachenfeldt, Sebastian, to Ivar Broman, February 2, 1943. Swedish letters, vol. 7, Ivar Broman's archive. LUL.

von Wachenfeldt, Sebastian, to Ivar Broman, n.d. Swedish letters, vol. 7, Ivar Broman's archive. LUL.

CHAPTER 7

Fetuses as Instruments of Health: Polio Vaccine and the Nation in the Postwar Period

Solveig Jülich and Isa Dussauge

Fetal tissue cultures have been widely used as a technique for medical research and vaccine development internationally and in Sweden since the mid-twentieth century. Increasingly, fetal tissue and cell cultures have also become controversial, and in some countries banned, because they are produced from the organs of aborted fetuses. Proponents have related to fetal tissue cultures as a valuable scientific tool, and opponents, as an ethically disputable bodily object contingent on abortions.[1]

This chapter aims to shed light on the establishment of fetal tissue cultures in medical research and practice in 1950s Sweden, most notably in the field of virology. During this period the medical field and surrounding debates were prime arenas for the shaping of tissue cultures' ethical status. The case of Sweden is highly interesting because of the country's early legislation on abortion, which, although restrictive, was an exception among many other Western countries: in Sweden, abortion was legal. In this context, prominent virologists established an infrastructure for supplying aborted fetuses to the national laboratory for vaccine development and research: the National Bacteriological Laboratory (NBL). Drawing on and comparing a wide range of unpublished archival sources and published materials, we examine how this infrastructure was built and communicated to the 'nation' in a time of crisis—the outbreak of polio—and the reasons why it failed to deliver the Swedish polio vaccine. We ask, in what way, if any, were the traffic and uses of aborted fetuses for scientific research publicly controversial?

In this chapter we use the term 'infrastructure' to highlight the pervasive yet (seemingly) invisible role that fetal tissue culture played in Swedish scientific research and vaccine development.[2] In order to understand how physicians and researchers involved in obtaining, collecting, and using fetal bodies from

1 Maynard-Moody, *Dilemma of the Fetus*; Banchoff, *Embryo Politics*.

2 Landecker, *Culturing Life*; Creager and Landecker, 'Technical Matters.'

 | DOI:10.1163/9789004703759_009

abortions balanced different values, we employ the concept of 'moral economy.'[3] We introduce the neologism 'uncontroversy' to show that no public debate concerning this practice arose.[4] This is not to say that the subject was not sensitive or uncomfortable, but rather that the virologists and other actors employed strategies to avoid transparency and public awareness about the establishment of the method to produce the vaccine. To highlight this, we draw on the intersection of reproduction studies and ignorance studies to demonstrate the dynamics of openness and secrecy at play in the communication of knowledge about fetal tissue to readers of newspapers and magazines in 1950s Sweden. In doing so, we reveal a strategic production of ignorance or 'selective ignorance' about risky abortions as a material source for the manufacture of the vaccine.[5]

A growing body of historical work has portrayed the biomedical use of human tissues as exploitative and unethical. Most prominently the story of the HeLa cell line, which was included in many research projects, including tests for the American polio vaccine in the early 1950s, has drawn attention to the lack of consent from patients even after guidelines for research were established in the 1960s and 1970s.[6] This also goes for (exceptional) Swedish abortion patients whose fetuses were prepared by virologists in Stockholm and then shipped across the Atlantic to the prestigious Wistar Institute in Philadelphia.[7] Duncan Wilson has, however, argued that 'it is unfair to claim that the non-consented use of human tissue was an injustice' since no one at the time objected—neither professionals nor journalists nor the public.[8] While we agree that more balanced histories are needed, our chapter shows that there were indeed controversies and secrecy involved in the building of an infrastructural supply of human tissues for the production of the Swedish

3 For a recent discussion of the concept of 'moral economy,' see Dussauge et al., 'On the Omnipresence,' 17–18.

4 According to *Merriam-Webster.com Dictionary*, the term 'uncontroversial' means 'not likely to be disputed or to cause strife or quarrel: not relating to or arousing controversy'; in other words, it refers to potential reactions, not events. When we write 'uncontroversy,' we simply mean that no controversy broke out even if there were contentious elements. See also Jülich's discussion in the epilogue of this volume.

5 Topçu and Maffi, 'Rethinking Ignorance Production.' On 'selective ignorance,' see Proctor, 'Agnotology,' 6–8; Burke, *Ignorance*, 12–13.

6 Skloot, *Immortal Life of Henrietta Lacks*; 'Culture of Consent.'

7 For this story, see Wadman, *Vaccine Race*, chap. 6.

8 Wilson, 'Troubled Past?,' 250.

polio vaccine. Crucially, both were related to values and issues specific to the context of abortion in Sweden.[9]

1 Fetal Tissue Cultures and Polio Epidemics

Tissue cultures have been in use in bacteriology since the early twentieth century. But viruses represented a new chapter. Unlike bacteria, viruses will not grow on lifeless media; they must be cultivated in living things. In addition, until the advent of electron microscopy, viruses were only detectable by indirect, non-visual means. Although embryologists and histologists had made many attempts to grow living human tissues, they were difficult to keep alive. Instead, early techniques were mainly established using animal tissues, especially chick embryos, and the results were extrapolated to humans.[10]

In the first half of the twentieth century the technique of 'passages' was used to cultivate viruses. In practice, this meant infecting animals or eggs with a virus, then harvesting infected materials to infect another animal. In the 1930s, virologists had succeeded in using tissue cultures to grow viruses and attenuate them, thus producing vaccines against yellow fever. However, the understanding of viruses' growth and their interactions with cells in cultures was still incomplete. The technique was demanding and expensive, and did not yield large quantities of viruses, which limited its utility in vaccine production.[11] While vaccines had been tested on institutionalized children and prisoners, the need for alternative methods was pressing. This was particularly urgent for virology, a discipline that was inclined toward diseases specific to humans.[12]

Therefore, in 1949, it was considered a major breakthrough when an American research group led by the virologist John Enders succeeded in keeping the polio virus alive and replicating in cultures of human fetal skin and muscle tissues. A large part of the living tissues used in these investigations came from therapeutic abortions, miscarriages, and other operations on patients at Boston hospitals. Through this association with polio, human cell culture technologies became a widely distributed and standardized research

9 The development of the Swedish polio vaccine has been analyzed by Axelsson, 'Cutter Incident.' However, he only briefly touches on the fact that the Swedish virologists used 'human embryos' (320).

10 Landecker, *Culturing Life*, 107–9.

11 Landecker, *Culturing Life*, 126.

12 Landecker, *Culturing Life*, 110–11.

tool. In 1954 Enders, together with his collaborators Thomas Weller and Frederic Robbins, traveled to Stockholm in order to receive the Nobel Prize in Physiology or Medicine.[13]

In Sweden, virologist Sven Gard had collaborated with Enders in the 1930s and was aware of his work. Gard had become a professor at the new department of virology at the Karolinska Institute in 1948, and he placed his desk, bench, and department in the premises of NBL in Stockholm. NBL was a national institution with broad responsibilities: its researchers, lab technicians, and veterinarians monitored and investigated epidemics and infectious agents on the behalf of the whole country. Attempts to produce vaccines were part of the NBL staff's research work, and the battle against polio had high priority.[14]

Sweden had long endured polio and was struck by one of its worst epidemics in 1953.[15] Yet public health initiatives were scarce, reflecting the limited tools available. For individuals and the authorities, it seemed impossible to protect oneself or others against polio. Prevention measures focused on isolating those who had become ill and disinfecting infected premises; in many ways people were left to their own devices.[16] The National Organization against Polio was created in 1946 by polio survivors, and by the 1950s, the organization was funding polio-related research (with money raised through many public fundraising campaigns).[17]

In the United States, the first effective polio vaccine was developed in 1952 by Jonas Salk. Large quantities of vaccine were needed, and it was prepared using monkey tissues as well as HeLa cells. Using human fetal tissues from abortions was hardly an option, considering the barriers to obtaining abortions at the time.[18] Following tests on small groups and a large field test, US authorities began the mass vaccination of children. In April 1955, alarming reports emerged: a number of patients had contracted polio and ten people died after

13 Landecker, *Culturing Life*, 121–25. As noted by Wadman, even if abortion was illegal in the United States at the time, 'therapeutic abortions' were conducted by licensed physicians. Enders and his team could acquire fetal tissues through informal contacts but only in smaller quantities. It was, in Robbins's recollection, 'not a reliable source.' See Wadman, *Vaccine Race*, 24–25; Robbins, 'Reminiscences of a Virologist,' 126.

14 Axelsson, 'Cutter Incident,' 316–17.

15 Axelsson, 'Cutter Incident,' 312.

16 Axelsson, *Höstens spöke*, 131–35.

17 Axelsson, *Höstens spöke*, 205–9.

18 Landecker, *Culturing Life*, 130, 135. According to Leslie Reagan, a wave of repression against abortion marked the 1950s in the United States. See Reagan, *When Abortion Was a Crime*, 162–63. From the early 1960s, as Wadman notes, American virologists lamented the lack of human fetal tissues for research and reached out to Swedish virologists for fetuses obtained from legal abortions. See Wadman, 'Medical Research,' 423–24.

being vaccinated with Salk polio vaccine from the Cutter pharmaceutical company—an episode later known as the Cutter Incident. It was discovered that a batch of this vaccine had not been properly inactivated, allowing live polio virus into the distributed doses. Security procedures were tightened, and the vaccination campaigns resumed. In a couple of years, the annual number of polio cases had dropped rapidly.[19]

Events in the United States were closely monitored by Swedish authorities and experts. But NBL's leaders were not content to simply wait for the American vaccine to be shipped. They were confident that Sweden could make its own contribution and play a leading role in the international vaccine race. In addition, even before the Cutter Incident, Gard had repeatedly expressed his distrust in Salk's vaccine, and he came to advocate for another type of inactivated vaccine. The Swedish vaccine, developed between 1952 and 1956, and used in mass vaccinations from 1957, was, according to its originators, much safer and more effective than the American one. It is still part of the Swedish national children's vaccination program.[20]

The development of the Swedish polio vaccine has often been portrayed as a success story, not least by the virologists themselves.[21] Yet a closer look into the activities of NBL during the crucial years around 1955 shows that the path chosen in Sweden—human instead of animal tissues—meant delay in launching the vaccination program and, ultimately, in the protection of the health and lives of Swedish citizens.

2 Building an Infrastructure of Supply

In 1952 a group of virologists in Stockholm took the initiative to develop a vaccine against polio. They included NBL's director, Gunnar Olin, and Gard at the Karolinska Institute's virology department, located within NBL; Astrid Fagraeus and Tore Wesslén at NBL; and Arne Svedmyr at the virology department of the Central Bacteriological Laboratory of Stockholm City.[22] The same year, Wesslén had established a method for fetal tissue cultures of polio viruses at

19 Oshinsky, *Polio*, esp. chaps. 12, 13.

20 Albert Sabin's oral polio vaccine, which was adopted globally from the early 1960s, was never used in Sweden. On the Swedish path to a vaccine, see Axelsson, *Höstens spöke*, chap. 5.

21 Lycke, 'Svenska poliovaccinet.'

22 Olin, 'Poliomyelitprofylax.' In 1954 Erik Lycke joined the group.

NBL. The hopes and the stakes were high. Sweden had a unique advantage over other nations: access to legal abortions.[23]

Still, the working conditions were a far cry from the facilities enjoyed by American researchers. By emphasizing the rapid development of the field of virology as well as the urgent need for a polio vaccine, Olin and Gard were able to increase funding for locations, equipment, and personnel. In 1952, NBL expanded its virus section to include a new unit for tissue culture, where Wesslén could work. Two years later funds were allocated for the construction of a new and significantly larger building to house the virus section and for the Karolinska Institute's virology department. Likewise, in 1952 the Central Bacteriological Laboratory of Stockholm City was equipped with new apparatus and instruments, including an electron microscope, to facilitate the method of tissue culture. Arne Svedmyr, who had returned to Sweden after two years as research fellow at Enders's laboratory in Boston, was recruited as its director. Nonetheless, even though conditions improved, the perceived lack of resources was constant.[24]

What proved to be the greatest difficulty in developing the vaccine, however, was acquiring aborted fetuses. The NBL virologists built upon a well-established precedent. As shown by previous international studies, the supply of human tissues has long functioned as a crucial infrastructure for research.[25] In Sweden, collegial networks of physicians and midwives sent fetuses from interrupted pregnancies to anatomy departments throughout the nineteenth and twentieth centuries. The number of fetal corpses increased after the decriminalization of abortion in 1938, when operations were performed at hospitals, establishing a closer link between clinics and laboratories.[26]

Even applied in a restrictive manner, the Swedish legislation allowed abortions on socio-medical indications since 1946—for instance, if a pregnancy might put a woman's physical or mental health at risk. In consequence, aborted, healthy fetal bodies were available in much larger numbers than in the United States and many other countries where abortions were permitted only on strictly medical grounds, or were simply illegal. Furthermore, long processing times for the applications meant that legal abortions in the second trimester

23 Wesslén, 'Vävnadsodlingstekniken inom poliomyelitforskningen,' 1686.

24 Swedish Parliament, 'Nr 128. Kungl. Maj:ts proposition', esp. 57–71; Stockholm City Council, 'Nr 143. Utlåtande angående anslag.'

25 Clarke, 'Research Materials and Reproductive Science.'

26 See the chapters by Franzén, Jülich, and Åhrén in this volume.

were quite common in Sweden; thus quite a number of aborted fetuses were large enough to be useful as research material.[27]

Many physicians, and especially gynecologists, were against abortion, unless the woman's life was at stake. Nevertheless, a moral economy was established in which both proponents and opponents of abortion supported the use of aborted fetuses for research that could improve conditions for the living. As Jülich has noted elsewhere, members of the Medical Research Council, and especially its committee on human fetal physiology and chemistry, emphasized Sweden's exceptional situation and considered that not using the aborted fetuses in medical research 'would be a remarkable waste of a unique scientific material.' A sense of urgency was also articulated: 'We do not know how long the current abortion law will last.'[28]

It has not been possible to find explicit statements of Swedish virologists' opinions on the abortion legislation. Yet their instrumental attitude toward the handling of aborted fetuses is striking. At meetings held as part of a 1953 state investigation on bacteriological sera and vaccines, several NBL experts discussed whether they should be using fetal tissues or available alternatives in research, diagnostics, and vaccine production. Bernt Malmgren, bacteriology professor at the Karolinska Institute, underscored Sweden's 'favorable situation' thanks to 'unique conditions' in the abortion legislation, and warned that it would be a 'serious malpractice, if we chose to use non-human tissue material.' He was skeptical toward moving state-controlled production to private pharmaceutical companies, which had shown interest in taking over the manufacture of the polio vaccine.[29] Wesslén, the tissue culture expert from NBL, underscored that only 10 percent of the country's available fetuses were used in vaccine production, implying that 90 percent remained an untapped resource. In turn, Gard pointed out that it was not possible at present to 'make use of the whole abortion frequency.'[30] He did not specify the obstacles but, as we discuss below, the Swedish abortion controversy would soon interfere with the planned upscaling of the infrastructure for polio vaccine.

There is no documentation of how the virologists acquired their very first fetal tissues, but by the end of 1952, NBL had established collaborations with women's clinics in the Stockholm region and was already planning for more. Within a year, NBL had a network of clinics supplying them with the fetuses they needed—five to ten each week. The providers were, first, Stockholm's

27 See Jülich's introduction to this volume.
28 Jülich, 'Fosterexperimentens produktiva hemlighet,' 17.
29 Malmgren, P.M. concerning the production of primarily virological vaccines.
30 Notes from meeting, October 30, 1954.

main abortion clinic at Sankt Erik's Hospital; then, by 1955, most gynecological clinics in Stockholm; and, after 1955, hospitals in an expanding radius: Södertälje, Eskilstuna, Västerås, Gävle. Slaughterhouses in Enskede and Uppsala provided amniotic fluid from cows, which was used as nutrients for the tissue cultures.[31] In the beginning, the transportation of fetal bodies was organized by taxi, owing to the irregular timing and necessary speed of the shipments. But taxis turned out to be very expensive, and NBL requested funding for a van and a driver for the task. Since they expected to need increasing quantities of fetal organs for laboratory use, sourced from providers within an increasing radius, this was said to be a more economically advantageous solution.[32]

At NBL and collaborating virus laboratories, these fetuses from women who had undergone abortion were used for polio activities.[33] Drawing on the work of Enders and his collaborators, the team of researchers and assistants developed methods for the culture of human tissue. Organs from the incoming fetuses were minced and mixed with solutions such as bovine amniotic fluid to provide a substrate in which viruses could thrive. Constantly moving roller tubes kept the cells alive. When polio virus was added, the cells died within twenty-four hours. In this way, the tissue cultures could be employed in diagnosing various types of polio as well as determining whether a person had immunity to them. In addition, fetal tissue cultures could be used to produce large quantities of virus and, in effect, develop a potent polio vaccine. The virus was inactivated with formaldehyde at a low temperature, and the antigenicity of the vaccine was tested by inoculation on guinea pigs. The use of human instead of monkey tissues and the technique for inactivation made the Swedish vaccine different from others that were developed during the same period, the most important of which was Salk's in the United States.[34]

In 1954, optimism ran high among NBL virologists: 'in our country we are fully "up to date" with the new approach to the study of different problems related to polio.' They were confident that 'Sweden [marched] on this field fully alongside other nations.'[35] The goal was to quickly produce a national vaccine against polio, made in Sweden and available in such quantities that the whole population could be vaccinated.[36] The laboratory was scaling up: in just a year, NBL established a new polio section, which in turn quickly divided into several

31 Reports of activities, 1953, p. 30; 1954–1955, p. 49; 1955–1956, p. 56.

32 Board of NBL, statement to the King in Council, May 21, 1955.

33 The research was funded by grants from King Gustaf V's 80th Anniversary Foundation, the National Organization against Polio, and the Swedish Medical Research Council.

34 Wesslén, 'Vävnadsodlingstekniken inom poliomyelitforskningen.'

35 Kling, 'Barnförlamningsprofylax,' 1388.

36 Swedish Parliament, 'Nr 206. Kungl. Maj:ts proposition,' 3–6.

specialized subsections. Soon the enterprise was running like a small factory, and the need for fetal tissues escalated.[37] However, expanding the supply chain would prove to be more difficult than envisioned.

The pros and cons of using human fetal organs and monkeys' organs in polio vaccine production were discussed by NBL representatives and officials as well as in Parliament. The main argument in favor of using human fetuses for a national vaccine was precisely that they were human, which—as NBL and the minister who pleaded its cause argued—minimized side effects such as hypersensitivity (*sensibilisering*). And human fetuses were cheap; their transportation was more or less the only cost.[38] (There is evidence that the pathologists who helped supply the fetal bodies got a symbolic wage, but this outlay seems to have been minor.[39]) Monkeys, in turn, were expensive, required care, might die on the way to Sweden or be infected and therefore unusable, and sometimes were difficult to acquire in the necessary quantities, since laboratories worldwide were participating in the polio vaccine race.[40]

Quite a few factors weighed against the use of human fetal tissues. They were already a scarce resource within NBL's polio department, where the diagnostic division and the vaccine production division fought over access to fetal tissues for their core activities.[41] Moreover, the parliamentary hearings acknowledged that the 'supply [of fetuses] always will be erratic and unpredictable,' whereas the buying and selling of monkeys 'facilitated a rational work strategy.' Therefore, in the autumn of 1955, the decision was taken to also use monkey tissues for the manufacture of the vaccine.[42] In 1957 monkey tissues were the primary source.[43] NBL abandoned fetal tissue cultures as a means of production for polio vaccine, but kept them as a standard tool for virological work.[44]

37 Reports of activities 1955–56, 55–59.

38 Board of NBL, statement to the King in Council, May 21, 1955; Swedish Parliament, 'Nr 206. Kungl. Maj:ts proposition.' See also notes from meeting, October 30, 1954.

39 Böttiger to Kaplan.

40 Board of NBL, statement to the King in Council, May 21, 1955. See also 'Svårt göra apnjurevaccin.'

41 Notes from meetings, October 21 and October 30, 1954.

42 Board of NBL, statement to the King in Council, September 21, 1955; Swedish Parliament, 'Nr 206. Kungl. Maj:ts proposition.'

43 Swedish Parliament, 'Nr 206. Kungl. Maj:ts proposition.'

44 'Human lung' cultures (fetal cell cultures) were used in epidemiological work such as the monitoring of sewage water and polio testing of adoptive children born abroad until at least the end of the 1970s. In many cases (when the culture is noted only as human lung) it is impossible to tell whether the tool used was fetal tissue cultures or cell lines. See various documents concerning polio, 1950–93.

These discussions demonstrate that the infrastructure that provided fetal tissues for research, diagnostics, and vaccine production was a standing item on the national agenda between 1952 and 1957. Yet annual activity reports, official letters, and government bills contain sparse information about the uses of aborted fetuses and whether vaccine production sparked any criticism among the larger public. The more outspoken report from the 1953 investigation on bacteriological sera and vaccines was classified as secret and thus accessible only to a restricted group. This measure indicates that the Government and NBL strove to control information about the making of the Swedish polio vaccine. As the next section will reveal, newspapers and magazines from the period do indeed suggest a tension between government secrecy and media interest.

3 The Nation against Polio

As previous research has taught us, infrastructures are invisible until they break.[45] An incident in Stockholm illustrates that this was also true of the virologists' supply chain. In March 1954 a local police station was contacted by the leading National News Agency regarding information received about four human fetuses found on a garbage heap next to the incinerator of Enskede slaughterhouse, on the outskirts of the city. Two police officers were immediately dispatched and conducted an on-site investigation. They reported that the fetuses were four to five months old and came from the Central Bacteriological Laboratory of Stockholm City. The incinerator of the virus department was out of order, and a substitute driver had mistakenly transported the packet containing the fetal corpses to the Slaughterhouse. The report was filed and a copy sent to Stockholm City Hospital Directorate, which took no action. Significantly, the news agency did not publish the sensitive story, which was not unusual when medical authorities were asked to comment beforehand.[46]

This series of events was indicative of the information policy at the time. Virologists were concerned about the publicity surrounding their work to develop a Swedish polio vaccine. They complained internally and to government officials about newspaper headlines giving the false impression among the public that the victory was already won.[47] Journalists, on the other hand, wanted full access to the story behind the development of the vaccine and

45 Bowker and Star, *Sorting Things Out*, 35.

46 Ouchterlony, statement from the chief of police. On the relationship between medical authorities and the media, see Jülich, 'Fosterexperimentens produktiva hemlighet.'

47 Olin, 'Poliomyelitprofylax,' 1693; Olin, 'Barnförlamningens förebyggande,' 11.

plans for the national vaccination program. 'Why do we get to know nothing?' a reporter wrote in May 1954. The research team that worked with the vaccine had surrounded itself with complete silence, and questions were left unanswered, according to the reporter.[48] Another article about six months later referred to 'impenetrable secrecy' and centralized control of publishing as principles governing vaccinations in the United States as well as in Sweden. NBL replied that it was necessary to 'give researchers the opportunity to carry out their investigations in peace and quiet.'[49] But in October 1956 an editorial in the same newspaper argued that it was high time that the 'hitherto very secretive department provided the public with the clearest possible information' on why the vaccination was delayed.[50]

Nevertheless, NBL and the Ministry of the Interior were dependent on the media for communication with the public. In the years 1952–57, reporters interviewed virologists in newspapers and magazines about the threat of polio and progress in the development of the new vaccine. Both the press and NBL representatives described polio epidemics in Sweden as escalating: 'In a few decades, the disease has changed character, now attacking people in their 70s and with ever more critical consequences.'[51] They portrayed fetal tissue cultures as virology's promising new tool, key to finding a safe and effective defense against polio. This was a pioneering scientific enterprise accelerated by an international race for polio vaccines, and therefore mobilized the best of Sweden's resources.[52]

At the end of 1952, NBL representatives were said to be optimistic about producing a Swedish vaccine. They were in possession of a potent 'weapon'—that is, the methodology of tissue cultures—but more resources, including laboratory facilities and personnel, were needed.[53] In an interview Sven Gard spoke of Swedish researchers' use of tissues from fetuses, adopting a specific metaphor: 'Here one can speak about the "front of the abortion medal."' By this he alluded to the Swedish expression 'the back of the medal,' meaning the ugly, unpleasant, or disadvantageous side of a thing or condition. In other words, there was a negative aspect to abortions; this was the back of the medal. The positive aspect was that aborted fetuses used for vaccine production could help save future lives.[54] That goal seemed distant. In 1953 Sweden endured one

48 Blaustein, 'Vaccination mot polio första juni.'
49 'Vaccinering mot polio nästa månad.'
50 'När får vi besked?'
51 Nordfeldt, 'Final mot polion?'
52 Bernholm, 'Professor Sven Gard i poliointervju.'
53 'Brist på medel binder forskare.'
54 Bernholm, 'Professor Sven Gard i poliointervju.'

of its worst polio epidemics, with more than five thousand cases registered, of which over three thousand had paralytic polio.

This crisis prompted the picture magazine *Se* (See) to publish a report, with photographs by Lennart Nilsson, on the work to develop a Swedish vaccine for polio at the laboratory in Huvudsta outside Stockholm. In typical fashion, the story had been created 'in collaboration with' NBL, and the images as well as the text had been 'reviewed and authorized by relevant research and health-care institutions.' Three spreads showed the different stages in the researchers' work of producing the vaccine at the 'sterile' laboratory. One of the images zoomed in on how fetal lung tissues were transferred from some kind of dissection table to a petri dish, and another displayed a cow's uterus from which amniotic fluid was tapped for growing the tissues in a test tube. Two pictures showed what a normal tissue culture looked like, and the same tissue culture after being infected with polio virus. However, nowhere on these pages was it mentioned that the tissues came from human fetuses. The reader had to flip through the magazine to the text-only section in the back, where the end of the article explained that the tissues came from legally aborted fetuses. Harder to miss was the spread in the middle announcing an article in the following issue that would focus on the struggle to prevent and cure polio, especially in young patients. In this way, the struggle to develop a vaccine (using aborted fetuses) was linked to concern for the lives of children.[55]

In April 1954 the press reported that the 'Swedish polio vaccine was now a fact.' It was only a matter of time before more than one hundred thousand children could be vaccinated. 'Two years of intense research had placed Sweden alongside the United States.'[56] In an interview Tore Wesslén, the scientist responsible for the 'research feat,' acknowledged the crucial contribution of the chemist Carola Neumüller, who (during a lunch when he was half-listening) had given him the idea of adding a small amount of glycerin to the formalin during the inactivation of the virus. Evidently, he had already injected himself with the polio vaccine and had not fallen ill. Yet the mass vaccinations had to be cancelled owing to 'not completely satisfying' results from test controls on monkeys. Only a small group of five hundred people in Stockholm was tested in the first round.[57] No negative side effects were registered, but because

55 Kjellström and Nilsson, 'Kampen mot polio, 1,' 41.

56 Blaustein, 'Polio-skydd för 100.000.'

57 Blaustein, 'Här har ni forskarbragden bakom poliovaccinet!'; Blaustein, 'Vaccination mot polio första juni.'

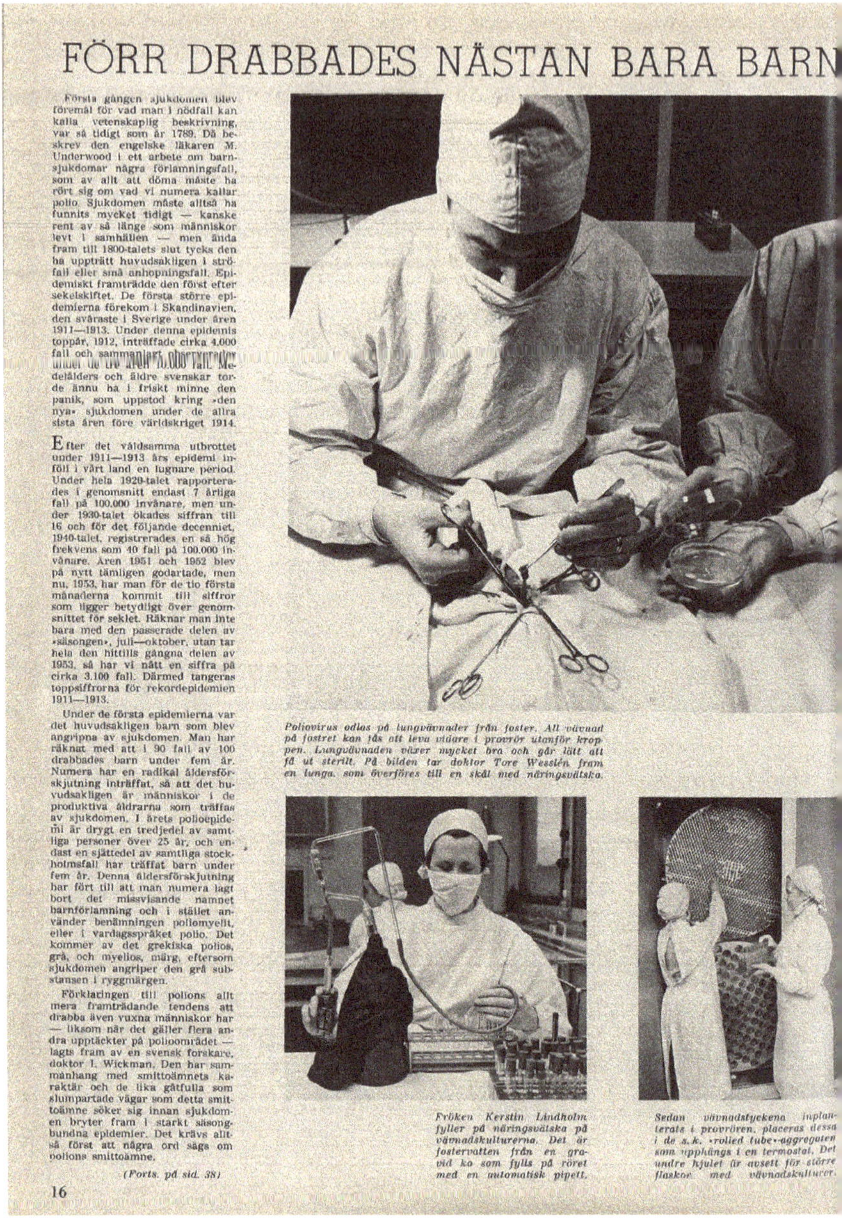

FÖRR DRABBADES NÄSTAN BARA BARN

Första gången sjukdomen blev föremål för vad man i nödfall kan kalla vetenskaplig beskrivning, var så tidigt som år 1789. Då beskrev den engelske läkaren M. Underwood i ett arbete om barnsjukdomar några förlamningsfall, som av allt att döma måste ha rört sig om vad vi numera kallar polio. Sjukdomen måste alltså ha funnits mycket tidigt — kanske rent av så länge som människor levt i samhällen — men ända fram till 1800-talets slut tycks den ha uppträtt huvudsakligen i ströfall eller små anhopningsfall. Epidemiskt framträdde den först efter sekelskiftet. De första större epidemierna förekom i Skandinavien, den svåraste i Sverige under åren 1911—1913. Under denna epidemis toppår, 1912, inträffade cirka 4.000 fall och sammanlagt observerades under de tre åren 10.000 fall. Medelålders och äldre svenskar torde ännu ha i friskt minne den panik, som uppstod kring »den nya» sjukdomen under de allra sista åren före världskriget 1914.

Efter det våldsamma utbrottet under 1911—1913 års epidemi inföll i vårt land en lugnare period. Under hela 1920-talet rapporterades i genomsnitt endast 7 årliga fall på 100.000 invånare, men under 1930-talet ökades siffran till 16 och för det följande decenniet, 1940-talet, registrerades en så hög frekvens som 40 fall på 100.000 invånare. Åren 1951 och 1952 blev på nytt tämligen godartade, men nu, 1953, har man för de tio första månaderna kommit till siffror som ligger betydligt över genomsnittet för seklet. Räknar man inte bara med den passerade delen av »säsongen», juli—oktober, utan tar hela den hittills gångna delen av 1953, så har vi nått en siffra på cirka 3.100 fall. Därmed tangeras toppsiffrorna för rekordepidemien 1911—1913.

Under de första epidemierna var det huvudsakligen barn som blev angripna av sjukdomen. Man har räknat med att i 90 fall av 100 drabbades barn under fem år. Numera har en radikal åldersförskjutning inträffat, så att det huvudsakligen är människor i de produktiva åldrarna som träffas av sjukdomen. I årets polioepidemi är drygt en tredjedel av samtliga personer över 25 år, och endast en sjättedel av samtliga stockholmsfall har träffat barn under fem år. Denna åldersförskjutning har fört till att man numera lagt bort det missvisande namnet barnförlamning och i stället använder benämningen poliomyelit, eller i vardagsspråket polio. Det kommer av det grekiska polios, grå, och myelios, märg, eftersom sjukdomen angriper den grå substansen i ryggmärgen.

Förklaringen till polions allt mera framträdande tendens att drabba även vuxna människor har — liksom när det gäller flera andra upptäckter på polioområdet — lagts fram av en svensk forskare, doktor I. Wickman. Den har sammanhang med smittoämnets karaktär och de lika gåtfulla som slumpartade vägar som detta smittoämne söker sig innan sjukdomen bryter fram i starkt säsongbundna epidemier. Det krävs alltså först att några ord sägs om polions smittoämne.

(Forts. på sid. 38)

Poliovirus odlas på lungvävnader från foster. All vävnad på fostret kan fås att leva vidare i provrör utanför kroppen. Lungvävnaden växer mycket bra och går lätt att få ut sterilt. På bilden tar doktor Tore Wesslén fram en lunga, som överföres till en skål med näringsvätska.

Fröken Kerstin Lindholm fyller på näringsvätska på vävnadskulturerna. Det är fostervatten från en gravid ko som fylls på röret med en automatisk pipett.

Sedan vävnadstyckena inplanterats i provrören, placeras dessa i de s.k. »rolled tube»-aggregaten som upphängs i en termostat. Det undre hjulet är avsett för större flaskor med vävnadskulturer.

16

FIGURE 7.1 Spread from the picture magazine *Se* (See) showing the production of polio vaccine at the NBL in Stockholm. On the *top* to the left: Tore Wesslén is extracting a lung from a human fetus. According to the text, fetal lungs were especially suited for cultivation since the cells grew rapidly and sterility was easy to maintain. On the *top* to the right: Preparator Annelise Zscheile showing a flask with virus substance to be used in vaccinations against polio. *Bottom* from left to right: an assistant is filling up nutrient fluid (amniotic fluid from a cow) on the test tubes with tissue cultures; two assistants are placing the tubes in the 'rolled tubes'; Astrid Fagraeus is immunizing a guinea pig against polio; technicians are adjusting the 'rolled tubes.' Photographer: Lennart Nilsson. From Kjellström and Nilsson, 'Kampen mot polio, 1,' 16–17. Courtesy of Lennart Nilsson Photography/SPL.

NU SLÅR POLION HÅRDAST MOT VUXNA

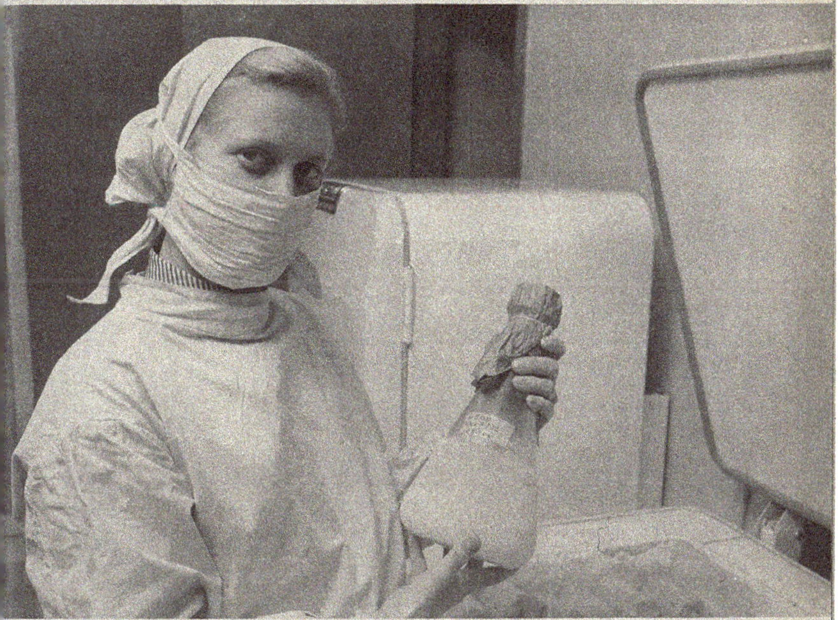

röken Annelise Zscheile visar en kolv med den virushaltiga vätska, som kall användas vid kommande vaccinationer på människor. Man arbetar nu å att få fram lämpliga metoder att avdöda virus. Vätskan kan nämligen spädas 00 miljoner gånger och fortfarande vara i stånd att infektera ett nytt provrör. ars innehåll sprutat in på en apa ger djuret barnförlamning på kort tid.

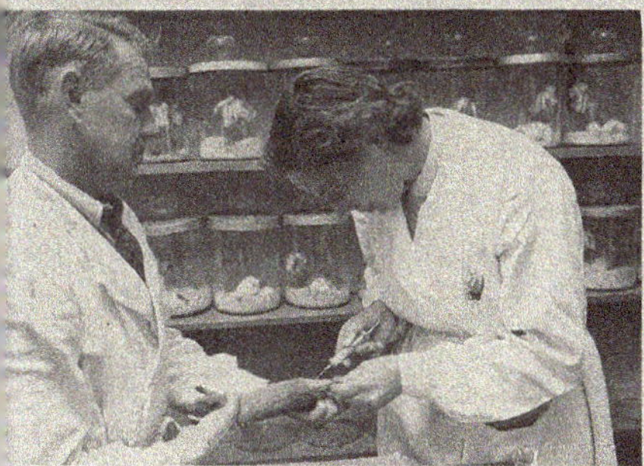

Docent Astrid Fagraeus immuniserar ett marsvin mot polio, assisterad av laboratoriebiträdet Jansson.

Inte bara läkare och laboratoriepersonal är viktiga länkar i forskningen. Teknikerna är lika oumbärliga. De flesta nya apparater för forskningen konstrueras och byggs på laboratoriets egna verkstäder. Maskinchefen Högberg och mekanikern Vallqvist arbetar här med insatser för »rolled tubes».

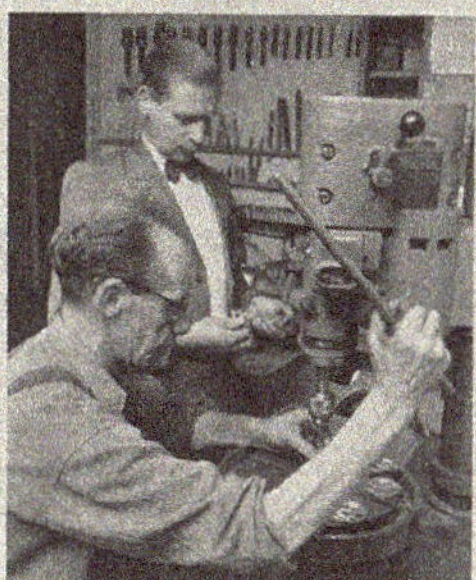

VÄND!

of the low prevalence of polio at the time, it was difficult to evaluate how effective the vaccine was.[58]

In early 1955 newspapers reported that an improved version of the Swedish polio vaccine had been developed. Since almost every article repeated the information in a similar way, the announcement was likely managed by authorities. Readers learned that the virus was now inactivated at a lower temperature than that suggested by Salk, which made the vaccine more effective. Above all, the Swedish vaccine was better than its American counterpart because it was produced from human material instead of tissues from other species (monkeys), thus reducing the risk of side effects.[59] The use of fetal tissues had been acknowledged before, but now it was presented in the media as a national advantage:

> Because of legal abortions, Sweden is in the quite unique situation, that polio researchers may use tissues from fetuses to produce vaccine. In the United States as well as Denmark, researchers are entirely dependent on kidney tissues from imported monkeys, which makes the vaccine more expensive. One may of course oppose, on emotional grounds, the method of 'making medicine' of unborn children, but concretely this means that the unborn support the living against a disabling, terrible disease.[60]

Once again legal abortions were weighed against polio vaccine, 'unborn children' against the future children of the nation. Within this moral economy, different values were enacted in a difficult balancing act.

A photomontage on the front page of Sweden's largest conservative daily showed individual portraits of the 'brain trust' responsible for the Swedish vaccine, against the background of the NBL location and buildings. Inside the newspaper, NBL's Astrid Fagraeus was interviewed. She emphasized that the achievement had not been possible without the support of a network of gynecologists at the women's clinics.

> In the fall of 1952, we had come so far as to scale up and organize our methods of tissue culture and the supply of the materials we had chosen, human fetal tissue. Our gynecologist colleagues were extraordinarily accommodating, this is something we want to emphasize. They are not

58 'Vaccinering mot polio nästa månad.'

59 Blaustein, '2.000 svenska barn börjar vaccineras på tisdag'; 'Svårt göra apnjurevaccin.'

60 'Svenska barn blir immuna i tre år.'

> happy to have to conduct legal abortions, but this way there is at least some blessing to it.[61]

According to Fagraeus, there were still 'unpredictable factors' that had to be resolved before mass vaccinations could begin. Most crucial, however, was the access to enough 'material.' Only tissues from humans and monkeys could be used.[62]

But within a week the scenario drastically changed, with reports that children had been affected by polio after mass vaccinations in the United States: the Cutter Incident.[63] Another phase of experiments and test controls started at the NBL laboratory. Soon it was announced that a new method had been developed, making it possible to create larger quantities of vaccine from the same volume of human fetal tissues (i.e., continuous cell cultures). Even so, production was limited, and NBL decided to also use kidney tissues from monkeys. For this reorganization they needed more funding, which the Government approved.[64] But success was long overdue; meanwhile, other countries, including Denmark, had already begun mass vaccinations using a version of the Salk vaccine. In 1956 a virologist at the Sahlgrenska University Hospital in Gothenburg spoke out in the press, describing the delayed vaccine as 'a national scandal.'[65] A schism became visible when the director of the National Board of Medicine pointed out that the production of the Swedish polio vaccine had 'in recent years suffered one setback after another.' The board had in every way tried to 'inspire and enthuse the bacteriological institute to take action in this area.' Importation of the American vaccine had to be considered—a measure which NBL's Gard opposed.[66]

Finally, in 1957, vaccinations of Swedish schoolchildren began, most of them with the Salk vaccine and only a few with the national version. After evaluating the program, Gard was quoted saying that he opposed further importation of foreign polio vaccine because its quality was poor. Instead, he emphasized the importance of producing sufficient quantities of domestic vaccine. The Swedish product was 'superior' to the American. This time human tissues were not mentioned—they were no longer used for vaccine production—but instead

61 Roque [pseud.], 'Svenska vaccinet av god klass.'

62 Roque [pseud.], 'Svenska vaccinet av god klass.'

63 'USA-larm för Salkvaccinet.'

64 'Poliovaccin massberedes'; 'Poliovaccinproduktionen ökas genom miljonanslag.'

65 'En riksskandal säger känd forskare.'

66 'Våraktion mot polion i farozonen.'

Gard highlighted the method of inactivating the virus, which according to him made the vaccine safer and more effective.[67]

Overall, the media contributed in making the polio vaccine into an uncontroversy. Newspapers and magazines mostly praised the virologists and their tireless work to save the future of the nation. However, they were also critical of the lack of information provided by the Government and NBL authorities. Official secrecy affected what could be written and how much knowledge readers could gain about the subject. In this way the media focus became the visible 'front of the abortion medal,' the positive aspects of using aborted fetuses for vaccine. But then the question remains: What was on the 'back of the medal'?

4 Abortion: an Unreliable Source

In the beginning, NBL advocated the exclusive use of aborted fetuses for the production of the Swedish polio vaccine. However, in the spring of 1955, monkey tissue was suddenly said to be an equivalent option, and soon it was also employed in practice. What was behind this change of course?

To find out we have to look into sources other than the news media. In a letter to the Stockholm City Hospital Directorate in 1956, the hospital director asked for more resources to be allocated to the Central Bacteriological Laboratory—NBL's collaborating partner. The virus department was in huge need of an extra laboratory assistant. The reason was that access to human fetuses that could be used for tissue cultures had been greatly reduced, and this situation was expected to become permanent. Hence the laboratory had to significantly expand the time-consuming task of the continuous culture of cells.[68] So far, this petition aligns with the media coverage but also emphasizes that something had drastically affected the supply of aborted fetuses. Records of proceedings from the Stockholm City Council reveal the cause for this shortage. Among descriptions of personnel and demands for funding appears a statement that the lack of access to human tissues resulted from the 'rather sharp decline in the number of legal abortions, and above all due to a change of surgical technique used for legal abortions.'[69] This information is not available in the newspapers.

---

67 'Svenskt vaccin utnyttjas vid vårens polioympningar'; 'Förskolebarnens tur att ympas mot polio'; 'Svenskt fabrikat av poliovaccin överlägset andra'; 'Svenskt preparat slår ut poliovaccinet.'

68 Pehrson, statement. It is not clear whether HeLa cells were used.

69 Stockholm City Council, 'Nr 258. Utlåtande med anledning,' 2002.

Asking why legal abortions decreased during the same period that NBL strove to scale up vaccine production takes us to the center of conflicts around abortion in Sweden. As we recall, in media coverage Astrid Fagraeus thanked gynecological colleagues who provided NBL with human fetuses even though they disliked conducting legal abortions.[70] In fact, most of them were against abortion except when the woman's life was in danger. Not all accepted the moral economy in which fetal lives were weighed against benefits for humanity. After the 1946 amendment to Swedish abortion law, which permitted abortion on socio-medical grounds, gynecologists as well as other physicians mobilized to rally support for stricter legislation.[71]

One of the strongest arguments for decriminalizing abortion in 1938 had been that illegal abortions were taking many women's lives. But what if legal abortions were also risky, even deadly? Then abortions should be avoided by every conceivable means, and instead social measures should be introduced to take care of the mother and the newborn child. This was the conclusion drawn by Erik Klintskog, a physician at the women's clinic at Sabbatsberg Hospital in Stockholm. On behalf of the National Board of Medicine, he had conducted a survey concerning mortality and morbidity related to legal abortions in Sweden in 1935–51, which he stated was the largest material in the world that was available for scientific analysis. A preliminary report was published in the Swedish medical journal *Svenska läkartidningen* in 1952. Klintskog stated that legal abortions were of two kinds: either abortion alone, or abortion combined with sterilization. Furthermore, sterilization was performed not only on eugenic grounds but also in several cases of 'weakness.' In the first instance sterilization was a condition for the interruption of pregnancy, but in the second instance the women themselves—many 'worn-out mothers'—often asked to be sterilized. In effect, the combination of abortion and sterilization was quite common. The numbers Klintskog presented were alarming. Mortality rates were at least twice as high in sterilization combined with abortion compared to abortion alone, and four times higher than those associated with childbirth.[72]

Klintskog's survey made the headlines, especially in newspapers published by left-wing parties. One read: 'High risk of death from sterilization

70 Roque [pseud.], 'Svenska vaccinet av god klass.'

71 Jülich, 'Picturing Abortion Opposition.'

72 During this period 35,000 women underwent legal abortions, of whom 10,300 were sterilized, and of these about 100 died in connection with the operation. See Klintskog, 'Om mortaliteten.' The National Board of Medicine required a report of every abortion that was conducted. It was primarily this group of data that Klintskog had used for his statistical survey.

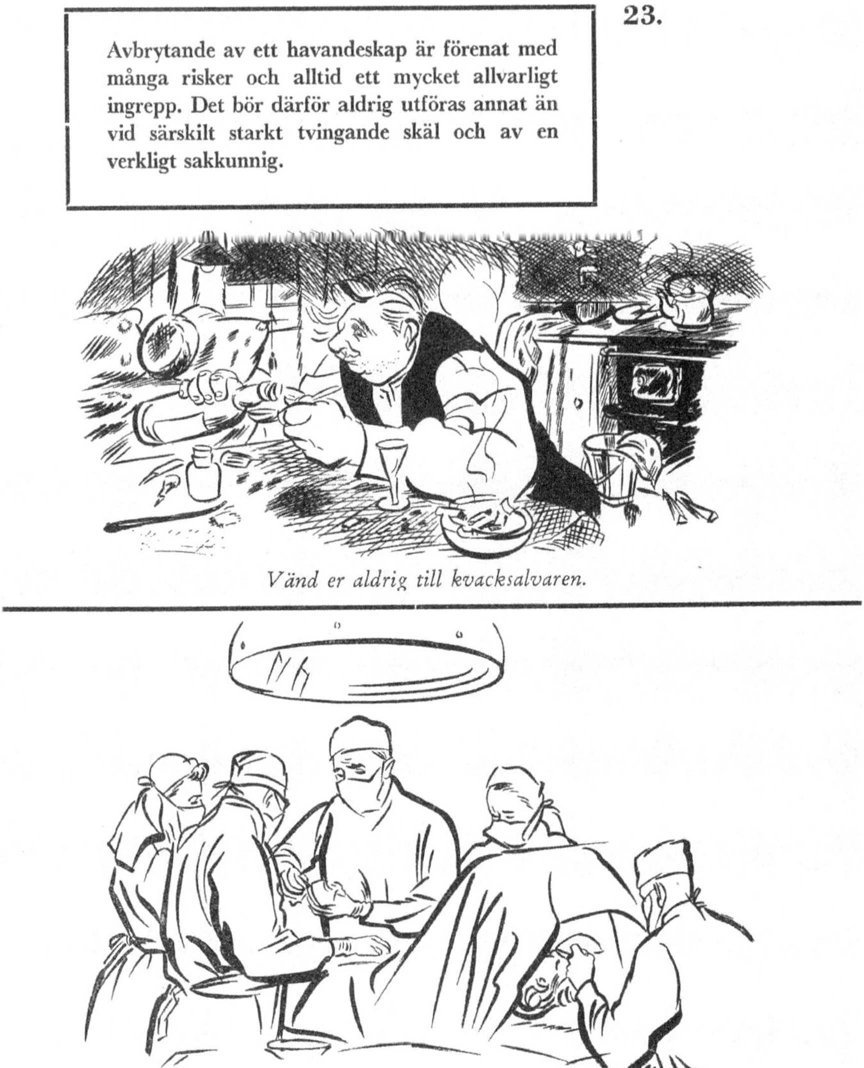
23.
Avbrytande av ett havandeskap är förenat med många risker och alltid ett mycket allvarligt ingrepp. Det bör därför aldrig utföras annat än vid särskilt starkt tvingande skäl och av en verkligt sakkunnig.
Vänd er aldrig till kvacksalvaren.
När läkaren avbryter ett havandeskap, sker detta genom operation.

FIGURE 7.2 Propaganda meant to illustrate the difference between illegal and legal abortions. Turning to a quack doctor and abortionist is associated with huge risks for the woman. When the physician performs the abortion this is done in a sanitized hospital setting where the patient is completely safe. The artist Margareta Sylwan made these drawings for a brochure that was produced and distributed by the National Board of Medicine. From Asklund and Lundberg, *Havandeskap, samhällets hjälp, abort*, 15. Reproduced with permission from the National Board of Health and Welfare and the family of Margareta Sylwan.

procedures.' Another was even more drastic: 'The sterilization condition for abortion is death for many women.'[73] In addition, Klintskog was interviewed by the picture magazine *Se*. In his responses he not only emphasized the risks associated with abortion but also spoke for 'the unborn.' He explained in detail how midterm and late abortions were performed by cesarean section, either vaginal or through the abdomen. In fact, the aborted fetuses were still alive and 'refused to die.' He claimed that '[f]etuses that are taken out through cesarean section have heartbeats for several hours.' It was an open question whether the physician who carried out the surgery was guilty of infanticide or not. In any case it was against the physician's primary ethical obligation to protect and safeguard life, according to Klintskog.[74]

The report included black-and-white photographs of embryos and fetuses by Lennart Nilsson. One covered a whole page, and the caption read: 'Does not everyone have the same right to be born and live in a democratic country? The picture shows one of those who was not asked: a fetus extracted during legal abortion at the age of five months.' (See figure 0.5 in the introduction of this volume.) A spread with four pictures of embryos and fetuses of different ages intended to illustrate '[t]he development of the fetus up to the point of viable life.' The caption under the photograph of the four-month-old fetus claimed that the face was already well developed and that 'fetuses at this stage show individual characteristics.' Below the captions, little boxes indicated how many out of every thousand legal abortions in Sweden were performed when the embryo or fetus was at each stage. Texts, pictures, and numbers combined to make specimens simulate human growth and life, encouraging readers to see connections between embryos, fetuses, and babies.[75]

Interestingly, whereas Klintskog's mortality numbers made headlines, Nilsson's fetal photographs were not much debated at the time. A few critical letters to the editor were included in the subsequent issue of *Se*, complaining of sensationalism, shock, and 'disgusting pictures.' The readers' revulsion suggests that there were no established visual conventions for seeing images of embryos and fetuses as 'babies.' The fact that Nilsson was not a scientist and lacked scientific credibility may also have played a part. In any case, it is not possible to know with certainty how Nilsson's photographs affected their viewers. There is no evidence to show whether the photographs persuaded women

73 'Dödsrisken stor vid steriliseringsingrepp'; 'Steriliseringskravet vid abort blir döden.'

74 Hillgren and Nilsson, 'Varför måste fostret dödas?'

75 Hillgren and Nilsson, 'Varför måste fostret dödas?' For a discussion, see Jülich, 'Picturing Abortion Opposition.'

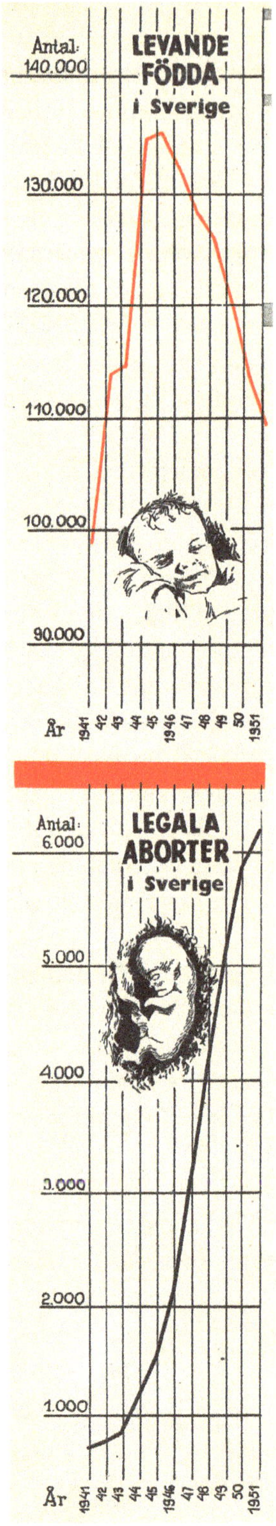

FIGURE 7.3

A graph showing (*top*) the number of live births in Sweden 1941–1951 and (*bottom*) the number of legal abortions during the same period. The drawing was included in a published interview with the physician Erik Klintskog who was critical of the Abortion Act. Unknown artist. From Hillgren and Nilsson, 'Varför måste fostret dödas?,' 14.

to forgo abortions or made physicians reject their applications, thus contributing to the low abortion rates in the 1950s.[76]

In contrast, Klintskog's descriptions of abortion surgery and statistics did have an impact. When a government committee published a report on the abortion issue in 1953, it included a summary by Klintskog, and the authors supported his conclusion that the combined abortion and sterilization operation posed a high risk to patients. Therefore, they recommended that sterilization no longer be a condition of abortion for eugenic reasons.[77] This too attracted a great deal of attention in the press. After reading the newspapers, women who had been granted abortions by the National Board of Medicine refused to have the surgery—that is, the small cesarean section. Nonetheless, not everyone was content with Klintskog's findings, not even those opposing abortion. Klintskog's colleagues were highly critical and insisted that his statistics were wrong.[78] But above all they were furious over his insinuation that members of the profession incorrectly stated medical reasons for abortions that actually had social grounds. This disloyalty had put them in a bad light in the eyes of the public. In a letter to the director general of the National Board of Medicine, Klintskog apologized for the damage he had caused, but also wrote that he 'had been taken by surprise by the inquisitorial attitude' among some colleagues and was bitter over their lack of appreciation for his difficult work.[79]

This detour through Swedish abortion conflicts can explain why NBL had to change direction in the development of its polio vaccine. The virologists had optimistically relied on legal abortions as a crucial part of their infrastructural supply. Gynecologists reluctantly collaborated, and the Government helped to keep the traffic confidential. Yet what NBL could not have foreseen is that Klintskog's survey and the media coverage, followed by the abortion committee report, led women to resist the current abortion practice by refusing to submit to sterilization (or refraining from applying for legal abortion). Even if there was no change in the law, the National Board of Medicine became more cautious, and from 1954 sterilization was less often a requirement for abortion.[80] Not only did the rate of abortions decrease but vaginal hysterotomies became less frequent. In effect, this created a shortage of human fetal tissues for vaccine research.

76 Jülich, 'Picturing Abortion Opposition.'

77 Swedish Ministry of the Interior, *Abortfrågan: Betänkande*.

78 The press coverage and women's refusal are mentioned by Ludvig Simon in his critical review, 'Yttrande över 1950 års abortutrednings betänkande.'

79 Klintskog to Engel.

80 On this change of praxis, see Tydén, *Från politik till praktik*, 241–44, 384–88. For a discussion of the abortion committee report, see Lennerhed, *Kvinnotrubbel*, esp. 72–76.

On the 'back of the medal' we find a controversial abortion method that risked women's lives and health. This precondition for the work of NBL was a closely guarded secret. Knowing this also puts the 'front of the medal' in a new light: How successful was the Swedish polio vaccine? One might wonder whether reliance on legal abortion ultimately delayed the launch of the national vaccine. As we have seen, when the infrastructure for supplying aborted fetuses failed in 1955, a complete reorganization of the production apparatus was necessary. It took time to adapt to monkey kidney tissues. Had this material been used earlier, or in combination with human tissues, the vaccine would probably have been ready earlier.[81]

In Sweden during the 1950s, few voices criticized the employment of human fetal tissues for the production of vaccines. Abortion was highly contested, but the use of aborted fetuses for scientific research was not publicly disputed; it was an uncontroversy. Responses began to change in the 1960s, when the media reported on medical experiments on living aborted fetuses as well as the use of fetal bodies for tissue cultures in virology and epidemiology. In the 1970s parliamentary politicians acted to regulate research involving fetuses. Finally, in 1995, the introduction of the Transplant Act regulated the use of aborted fetuses for medical research and vaccine production for the first time. From that point, the consent of the woman was required.[82]

5 Conclusion

We have described how an infrastructure supplying aborted human fetuses for vaccine research and production was built in Sweden during the 1950s. Swedish abortion legislation was a crucial condition for the development of a national polio vaccine. Access to human fetal material was the key factor for the group of virologists who envisioned a cheaper, safer, and more effective vaccine than the American one, produced using monkey tissues. In this process virology was established as an academic subject, and the National Bacteriological Institute and the virology department of the Karolinska Institute expanded thanks to increased government resources in a time of crisis. But in the end, the infrastructure failed to deliver. Conflicts over abortion interfered with ambitions for a national vaccine, and monkey tissues became the only alternative.

81 Indeed, this has belatedly been implied by one of Gard's coworkers. See Norrby, 'Segern över polio.'

82 Swedish Ministry of Health and Social Affairs, *Aborterade foster*. See also the introduction in this volume and the chapters by Tinnerholm Ljungberg and Björklund.

By focusing on the Swedish case, this chapter has contributed to the history of tissue culture in several ways. First, we have highlighted how a moral economy developed around the use of aborted fetuses for scientific research in Sweden. Above all, this was the case for the physicians at women's clinics who collected and sent the material to virologists and other researchers. Many gynecologists were against abortion in the 1950s and well into the 1960s. But instead of throwing away the material from abortions, they preferred to use it for research activities that could improve the human condition. The virologists were obviously sympathetic to their colleagues' concerns': the polio vaccine was the 'front of the abortion medal.'

Second, the use of human fetal tissues for vaccine research and production was an uncontroversy in Sweden in the 1950s, i.e. no public controversy broke out. However, we have shown that the lack of public debate about the infrastructural use of fetal tissues for the polio vaccine was not simply because this practice may have been seen as unproblematic. Secrecy imposed by the Government and authorities strictly limited reporting on how the vaccine was produced and the origins of the tissue cultures. When they did discuss these questions, journalists downplayed the human material and celebrated the work of the researchers, always respecting their medical and scientific sources. For general readers of newspapers and magazines, it must have been easy to miss these crucial details about virologists' work. Thus, a form of selective ignorance was produced around the manufacture of the Swedish polio vaccine.

Third, and relatedly, we found no clear evidence that people were upset because they thought that aborted fetuses were persons with rights. Rather, the process was (potentially) controversial due to its link to legal abortions, which in turn were seen as problematic in several ways. Abortion-critical physicians were convinced that the National Board of Medicine permitted abortions on the wrong grounds and too easily. Women who had been granted abortions refused to undergo the 'small cesarean section' because it was too risky. Fewer abortions were performed, and the use of hysterotomy declined. These incidents had unforeseen consequences for the expansion of an infrastructural supply of aborted fetuses to NBL. The grand project of developing a Swedish national polio vaccine with human fetal tissues failed.

Bibliography

Asklund, Lis, and Willy Maria Lundberg. *Havandeskap, samhällets hjälp, abort: Folkskrift i abortfrågan*. Stockholm: Medicinalstyrelsen, 1947.

Axelsson, Per. 'The Cutter Incident and the Development of a Swedish Polio Vaccine, 1952–1957.' *Dynamis* 32, no. 2 (2012): 311–28.
Axelsson, Per. *Höstens spöke: De svenska polioepidemiernas historia.* Stockholm: Carlsson, 2004.
Banchoff, Thomas F. *Embryo Politics: Ethics and Policy in Atlantic Democracies.* Ithaca, NY: Cornell University Press, 2011.
Bernholm, Bernt. 'Professor Sven Gard i poliointervju.' *Expressen*, December 2, 1952.
Blaustein, Eric. 'Här har ni forskarbragden bakom poliovaccinet!' *Expressen*, April 3, 1954.
Blaustein, Eric. 'Polio-skydd för 100.000.' *Expressen*, April 2, 1954.
Blaustein, Eric. '2.000 svenska barn börjar vaccineras på tisdag.' *Expressen*, March 6, 1954.
Blaustein, Eric. 'Vaccination mot polio första juni.' *Expressen*, May 27, 1954.
Bowker, Geoffrey C., and Susan Leigh Star. *Sorting Things Out: Classification and Its Consequences.* Cambridge, MA: MIT Press, 1999.
'Brist på medel binder forskare i arbetet på vaccin mot polio.' *Svenska Dagbladet*, November 25, 1952.
Burke, Peter. *Ignorance: A Global History.* New Haven, CT: Yale University Press, 2023.
Clarke, Adele E. 'Research Materials and Reproductive Science in the United States, 1910–1940.' In *Physiology in the American Context 1850–1940*, edited by Gerald L. Geison, 323–50. New York: Springer, 1987.
Creager, Angela N. H., and Hannah Landecker. 'Technical Matters: Method, Knowledge, and Infrastructure in Twentieth-Century Life Science.' *Nature Methods* 6, no. 10 (2009): 701–5.
'A Culture of Consent.' *Nature* 498 (June 27, 2013): 407.
'Dödsrisken stor vid steriliseringsingrepp.' *Arbetartidningen*, June 28, 1952.
Dussauge, Isabelle, Claes-Fredrik Helgesson, Francis Lee, and Steve Woolgar. 'On the Omnipresence, Diversity, and Elusiveness of Values in the Life Sciences and Medicine.' In *Value Practices in the Life Sciences and Medicine*, edited by Isabelle Dussauge, Claes-Fredrik Helgesson, and Francis Lee, 1–28. Oxford: Oxford University Press, 2015.
'En riksskandal säger känd forskare om uteblivet vaccin.' *Ny Tid*, September 21, 1956.
'Förskolebarnens tur att ympas mot polio.' *Dagens Nyheter*, March 26, 1957.
Hillgren, Karl E., and Lennart Nilsson. 'Varför måste fostret dödas?' *Se*, no. 28, July 10–16, 1952, 13–17.
Jülich, Solveig. 'Fosterexperimentens produktiva hemlighet: Medicinsk forskning och vita lögner i 1960- och 1970-talets Sverige.' *Lychnos* (2018): 10–49.
Jülich, Solveig. 'Picturing Abortion Opposition in Sweden: Lennart Nilsson's Early Photographs of Embryos and Fetuses.' *Social History of Medicine* 31, no. 2 (2018): 278–307.

Kjellström, Nils, and Lennart Nilsson. 'Kampen mot polio, 1: Forskarna skönjer målet.' *Se*, no. 45, November 5–11, 1953, 14–21, 38–41.

Kling, Carl. 'Barnförlamningsprofylax: Discussion.' *Nordisk medicin* 52, no. 40 (1954): 1388.

Klintskog, Erik. 'Om mortaliteten vid de legala aborterna utförda i Sverige 1935–1951.' *Svenska läkartidningen* 49, no. 26 (1952): 1691–99.

Landecker, Hannah. *Culturing Life: How Cells Became Technologies*. Cambridge, MA: Harvard University Press, 2007.

Lennerhed, Lena. *Kvinnotrubbel: Abort i Sverige 1938–1974*. Möklinta: Gidlunds, 2017.

Lycke, Erik. 'Svenska poliovaccinet: En framgångssaga.' *Läkartidningen* 110, no. 43–44 (2013): 1937–39.

Maynard-Moody, Steven. *The Dilemma of the Fetus: Fetal Research, Medical Progress, and Moral Politics*. New York: St. Martin's Press, 1995.

Merriam-Webster.com Dictionary. 'Uncontroversial.' Accessed April 15, 2024, https://www.merriam-webster.com/dictionary/uncontroversial.

'När får vi besked?' *Expressen*, October 7, 1956.

Nordfeldt, Stig. 'Final mot polion?' *Aftonbladet*, February 2, 1954.

Norrby, Erling. 'Segern över polio—en triumf för vetenskapen.' *Läkartidningen* 114, no. 38 (2017): 1542–43.

Olin, Gunnar. 'Barnförlamningens förebyggande: Förutsättningar och möjligheter.' *Polio* 4, no. 2 (1954): 1–11.

Olin, Gunnar. 'Poliomyelitprofylax.' *Nordisk medicin* 52, no. 49 (1954): 1689–93.

Oshinsky, David M. *Polio: An American Story*. New York: Oxford University Press, 2005.

'Poliovaccin massberedes: Framställning om anslag.' *Svenska Dagbladet*, May 24, 1955.

'Poliovaccinproduktionen ökas genom miljonanslag.' *Svenska Dagbladet*, June 4, 1955.

Proctor, Robert N. 'Agnotology: A Missing Term.' In *Agnotology: The Making and Unmaking of Ignorance*, edited by Robert N. Proctor and Londa Schiebinger, 1–33. Stanford, CA: Stanford University Press, 2008.

Reagan, Leslie J. *When Abortion Was a Crime: Women, Medicine, and Law in the United States, 1867–1973*. Berkeley: University of California Press, 1997.

Robbins, Frederick C. 'Reminiscences of a Virologist.' In *Polio*, edited by Thomas M. Daniel and Frederick C. Robbins, 121–34. Rochester, NY: University of Rochester Press, 1997.

Roque [pseud.]. 'Svenska vaccinet av god klass.' *Svenska Dagbladet*, April 21, 1955.

Simon, Ludvig. 'Yttrande över 1950 års abortutrednings betänkande.' *Svenska läkartidningen* 51, no. 9 (1954): 485–96.

Skloot, Rebecca. *The Immortal Life of Henrietta Lacks*. New York: Crown, 2010.

'Steriliseringskravet vid abort blir döden för många kvinnor.' *Arbetaren*, June 28, 1952.

Stockholm City Council. 'Nr 143. Utlåtande angående anslag till inventarieutrustning för sjukhusdirektionens bakteriologiska centrallaboratorium.' In *Stockholms*

stadsfullmäktiges handlingar. Collection 3, Vol. 1. *Stadskollegiets utlåtanden och memorial*, 1115–22. Stockholm: Stockholms stadsfullmäktige, 1951.
Stockholm City Council. 'Nr 258. Utlåtande med anledning av motion angående inrättande av ytterligare laboratristjänster vid bakteriologiska centrallaboratoriet.' In *Stockholms stadsfullmäktiges handlingar*. Collection 3, Vol. 2. *Stadskollegiets utlåtanden och memorial*, 2001–2006. Stockholm: Stockholms stadsfullmäktige, 1956.
'Svårt göra apnjurevaccin: Svensk avdödning jämnare.' *Dagens Nyheter*, April 23, 1955.
'Svenska barn blir immuna i tre år.' *Aftonbladet*, April 13, 1955.
'Svenskt fabrikat av poliovaccin överlägset andra.' *Dagens Nyheter*, September 19, 1957.
'Svenskt preparat slår ut poliovaccinet från USA.' *Svenska Dagbladet*, September 19, 1957.
'Svenskt vaccin utnyttjas vid vårens polioympningar.' *Dagens Nyheter*, February 1, 1957.
Swedish Ministry of Health and Social Affairs. *Aborterade foster, m.m.: Betänkande*. SOU 1991:42. Stockholm: Allmänna förlaget, 1991.
Swedish Ministry of the Interior. *Abortfrågan: Betänkande*. SOU 1953:29. Stockholm: Inrikesdepartementet, 1953.
Swedish Parliament. 'Nr 128. Kungl. Maj:ts proposition till riksdagen angående vissa anslag till statens bakteriologiska laboratorium m.m.; given Stockholms slott den 5 mars 1954.' In *Bihang till riksdagens protokoll 1954*. Collection 1, Vol. 11. *Kungl. Maj:ts propositioner nr 112–130*, 1–73. Stockholm: Riksdagen, 1954.
Swedish Parliament. 'Nr 206. Kungl. Maj:ts proposition till riksdagen angående anslag för tillverkning av polioympämne m.m.; given Stockholms slott den 14 oktober 1955.' In *Bihang till riksdagens protokoll 1955*. Collection 1. *Kungl. Maj:ts propositioner nr 200–217*, 1–14. Stockholm: Riksdagen, 1955.
Topçu, Sezin, and Irène Maffi. 'Rethinking Ignorance Production in the Field of Reproductive Biomedicine: An Introduction.' *Reproductive Biomedicine and Society Online* 14 (2022): 216–21.
Tydén, Mattias. *Från politik till praktik: De svenska steriliseringslagarna 1935–1975; Rapport till 1997 års steriliseringsutredning*. Stockholm: Fritzes offentliga publikationer, 2000.
'USA-larm för Salkvaccinet.' *Morgon-Tidningen*, April 28, 1955.
'Vaccinering mot polio nästa månad.' *Expressen*, January 6, 1955.
'Våraktion mot polion i farozonen.' *Dagens Nyheter*, September 25, 1956.
Wadman, Meredith. 'Medical Research: Cell Division.' *Nature* 498 (June 27, 2013): 422–26.
Wadman, Meredith. *The Vaccine Race: Science, Politics, and the Human Costs of Defeating Disease*. New York: Viking, 2016.
Wesslén, Tore. 'Vävnadsodlingstekniken inom poliomyelitforskningen.' *Nordisk medicin* 52, no. 49 (1954): 1685–86.

Wilson, Duncan. 'A Troubled Past? Reassessing Ethics in the History of Tissue Culture.' *Health Care Analysis* 24, no. 3 (2016): 246–59.

Archival Sources

Board of NBL. Statement to the King in Council, May 21, 1955. E1a:1440, Ministerial act, June 3, 1955, no. 78. Main archive 1932–1974, MI.

Board of NBL. Statement to the King in Council, September 21, 1955. E1a:1474, Ministerial act, October 14, 1955, no. 40. Main archive 1932–1974, MI.

Böttiger, Margareta, to Dr. B. Kaplan, May 25, 1960. Ö3a:24, Documents concerning polio 1950–1993. NBL 1962–1993.

Klintskog, Erik, to Arthur Engel, November 5, 1952. EII:4. Director general, Incoming correspondence 1952–1953. NBM.

Malmgren, B. P.M. concerning the production of primarily virological vaccines, November 30, 1954. Copy. Investigation on bacteriological sera and vaccines (1953–). NAS, Stockholm.

Notes from meeting, October 21, 1954. Investigation on bacteriological sera and vaccines (1953–). NAS, Stockholm.

Notes from meeting, October 30, 1954. Investigation on bacteriological sera and vaccines (1953–). NAS, Stockholm.

Ouchterlony, F. Statement from the chief of police concerning the slaughterhouse's incineration of four human fetuses sent by accident, March 30, 1954. Dnr 1954–264. E1a, Incoming correspondence. Stockholm City Hospital Directorate Archive. SCA.

Pehrson, Gösta. Statement on motion regarding the establishment of additional laboratory services at the Central Bacteriological Laboratory, March 5, 1956. F1:2. Central Bacteriological Laboratory of Stockholm City. SCA.

Reports of activities 1953–1956. E8:2 (1953–1959). Reports of the activities at NBL. Health Care Bureau 1915–1967. NBM.

Various documents concerning polio. Ö3a:7, Documents concerning polio 1950–1993. NBL 1962–1993.

CHAPTER 8

The Moral Imperative of Fetal Research: Framing the Scientific Use of Aborted Fetuses in the 1960s and 1970s

Helena Tinnerholm Ljungberg

During the 1950s and 1960s, a new area of medical research developed in Sweden. The country's comparatively liberal abortion law and financial support from research-funding agencies created a productive environment for experiments on human fetuses. Gynecologists, endocrinologists, and pediatricians conducted research on material from legal abortions as well as on pregnant female and infant patients without attracting much attention from society at large. Medical representatives and authorities argued in favor of using aborted fetuses that would otherwise be thrown away and destroyed.[1] According to some researchers, there was even a moral imperative to make the most of this 'medical waste,' which would help to further scientific knowledge on prenatal life. Increasingly, however, these practices came under debate in both the media and parliamentary politics, and in the 1970s they became entangled with public debates on the ethics of medical research on human subjects.

Most researchers interested in histories of fetal research on abortion material have focused on the United States and United Kingdom.[2] What is apparent from previous historical scholarship, and this chapter, is that over time certain uses of fetal material became the cause of greater controversy than others, and in some cases Sweden's liberal abortion laws, the research, and researchers themselves played a part.[3] Above all, I am interested in how these medical practices have been understood and framed in discussions about research ethics, especially in relation to the new demands for ethical review placed on

1 Jülich, 'Fosterexperimentens produktiva hemlighet'; Jülich and Tinnerholm Ljungberg, 'Från medicinskt avfall.'

2 Dubow, *Ourselves Unborn*; Schoen, *Abortion after* Roe; Morgan, *Icons of Life*; Pfeffer and Kent, 'Framing Women, Framing Fetuses'; Wilson, 'Ex Utero.' One important exception to this focus on the Anglo-American context is Maria Fannin's study of the Kyoto collection of embryologic material, established in 1961. Fannin, 'Making an "Embryological Vision."'

3 See Schoen, *Abortion after* Roe, chap. 2; Dubow, *Ourselves Unborn*, chaps. 2, 3; Morgan, *Icons of Life*, chap. 7.

 | DOI:10.1163/9789004703759_010

research with human subjects.[4] In this way, the Swedish case provides fresh historical perspectives on the international development of fetal knowledge production and adds to the call for 'more nuanced empirical studies' on the history of research ethics.[5]

The aim of this chapter is to trace Swedish fetal politics on a local and national level, with a focus on the framing of aborted fetuses as research material in the late 1960s and early 1970s.[6] Moreover, by providing examples of how Swedish fetal research was framed in other national contexts during this period, I highlight both more general tendencies and national particularities of the Swedish practices and policies. The analysis draws on material from the archives of medical organizations that were engaged in research ethics. Publicly available material from research ethics committees (RECs) provides valuable sources that give insight into the medical community's internal discussions.[7] In order to chart the changing landscape of fetal politics in Sweden, I analyze how various actors, such as researchers, members of RECs, parliamentary politicians, and critical voices framed and problematized these practices. In seeing this strand of research as a potential policy problem, I build on Sheila Jasanoff's discussion of *framing*, and the application of this concept by Naomi Pfeffer and Julie Kent in their study of British policies on the use of fetuses in medicine. In line with Jasanoff's concept of *ontological surgery*, I also discuss varying perceptions of fetuses as research material, and their ontological and moral status.[8] The concept of ontological surgery implies that, before one can decide whether, for example, fetal research is moral or not, it must be determined 'how to describe and characterize the problematic entities whose natures must be fixed as a prelude to ethical analysis.'[9] Jasanoff uses the example of the boundary drawing performed by the British Warnock

---

4 For more on the origins and early development of the research ethics committees in Sweden, see Tinnerholm Ljungberg, 'Regulating Research.'

5 Jacobs and Tinnerholm Ljungberg, 'How Ethics Travels,' 265; see also Jacobs, *Ethics by Committee*, 4.

6 The decision to study the Swedish debates and regulations surrounding fetal research and to include material relating to a local, national, and international context, is in line with Thomas Banchoff's comparative analysis of four nations' diverse 'embryo politics.' His analysis demonstrates how national policies and ethical discussions occurred within and in relation to international developments in embryo research. See Banchoff, *Embryo Politics*.

7 This archival access to the Swedish RECs' assessments of research on aborted fetuses in Sweden can be compared with the situation in the United Kingdom, where in 2007 there was 'no public record of research projects using aborted fetuses that they [RECs] have approved.' See Pfeffer and Kent, 'Framing Women, Framing Fetuses,' 434.

8 Jasanoff, 'Making the Facts of Life,' 77; Pfeffer and Kent, 'Framing Women, Framing Fetuses.'

9 Jasanoff, 'Making the Facts of Life,' 61.

committee in 1984, when research was restricted to in-vitro embryos younger than fourteen days. She describes how this 'ontological surgery succeeded here because the steady hand of experienced ethicists guided the knife blade.'[10] By using these concepts, this chapter will illustrate how the fetus was located at the center of an ongoing and conflictual process that actualized the dichotomies of the human and nonhuman, life and death.

To begin with I outline the debates on the status of the fetus in Sweden in the early 1960s and early reactions to the proposal of establishing ethical assessments of medical research. This account provides a starting point for understanding the further development of policies and praxis in relation to medical research on aborted fetuses. Thereafter, I demonstrate how fetal research was framed through the assessments of local ethics committees. The last two sections include an international outlook and an analysis of the national and parliamentary debate on these matters in Sweden.

1 From the 'Most Highly Regarded Researchers' to a New System of Ethics Committees

In the first half of the twentieth century research on fetuses was not seen as a controversial issue within the medical community. Aborted fetuses were framed as important resources that could be beneficial in the pursuit of a polio vaccine or to further endocrinological knowledge on prenatal development.[11] In the latter instance, various methods were used, including perfusion studies. Perfusion was a method used to oxygenate aborted fetuses still attached to the placenta, so that researchers could track the hormonal exchanges between the two entities. In order to acquire intact fetal material, fetuses were removed either through the abdomen or the uterus of the pregnant woman. This specific abortion method was sometimes referred to as the 'small cesarean section.'[12] The use of whole fetuses, however, soon spurred public controversy. By following these debates, I investigate how boundaries between life and death, and viability and nonviability, were reshaped through the perfusion studies.[13]

10 Jasanoff, 'Making the Facts of Life,' 64.

11 See Jülich and Dussauge's chapter in this volume.

12 Jülich, 'Fosterexperimentens produktiva hemlighet,' 18.

13 The concept of 'viability' can be traced back to nineteenth-century medicine, but during the 1960s and 1970s the concept became closely interlinked with matters relating to abortion and the maximum time limit for the procedure. See Swedish National Council on Medical Ethics, *Livstecken efter sen abort.* See also Svärd and Tinnerholm Ljungberg, 'Fetal and Animal Research' for a discussion on viability in the Swedish political debates of the

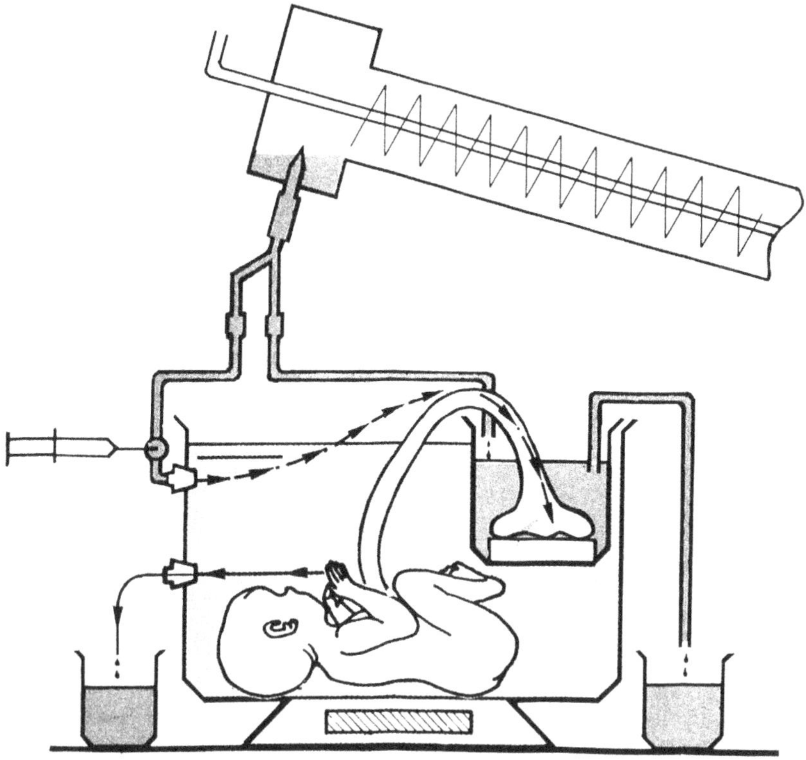

FIGURE 8.1 Schematic illustration of 'nonviable' fetus in perfusion apparatus. From Johannisson, 'Befolkningstillväxten måste mötas,' 8.

In the early 1960s, fetal research started to attract attention outside the medical community. The Swedish press reported on the use of aborted fetuses, and the matter became a subject of parliamentary debates.[14] These discussions concerned both the lawfulness and the ethics of the use of fetuses in a scientific setting. The Swedish minister of justice stated that no laws had been circumvented by the disputed research. The minister's statement also illustrated a recurring frame in which fetal research could be described as an ethical gray area—not illegal but still somewhat problematic from an ethical perspective. However, the minister of justice gave legitimacy to the research when he concluded that it had been performed by the "most highly regarded researchers," who had been granted funding for several years by respected bodies like the

1970s and 1980s. For a contemporary ethnographic study of viability in relation to personhood, in the context of hospital births, see Christoffersen-Deb, 'Viability.'

14 Jülich, 'Fosterexperimentens produktiva hemlighet.'

Swedish Medical Research Council and its counterpart in the United States, the National Institutes of Health (NIH).[15] The matter of the lawfulness and ethics of fetal research stayed off the parliamentary agenda for the rest of the decade, but it became much more visible to a broader public in the Swedish press. However, the legitimacy of fetal research would soon be guaranteed by a new entity within the medical community—the local RECs.

In February 1966, the medical university of Stockholm, the Karolinska Institute (KI), received a memo from Surgeon General William H. Stewart.[16] He stated that all research on human subjects receiving money from the NIH must henceforth be reviewed by a local ethical committee. Behind this decision was the evolution and expansion of an earlier local ethics committee at the Clinical Central Research Hospital in Bethesda, Maryland.[17] This decision by the NIH thus affected US-affiliated medical research departments in several countries, including Sweden and the United Kingdom, and would in due course also affect research projects that made use of human fetuses.[18] The memo prompted the rapid formation of the first formal Swedish committee at the medical faculty at the KI. Correspondence between the NIH and KI bears witness to intense communication during the formation of the REC. This suggests that the new ethics committee was eager to fulfill its role and ensure KI's ability to receive funding from the NIH.[19] A number of other formal RECs soon followed—for example, at Lund University in 1969—and at Gothenburg University a working group acted as a committee in early 1968. Within a few years there were ethical committees at every medical faculty across the country. The foundation for this new form of local review was spurred by the NIH in its capacity as a research funder, but as we will see, it soon became a naturalized medical-scientific practice.

In 1966 and 1967, the REC at the KI formalized and started to assess applications. The aim of this new practice was, according to the NIH, to make sure that research subjects gave their informed consent before participating in medical research, and to assess both 'risks and potential medical benefits' of proposed medical studies.[20] The NIH further demanded that the constitution of these new committees be accounted for, requesting details such as 'the numbers of members and the professional or public interests they reflect.'[21] In January

15 Swedish Parliament, 'Svar på interpellation av herr Gustafsson,' 38.
16 Surgeon general, Public Health Service, to the heads of institutions.
17 Stark, *Behind Closed Doors*.
18 Hedgecoe, '"A Form of Practical Machinery."'
19 See, for instance, Gordon to Holmstedt.
20 Angelone to Bergström.
21 Angelone to Bergström.

DEPARTMENT OF HEALTH, EDUCATION, AND WELFARE
PUBLIC HEALTH SERVICE

NATIONAL INSTITUTES OF HEALTH
BETHESDA, MD. 20014
AREA CODE 301 TEL: 656-4000

March 17, 1967

FOLKE

Dr. Bo Holmstedt
Professor of Pharmacology
Karolinska Institutet
Stockholm 60, Sweden

Dear Dr. Holmstedt:

It was a pleasure to discuss with you on the telephone today my request of February 24, 1967, for additional information in relation to the statement of assurance concerning investigations involving human subjects, submitted January 30 for the Karolinska Institutet.

A reply substantially as follows would, I feel certain, be acceptable to our reviewers:

> Our reviewing committee studies the written protocol or discusses the protocol in person with the investigator and decides whether his provisions are adequate for protecting the rights and welfare of the human subjects in his investigation, whether his methods of securing the consent of the subjects to participate in the investigation are appropriate, and whether the potential benefits of the investigation outweigh the risks. The committee employs as its criteria for these judgments the principles of the Declaration of Helsinki. The committee conveys its advice to the investigator through personal discussion with him.
>
> The professional staff and facilities of the Karolinska Institutet are available if needed for the subjects.

Sincerely yours,

D. T. Chalkley, Ph.D. for

Mordecai H. Gordon, Ph.D.
Special Assistant to the Director
Division of Research Grants

FIGURE 8.2 Correspondence between the NIH and KI reveals a part of the extensive communication between the two organizations. In this letter from 1967, KI receives advice on how to describe the work performed by their REC in future contacts with the NIH. 'Folke' (Sjöqvist) was the name of the secretary of the KI committee. Source: Gordon to Holmstedt.

1967, the KI committee consisted of seven professors and one associate professor. One of the professors was a specialist in gynecology and obstetrics, and another specialized in pediatrics.[22] The committee's composition was justified by the argument that members represented the disciplines that might produce 'research projects that demand thorough assessments' and that trials including children and pregnant women were considered to carry 'specific ethical problems.'[23] The policy from the NIH thus sparked a new ethical practice in Sweden, which meant that researchers collectively reviewed proposals for research projects involving human subjects, and assessed them from an ethical standpoint.

2 Local Ethical Review of a Planned International Program on Fetal Research

It was not long before the committee at the KI assessed its first application on fetal research. In the autumn of 1967, an application titled 'Human Fetal Development: An Interdisciplinary Study' was discussed at a meeting.[24] The Swedish applicants, led by the professor of pediatrics John Lind, were working with researchers from Yugoslavia and Japan (including the individual behind what would become known as the Kyoto collection).[25] This collaboration had been initiated by the American Association for the Aid of Crippled Children (AACC), a private foundation and grant-making organization established in 1899.[26] The AACC had previously funded research projects in Sweden, including those conducted by Lind and his colleagues. Additionally, since 1961 they had helped fund a laboratory in Stockholm for collecting and distributing fetal material transnationally.[27] The Stockholm-based collection was described in

22 'Institutional Assurance on Investigations.'

23 Sjöstrand and Sjöqvist, 'Etiska kommittén,' 24.

24 Lind et al., 'Human Fetal Development.' English in original.

25 The application mentions cooperation with M. Yasuda in Kyoto, Japan. This is probably the same Mineo Yasuda who was coauthor of at least one article based on research on the Kyoto collection, funded by both NIH and AACC; namely, Nishimura et al., 'Normal and Abnormal Development.' See also Fannin, 'Making an "Embryological Vision."' The Kyoto collection has been described as the 'largest collection of embryos in the world' by Fannin et al., 'Introduction,' 9.

26 Today the AACC is known as the Foundation for Child Development.

27 'Three Year Report.'

1967 as containing 'about 350 specimens stored in different fixatives and from which ca. 5000 blocks from most organs and tissues are available in paraffin.'[28]

This collection of fetal material was an important feature of the application. In 1967, the AACC was planning the international Human Fetal Development program, in which Swedish material played an important part. They were also planning to request co-funding from the NIH.[29] The program was internally motivated by the fact 'that alternative methods of birth control might hamper the supply of fetuses in the future and negate the great potential for research presently available.'[30] This statement only becomes understandable in light of the specific conditions for medical researchers in various countries, especially abortion legislation and practices.

The overall aim of the program was to investigate the factors causing prenatal mortality and spontaneous abortions. The proposed international, collaborative research program was divided into several national sub-studies, but they all planned to use material acquired from legal abortions. But the Swedish applicants also highlighted the importance of the rare, and soon to be even rarer, material that was claimed to be necessary to produce new knowledge: intact fetal material from late abortions. A memo to the Boards of Directors of the AACC stated that whole fetuses were about to become a scarce resource owing to 'new abortive techniques which macerate the fetus.'[31] It was the availability of this kind of intact fetal material from the second trimester that framed Swedish participation in the program as crucial, since the fetal material from Zagreb and Kyoto was mainly from earlier pregnancies (up to week ten). Lind argued as follows, in his application:

> Since Sweden is one of the few countries in the world where late induced abortions are performed the material sampled in Stockholm will be composed of late abortions to as great an extent as possible. However, relatively more early abortions are being performed and within a few years late abortions will be very rare also in Sweden. This prompts us to take care as soon as possible of this valuable material.[32]

The availability of this exceptional material (from a global perspective) was explained by the combination of Swedish abortion laws and the fact that

28 Lind et al., 'Human Fetal Development.'
29 Meetings of the Council, 7.
30 Executive committee minutes, 2.
31 Memo on Human Fetal Development.
32 Lind et al., 'Human Fetal Development.'

the project could use certain methods that resulted in material 'in very good condition' (the memo mentions the 'Caesarean section,' referring to the same procedure that was used to collect fetuses for perfusion studies).[33] This collecting process was described in some detail, specifying that researchers would be allowed into 'the operation room,' which meant that 'all necessary steps for the preparation of the material (deep-freezing, fixation, perfusion etc.) can be undertaken without delay.'[34] This material could later be compared with 'tissues from stillborn babies and fetuses of various ages' that were said to be 'easily available at the Karolinska Hospital.'[35] What is remarkable about this application, besides its level of concrete detail, is that it describes Swedish fetal research as unique in an international context, and that this research was supported financially by the AACC, with the hope of receiving even more funding from the American NIH. Moreover, it illustrates a medical and scientific framing of fetal research, in which the fetus is cast as pivotal research material in the search for new and valuable scientific knowledge.

The application also contained an appendix regarding the ethical aspects of the proposed research, described by the applicant as an excerpt from the AACC's opinion on the use of fetal material in research.[36] These three pages are dense with interesting ethical considerations, as in the following comparison between autopsies of executed criminals and abortion material:

> The situation is entirely similar to that involving autopsies of executed criminals or of murder victims. The autopsy does not justify capital punishment nor condone the crime. Neither does the use of tissue from human embryos imply either approval or disapproval of abortion. The fact is that large numbers of abortuses are available for reasons entirely unrelated to this proposed study. The use of these embryos will yield an understanding of certain human diseases obtainable in no other known way. In this instance it is morally imperative that the proposed study be attempted.[37]

33 Lind et al., 'Human Fetal Development.'
34 Lind et al., 'Human Fetal Development.'
35 Lind et al., 'Human Fetal Development.'
36 Appendix to 'Human Fetal Development.' English in original. According to the covering letter from the applicants, this text is from the Association for the Aid of Crippled Children's 'Viewpoints on research on human fetuses' (Synpunkter på forskning på mänskliga foster).
37 Appendix to 'Human Fetal Development.'

The claim that the material was so valuable that neglecting to study it would be immoral was also echoed in the application, articulating a frame in which the aims of fetal research override other possible ethical concerns. Moreover, the appendix discussed whether it was immoral to use fetal material from abroad that was not admissible in the United States. On that matter, it offered an analogy with global trade: 'Cheap labor has never prevented the import of products from countries less developed than ours.'[38] That said, the level of development within countries that would supply the fetal material was also discussed. These countries, it stated, were not generally associated with lower 'cultural development'; on the contrary, they were claimed to be advanced cultures, and even representative of the 'ones from which our own culture is a derivative.'[39] Thus the national variations in fetal research could be framed as differing, but not necessarily problematic or immoral.

The committee at the KI seems to have discussed the Human Fetal Development project at length. Various aspects of the proposed research were brought up, such as the status of the fetuses as research material, definitions of fetuses versus newborns, and whether the aborted fetuses would be kept alive. One member of the board clearly stated that the practice of 'organ preparation is O.K.,' but underscored that keeping fetuses alive was unethical.[40] Another member pointed out that fetuses could sometimes survive after being delivered in week twenty-six.[41] The timing of the termination, but also the development of the fetus, was an important marker between usable and nonusable material, and between 'pre-viable' and 'viable' fetuses in the committee's discussions on fetal research.[42] One of the committee members made this distinction explicit by stating that research on 'dead children and fetuses' did not pose a problem, but in the cases with 'live fetuses, which had reached such a level of development that they possibly could live on after an eventual abortion' the ethical considerations would be different.[43]

When discussing this project, the REC at KI drew certain limitations. These limitations can be regarded as a form of ontological surgery, through which certain fetuses were cast as ethically usable research material, while those

38 Appendix to 'Human Fetal Development.'

39 Appendix to 'Human Fetal Development.'

40 Minutes from meeting, November 13, 1967, 3.

41 Minutes from meeting, November 13, 1967, 3.

42 See Jülich's introduction to this volume for more on viability in relation to abortion. During this time the Abortion Act of 1974 was in preparation, and it would strictly forbid abortion if the fetus could be considered viable. See also Jülich and Tinnerholm Ljungberg, 'Från medicinskt avfall.'

43 Forsberg to Sjöstrand.

from other developmental stages were not. The committee urged the applying principal investigator to clearly state that the planned research would 'not affect the choice of abortion technology nor the timing of the abortion. Furthermore, it should be clearly stated that the fetuses will not be kept alive after the abortion by artificial measures.'[44] The meaning of this prohibition on 'keeping fetuses alive' becomes ambiguous in light of the fact that the KI committee later approved the use of the perfusion technique in at least two cases. Besides these limitations placed by the committee, there is no evidence of the approval or rejection of the proposed research project in its entirety in the archives at the KI. However, it is clear that discussions on the project continued when the principal applicant was invited to an REC meeting in December 1967.[45] Furthermore, in the spring of 1968 the project was discussed for the last time, when part of the proposed research that included the use of an isotope on newborns was not approved by the Isotope Committee at the Karolinska Hospital, and accordingly was not approved by the REC at KI.[46]

Within the AACC there was great optimism around the Human Fetal Development program in late 1967. But this optimism faded in early 1968, when a committee of AACC consultants that had reviewed the program had found that it was neither approvable nor up to the presumed standards of projects funded by the NIH.[47] One of the reasons was that the proposed application highlighted the method and the unique material, without clearly presenting the possible scientific results. The Human Fetal Development program did not evolve further and thus did not submit an application to the NIH; instead the AACC decided in late 1969 to give a twenty-eight-month terminal grant to the participating laboratories.[48]

3 Ethical Reviews of Perfusion Studies and the Question of Research on Live Fetuses

In the years that followed, the most publicly debated fetal research practice in Sweden concerned the so-called perfusion technique.[49] At least three applications sent to the REC at KI were for projects explicitly planning to use this

44 Sjöstrand to Lind.
45 Sjöstrand to Lind.
46 Minutes from meeting, March 25, 1968; Isotope Committee to Ethics Committee.
47 Amoroso, report.
48 Meeting of the Executive Board.
49 Jülich, 'Fosterexperimentens produktiva hemlighet.'

technique. In one example from 1969, the technique was motivated by the need for more knowledge of fetuses, and it was stated that previous results had helped 'a great number of children every year.'[50] The applicants, Egon Diczfalusy and Nils Wiqvist, described how they had set some boundaries; for example, they would only use fetuses of a gestational age of sixteen to twenty weeks, and fetuses weighing less than 250 grams. Moreover, they assured readers that 'breathing movements or gasps never occur at this stage of development.'[51] The KI committee approved this application—that much is evident from its assessment—but any discussion that members had about it left no paper trail. We may assume that they thought the ethical considerations were at least not objectionable enough for the application to be rejected.

Another planned perfusion study was approved in November 1970, which also involved aborted fetuses from weeks sixteen to twenty. The use of fetal material in this research project was motivated by the possibility of gaining knowledge about whether and how pharmaceuticals were transferred from the mother's body into the fetus. Parallels with the thalidomide scandal were drawn to stress the importance of the research.[52] This trial was also approved by the REC. It is noteworthy that three years later, in 1973, two of the three applicants sent a letter to the REC, stating that the perfusions 'neither had nor would be carried out since a new method has been developed' for the study of the transference of pharmaceuticals. This method involved taking blood samples from newborns in cases where pregnant women had been ill and therefore had been given medications on therapeutic grounds.[53] This is the only example I have found in the REC's archives of scientists explicitly withdrawing a research application or writing to explain that their research had not been conducted. One possible reason behind this shift in approach might have been the intense public debate on fetal research and perfusion technology in 1973. In this context it might have seemed important to state on record that the trials had not been carried out.

In December 1973 the REC at the KI received a letter from a liberal parliament member, Kerstin Anér, asking whether the committee had made any comments on research involving 'living fetuses' between 1971 and 1973.[54] The committee's very short answer stated that no comments had been made, nor

50 Diczfalusy and Wiqvist, *Försök på previabla foster*, 3.

51 Diczfalusy and Wiqvist, *Försök på previabla foster*, 3.

52 Johannisson, Rane, and Sjöqvist, research application.

53 Rane and Sjöqvist to the REC at KI.

54 Anér to the secretary of REC at KI. Kerstin Anér was an active advocate for the regulation and control of the scientific use of both fetal material and animal experiments in the early 1970s. See Svärd and Tinnerholm Ljungberg, 'Fetal and Animal Research.'

had the secretary found 'any research project concerning experiments on living fetuses' during the stated period.[55] Neither of the letters defined what was meant by 'live fetuses,' and it would be interesting to see how the ethics committee would have replied, had Anér not limited her question to those specific years. About a week after the committee's reply, Anér wrote a new parliamentary bill on fetal research, in which she referenced new policies that had been published in Britain. In light of this international development, she problematized the lack of corresponding national regulations in Sweden.[56] Among the solutions she proposed was that REC's assessments of fetal research should 'treat fetuses not like animals, but as patients' and that the point at which fetuses were deemed nonviable, and therefore usable, should be set below twenty weeks' gestational age.[57]

Overall, the REC assessments analyzed here illustrate that fetal research provoked internal debate, and that researchers wrote to or visited the REC to justify their research. But, at the same time, there were few restrictions placed on this research by the committees. Neither was there any cohesive discussion on the ethics of fetal research by these organizations. Instead, various criteria were adopted to distinguish between fetuses that were admissible or inadmissible for use—such as weight, length, gestational age, and level of development—and these criteria were actualized on a case-by-case basis.

4 Swedish Fetal Research Debated Internationally

Assessments of the perfusion technique took place alongside growing public debate on fetal research in various national contexts, in which Sweden was often used as an example. In response to this increased public attention, communication was initiated between the medical community, politicians, and governmental authorities. In May 1970, the UK Government appointed an advisory group to investigate fetal research. The main reason for taking this step was allegations circulating in the British press 'that live aborted fetuses were being sold for medical experiments' and 'being kept alive by heart-and-lung machines.'[58] The group came to be known as the Peel Advisory Group, after its chair, Sir John Peel. Peel had previously played an active and diplomatic role, as president of the Royal College of Obstetricians and Gynecologists, in the

55 Andersson to Anér.
56 Swedish Parliament, 'Nr 30 av fru Anér,' 13.
57 Swedish Parliament, 'Nr 30 av fru Anér,' 13.
58 Pfeffer and Kent, 'Framing Women, Framing Fetuses,' 433.

process leading to the passage of the United Kingdom's Abortion Act.[59] Back in Sweden, the Parliamentary Ombudsman Alfred Bexelius began investigating the matter of fetal research in 1969, after receiving letters from concerned citizens. In order to answer these complaints, Bexelius had appointed members of the Scientific Council of the National Board of Health and Welfare (NBHW) to investigate the matter.[60] He concluded in the summer of 1970 that he had not discovered any wrongdoing and that no further action was necessary.[61] Some of the written statements from Bexelius's investigation eventually surfaced in Britain when Sir John Peel started to collect knowledge and evidence from outside the country and turned to the United States and Sweden.[62] The committee was seeking 'factual, unemotive information' and decided to approach the director general of the Swedish NBHW, Bror Rexed.[63] The evidence submitted from Sweden included a letter from Professor Axel Ingelman-Sundberg, a member of what was called the NBHW's research council in the correspondence. He described the Swedish praxis:

> Where foetuses do not fulfil the criteria for live-born infants according to the regulations, or have not reached a size, or come from a stage of pregnancy where they would not be regarded as still born infants, they can, as in the case of tumours, etc. be examined for the cause of death or used in research and teaching. This practice is of long standing and does not require the mother's consent.[64]

This view on consent was shared by several of the other individuals who submitted evidence to the committee.[65] In the end, the recommendations from the Peel report aligned with this view on consent and stated that fetal material could be used as long as there were no explicit objections and that asking women for permission 'could be an unnecessary source of distress.'[66] Previous research has depicted this approach to consent as only giving 'modest

59 Sheldon et al., *Abortion Act 1967*.
60 Brereton to Peel.
61 Jülich, 'Fosterforskningens produktiva hemlighet,' 33.
62 Brereton to Peel.
63 Peel to Gray.
64 Ingelman-Sundberg to the Ministry of Social affairs.
65 United Kingdom Department of Health and Social Security, *Use of Fetuses*. See also Pfeffer and Kent, 'Framing Women, Framing Fetuses,' 438.
66 United Kingdom Department of Health and Social Security, *Use of Fetuses*, 9, 12. See also Sheldon et al., *Abortion Act 1967*, 55.

weight [...] to women's wishes.'[67] Overall, the controversy about consent is an illustrative example of ontological surgery: depending on the understanding and categorization of fetal material (here as an unwanted body part, or even a malicious intruder, comparable with a tumor), certain implications follow. In this case, what followed from the comparison was that consent was not deemed necessary.

Another link between the Peel Advisory Group and Sweden was established by a member of the group, Sir Harold Himsworth, who discussed Diczfalusy and his research in discussion with the headquarters of the British Medical Research Council. He said that 'he had recently had the opportunity of speaking (in Geneva) with Dr Diczfalusy [...] and learned that he had done some 200 experiments on "non-viable but not completely dead" fetuses (i.e. "heart beating but no respirations of course").'[68] The memo further depicted a situation in which 'the use of the whole "semi-viable" fetus' was considered a 'particularly "sensitive" aspect.' But even though these were described as very sensitive issues, cautionary opinions were expressed defending research on fetal material: if 'the use of live whole fetuses had no scientific justification and it accordingly became prohibited by law, that law would be difficult to undo later should a scientific justification develop.'[69] In 1972, the Peel report concluded that research involving the whole previable fetus had been carried out after delivery in certain countries' under 'stringent precautions,' placing this sensitive research outside Britain and, implicitly, in Sweden.[70]

Swedish fetal research also became subject to a heated public debate in the United States. In April 1973, the *Washington Post* ran a series of articles on the medical use of fetuses, which became a major talking point.[71] These articles were later described as the 'American public's first introduction to fetal research.'[72] Sweden was depicted as a nation where abortion was less controversial than in the United States, and where foreign research funding and researchers related to this area of expertise were welcomed with open arms. One researcher interviewed for the series described a situation in which 'some U.S scientists are going to Sweden and Japan or other countries to do such research and doing so with the help of their NIH funds.'[73] The aspect

67 Sheldon et al., *Abortion Act 1967*, 55.
68 Note on call from Sir Harold Himsworth.
69 Note on call from Sir Harold Himsworth.
70 United Kingdom Department of Health and Social Security, *Use of Fetuses*, 3.
71 Cohn, 'Live-Fetus Research Debated'; Cohn, 'Scientists and Fetus Research.'
72 Sarkos, 'Fetal Tissue Transplant Debate.'
73 Cohn, 'Live-Fetus Research Debated.'

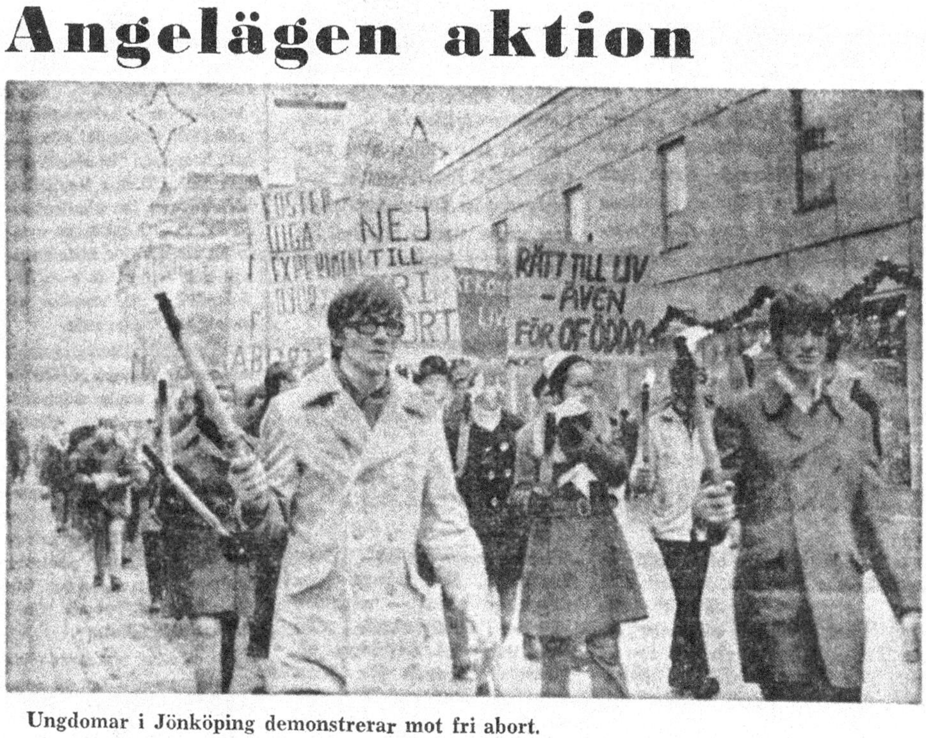
Angelägen aktion
NEJ
RÄTT TILL LIV
-ÄVEN
Ungdomar i Jönköping demonstrerar mot fri abort.

FIGURE 8.3 'Urgent action.' Christian youth protesting against plans on free abortion and fetal experimentation. Demonstration in Jönköping, Sweden, 1969. From 'Angelägen aktion.'

that was presented as most troubling in these articles was research that seemingly was 'keeping fetuses alive [...] by artificial means.'[74] One scientist was quoted as saying that he knew the 'NIH has funded such work in Sweden, at the famous Karolinska Institute.'[75] The *Washington Post* articles presented Swedish research as the extreme example in these discussions. They also revealed that funding, researchers, and demands for local ethical reviews had traveled from the United States to Sweden, thus setting the stage for Swedish policy debates and practices.

74 Cohn, 'Scientists and Fetus Research.'
75 Cohn, 'Scientists and Fetus Research.'

5 Medical Research Ethics on the Parliamentary Agenda in the Early 1970s

Following intense discussion in the media and protests, even more members of the Swedish Parliament started to problematize the use of fetuses in medical trials and called for political action.[76] In the early 1970s, a public debate also arose in the Swedish press, that drew attention to the framing of the fetus.[77]

In January 1974, parliamentary politicians claimed that further regulation of fetal research was needed, and the matter was delegated to the Parliamentary Committee on Education. This committee published a report in November 1974, stating that all research on humans, including fetuses, should be assessed by a local REC and that the medical community should consider including lay members in these committees.[78] In the 1970s, one important means of mollifying critics was to reassure them that the medical faculties' newly institutionalized RECs would 'guarantee that the ethical aspects of the fetal experiments had been taken into account.'[79]

The medical community proved responsive to these new demands for ethical review of fetal research. The Swedish Medical Research Council arranged a conference in December 1974, in which they decided to agree with the Parliamentary Committee on Education's statement that all research involving aborted fetuses should be pre-reviewed.[80] The conference centered on questions of medical research ethics in general, and research on aborted fetuses in particular. Participants discussed the need to obtain consent from research subjects, noting that written consent should be required from adults, with an exception being the case of aborted fetuses. It was not considered necessary to ask the woman for consent to use the material from her abortion. Similar discussions also took place at the local RECs: the committee in Gothenburg decided in December 1974 that they should, from now on, assess all research projects involving fetuses. This decision was taken while approving a research project using fetuses no older than twelve weeks, and after reassurances that the researcher did not plan to keep them alive.[81] In February 1975, the Swedish Medical Research Council decided that all medical research involving humans

76 Swedish Parliament, 'Nr 1364 av herr Carlshamre,' 1.
77 Jülich, 'Fosterexperimentens produktiva hemlighet.'
78 Swedish Parliament, 'Nr 35. Utbildningsutskottets betänkande.'
79 Jülich, 'Fosterexperimentens produktiva hemlighet,' 38.
80 Danielsson, notes.
81 Minutes from meeting, December 10, 1974, 2.

should be assessed by an ethics committee, regardless of where the funding came from.[82]

In less than ten years, what had started as a demand from the NIH became a policy supposedly applicable to all research on humans in Sweden. In close connection to public and political debates on the medical use of aborted fetuses, medical research ethics had developed from a question primarily relevant to the individual researcher responsible for the project to a matter for a medical ethics committee. Nonetheless, the problem of fetal research was repeatedly elevated to the level of politics in the 1970s. Criticism of fetal research challenged the medical community by bringing medical research ethics into the Swedish parliamentary agenda, but it did not result in new laws. Instead, the RECs that had been formed in response to the NIH's demands met with appreciation from political and governmental representatives and managed to retain authority over questions of research within the medical community. This situation lasted until 1974, when the Parliamentary Committee on Education, after a debate on the ethics of fetal research, announced that lay members should be included in the RECs to achieve increased legitimacy and transparency.

6 Conclusion

This chapter has moved from the local via the international to the national debate about Swedish fetal research. But this seemingly straightforward organization needs to be disassembled—since the matter of Swedish research ethics and the scientific use of fetuses is best read as an intricate history of recurring linkages between all three levels. During the 1960s and 1970s, research funding, projects, materials, and researchers themselves traveled and cooperated internationally with the collective and global aim of furthering knowledge on prenatal life and death.

Concerns about the ethics of using aborted fetuses for these aims traveled as well. Swedish debates and practices did not occur in a vacuum; these matters were simultaneously addressed abroad, where different discursive frames were employed. These debates and policies, according to Banchoff, are best described as containing 'transnational linkages' but retaining an emphasis on the 'primacy of the national.'[83] In this chapter we can see the same tendencies toward national particularity. But during

82 Swedish Medical Research Council to Zetterström, et al.

83 Cf. Banchoff, *Embryo Politics*.

the 1960s and before RECs became a topic in parliamentary debates, research ethics concerning fetal knowledge production is best described as a local responsibility, embodied and executed by the very recently institutionalized RECs. The interconnection between research on fetal material and research ethics committees in Sweden thus provides an interesting case, thanks not least to relatively numerous and openly accessible archival traces.

Swedish fetal politics contained diverging frames, at the national and the local levels, that organized the understanding of fetal research in the 1960s and early 1970s. These concerned whether and how fetuses could (or even should) be used in medical research. The medical community, represented by both researchers involved in fetal research and RECs, framed fetuses as indispensable research material. Some even stated that it was a moral imperative to conduct fetal research. However, boundaries were also set, limiting the use of some fetuses, and differentiating between younger, smaller, nonviable fetuses and older fetuses approaching viability. These various ways of framing usable versus nonusable abortion material could be read as a form of ontological surgery—depending on the status of the fetus, different moral obligations followed. Fetal research was thus controversial, but if it was to be performed, various parties agreed on the necessity of increased control over the use of fetal material by research ethics committees.

Bibliography

'Angelägen action.' *Dagen*, December 17, 1969.

Banchoff, Thomas. *Embryo Politics: Ethics and Policy in Atlantic Democracies*. Ithaca, NY: Cornell University Press, 2011.

Christoffersen-Deb, Astrid. 'Viability: A Cultural Calculus of Personhood at the Beginnings of Life.' *Medical Anthropology Quarterly* 26, no. 4 (2012): 575–94.

Cohn, Victor. 'Live-Fetus Research Debated.' *Washington Post*, April 10, 1973.

Cohn, Victor. 'Scientists and Fetus Research.' *Washington Post*, April 15, 1973.

Dubow, Sara. *Ourselves Unborn: A History of the Fetus in Modern America*. New York: Oxford University Press, 2011.

Fannin, Maria. 'Making an "Embryological Vision of the World": Law, Maternity and the Kyoto Collection.' In *Reproductive Geographies: Bodies, Places and Politics*, edited by Marcia R. England, Maria Fannin, and Helen Hazen, 17–30. London: Routledge, 2018.

Fannin, Maria, Helen Hazen, and Marcia R. England. 'Introduction: A Call for Reproductive Geographies.' In *Reproductive Geographies: Bodies, Places and Politics*, edited by Marcia R. England, Maria Fannin, and Helen Hazen, 1–14. London: Routledge, 2018.

Hedgecoe, Adam. '"A Form of Practical Machinery": The Origins of Research Ethics Committees in the UK, 1967–1972.' *Medical History* 53, no. 3 (2009): 331–50.

Jacobs, Noortje. *Ethics by Committee: A History of Reasoning Together about Medicine, Science, Society, and the State*. Chicago: University of Chicago Press, 2022.

Jacobs, Noortje, and Helena Tinnerholm Ljungberg. 'How Ethics Travels: The International Development of Research Ethics Committees in the Late Twentieth Century.' *European Journal for the History of Medicine and Health* 78, no. 2 (2021): 257–65.

Jasanoff, Sheila. 'Making the Facts of Life.' In *Reframing Rights: Bioconstitutionalism in the Genetic Age*, edited by Sheila Jasanoff, 59–83. Cambridge, MA: MIT Press, 2011.

Johannisson, Elisabeth. 'Befolkningstillväxten måste mötas med nya medel för födelsekontroll.' *Forskning och framsteg* 6, no. 4 (1971): 5–11.

Jülich, Solveig. 'Fosterexperimentens produktiva hemlighet: Medicinsk forskning och vita lögner i 1960- och 1970-talets Sverige.' *Lychnos* (2018): 10–49.

Jülich, Solveig, and Helena Tinnerholm Ljungberg. 'Från medicinskt avfall till rättighetsinnehavare: Framväxten av värdekonflikter kring aborterade foster i Sverige.' *Tidskrift för genusvetenskap* 40, no. 3–4 (2019): 33–54.

Morgan, Lynn M. *Icons of Life: A Cultural History of Human Embryos*. Berkeley: University of California Press, 2009.

Nishimura, Hideo, Kiichi Takano, Takashi Tanimura, and Mineo Yasuda. 'Normal and Abnormal Development of Human Embryos: First Report of the Analysis of 1,213 Intact Embryos.' *Teratology* 1, no. 3 (1968): 281–90.

Pfeffer, Naomi, and Julie Kent. 'Framing Women, Framing Fetuses: How Britain Regulates Arrangements for the Collection and Use of Aborted Fetuses in Stem Cell Research and Therapies.' *BioSocieties* 2, no. 4 (2007): 429–47.

Sarkos, Chrysso B. 'The Fetal Tissue Transplant Debate in the United States: Where Is King Solomon When You Need Him.' *Journal of Law & Politics* 7, no. 2 (1990): 379–416.

Schoen, Johanna. *Abortion after* Roe. Chapel Hill: University of North Carolina Press, 2015.

Sheldon, Sally, Gayle Davis, Jane O'Neill, and Clare Parker. *The Abortion Act 1967: A Biography of a UK Law*. Cambridge: Cambridge University Press, 2022.

Sjöstrand, Torgny, and Folke Sjöqvist. 'Etiska kommittén vid Karolinska Institutet: Tillkomst och erfarenheter.' *Läkartidningen* 68, no. 1 (1971): 21–25.

Stark, Laura. *Behind Closed Doors: IRBs and the Making of Ethical Research*. Chicago: University of Chicago Press, 2012.

Svärd, Per-Anders, and Helena Tinnerholm Ljungberg. 'Fetal and Animal Research in Sweden: The Construction of Viable Lives in Regulatory Policy Debates, 1970–1980.' *Studies in History and Philosophy of Science, Part A* 89 (2021): 248–56.

Swedish National Council on Medical Ethics. *Livstecken efter sen abort*. Stockholm: Statens medicinsk-etiska råd, 2019.

Swedish Parliament. 'Svar på interpellation av herr Gustafsson i Borås ang. vissa vetenskapliga undersökningar i samband med abortoperationer.' In *Riksdagens pro-*

tokoll. Vol. 4. *Andra kammarens protokoll 1960*, no. 21, 38–42. Stockholm: Riksdagen, 1960.

Swedish Parliament. 'Nr 35. Utbildningsutskottets betänkande med anledning av motioner angående medicinsk forskning på abortfoster.' *Riksdagens protokoll*. Collection 14, Vol. E11. *Utbildningsutskottets betänkanden och yttranden nr 1–39*, 1–19. Stockholm: Riksdagen, 1974.

Swedish Parliament. 'Nr 30 av fru Anér angående individens okränkbarhet.' In *Riksdagens protokoll*. Collection 3, Vol. D1. *Motioner nr 1–278*, 9–14. Stockholm: Riksdagen, 1974.

Swedish Parliament. 'Nr 1364 av herr Carlshamre angående nyttjandet av levande abortfoster inom forskningen.' In *Riksdagens protokoll*. Collection 3, Vol. D5. *Motioner nr 1278–1598*, 1. Stockholm: Riksdagen, 1974.

Tinnerholm Ljungberg, Helena. 'Regulating Research: The Origins and Institutionalization of Research Ethics Committees in Sweden.' *European Journal for the History of Medicine and Health* 78, no. 2 (2021): 267–86.

United Kingdom Department of Health and Social Security. *The Use of Fetuses and Fetal Material for Research: Report of the Advisory Group*. London: HMSO, 1972.

Wilson, Emily K. 'Ex Utero: Live Human Fetal Research and the Films of Davenport Hooker.' *Bulletin of the History of Medicine* 88, no. 1 (2014): 132–60.

Archival Sources

Amoroso, Emmanuel C. Report from meeting of the Scientific Review Committee by Dr. Emmanuel C. Amoroso to the President of the AACC, Dr. Robert J. Slater, Meeting of the Board of Directors, January 16, 1968. Administration, Series 1—Board of Directors Meetings, Subseries 1. FCD.

Andersson, Sven, to Kerstin Anér, January 2, 1974. Copy. A1:5. KIREC.

Anér, Kerstin, to the secretary of REC at KI, December 12, 1973. A1:5. KIREC.

Angelone, Luis, executive secretary, NIH, to Sune Bergström, dean at the medical faculty, KI, April 12, 1966. A1:1 1967–1968. KIREC.

Appendix to 'Human Fetal Development.' A1:1 1967–1968. KIREC.

Brereton, D., to Sir John Peel, March 18, 1971. Peel Committee: Evidence from various bodies, MH 160/732. NA.

Danielsson, Henry. Notes taken at the conference, December 18, 1974, by Henry Danielsson, assistant secretary, February 7, 1975. Ö4:7. SSM.

Diczfalusy, Egon, and Nils Wiqvist. *Försök på previabla foster*, 1969. A1:2 1969–1970. KIREC.

Executive committee minutes, June 24, 1968. Administration, Series 1—Committees, Subseries 2. FCD.

Forsberg, Arne, to Torgny Sjöstrand, November 1, 1967. A1:1 1967–1968. KIREC.

Gordon, Mordecai H., to Bo Holmstedt, March 17, 1967. A1:1 1967–1968. KIREC.

Ingelman-Sundberg, Axel, to the Ministry of Social Affairs, August 19, 1969. Peel Committee: Evidence from various bodies, MH 160/732. NA. [The English version of the letter in the NA has been lightly summarized.]

'Institutional Assurance on Investigations Involving Human Subjects, Including Clinical Research.' Draft, January 27, 1967. A1:1 1967–1968. KIREC.

Isotope Committee, Karolinska Hospital, to the Ethics Committee, KI, March 11, 1968. A1:1 1967–1968. KIREC.

Johannisson, E., A. Rane, and F. Sjöqvist. Research application. Appendix to meeting, November 17, 1970. A1:2 1969–1979. KIREC.

Lind, John, et al. 'Human Fetal Development: An Interdisciplinary Study,' research application to the NIH, October 23, 1967. Appendix to REC meeting, November 23, 1967. A1:1 1967–1968. KIREC.

Meeting of the Executive Board of the AACC, December 15, 1969. Administration, Series 1—Committees, Subseries 2. FCD.

Meetings of the Council, April 17, 1967. Series 1 Administration, subseries 1 Administration: Board of Directors Meetings. FCD.

Memo on Human Fetal Development, attached to the minutes of the Meetings of the Boards of Directors, November 21, 1967. Administration, Series 1—Board of Directors Meetings, Subseries 1. FCD.

Minutes from meeting of the REC at KI, March 25, 1968. A1:1 1967–1968. KIREC.

Minutes from meeting, December 10, 1974. A1:1 1970–1977. Minutes from the Research ethical committee, Research ethical committee. GUA.

Minutes from meeting, November 13, 1967. A1:1 1967–1968. KIREC.

Note on call from Sir Harold Himsworth, April 24, 1971. Medical Research Council (S Series): Foetal tissues, FD 23/1901. NA.

Peel, Sir John, to J. A. B. Gray, secretary of the Medical Research Council, August 1970. Medical Research Council (S Series): Advisory Group on the Use of Foetal Tissue, FD 23/3419. NA.

Rane, Anders, and Folke Sjöqvist, to the REC at KI, received November 9, 1973. Appendix to meeting, December 14, 1973. A1:5. KIREC.

Sjöstrand, Torgny, to John Lind, n.d. Appendix 1, meeting December 6, 1967. A1:1 1967–1968. KIREC.

Surgeon General, Public Health Service, to the heads of institutions conducting research with public health service grants, February 8, 1966. A1:1 1967–1968. KIREC.

Swedish Medical Research Council to R. Zetterström, S. Alsen, A. Rosén, B. Gustafsson, G. Dahlström, E. Bárány, M. Holmdahl, G. Ström, L. Thorén, and B. Lannering, et al., April 7, 1975. Ö4:7 SSM.

'Three Year Report Association for the Aid of Crippled Children for the Fiscal Years 1964–65, 1965–66, 1966–67,' n.d. Annual Reports, Series 2. FCD.

CHAPTER 9

From the Laboratory to the Parliament: Valuing Abortion Pills in the 1960s

Morag Ramsey

Throughout 1965, the physician and researcher Lars Engström conducted clinical trials of abortion pills on roughly fifty women. The women had applied for abortions, gone through a series of interviews and medical examinations, and received legal permission for abortion from the state.[1] When they went into the women's clinic for their legal abortion, they were then included in Engström's clinical trial and administered doses of the compound F6103. On average, the women were hospitalized for five days and experienced varying degrees of discomfort and bleeding. To determine whether F6103 had caused an abortion, Engström examined vaginal bleeding and tissues obtained by scraping the women's uteruses, as well as using hormonal assays to measure HCG levels in the urine.[2]

Various factors were involved in determining the stage of pregnancy and then the success of the abortion attempt. The women had made assessments of their own reproductive lives, either through local laboratory pregnancy testing services or by other means, and concluded that they were pregnant.[3] In enrolling the women in the trial, Engström collaborated with other professionals, such as psychiatrists, social workers, and gynecologists, who interviewed the women not only to judge the merits of their applications for legal abortion, but also the length of their pregnancy.[4] Engström wanted to design an abortion method to be used in early pregnancy and required suitable trial participants. However, determining the length of a pregnancy was a complex affair biologically, legally, and technically.

Scholarship on abortion pills mainly focuses on the use of the compound RU486, a method that is often attributed to French research efforts in the

1 Ramsey, 'Swedish Abortion Pill,' 71, 72.

2 Ramsey, 'Swedish Abortion Pill,' 78.

3 Ramsey, 'Swedish Abortion Pill,' 73.

4 Ramsey, 'Swedish Abortion Pill,' 73, 74. For a more comprehensive look at the experiences of the trial participants, see Ramsey, 'Swedish Abortion Pill,' 62–85.

 | DOI:10.1163/9789004703759_011

1980s.[5] However, what is not well known is the decades of research in Sweden that played an important role in RU486's success, with Engström's first trials paving the way for further experiments. Yet conducting clinical trials of abortion pills in Sweden was not without its difficulties, and this chapter examines how abortion-pill research forced discussions of reproductive processes on the Swedish Parliament, revealing how technological development impacted understandings of abortion, and vice versa. Specifically, I use an official investigation into the research and the subsequent parliamentary proceedings. Examining clinical trial applications, legal documents and opinions, and parliamentary discussions reveals how abortion, reproductive technologies, and the law were understood and negotiated in Sweden during the mid-1960s.

To study the different constructions of reproduction, particularly of abortion, I borrow methods from valuography, a theoretical approach that emphasizes the construction of values.[6] Examining the construction of values prevents an analysis that attributes specific deterministic positions to actors. In line with methods from valuography, I do not consider values to be predetermined but instead see them as being made through practices. By examining the varied practices of abortion-pill research, a large network of different actors and activities emerges, allowing an appraisal of how these actors made new values and understandings through their interactions. In this chapter, I examine how different actors in the research network understood reproduction, how they negotiated over these understandings, and how they created a new way of valuing the often polarizing procedure of abortion.

In addition to examining the making of values, this chapter builds on previous research that has shown how reproductive research and technologies have been handled differently depending on national context. The laws, education system, scientific community, and pharmaceutical incentives, for instance, impact the conditions for research and innovation.[7] How reproduction is understood and constructed also plays an important role in its regulation. For example, in their work, Sarah Franklin and Marta Kirejczyk showed the intricate processes of regulating in vitro fertilization (IVF) and embryo research in the United Kingdom and the Netherlands respectively.[8] In the United Kingdom, creating certainty around biological processes guided the making

5 Campbell, 'Making Sense,' 121; Clarke and Montini, 'Many Faces of RU486,' 47; Joffe and Weitz, 'Normalizing the Exceptional,' 2553.

6 Dussauge, Helgesson, and Lee, *Value Practices*.

7 See, e.g., Nordlund, 'Hormones for Life?,' 212–13; Clarke, *Disciplining Reproduction*.

8 Franklin, 'Rethinking Reproductive Politics,' 115; Kirejczyk, 'Parliamentary Cultures and Human Embryos,' 908.

of legislation, while the same effect did not occur in the Netherlands.[9] As I will demonstrate, the case of abortion-pill research in the 1960s also blurred boundaries, mainly between what the historical actors considered to be anticonception and antidevelopment technologies (technologies that prevent a pregnancy and those that end a pregnancy) and demanded that the Swedish Parliament make decisions on unstable biological, legal, and technical subjects.[10]

As this chapter will show, the terminology and concepts surrounding abortion-pill research shifted. The researchers involved referred to their work on the A-pill, the abortion pill, the M-pill, or the menstruation pill and also likened the capsules to morning-after pills.[11] Heather Munro Prescott has shown similar shifts in terminology surrounding emergency contraceptives—which went from 'post coital contraception' to 'morning-after pill.'[12] How reproductive technologies have been branded has not always been accurate and has led to confusion over the intended effects.[13] While ambiguity surrounded the technology in this chapter, the main intention of the researchers was to end pregnancies, and the use of 'abortion pill' as a concept was consistently linked to F6103.

This chapter begins by giving an overview of the main motivations and contexts for abortion-pill research. The second section introduces the case of F6103 and the legal dilemma researchers faced in conducting clinical trials on pregnant women. The third section centers on the legislative process in Parliament spurred by the clinical trials. It examines the different ways reproduction was understood and the practices that made a new abortion value. Finally, the broader significance of these Swedish abortion trials in a postcolonial context is discussed in the conclusion.

---

9 Kirejczyk, 'Parliamentary Cultures and Human Embryos,' 908–10.

10 Some of the historical actors used the Swedish term 'anticonception' (*antikonception*) or 'pregnancy prevention' (*graviditetsförhindrande* or *graviditetsförbyggande medel*), which I refer to as anticonception technologies, and they broadly spoke of technologies that prevented the development of fertilized eggs (*hindra utvecklingen av befruktat ägg*) or more legally spoke of fetal displacement (*fosterfördrivning*), which I refer to as antidevelopment technologies.

11 Ramsey, 'Swedish Abortion Pill,' 106–9.

12 Prescott, *Morning After*, 2.

13 Prescott, *Morning After*.

1 Motivations and Contexts for Abortion-Pill Research

The Swedish state's increasing involvement with abortion during the twentieth century created incentives to support the development of new abortion technologies. As the decades passed, more motivations for abortion were recognized by law, and more women were able to apply for abortions. Sweden first legalized abortion with the 1938 Abortion Act, which allowed abortion on medical, humanitarian, and eugenic grounds.[14] This meant that abortion could be permitted if a woman's life was in danger, if there was risk of hereditary disease, or if the pregnancy was the result of rape or incest.[15] The act would be amended during the following decades, once in 1946 to include socio-medical grounds, and then again in 1963 to include fetal damage.[16] Legal abortions, with the exception of emergency cases, could only be performed at hospitals by a physician on staff.[17]

From the 1930s onward the state carried out a series of official government inquiries to provide updated information on the abortion situation nationally, in which abortion methods were also reviewed.[18] According to the 1965 Abortion Committee, between 1959 and 1963, 9 out of 15,505 abortion procedures resulted in the woman's death.[19] This proportion was contextualized as high in comparison to other countries that used early abortion operations as acceptable birth control methods, although numbers were also seen to be decreasing in Sweden.[20] The committee's report suggested that lower death rates could be attributed to both conducting abortions earlier in pregnancy and a lower frequency of abortions due to serious medical reasons.[21] Although deaths were considered to be rare, the report still stressed the need to continuously monitor the situation.[22] The committee felt a responsibility to control and assess legal abortions in order to offer safe abortion procedures.[23]

14 Lennerhed, 'Troubled Women,' 89.
15 Lennerhed, 'Troubled Women,' 91.
16 For a comprehensive examination of the thalidomide scandal see Maria Björklund's contribution to this volume.
17 Swedish Ministry of Justice, *Rätten till abort*, 109.
18 Swedish Ministry of Health and Social Affairs, *Yttrande i abortfrågan*; Swedish Ministry of Justice, *Betänkande med förslag*; Swedish Ministry of Health and Social Affairs, *Betänkande i abortfrågan*; Swedish Ministry of the Interior, *Abortfrågan: Betänkande*.
19 Swedish Ministry of Justice, *Rätten till abort*, 49.
20 For a further look at debates around abortion safety in the preceding years, see the section 'Abortion: An Unreliable Source,' in Jülich and Dussauge's contribution to this volume.
21 Swedish Ministry of Justice, *Rätten till abort*, 50.
22 Swedish Ministry of Justice, *Rätten till abort*, 50.
23 Swedish Ministry of Justice, *Rätten till abort*, 50.

By the time researchers began their clinical trials in the 1960s, abortion had been legal in various ways for over twenty-five years. The state provided and regulated legal abortion, and there was also an active Abortion Committee that would involve itself in the legal dilemma of abortion-pill research. However, abortion was still a controversial issue. Heated coverage about the ethical ramifications of conducting abortions was printed in major newspapers.[24] Abortion was far from a benign public topic, but there were still legal spaces from which to work with abortion, both in practice and research. The state was invested in providing legal abortions, and developing new abortion techniques could improve family planning efforts both in Sweden and abroad.

During the twentieth century, Sweden, among other countries, was preoccupied with population growth, both nationally and internationally.[25] Population concerns were not new state phenomena of the 1960s—a well-known publication by Gunnar and Alva Myrdal, *Crisis in the Population Question*, was published in 1934. In their book, the Myrdals framed the declining birth rate in Sweden as a crisis.[26] However, by the 1960s the emphasis shifted to global overpopulation.[27] Family planning was seen as a multifaceted tool: it could both increase national populations and reduce global overpopulation.

The Swedish International Development Cooperation Agency (SIDA) was in charge of family planning and population control initiatives.[28] Family planning involved various measures, such as distributing contraceptives, opening clinics, and circulating educational materials on sex.[29] Publications from the mid-1960s show SIDA's interest in incorporating research into its family planning strategies. A 1966 publication contained several sections that the agency saw as key to family planning's success, and research was one of the areas that SIDA thought could be developed further.[30] SIDA assumed that expanding research would lead to a better understanding of the effects of family planning in a given region. These research areas included demography, sociology, and economics, but also, and most importantly for abortion-pill concerns, reproductive questions.[31] While this intention to expand reproductive research did not explicitly refer to the development of abortion techniques, it does illustrate how reproductive research was of interest to the state. As will be demonstrated

24 Jülich, 'Picturing Abortion Opposition in Sweden,' 286–90.
25 Berg, 'Suitable Country,' 299.
26 Ekerwald, 'Modernist Manifesto,' 542.
27 For a broader look at population concerns in this era, see Bashford, *Global Populations*.
28 'Main views.'
29 Thoradeniya, 'Altruism, Welfare, or Development Aid?,' 435, 456.
30 'Main views,' 1.
31 'Main views.'

through a discussion of the parliamentary debate, this interest in population control was an important part of valuing abortion pills.

As several chapters in this volume have shown, the state also supported various forms of research on human fetuses. Because of the Abortion Act of 1938, research that involved fetal tissue was relatively easy to facilitate.[32] Already in 1960, how fetuses were to be considered—as alive, dead, or comparable to organs used in transplants—was debated in the Swedish Parliament. Throughout the 1960s, the National Board of Medicine equated fetal tissue to other types of tissue, which was considered an objective and scientific assessment.[33] Before abortion-pill research began, fetal knowledge production and reproductive materials had been important to the state. Not insignificantly, abortion-pill development was compatible with existing population concerns and with research practices.

Abortion, reproduction, and population were state issues, and while there was consensus over some reproductive aspects, others remained problematic. When two researchers approached the National Board of Medicine with a proposed clinical trial for abortion pills, the responses varied. Closely examining the legal and political practices, including the constructions of abortion, fetus, and various reproductive processes, shows how consensus was met over the debated topic of abortion.

2 The Legal Dilemma

In April 1966, Engström wanted to follow up on his 1965 pilot study of F6103. His first trial had occurred within the existing medical system, and the women had already been evaluated and deemed worthy of abortions, but Engström now wanted to test F6103 on women in very early pregnancy. This required some adjustments. With Åke Hanngren as a coapplicant, Engström submitted a new clinical trial application to the National Pharmaceutical Laboratory (NPL). In the 1960s, clinical trials of drugs in Sweden were monitored and regulated by NPL and the National Board of Medicine.[34] Researchers were required to submit applications and to wait for approval before conducting human clinical trials. However, no formal ethical review of the project was necessary. As Helena Tinnerholm Ljungberg describes, it was not until 1966 that the first

32 Jülich, 'Fosterexperimentens produktiva hemlighet,' 16.

33 Jülich, 'Fosterexperimentens produktiva hemlighet,' 22.

34 Ramsey, 'Swedish Abortion Pill,' 64–67.

research ethics committee was established in Sweden.[35] Abortion-pill research first occurred ahead of the emergence of research ethics committees, and while under other types of review, Engström's research did not become a part of the new research ethics committee process.

Engström and Hanngren wanted to test the compound F6103 as an early medicinal abortifacient (*medikamentellt tidigabortivum*) and as a pregnancy-prevention agent.[36] The trial would be held at the women's clinic at Karolinska Hospital, and the researchers looked to test F6103 on women who, as they described, had missed their menstruation. Considering the legal restrictions governing abortions, there were numerous steps in finding the right women for the trials. They wanted women who were early in their pregnancy, while also having official permission for an abortion. The logistics of finding enough women who met these criteria were problematic. As Engström discovered in 1965, running trials on pregnant women required collaborating with many different actors who regulated legal abortion. This process, with social workers, psychiatrists, and gynecologists, slowed down the pace of the trial. Subsequently, the researchers turned to the National Board of Medicine for guidance.[37] In turning to the board, Engström and Hanngren were mainly curious about two things: could they develop a smoother system for finding women for these trials, and would this particular type of clinical trial be legal?[38]

By the 1960s, Sweden had two fundamental legal grounds that applied to abortion: the Swedish Penal Code, chapter 3, section 4; and the Abortion Act.[39] With the 1734 codification of Swedish law, a criminal law provision sentenced abortion providers to death, although it seems this punishment was never carried out.[40] Over the years the punishments changed, and by the 1920s abortion providers were incarcerated.[41] In 1939 the Abortion Act came into force, and here the focus was not on punishment, but rather on the specific circumstances where abortion could be provided legally. At that point, the Swedish Penal Code was put into dialogue with the Abortion Act. By the 1960s, abortion was legal in certain circumstances, but it was not legal across the board. Engström and Hanngren wanted to conduct their trials within the legal parameters.

Certain concepts guided the laws surrounding abortion from the 1700s until the 1960s. Of particular interest to lawmakers were the concepts of fetus,

35 See Tinnerholm Ljungberg's chapter in this volume.
36 Application for permission.
37 Application for permission.
38 Application for permission.
39 Thornstedt to NBM, 2.
40 Thornstedt, 'The Beginning and the End,' 229.
41 Swedish Ministry of Health and Social Affairs, *Betänkande i abortfrågan*.

conception, and implantation. The Swedish term *foster*, which is translatable to the English term 'fetus,' had been in use in various ways since at least 1613 and is linguistically related to the Swedish term for birth (*föddes*).[42] The Penal Code chapter 3, section 4, made it unlawful to abort or kill a fetus by internal or external means.[43] In 1734 the law did not specify stages of fetal development, although there was discussion of when the fetus had truly 'come to life,' which could be interpreted as a reference to quickening.[44] By 1864 there was discussion calling for penal measures to be taken even during early stages of fetal development.[45] By 1906, a legal statement defined fetal displacement as occurring after the egg cell was fertilized.[46] In this legal statement, the author noted that medical terminology may use the word 'embryo,' but it was not a legally relevant term. Legally, a fetus (*foster*) was considered to exist as soon as an egg was fertilized.[47] The specifics of conception, implantation, and fetal development, concepts which had historically shifted, would play a central role in the discussions of testing F6103. As will be illustrated, in the mid-1960s it was especially difficult to come to consensus over how to define the concept of a fetus—making policy decisions on reproductive technologies confusing.

The importance of managing the perceived overpopulation issue would also be brought into the discussion of abortion-pill development. During the 1960s, Swedish newspapers reported on 'the child bomb' and the 'population explosion,' and coverage showed concern over starvation rates (see figure 9.1).[48] Engström himself discussed overpopulation in the press, and there were efforts to organize experts around population issues.[49] Various government employees were invested in this topic, and there were those who also wanted to ensure the success of the abortion-pill trials.

For instance, in an internal note, two employees of the National Board of Medicine, Gunnar af Geijerstam and Arthur Engel, commented on the case of F6103. Geijerstam, a gynecological expert working at the board, wrote to its legal bureau, describing a web of actors who were interested in the

42 *Svensk ordbok*, s.v. 'foster.'

43 Thornstedt, 'The Beginning and the End,' 228.

44 Thornstedt, 'The Beginning and the End,' 229. For a discussion of quickening, see Runesson's chapter in this volume.

45 Thornstedt, 'The Beginning and the End,' 229.

46 Thornstedt to NBM, 2, 4.

47 Thornstedt to NBM.

48 Heng [pseud.], 'Optimism i kampen mot befolkningsökning'; 'Världskongress söker vapen mot "barnbomben"'; Schoug [pseud.], 'Större svensk insats.'

49 Wiqvist and Westin, *Fertility and Sterility*.

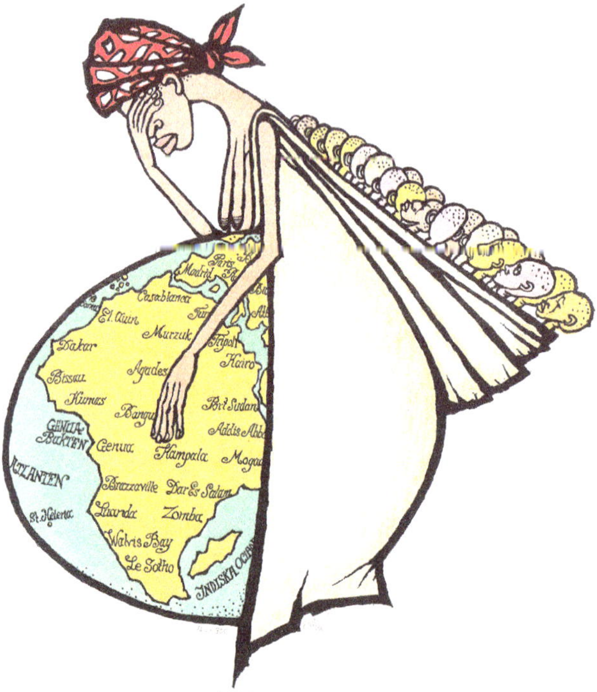

FIGURE 9.1
This famous image drawn by political cartoonist Ewert Karlsson in 1966 illustrates 'Mother Earth' as a woman with a pregnant stomach that appears as a globe and with a sack full of children on her back. The globe mainly shows Africa and the woman is covering her eyes with her hand. The image did not have accompanying text, but this portrayal of an exhausted earth, with many presumably hungry children, would have resonated with a Swedish public who was used to rhetoric of a population bomb and the subsequent starving foreign peoples. Moder Jord, 1990 ©Ewert Karlsson, EWK/ Bildupphovsrätt 2024. Photo courtesy of the EWK Archive, Museum of Work.

'very delicate legal decision' of testing F6103.[50] According to this note, the minister of social affairs, the director general of the National Board of Medicine, the 1965 Abortion Committee's chairman, the state secretary, and a lawyer from the Social Department had a meeting regarding F6103. The director general of the National Board of Medicine, Arthur Engel, stressed that the trials were of utmost importance and expressed support for their implementation. In this meeting it was suggested that a legal expert be employed to look into the issue.[51]

Shortly thereafter, the National Board of Medicine employed Hans Thornstedt, a professor of criminal law at Stockholm University, to investigate whether the trials conflicted with the existing law.[52] The clinical-trial application stated that the researchers wished to test F6103 as an abortifacient and as a pregnancy-prevention agent. To Thornstedt, the Abortion Act of 1938 clearly indicated that tests of an early abortion method would not be legal and required

50 Handwritten note.
51 Handwritten note.
52 Thornstedt and Andersson, *Festskrift till Hans Thornstedt*, 5.

little interpretation.[53] But whether F6103 acted as a preventative method was another question. From Thornstedt's understanding of the researchers' application, the contraceptive aspect of F6103 required that the fertilized egg not be implanted in the uterus. F6103 was supposed to inhibit progesterone metabolism in the ovaries, thus making the uterus membrane ill-suited for implantation. Thornstedt saw his primary task as determining whether this use of the compound was to be considered an abortion, 'which may be undertaken only under certain conditions provided for in the Abortion Act, or if it is to be compared to contraceptive measures, which are in principle allowed.'[54] That the researchers would be testing two aspects of F6103 opened up the possibility that the part of their trial concerned with preventing pregnancy could be conducted legally. Anticonception technologies could more easily fall within existing legislation.

In his work, Thornstedt investigated how the legal tradition had treated the concept of fetus, as the penal law explicitly focused on aborting or killing fetuses. Thornstedt's focus on the precise legal definitions of fetus would determine whether Engström and Hanngren were actually harming a fetus with the use of F6103, or if they were using the compound on women before a fetus was thought to exist. Ultimately, Thornstedt concluded that the legal tradition indicated that a fetus was a fertilized egg.[55] From his reading of the law and the researchers' application, this meant that clinical trials of F6103 conflicted with the Penal Code in both instances.[56]

However, in his report Thornstedt also discussed the possibility of conducting the research regardless of the law, relying on grounds for impunity. In this context, Thornstedt explained that due to conflicting interests, the legal grounds could still support actions that might otherwise be illegal. He presented the conflicting interests associated with F6103 as harming fetuses versus creating means to control overpopulation, which he framed as a humanitarian issue.[57] As he was employed by state actors who supported this research, it seems likely that the National Board of Medicine explicitly explained their interests in F6103 as being connected to overpopulation.

Newspapers reported on these developments. While there were prospects of developing a new abortion technology soon, controversial aspects were highlighted, and Engström pronounced in a newspaper article that 'Life first

53 Thornstedt to NBM, 1.
54 Thornstedt to NBM, 2.
55 Thornstedt to NBM, 5.
56 Swedish Parliament, 'Nr 18. Kungl. Maj:ts proposition,' 4.
57 Thornstedt to NBM, 16.

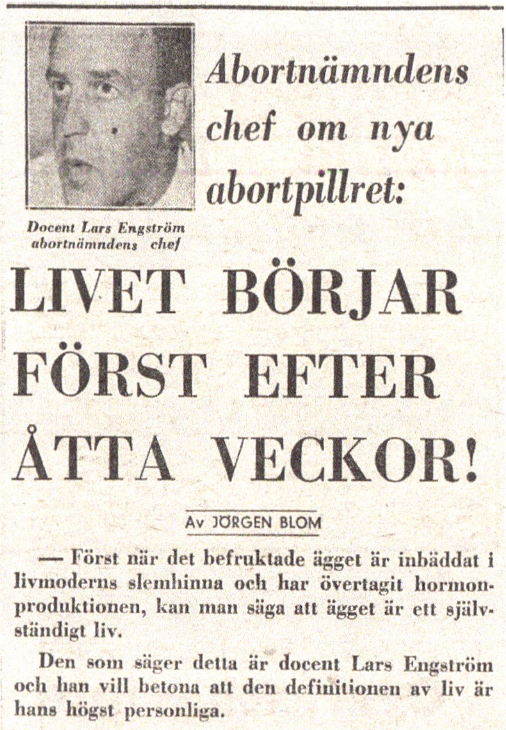

Abortnämndens chef om nya abortpillret:

Docent Lars Engström abortnämndens chef

LIVET BÖRJAR FÖRST EFTER ÅTTA VECKOR!

Av JÖRGEN BLOM

— Först när det befruktade ägget är inbäddat i livmoderns slemhinna och har övertagit hormonproduktionen, kan man säga att ägget är ett självständigt liv.

Den som säger detta är docent Lars Engström och han vill betona att den definitionen av liv är hans högst personliga.

FIGURE 9.2
In the midst of Engström's research, national newspapers ran coverage of the trials. Here, *Aftonbladet* reported on Engström explaining biological processes that led to 'life,' introducing the public to concepts such as 'fertilized egg,' 'uterine lining,' and 'hormone production.' From Blom, 'Livet börjar först efter åtta veckor!' Courtesy of *Aftonbladet*.

begins after eight weeks.'[58] Here, he stated that life began when a fertilized egg was 'embedded in the lining of the uterus and had taken over hormone production.'[59] The paper added that these were Engström's own personal views, separating Engström from organizations to which this definition could be attributed by association. 'Life' was an additional concept that was brought into the abortion-pill discussions. By Engström's logic, abortive technologies used before eight weeks would not interact with anything considered alive.

In approaching the National Board of Medicine, these two researchers sparked a larger discussion of the potentiality of their work and mobilized various organizations to work in their favor. This network of actors acknowledged the 'delicate' legal situation, but, as will be discussed further, they also worked to enable the research within a new legal framework. While the proposed experimental work constituted a crime, the potential value of such work in improving family planning initiatives abroad weighed heavily in its

58 Engström, 'Livet börjar.'
59 Engström, 'Livet börjar.'

favor.[60] While Thornstedt did not recommend conducting the clinical trials on grounds of impunity, he did offer another solution. In his report, he suggested a legal amendment be made in order to support the clinical trial.[61]

3 Debating Abortion-Pill Research

After receiving Thornstedt's findings, the National Board of Medicine agreed that new legislation should be created. This required submitting a bill through the Department of Justice to the Swedish Parliament, who would then decide whether to pass the bill, subsequently making a new law. In October 1966, the board submitted an official letter regarding the issue of testing certain means of birth control, which included Thornstedt's analysis, to the Department of Justice.[62]

In the bill the National Board of Medicine outlined that research with F6103 had been seen to conflict with the Penal Code on abortion and that a legislative amendment was required to properly and legally govern such scientific endeavors.[63] In response to this suggestion, the 1965 Abortion Committee was asked to give a referral. In its assessment the definitions brought forth by Thornstedt concerning fetus, conception, and implantation were seen as worth discussing. Members of the Abortion Committee perceived recent medical advancements to be the reason such questions were now pertinent.[64] They stated that technologies and innovations in science had only lately permitted the prevention of fertilization, and for this reason there was still ambiguity surrounding definitions. The Abortion Committee considered the question of whether there was a legal difference between anticonception and antidevelopment to be part of its own investigative interests. However, it had not established a final position on these issues.[65]

Nevertheless, the committee was inclined to allow the reproductive research described by the National Board of Medicine. The description of the Abortion Committee's referral stated,

60 Thornstedt to NBM, 16.
61 Thornstedt to NBM, 16.
62 Swedish Parliament, 'Nr 18. Kungl. Maj:ts proposition.'
63 Swedish Parliament, 'Nr 18. Kungl. Maj:ts proposition,' 4.
64 Swedish Parliament, 'Nr 18. Kungl. Maj:ts proposition,' 4.
65 Swedish Parliament, 'Nr 18. Kungl. Maj:ts proposition,' 4.

> An agent whose use would cause early pregnancy to be discontinued without surgery, must be seen as a major advancement. What seems to be the most important, however, is the importance of such an agent for family planning. In all endeavors to assist developing countries, one of the more important elements must be to help master the overpopulation problem. Although this problem is not relevant in our country it is internationally so significant that Sweden too should help in approaching its solution by making an easy and effective means of birth control available.[66]

The 1965 Abortion Committee was convinced that the family-planning value of developing new methods for birth control was sufficient to motivate supporting new legislation. Until this point, abortion had been understood as a technique that required skilled labor, which complicated attempts at exporting abortion as a birth-control method. An abortion pill, however, would make this a possibility. While the issue of definitions, particularly of the difference between anticonception and antidevelopment, was of importance, it did not have to be entirely settled. The Abortion Committee would still support the reproductive research put forth by the National Board of Medicine. However, not all the committee members saw the research favorably.

A separate letter written by Astrid Kristensson, a jurist and member of the committee from the Conservative Party, argued that the law should be specifically worded to allow testing of substances that affected the uterus, so that implantation would be prevented, or substances that destroyed fertilized eggs immediately before or right at implantation. According to Kristensson, whether to allow testing of substances that 'in a real sense' interrupt the pregnancy was more dubious.[67] While recent scientific advances had created uncertainty around reproduction for some, for others pregnancy and abortion were straightforward. Kristensson had a clear idea of what research she could support, and it came down to fertilized eggs being implanted in the uterus.

By January 1967 government bill 18 was put forward to the Swedish Parliament.[68] By February 7, 1967, three separate motions were sent to the

66 Swedish Parliament, 'Nr 18. Kungl. Maj:ts proposition,' 5.

67 Swedish Parliament, 'Nr 18. Kungl. Maj:ts proposition,' 6.

68 Following this, Parliament members had the opportunity to respond to the bill through motions that they submitted to the chambers, with all processes and documents being reviewed by a smaller legal committee that reflected the political representation in Parliament. This committee had the opportunity to create a legal opinion that would then again go to the chambers for appraisal. If a majority voted the bill through, it would become a new law.

Parliament's second chamber in response to the bill. The motions outlined several aspects that four Parliament members, supported by signatories representing the Liberal People's Party, the Center Party, and the Conservative Party, saw as needing to be addressed.

A member of the Liberal People's Party submitted a motion maintaining that pregnancy must be considered the point when a fertilized egg is implanted and that research should respect this limit.[69] The motion summarized that the law on clinical trials of certain methods for birth control should impose time limits and that the research should not disrupt pregnancy.[70] From the Conservative Party, similar concerns over the sanctity of life were brought forth. A Conservative Party member wrote that while he could see the importance of such research, especially for overpopulation issues, he could not support trials that interrupted pregnancy.[71] In addition, such work was also seen to conflict with medical ethics.[72] A motion submitted by the Center Party also focused on the significance of such research for international reasons, especially related to overpopulation and limited global resources. The authors weighed the benefits of clinical trials in the face of protecting life. They concluded that research could be permitted if the women involved gave written consent, and if they were to be granted abortion for medical reasons.[73]

These motions highlighted concerns with the bill. Two agreed that the research was important, especially for international family planning, but struggled with the implications when it came to protecting lives. While testing birth control methods was seen as acceptable, for several members of the Liberal People's Party and the Conservative Party the limit of this acceptability was disturbing the implantation of a fertilized egg. Again, the boundary between anticonception and antidevelopment was raised as an important distinction for those who wanted to protect fetuses, and this issue would persist throughout the bill review process.

On April 5, 1967, the second parliamentary chamber met to discuss the potential change in legislation. Those who spoke outlined the sensitive nature of such a change, and a member from the Conservative Party commented that it reflected an ideological standpoint.[74] He stated that the signatories of his party's motion did not oppose birth control research—instead, they saw it as

69 Swedish Parliament, 'Nr 855. Av herr Gustafsson,' 7.
70 Swedish Parliament, 'Nr 855. Av herr Gustafsson,' 7.
71 Swedish Parliament, 'Nr 857. Av herr Åkerlind,' 10.
72 Swedish Parliament, 'Nr 857. Av herr Åkerlind,' 10.
73 Swedish Parliament, 'Nr 856. Av herrar Lindberg och Johansson,' 8.
74 Swedish Parliament, 'Lag om klinisk prövning,' 93.

crucial for solving global nutritional issues and starvation. But they did not want to fail defenseless fetuses.[75] The Conservative Party member was satisfied that the research would focus on finding means to interrupt development prior to implantation. As this was the case, he reported that the signatories were willing to accept the practical boundary established in medicine that saw pregnancy as beginning at implantation.[76]

The Conservative Party member noted, however, that such trials might inevitably involve women who were already in the early stages of pregnancy. Furthermore, there was the matter of testing substances on women whose pregnancies were more advanced, and he struggled with this possibility.[77] A member from the Center Party followed suit by outlining the importance of such research and its conflicts with the abortion laws but insisted that he would not reject the bill and rather hoped a new law would consider implantation as a boundary.[78]

One of the authors of the Liberal People's Party motion professed that the entire matter would have been easier to analyze if there were consensus on the definition of a fetus. He noted that lawyers considered the fetus to exist when an egg cell had been fertilized, while gynecologists' definition centered on implantation. The Liberal People's Party member said,

> here one thus meets an unresolved boundary issue. There should be consensus among medical professionals and other professionals, including ethicists, of when pregnancy begins, before it is requested that legislators take a position on such an important issue. It is not now, and we must act in the best sense of the day.[79]

While some members of the Parliament had strong feelings about when pregnancy began, namely at implantation, there was no absolute consensus from experts.

Even if the majority had agreed on implantation as a significant threshold, there would have been other difficulties. The Liberal People's Party member remarked that several elements outlined in the motions had been deemed unreasonable, such as certainty that substances would only be tested before implantation. It was difficult to track this point with accuracy, and experts

75 Swedish Parliament, 'Lag om klinisk prövning,' 93.
76 Swedish Parliament, 'Lag om klinisk prövning,' 93.
77 Swedish Parliament, 'Lag om klinisk prövning,' 93.
78 Swedish Parliament, 'Lag om klinisk prövning,' 96.
79 Swedish Parliament, 'Lag om klinisk prövning,' 96.

had stated there was a four-to-six-day range that varied by individual.[80] As the researchers were looking to design a technology to be used in early pregnancy, and there were variations between individuals, it was hard to know at what point the substance would act. It was difficult to establish biologic certainty, just as it was difficult to establish how the proposed technology worked.

A member from the Social Democrats who supported the research initiative used the ambiguity around the research to further his point that it should be conducted. He said that those who were worried about whether the compound acted on an implanted fertilized egg or not were 'to some extent fighting with windmills, because they do not yet know how these substances actually work in this respect. [... I]t is to find this out which has opened this opportunity for scientific examination.'[81] While some supporters of the research emphasized its international value as a family planning method, others pointed to the ambiguity of the abortion pill. Without conducting the research, the boundary issue between anticonception and antidevelopment would be no closer to being solved. In this ambiguous sense, it was also possible that the compound would, in some cases, act before implantation, making it a more appealing technology for those opposed to harming fetuses.

The bill was also discussed in the first parliamentary chamber. Ingrid Segerstedt Wiberg, from the Liberal People's Party, and the Social Democrat justice minister Herman Kling debated the merits of the research.[82] Segerstedt Wiberg was not happy with how the matter had been handled, and she connected it to a discussion from the previous year, when, according to her, a decision about intrauterine devices (IUDs) had been made erroneously. Segerstedt Wiberg thought that IUDs conflicted with the Penal Code and that allowing their use had set a poor precedent.[83] Kling disagreed, seeing IUDs as contraceptives and not devices that displaced fetuses. For some, the research on F6103 was considered to be related to IUDs in its function, but to others this was a fallacy. As Kling stated, the IUD was to be used before sex, and the abortion pill afterward.[84]

When discussed in Parliament, F6103 illustrated the instability of the key concepts anchoring the debate. Some people held firm beliefs about when reproductive phases began, while others did not. Some struggled with technologies that acted on fertilized, implanted eggs, while others maintained it was

80 Swedish Parliament, 'Lag om klinisk prövning,' 96.
81 Swedish Parliament, 'Lag om klinisk prövning,' 102.
82 Swedish Parliament, 'Granskning av statsrådsprotokoll.'
83 Swedish Parliament, 'Granskning av statsrådsprotokoll,' 7.
84 Swedish Parliament, 'Granskning av statsrådsprotokoll,' 22.

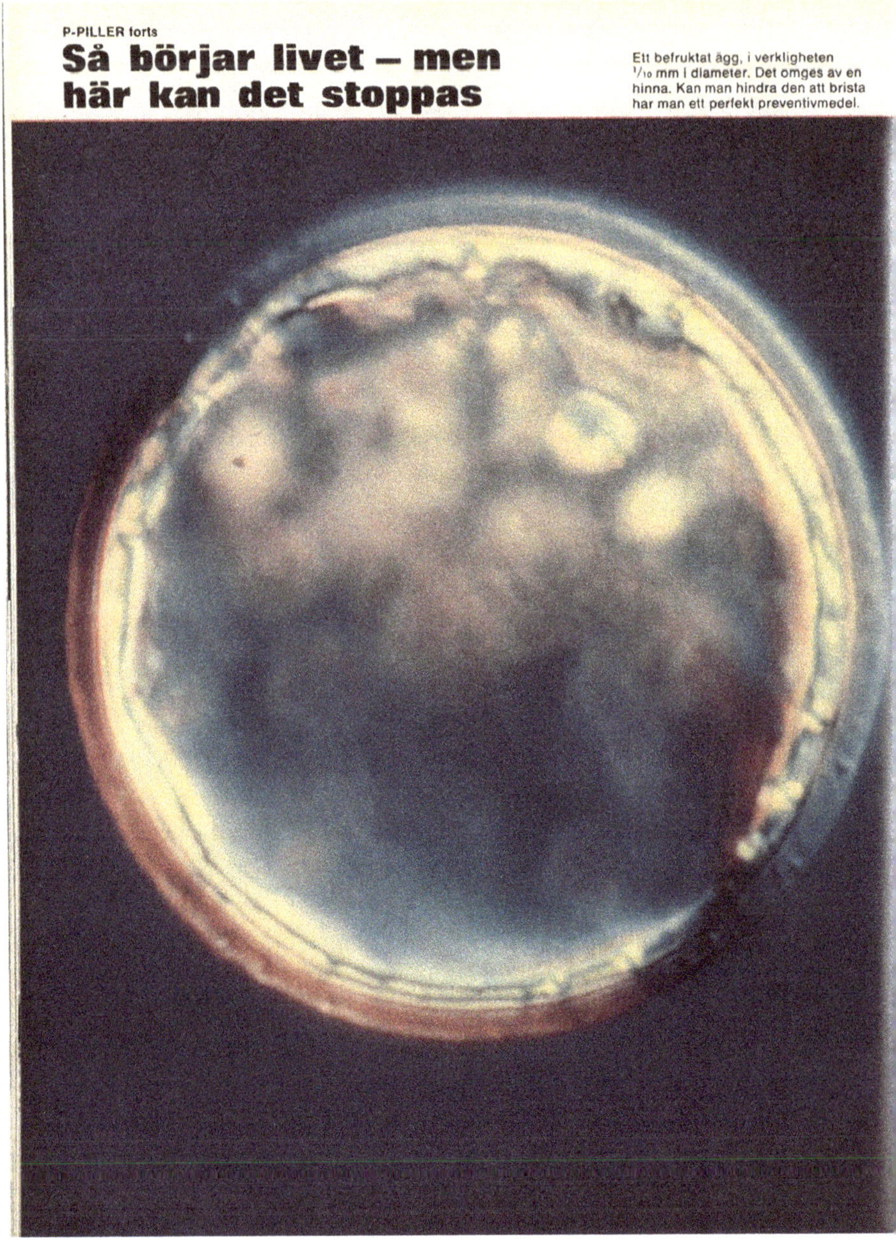

P-PILLER forts

Så börjar livet – men här kan det stoppas

Ett befruktat ägg, i verkligheten 1/10 mm i diameter. Det omges av en hinna. Kan man hindra den att brista har man ett perfekt preventivmedel.

FIGURE 9.3 The idea of developing a once-a-month contraceptive pill spread in the popular imagination. In this issue of *Se* (See), the magazine focused on research on early conception that was occurring in Uppsala, connecting this work to the possibility of making abortion-pills. In the piece, they reported on how the photographer Lennart Nilsson had taken images of the process of eggs fertilizing. Nilsson was well known for publishing photos of fetuses in *Life* magazine and then in the book *A Child Is Born* in the mid-1960s. How early conception worked and whether it could be photographed in action also piqued Nilsson's interest. From Fröberg and Nilsson, 'Unika SE-bilder visar,' 52–53. Courtesy of Lennart Nilsson Photography/SPL.

Annars händer detta: hinnan går sönder av cellernas rörelser. Finns hinnan kvar kan inte ägget fastna i livmodern.

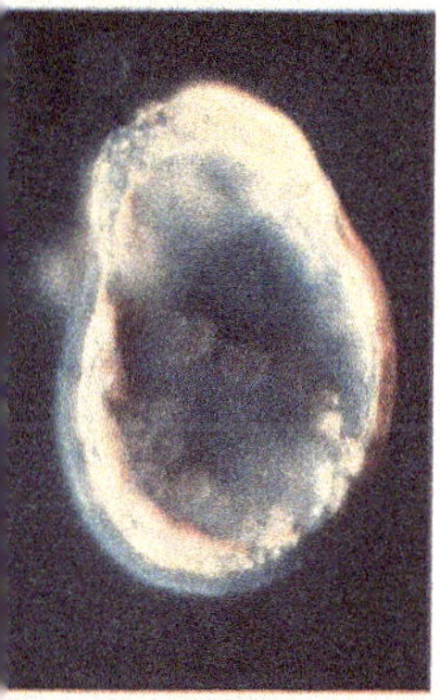

Rörelserna hos cellerna i ägget gör att det alltmer kryper ur sitt skal. Forskarna kallar ägg i detta stadium blastocyst.

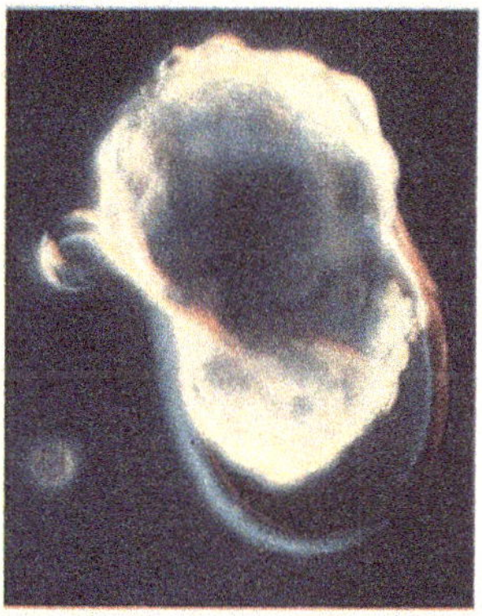

"Kläckningen" tar ungefär ett dygn. Sedan kan ägget fastna på livmoderns slemhinna och få näring via små blodkärl.

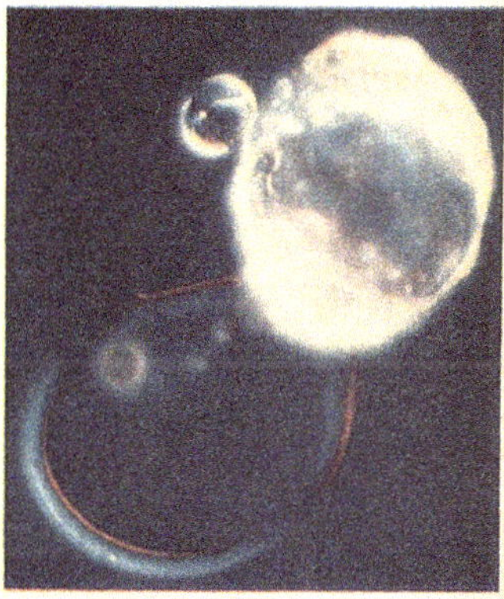

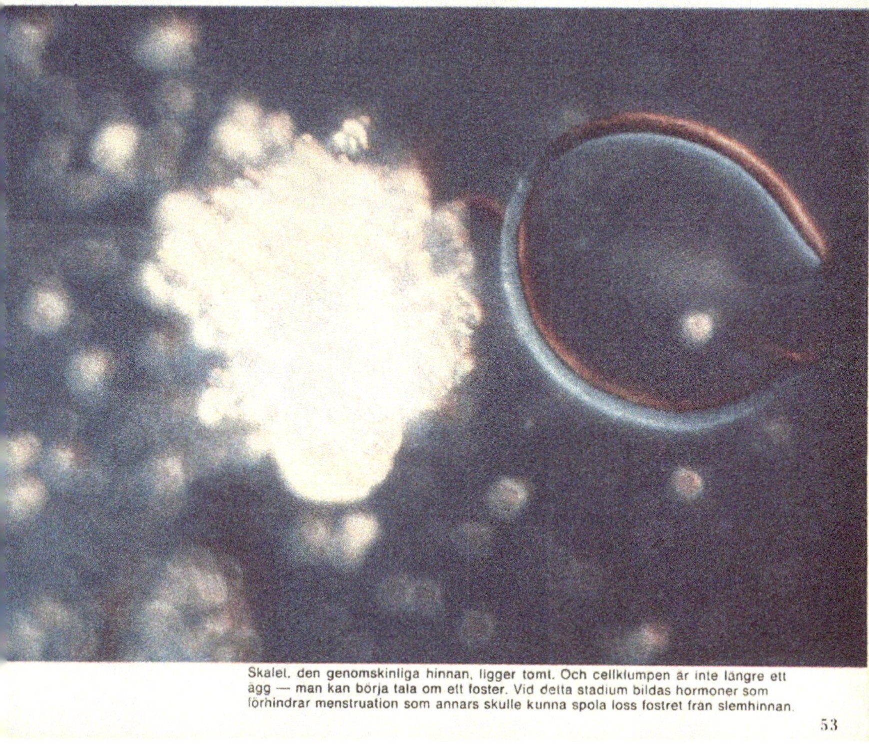

Skalet, den genomskinliga hinnan, ligger tomt. Och cellklumpen är inte längre ett ägg — man kan börja tala om ett foster. Vid detta stadium bildas hormoner som förhindrar menstruation som annars skulle kunna spola loss fostret från slemhinnan.

impossible to tell whether this occurred. The biological phases were unstable, and the technology was not fully understood. In addition, the law was up for interpretation. While Segerstedt Wiberg saw IUDs, and subsequently F6103, as conflicting with the Penal Code, Kling did not.

Signatories of the three motions dominated the discussion in April. However, they were far from a majority. Altogether, sixteen Parliament members signed the motions, signaling dissatisfaction with the original bill. While there was dissonance over what boundaries to draw around such research, there was still space for compromise and agreement. The one overarching position that most members agreed on was that they should support measures to address overpopulation. The research was seen to align with this end, but also presented ideological concerns. While birth-control development was generally viewed positively, several members saw abortion-pill development as problematic.

Many members who felt uneasy about this research positioned it against their own moral concern with protecting fetuses, but there were also logistic issues. The potential for birth defects, as with thalidomide, was viewed as a serious drawback in both supporting and rejecting the bill.[85] Who should be eligible for the trials was also seen as an important question. Should it be anyone, or women who already had permission for abortion? If this research was approved, what phase of pregnancy was then permissible to interrupt? These questions were not clearly answered in the discussion and process of passing the legislation. In the end, the bill was voted through despite these initial concerns voiced in the motions. The majority in Parliament supported it, and the state was interested in promoting family planning abroad—reproductive research could ease these efforts.

On May 12, bill 18 was written as the Law of Clinical Trials of Certain Means of Birth Control.[86] The law states, 'In order to find suitable means of birth control, clinical examination may be undertaken, after being granted special permission, which may inhibit the development of fertilized eggs in women.'[87] It came into effect June 6, 1967, creating clarity for the researchers working on abortion-pill trials, opening up possibilities for other researchers, and establishing the National Board of Medicine as the governing body.

In this instance, the introduction of a new technology—abortion pills—into Swedish reproductive research created the opportunity for the making of a new value. A technology that could be administrated in pill form opened up new possibilities for family planning initiatives, and many actors clearly

85 Swedish Parliament, 'Lag om klinisk prövning,' 105.
86 Swedish Code of Statutes, 'Lag om klinisk prövning.'
87 Swedish Code of Statutes, 'Lag om klinisk prövning.'

saw abortion pills serving a purpose beyond Swedish borders. Overpopulation concerns spanned party lines, and the topic was not as polarizing as abortion. The ambiguity of the research also meant that those who opposed abortion could still argue the strengths of fighting global starvation without overtly condoning abortion technologies. These practices—legal discussions, investigations, writing a bill, and parliamentary discussions—introduced a new way of valuing abortion pills and, subsequently, abortion. Abortion was worth pursuing as a family planning strategy.

However, optimism over the new research regulations would eventually turn to pessimism. F6103 was not as promising an abortifacient as scientists once hoped. By 1968, Engström warned against putting too much stock in the compound's abortive abilities. In an article published in the *International Planned Parenthood Federation's Medical Bulletin*, Engström mused that the effects seen in animal studies did not seem to be transferable to humans.[88] By 1970, the main researchers involved with the compound stopped pursuing its abortive qualities—F6103 was a dead end. But the research left lasting effects on how abortifacients were regulated for clinical use, opening up the field for other researchers and chemical compounds as well as energizing the popular imagination (see figure 9.3).

4 Conclusion

As other scholars have illustrated, abortion is not always polarized in a pro-life and pro-choice dichotomy.[89] Examining the passage of bill 18 illustrates how a new abortion value was made in Sweden in the 1960s. This chapter has shown a wide variety of actors involved in abortion-pill research—including many outside the clinic or laboratory setting. Meetings, legal investigations, governmental bills, parliamentary discussions, and the passage of legislation were also practices in the abortion-pill network. While familiar ideological standpoints around abortion were present in the parliamentary process, such as the stance of defending fetuses, examining the varied actors and practices makes visible more nuanced negotiations over the research.

Biological, technological, and legal definitions were an important part of the discussions over F6103. In particular, the boundary between anticonception and antidevelopment was key for those who professed ideological concerns with the research. However, there was uncertainty over the biological processes, the technology's supposed function, and the legal conditions. Owing

88 Engström, 'Swedish Post-Conception Pill.'

89 See, e.g., Campbell, 'Making Sense'; Clarke and Montini, 'Many Faces of RU486.'

to these uncertainties, maintaining and respecting such a boundary was perceived to be difficult. However, this ambiguity over the terms of the research opened up room for negotiation. In this sense, the interpretability and ambiguity of the technology was a strength used in discussing the merits of the research. The few who opposed research that 'interfered with pregnancy in a real sense' were met with statements over its ambiguity. Before the research was conducted, no one could tell what it actually did, and there was a possibility that the boundary between anticonception and antidevelopment could be preserved.

Alongside this ambiguity, there was also interest in providing solutions to a perceived global overpopulation problem, which was used to explain the relevance of the research. The state was invested in abortion services in Sweden but was also increasingly interested in family planning projects abroad. An abortion pill was seen to have the potential to make abortion exportable and would consequently be an asset for family planning initiatives. As this chapter has shown, bill 18 passed because various state actors were invested in and supported the research. The National Pharmaceutical Laboratory and the National Board of Medicine monitored the researchers, which permitted the involvement of various agencies and individuals, such as the Abortion Committee, the state secretary, and the Social Department. The director general of the National Board of Medicine professed a personal interest in the case of F6103. Even before the compound was brought to the Department of Justice, different actors had been involved in setting its legal trajectory.

In her work, Nelly Oudshoorn has showcased the difficulties of conducting clinical trials of the oral contraceptive pill in the United States.[90] The principal researchers, John Rock and Gregory Pincus, struggled to find participants and the right parameters for their trials. During the 1950s, testing contraceptives in Massachusetts was against the law, but unlike the Swedish researchers in this chapter, Rock and Pincus did not petition their government for change. Instead, they turned to Puerto Rico.[91] In contrast to Sweden, the American state was not invested in securing conditions for reproductive research.

The case of abortion-pill testing in Sweden complicates the widespread perception that in this era medical trials were being run on women of color, only to benefit white women.[92] While clinical trials of contraceptives were indeed

90 Oudshoorn, *Beyond the Natural Body*, 112–37.

91 It was not necessarily easy to find trial participants in Puerto Rico, as described in Oudshoorn's book and in Lara Marks's work, but the law did not forbid testing contraceptives. Oudshoorn, *Beyond the Natural Body*, 122; Marks, 'Human Guinea Pigs?,' 267.

92 In her work, Lara Marks has challenged the idea that women were simply uninformed guinea pigs and points to the high level of cooperation needed in contraceptive pill trials. Marks, 'Human Guinea Pigs?,' 264; Oudshoorn, *Beyond the Natural Body*, 136.

done on women of color, here we see a reversal. What might seem notable is the willingness to experiment with Swedish women's bodies, among all the biological and legal uncertainty, when there has been an assumption that white bodies would not be experimented on for the sake of a technology primarily designed to be used by people of color. Yet these trials still contributed to what Oudshoorn describes as 'cultural imperialism,' as they were intimately enmeshed with overpopulation worries and controlling the reproduction of women in what was described as 'the developing world.'[93]

In this way, the Swedish case contributes to discussions on postcolonial power dynamics—regardless of uncertainty over the technology, the biology, and the law, abortion-pill research was to be accommodated. It did not, in the end, deviate from the broad goal of curbing population growth. However, the complex relationships between many actors in the research network, the various ways power shifted over the course of clinical testing in Sweden, and the legal system of abortion care resist the oversimplification of these trials as either good or bad.[94] The debates among policymakers who were worried they did not understand the very mechanisms they were asked to make policy on capture the messy process of technological development. In this, and many cases, ethical concerns emerged when people were confronted with a new technology, and many who partook in discussions over abortion-pill research were not, in fact, experts in the fields of reproduction or law.

Sweden's approach to clinical-trial regulation, parliamentary procedures, and foreign aid played a significant part in creating acceptability around abortion pills. After the passage of bill 18, clinical trials on pregnant women were possible, and further reproductive research followed.[95] Swedish researchers would go on to test other compounds, among them prostaglandins—the next promising abortifacient.[96] With the supportive infrastructure around clinical testing, Sweden also became internationally appealing as various actors from the World Health Organization, SIDA, and the Ford Foundation looked to establish an international research center.[97] In the 1980s, Swedish researchers would collaborate with Étienne-Émile Baulieu, helping to make RU486 a feasible abortifacient.[98] Today, the vast majority of abortions performed in Sweden

93 Oudshoorn, *Beyond the Natural Body*, 136. Oudshoorn explains that since the contraceptive pill was mainly meant for populations in 'underdeveloped countries,' it was a form of cultural imperialism.

94 For a more thorough examination of the impact of abortion-pill trials in Sweden, see Ramsey, 'Swedish Abortion Pill,' 192–202.

95 Ramsey, 'Swedish Abortion Pill,' 110, 113.

96 Ramsey, 'Swedish Abortion Pill,' 113.

97 Ramsey, 'Swedish Abortion Pill,' 144–8.

98 Ramsey, 'Swedish Abortion Pill,' chap. 7.

are medically induced, with 75 percent of all abortions occurring at home.[99] Valuing abortion as an exportable family planning method in the 1960s contributed to the making of a technology that today embodies different values, including, for many, that of individual choice.

Bibliography

Bashford, Alison. *Global Populations: History, Geopolitics, and Life on Earth.* New York: Columbia University Press, 2013.

Berg, Annika. 'A Suitable Country: The Relationship between Sweden's Interwar Population Policy and Family Planning in Post-independence India.' *Berichte zur Wissenschaftsgeschichte* 33, no. 3 (2010): 297–320.

Blom, Jörgen. 'Livet börjar först efter åtta veckor!' *Aftonbladet* October 15, 1966.

Campbell, Patricia. 'Making Sense of the Abortion Pill: A Sociotechnical Analysis of RU486 in Canada.' *Health Sociology Review* 27, no. 2 (January 2018): 121–35.

Clarke, Adele E. *Disciplining Reproduction: Modernity, American Life Sciences, and 'The Problems of Sex.'* Berkeley: University of California Press, 1998.

Clarke, Adele E., and Teresa Montini. 'The Many Faces of RU486: Tales of Situated Knowledges and Technological Contestations.' *Science, Technology & Human Values* 18, no. 11 (Winter 1993): 42–78.

Dussauge, Isabelle, Claes-Fredrik Helgesson, and Francis Lee, eds. *Value Practices in the Life Sciences and Medicine.* Oxford: Oxford University Press, 2015.

Ekerwald, Hedvig. 'The Modernist Manifesto of Alva and Gunnar Myrdal: Modernization of Sweden in the Thirties and the Question of Sterilization.' *International Journal of Politics, Culture, and Society* 14, no. 3 (2001): 531–61.

Engström, Lars. 'Livet börjar först efter åtta veckor.' *Aftonbladet,* October 15, 1966.

Engström, Lars. 'The Swedish Post-Conception Pill.' *IPPF Medical Bulletin* 2, no. 2 (1968): 923.

Franklin, Sarah. 'Rethinking Reproductive Politics in Times, and Time in UK Reproductive Politics: 1978–2008.' *Journal of the Royal Anthropological Institute* 20, no. 1 (2014): 109–25.

Fröberg, Anders S., and Lennart Nilsson. 'Unika SE-bilder visar: Så kan vi få det perfekta p-pillret.' *Se* no. 49, December 3, 1970, 52–53.

Heng [pseud.]. 'Optimism i kampen mot befolkningsökning.' *Svenska Dagbladet,* June 16, 1966.

99 As of 2022, 96 percent of abortions were done medically. Socialstyrelsen, 'Statistik om aborter,' 3.

Joffe, Carole, and Tracy Weitz. 'Normalizing the Exceptional: Incorporating the "Abortion Pill" into Mainstream Medicine.' *Social Science & Medicine* 56, no. 12 (2003): 2353–66.

Jülich, Solveig. 'Fosterexperimentens produktiva hemlighet: Medicinsk forskning och vita lögner i 1960- och 1970-talets Sverige.' *Lychnos* (2018): 11–49.

Jülich, Solveig. 'Picturing Abortion Opposition in Sweden: Lennart Nilsson's Early Photographs of Embryos and Fetuses.' *Social History of Medicine* 31, no. 2 (2018): 278–307.

Kirejczyk, Marta. 'Parliamentary Cultures and Human Embryos: The Dutch and British Debates Compared.' *Social Studies of Science* 29, no. 6 (1999): 889–912.

Lennerhed, Lena. 'Troubled Women: Abortion and Psychiatry in Sweden in the 1940s and 1950s.' In *Transcending Borders: Abortion in the Past and Present*, edited by Shannon Stettner, Katrina Ackerman, Kristin Burnett, and Travis Hay, 89–100. Cham: Springer International, 2017.

Marks, Lara. 'Human Guinea Pigs? The History of the Oral Contraceptive Clinical Trials.' *History and Technology* 14, no. 4 (1999): 263–88.

National Board of Health and Welfare. 'Statistik om aborter.' Statistik och data. Accessed June 1, 2023. https://www.socialstyrelsen.se/globalassets/sharepoint-dokument/artikelkatalog/statistik/2023-5-8521.pdf.

Nordlund, Christer. 'Hormones for Life? Behind the Rise and Fall of a Hormone Remedy (Gonadex) against Sterility in the Swedish Welfare State.' *Studies in History and Philosophy of Science Part C: Studies in History and Philosophy of Biological and Biomedical Sciences* 69, no. 1 (2007): 191–216.

Oudshoorn, Nelly. *Beyond the Natural Body: An Archeology of Sex Hormones.* London: Routledge, 1994.

Prescott, Heather Munro. *The Morning After: A History of Emergency Contraception in the United States.* New Brunswick, NJ: Rutgers University Press, 2011.

Ramsey, Morag. *The Swedish Abortion Pill: Co-producing Medical Abortion and Values, ca. 1965–1992.* Uppsala: Uppsala University, 2021.

Schoug [pseud.]. 'Större svensk insats krävs i kamp mot överbefolkning.' *Dagens Nyheter*, July 17, 1966.

Svensk ordbok, s.v. 'foster.' Accessed May 12, 2023. https://svenska.se/so/.

Swedish Code of Statutes. 'Lag om klinisk prövning av vissa medel för födelsekontroll.' In *Svensk författningssamling*. SFS 1967:185. Stockholm: Svensk författningssamling, 1967.

Swedish Ministry of Health and Social Affairs. *Betänkande i abortfrågan.* SOU 1944:51. Stockholm: Socialdepartementet, 1944.

Swedish Ministry of Health and Social Affairs. *Yttrande i abortfrågan.* SOU 1937:6. Stockholm: Socialdepartementet, 1937.

Swedish Ministry of the Interior. *Abortfrågan: Betänkande*. SOU 1953:29. Stockholm: Inrikesdepartementet, 1953.

Swedish Ministry of Justice. *Betänkande med förslag till lagstiftning om avbrytande av havandeskap*. SOU 1935:15. Stockholm: Justitiedepartementet, 1935.

Swedish Ministry of Justice. *Rätten till abort*. SOU 1971:58. Stockholm: Justitiedepartementet, 1971.

Swedish Parliament. 'Lag om klinisk prövning av vissa medel för födelsekontroll.' In *Riksdagens protokoll*. Vol. 3. *Andra kammarens protokoll 1967*, no. 17, 93–98, 101–106. Stockholm: Riksdagen, 1967.

Swedish Parliament. 'Granskning av statsrådsprotokoll.' In *Riksdagens protokoll*. Vol. 3. *Första kammarens protokoll 1967*, no. 33, 3–22. Stockholm: Riksdagen, 1967.

Swedish Parliament. 'Nr 18. Kungl. Maj:ts proposition till riksdagen med förslag till lag om klinisk prövning av vissa medel för födelsekontroll; given Stockholms slott den 13 januari 1967.' In *Bihang till riksdagens protokoll 1967*. Collection 1, Vol. 5. *Kungl. Maj:ts propositioner nr 2–21*, 1–10. Stockholm: Riksdagen, 1967.

Swedish Parliament. 'Nr 855. Av herr Gustafsson i Borås m.fl., i anledning av Kungl. Maj:ts proposition nr 18, med förslag till lag om klinisk prövning av vissa medel för födelsekontroll.' In *Bihang till riksdagens protokoll 1967*. Collection 4, Vol. 3. *Motioner i andra kammaren nr 760–1065*, 7. Stockholm: Riksdagen, 1967.

Swedish Parliament. 'Nr 856. Av herrar Lindberg och Johansson i Skärstad, i anledning av Kungl. Maj:ts proposition nr 18, med förslag till lag om klinisk prövning av vissa medel för födelsekontroll.' In *Bihang till riksdagens protokoll 1967*. Collection 4, Vol. 3. *Motioner i andra kammaren nr 760–1065*, 8–9. Stockholm: Riksdagen, 1967.

Swedish Parliament. 'Nr 857. Av herr Åkerlind m.fl., i anledning av Kungl. Maj:ts proposition nr 18, med förslag till lag om klinisk prövning av vissa medel för födelsekontroll. In *Bihang till riksdagens protokoll 1967*. Collection 4, Vol. 3. *Motioner i andra kammaren nr 760–1065*, 10–11. Stockholm: Riksdagen, 1967.

Thoradeniya, Darshi. 'Altruism, Welfare, or Development Aid? Swedish Aid for Family Planning in Ceylon.' *East Asian Science, Technology and Society: An International Journal* 10, no. 4 (2016): 423–44.

Thornstedt, Hans. 'The Beginning and the End of Life from the Perspective of Swedish Criminal Law.' *Scandinavian Studies of Law* 14 (1970): 225–49.

Thornstedt, Hans, and Madeleine Andersson. *Festskrift till Hans Thornstedt*. Stockholm: Norstedt, 1983.

'Världskongress söker vapen mot "barnbomben."' *Svenska Dagbladet*, May 25, 1966.

Wiqvist, Nils, and Björn Westin, eds. *Fertility and Sterility: Proceedings of the Fifth World Congress, June 16–22*. Stockholm: International Congress Series, 1966.

Archival Sources

Application for permission for clinical trials of the substance F6103 (Ferrosan) used as an early medicinal abortifacient and pregnancy-prevention agent, April 1966. F7:8 (1966). Common matters. Documents concerning clinical trials. NPL.

Handwritten note, n.d. F7:6 (1965–1966). Common matters. Documents concerning clinical trials. NPL.

'Main views on Swedish family planning in developing countries,' n.d. FXXXI:4 (1952–1967). Director General Engel's documents arranged by subject. NBM.

Thornstedt, Hans, to NBM, September 30, 1966. D:nr LU 203. EII:22 (1966). Law and investigation bureau. NBM.

CHAPTER 10

Thalidomide in the Welfare State: Rehabilitation and Contested Normality

Maria Björkman

In the early 1960s, the unexpected consequences of the drug thalidomide (in Sweden sold as Neurosedyn) challenged the medical community. Since 1959, thalidomide had been prescribed to pregnant women to help them combat morning sickness, anxiety, and insomnia.[1] It was manufactured by the licensed pharmaceutical company Astra AB.[2] Embryos exposed to the drug during vulnerable periods of gestation displayed, if they survived until birth, various degrees of disability—shortened or absent limbs, facial paralysis, sight or hearing loss, or disorders of internal organs. This resulted in a heterogeneous group of infants with disabilities, many of them requiring intervention from internal medicine, surgery, and orthopedics.[3]

Prior to the 1960s, Swedish children born with severe disabilities were often permanently institutionalized.[4] This measure was intended to ensure that they were cared for according to medical standards, as well as to ease the strain on the family, for whom the care of a child with special needs could be difficult. Although some of the parents of children affected by thalidomide reportedly were encouraged by physicians to leave their children at an institution and forget about them, the rehabilitation program argued in favor of family care.[5]

The question whether severe disability could be a part of a fulfilling life was raised in a heated media debate. Eventually, the thalidomide scandal resulted in a revised Abortion Act, in which abortion was permitted if fetal damage from pharmaceuticals, or birth defects caused by e.g. rubella, could be expected.[6] In order to detect harmful pharmaceutical agents and prevent similar scandals in the future, it also resulted in a register of congenital malformations.[7] Helena

1 For a comprehensive overview of thalidomide studies, see Chisholm, *Life after the Scandal.*

2 Board of Medicine, statement, 2–3.

3 Avignon, Hellgren, and Juhlin, 'Thalidomidskadade barn,' 2786.

4 Persson Bergvall and Sjöberg, *Åratal: Ur handikapphistorien*, 22.

5 Juhlin, 'Neurosedynbarnens problem—främst föräldrarnas problem,' 1–2.

6 Lennerhed, 'Sherri Finkbine Flew to Sweden,' 25–45.

7 See Lee's chapter in this volume.

 | DOI:10.1163/9789004703759_012

Tinnerholm Ljungberg also argues that the thalidomide scandal was used to justify the need for more fetal research and knowledge production.[8]

Apart from motivating such preventive measures, the surviving children challenged social attitudes toward normality and disability.[9] Therefore, it is important to study the intense medical as well as sociopolitical attention that was directed at the surviving infants, in the form of their rehabilitation. This chapter focuses on the latter issue, investigating how the Swedish rehabilitation program was organized and implemented, and illuminating how understandings of the children and their needs shifted between various authorities and organizations as well as over time. The central actors involved in managing the program were the National Board of Medicine; institutions that carried out treatment and care, like the Eugenia Home, an educational boarding institution established in 1879 for children with severe physical disabilities and the first thalidomide patient organization, Society for the Neurosedyn Affected, founded by parents of affected infants in early 1962.

The Swedish authorities' actions in response to the affected children were guided by the principle of *normalization*, a concept later used within both the disability movement and disability studies. Normalization in this setting meant that infants and children should be able to live as normally as possible, despite their disabilities. In analyzing the rehabilitation program, I argue that its 'normalization' also carried an implicit understanding that the body to strive for was an able body. This, in turn, made the rehabilitation program heavily reliant on technological aids.

The aim for 'normality' made the rehabilitation program a complex arena where interactions, conflicts, and negotiations between medical professionals, the children, and their parents took place, ultimately challenging the dominant medical model of disability. The term 'medical model' is often used to describe how disability was (and sometimes still is) explained as an impairment or defect of the individual, which required interventions to 'solve' the problem, with the ultimate goal of normalization.[10]

The biopolitical concepts 'technologies of normalization' and 'self-governance' have been used to describe practices of normalization. Using these concepts, the chapter analyzes aspects of rehabilitation which aimed at correcting and adjusting the bodies of the children. In discussing technologies

8 See Tinnerholm Ljungberg's chapter in this volume.

9 Paulsson, *'Dom säger.'*

10 The medical model is often contrasted with the social model of disability. In the social model, it is a nonaccessible environment that causes much of the disability, rather than its being inherent within the individual. See Haegele and Hodge, 'Disability Discourse.'

of normalization, Abram Anders emphasizes the biopolitical risks modern societies face from 'the continued intensification of power relations through increasingly invasive [...] mechanisms of rehabilitation.' This mode of bio-power (an aspect of biopolitics) 'is a form of power that makes individuals subjects [...] to someone else by control and dependence, and tied to his own identity by a conscience or self-knowledge.'[11]

Drawing on rich public, although partly classified, archival material makes it possible to follow the rehabilitation program in detail, through board minutes, legal documents, parliamentary reports, and not least the medical files of affected individuals. To complement the public records, I have studied the archive of the Society of the Neurosedyn Affected, professional journals, documentaries, and popular books. The latter two categories have been used to gather information about the personal views of affected individuals, which are otherwise difficult to discern in the archival material, as illustrated by the case of 'M,' mentioned below.

Previous historical research on thalidomide has mainly focused on its legal, medical, and policy consequences. One strand of research has illuminated how thalidomide contributed to new ways of standardizing birth defects, to the monitoring and prediction of pharmaceutical risks, and to legal issues for companies that produced and licensed the drug.[12] Others have analyzed how thalidomide effects contributed to new or rewritten abortion clauses.[13] By comparison, the rehabilitation and care of affected children call for more attention. Canadian research argues that the physical presence of thalidomide affected ultimately helped counteract cultural 'fears of difference.'[14] Research on the thalidomide scandal in the United Kingdom has shown that the affected children sparked public discussions on 'normality,' as well as the needs of children with disabilities in a more general sense in society.[15] A few studies have used oral history methods to explore lived experiences of affected individuals.[16] In the Swedish context, an interview study portraying the experiences of young thalidomide affected with leg prostheses was published by Karin Paulsson in

11 Anders, 'Foucault and "the Right to Life."'

12 Ceccoli, 'Divergent Paths to Drug Regulation'; Moro and Invernizzi, 'Thalidomide Tragedy'; Quirke, 'Impact of Thalidomide,' 137–52. See also Lee's chapter in this volume.

13 Chisholm, 'Curious Case of Thalidomide'; Klausen and Park, '"Are We Going to Stand By"'; Parker, 'From Immorality to Public Health'; Lennerhed, 'Sherri Finkbine'; Löwy, *Imperfect Pregnancies*, chap. 3.

14 Chisholm, *Life after the Scandal*, 11–111.

15 Sewell, '"If One Member of the Family,"' 50. For the American case, see also Roskies, *Abnormality and Normality*.

16 Chisholm, *Life after the Scandal*; Blue, 'Adapting to Life.'

1995.[17] The rehabilitation program has not, however, been studied from a biopolitical perspective in relation to the Swedish welfare state.[18]

In the early 1960s, Sweden was rapidly becoming a modern welfare society. Unaffected by World War II and with a burgeoning economy and progressive tax system, the country launched several social welfare reforms, including general health insurance as well as generous additions to the pension system. The general health insurance meant that a large proportion of health-care facilities—clinics for mothers and children, hospitals, as well as institutions for people with mental and physical disabilities, operated by the state, county councils, or municipalities—were subsidized for citizens, contributing to the early discovery of the thalidomide-affected infants.[19]

In the sections that follow, I first provide an overview of the Swedish thalidomide case and the general actions taken by the National Board of Medicine. The focus will then turn to details of the rehabilitation program, as well as exploring how the aims for normalization were carried out. A concluding discussion on some consequences of normalization will close the chapter.

1 The Unfolding Scandal

During the 1950s, several cases of institutional maladministration were criticized in the media, and a successive shift in attitudes toward a greater emphasis on individual autonomy can be noted in public debates, and sometimes also in institutional practice.[20] However, as we shall see in the following account of the National Board of Medicine, this change was not unambiguously reflected by public authorities and their experts.

The National Board of Medicine first became aware of the risks of Neurosedyn on November 27, 1961, when a Swedish newspaper published a brief piece on the German withdrawal of the drug from the market due to fetal injuries.[21] Two days later, the National Board of Medicine requested that Astra warn Swedish physicians of this risk, asking them not to prescribe the compound to pregnant women until 'full clarity' had been reached.[22] Even though causality

17 Paulsson, *'Dom säger.'*

18 However, see Björkman, 'Cost of Normalization.'

19 Lindqvist, 'Swedish Disability Policies.'

20 Björkman, *Vård för samhällets bästa*; Swedish Ministry of Health and Social Affairs, *Barnen som samhället svek*; Lundmark, *'Lappen är ombytlig'*; Tydén, *Från politik till praktik*; Grunewald, *Från idiot till medborgare*.

21 Board of Medicine, statement, 6–7.

22 Astra AB to Swedish physicians, December 1961.

had not yet been established between the anomalies and thalidomide, in a meeting with his experts on December 12, the board's director general, Arthur Engel, decided that the sale of thalidomide should be stopped. During the following week, all pharmacies and hospitals halted sales and returned the products.[23] Despite these actions, no public warning was given.

The Society for the Neurosedyn Affected reacted strongly to this failure to warn the public. From the start, they had two immediate aims: to find all the affected children in Sweden, and to make the dangers of thalidomide public. According to a later statement by the journalist Nils Lalander, the press, in a silent agreement with the National Board of Medicine, had promised not to cover the topic until greater certainty was reached.[24] However, the society used personal contacts to persuade the Christian newspaper *Dagen* to cover the story two months after the drug's withdrawal. The rest of the media followed suit. The society thought that if the National Board of Medicine had acted promptly, children could have been saved from injuries. Accordingly, it filed a complaint with the Parliamentary Ombudsman, demanding an investigation.[25] The parliamentary ombudsman, appointed by the Swedish Parliament to ensure that public authorities followed laws and regulations, demanded an answer from the National Board of Medicine. The board answered the complaints in a memorandum stating that it had acted correctly in every step of the process.[26] The board explained that because of the drug's withdrawal, and the information given to physicians, no public warning was considered necessary. Additionally, alarming publicity could have been frightening for pregnant women.[27]

During the months following the withdrawal, the National Board of Medicine received information from hospitals about infants affected by the compound.[28] In 1962, the board developed a rigorous procedure for finding affected infants, classifying their injuries, and organizing their immediate care.

23 Board of Medicine, statement, 8–9.

24 See his account in Lalander, *Svenska miljöskandaler*, 43–44; Yllner, *Bara en liten vit sömntablett*, 62.

25 Board of Medicine, statement. See also Society for the Neurosedyn Affected, 'Neurosedyn.'

26 Board of Medicine, statement.

27 Board of Medicine, statement, 9. In 2003, the scandal was investigated again, now by the Chancellor of Justice, to determine whether the Swedish authorities had managed the case correctly. The investigation concluded that they had, and that it was unfortunate, but not illegal, that the National Board of Medicine did not immediately launch a public warning. See Swedish Chancellor of Justice, Justitiekanslerns utlåtande angående neurosedynkatastrofen.

28 Board of Medicine, statement, 9.

They also dealt with preventing future pharmaceutical disasters and assessing the needs of the affected infants. To grasp the magnitude of the scandal, the board launched an investigation, led by the pediatrician Jan Winberg. To provide material, all maternity wards were ordered to start registering newborns with anomalies, and to send the list monthly to the board for evaluation. Previously they had been obliged to send yearly reports.[29]

These procedures signal the beginning of the National Board of Medicine's search for all those affected, as well as the stricter regulation of pharmaceuticals. The goal of finding all affected infants was to enroll them in a program of rehabilitation. In the following, we will see how institutional structures were established in order to locate, diagnose, and treat the affected, but also to produce statistics to estimate the future need for interventions. The board was the main actor in these initiatives, and Engel was personally involved in their administration. An institutional network was established to monitor events, appointing a range of experts who worked together on addressing the alarming reports and dealing with the affected children.

According to Winberg's investigation, 102 affected children were born between January 1960 and February 1962. Of these, only fifty-three survived. From March to September 1962, another twenty-nine affected children were born, of whom 50 per cent were estimated to survive infancy.[30] Among the survivors, it was estimated that around forty children were in need of part- or full-time institutional care.[31]

In case any children had been missed at maternity wards, the National Board of Medicine sent out information to all physicians in charge of regional institutions for cerebral palsy. These care and educational institutions were chosen due to the fact that they already had expertise in pediatrics, audiology, speech therapy, orthopedics, and child rehabilitation, and catered to every region in Sweden. By obliging the physicians in charge to make sure that every infant not yet introduced into the emerging program of care and rehabilitation was traced and registered, the National Board of Medicine ensured the enrolment of all affected.[32] Correspondence from the board contained the information cards of all known affected children born in each region between January 1, 1960, and February 28, 1962. The register was handled by the Eugenia Home.

29 For an account of how the anomalies were defined, measured, and classified, including the difficulties of each of these steps, see Lee's chapter in this volume.

30 Board of Medicine, supplement.

31 Board of Medicine, memorandum on the care, 1.

32 Board of Medicine, memorandum on the care, 1.

These measures led to the registration of an additional number of children in the rehabilitation program.[33]

The discovery that a compound considered harmless could be extremely toxic raised several questions. One was whether other medicines on the market posed similar threats. To address this uncertainty, the National Board of Medicine added other medicines to Winberg's investigation list.[34] Later, the board summarized these efforts, stating that demands on the public pharmaceutical bureau for investigations of new compounds were high. To meet the increased workload, a special unit was installed, which focused on active risk surveillance by surveying pharmaceutical literature and indexing the side effects of drugs.[35] The board also took part in international efforts to track the effects of drugs. In 1963, the World Health Organization started to issue 'drug warnings' from each country to the member states, an activity that Sweden contributed to. Sweden also engaged in the newly established European organization for drug toxicity. Additionally, information was shared within the Nordic countries, and an exchange was established with the US Food and Drug Administration.[36]

In West Germany, as in Sweden, policies for regulation were established through the collaboration of the Government, the pharmaceutical industry, and the medical profession. In the United States, however, the Food and Drug Administration had authority over the other parties. Compared to West Germany and Sweden, the US outcome for thalidomide was considerably different, since approval of the compound was delayed owing to lack of proof that it was nontoxic.[37]

In Sweden, clinical trials of new drugs became strictly regulated in 1964, and thereafter companies had to apply to the State Pharmaceutical Laboratory for permission, with a careful plan of the testing procedure.[38] Due to the risks associated with new drugs, physicians also needed quick and efficient ways of reporting side effects to the National Board of Medicine. A group of experts were appointed to investigate how this could be achieved.[39] As mentioned earlier, another effect of thalidomide was the revision of the Swedish Abortion Act. Previously, the Abortion Act had allowed the abortion of fetuses with a high risk of severe inherited malformations or disease. Now it was also

33 Board of Medicine, memorandum on the care, 19–20.
34 Board of Medicine, memorandum on the care, 9–10.
35 Board of Medicine, memorandum on the care, 13–14.
36 Board of Medicine, memorandum on the care, 15–16.
37 Daemmrich, 'Tale of Two Experts.'
38 Board of Medicine, statement, 16.
39 Board of Medicine, statement, 15.

permitted when the fetus had risks of noninherited anomalies or disease.[40] In this way, thalidomide contributed to regulations that went far beyond the compound's direct effects.

To summarize, thalidomide demonstrated the risks of modern medicine, not only to individuals, but also, in aggregate, to populations. The statistics produced in response served to protect the population and strategically decrease the risk of similar scenarios. From a biopolitical perspective, the establishment of new routines of drug testing and regulation, as well as the system of reporting suspected side effects through new and existing infrastructures, can all be considered powerful technologies of normalization at the population level in the welfare state. In the following, we will shift to the rehabilitation program and examine how these practices played out in individual treatment.

2 Normalization and Rehabilitation at the Eugenia Home

In 1961 children affected by thalidomide were treated in hospitals, orphanages, or boarding schools for children with disabilities, like the Eugenia Home. Early on, the National Board of Medicine emphasized the importance of centralizing care. The argument was that the resources of staff and equipment would be best used in a small number of units, which would be able to build expertise on the particular needs of these children. Those who could not be cared for by the regional institutions were treated at the Eugenia Home.[41] It was decided that the Eugenia Home needed a counsellor to communicate information to the parents, and in 1962, Inga-Maj Juhlin was hired to this position.[42] She was also assigned the task of establishing the national register of children affected by thalidomide. In this she was guided by Winberg, the physician who performed the investigation.[43]

As previously mentioned, the key concept guiding the approach of the National Board of Medicine, care institutions, political parties, teachers, and parents toward these children was *normalization*. A large proportion of Swedish disability research has been focused on the process of normalization for people with intellectual disabilities, which took place from the end of the 1960s. This process aimed to allow these individuals to live as normal lives as possible, in terms of housing as well as opportunities for forming close social

40 Swedish Parliament, 'Nr 100. Kungl. Maj:ts proposition.'
41 Board of Medicine, memorandum on the care, 1.
42 Juhlin, *Rikskuratorn*, 17–19.
43 Board of Medicine, statement, 19.

relations and for employment.[44] The normalization principle led to the abandonment of lifelong institutionalization for several patient categories, and to modernized institutions for those who still needed constant care—changes that are usually described as the start of the modern disability movement in Sweden.[45] The thalidomide case sheds light on a previously understudied group in the Swedish history of disability: those with physical disabilities.

The pediatrician Karl Grunewald, head of the National Board of Medicine's division for the care of people with intellectual disabilities, was responsible for monitoring institutions and facilities for these individuals during the 1960s and 1970s. In an overview of the development of normalization in this context, he argued that there was a lingering opinion among physicians that children with disabilities posed a strain on their families and needed to be institutionalized. According to Grunewald, a common recommendation from pediatricians was to leave the child at an institution and 'forget them.' However, he claimed that most parents, with encouragement and enough societal support, wanted to raise their children at home.[46]

A 1963 journal article by Juhlin, the Eugenia Home counsellor, is representative of the dominant way of reasoning within the program. She emphasized the children's need to have a 'normal upbringing.' The children were to be 'anchored' within a family in order to form deeper connections with others. The opinion on children with intellectual disabilities that Grunewald recalled hearing from pediatricians seems to have been expressed about thalidomide-affected children too; in her article Juhlin condemned the recommendation some parents had received from physicians: to forget about their children and leave them at an institution. Juhlin argued that forgetting a child was both an impossible task for the parents and harmful for the child.[47]

However, the pursuit of normalization also meant adjustments imposed on the children themselves, in the form of prosthetic limbs, surgery, and hearing and speech training. In 1963, the Eugenia Home was rapidly expanding its resources in this regard. An activity therapist, a medical nurse, and a physical therapist were employed. Staff attempted to find a bandage maker, but owing to a lack of applicants, the position remained vacant. Furthermore, the consultant hours for a child psychiatrist had been increased. A phoniatrician and an audiologist were available as consultants.[48] To coordinate treatments, the staff

44 Grunewald, *Från idiot till medborgare*.
45 Grunewald, *Från idiot till medborgare*, 30–31; Holme, 'Disability, Identity and Ageing,' 37.
46 Grunewald, *Från idiot till medborgare*, 227–28.
47 Juhlin, 'Neurosedynbarnens problem,' 1–2.
48 Board of Medicine, supporting data, 2.

was organized in teams: pediatric, orthopedic, psychiatric, and rehabilitation.[49] At the end of 1963, around one hundred children were registered, and the counsellor had been in contact with the parents or caregivers to seventy of them. She advised them on where to get treatment and on how to apply for financial help to make their existing home accessible for the child. She searched for foster parents and educated parents or carers before discharging the children.[50] Eventually, 'real' homes were assigned to all children at the Eugenia Home—if not with their biological families, in foster care or as adoptees, according to Juhlin's account.[51]

At the Eugenia Home, every child received between forty-five and sixty minutes of physical therapy each day, in a schedule including play school, exercise, outdoor activities, meals, naptime, and medical treatments.[52] The hearing impaired were given audiological training by a specially qualified preschool teacher, and also saw a play and activity therapist. Deaf children received sixty to ninety minutes of group training each day, and thirty to sixty minutes of individual training.[53] From the end of 1963, the specialized preschool teacher for the hearing impaired provided ten hours of weekly training, partly in the children's day room. This enabled other employees to learn audiology strategies while assisting the children. The phoniatric consultant created individualized programs for children in need of speech training.[54] Each child was also assessed by the child psychiatrist during their stay. The children's psychological development was monitored by the staff, with the help of the psychiatrist's discussions with the parents. On top of this, each child also had play and activity therapy, both individually and in a group.[55]

The situation for children outside the Eugenia Home was not as uniform, and according to the Society for the Neurosedyn Affected, not all of them were sufficiently examined, resulting in an unequal situation in which some children's needs went unknown. This disparity became pressing when the children were nearing the age when they would attend primary school. When a government body for disability issues was constituted in 1965, one of its first tasks was to launch a public investigation into the situation of people with disabilities in Sweden, including children affected by thalidomide.[56] In a letter to the

49 Board of Medicine, supporting data, 3.
50 Board of Medicine, supporting data, 5.
51 Juhlin, *Rikskuratorn*, 99–105.
52 Board of Medicine, supporting data, 2.
53 Board of Medicine, supporting data, 2–3.
54 Board of Medicine, supporting data, 3.
55 Board of Medicine, supporting data.
56 Persson Bergvall and Sjöberg, *Åratal*, 51.

investigators, the society advocated a 'comprehensive medical investigation,' including 'social, medical, mental and intellectual' factors. This, according to the society, was necessary to find out whether the 'parents and children's mental and intellectual equipment' was sufficient for successful local schooling. According to the society, local schools, which required adjustments and new equipment, could not be properly prepared unless all the affected children had been thoroughly studied.[57]

The program at the Eugenia Home and the actions taken by the society to enhance the investigation and treatment of affected children outside the institution suggest that rehabilitation, with its extensive training programs that took up much of the children's day, was not only tolerated or accepted by the parents, but desired. According to Abram Anders, the biopolitical risks faced by modern societies include rehabilitation that becomes increasingly 'invasive,' thus subjugating individuals by controlling them to the point that the rehabilitation becomes tied to their own identity.[58] This risk does not seem to have been perceived by the parents. Instead, the society asked for thorough studies of all the affected children in order to organize schooling and standardize rehabilitation. Below, we will see how this attitude, over time, was modified by both the children and their parents.

Prosthetic limbs formed a substantial part of the technical equipment demanded by the society. In general, much hope was placed on the promises of prosthetic limbs, by the society, individual parents, and the rehabilitation program. That the children deviated from existing norms of physical appearance was obvious. When interviewing thalidomide-affected adults, psychologist Karin Paulsson found that they recalled an intense focus on prosthetic limbs, due in part to the expectations of increased mobility, but also because prosthetic limbs made them look more 'normal.'[59]

As the Swedish experience in prosthetic technology was limited, a state-funded delegation went to West Germany to study its development.[60] The delegation visited specialized care units for children with thalidomide disabilities in Heidelberg and Münster, and upon their return reported to the minister of the interior. In their report, they stressed that the advanced prosthetic technology of West Germany was a result of research grants from German state

57 Society for the Neurosedyn Affected to Swedish Government Commission on Disability Issues.

58 Anders, 'Foucault and "the Right to Life."'

59 Paulsson, *'Dom säger.'* For a discussion of normality in relation to thalidomide prosthetics, see also McEnroe, *Medicine*, 32–34.

60 'Avancerad behandling,' 25; Board of Medicine, supporting data, 5.

authorities. It was also reported that West Germans had an optimistic view of the affected children's future. As in Sweden, prosthetic limbs contributed to this sense of optimism.[61]

At the Norrbacka Institute, close to the Eugenia Home, individual splints and bandages were constructed. Children with affected legs were initially given 'stilt' prosthetics that were used to practice balancing while standing. Later, more sophisticated prosthetics that mimicked 'natural legs and feet' were developed. In collaboration with the Royal Institute of Technology, advanced prosthetic arms were also developed. Since some children lacked mobility in their arms, their artificial hands needed to be directed by power sources other than arm movements in order to perform.[62] For children who had hands, fingers, or parts of fingers, the Eugenia Home pediatrician Marcel d'Avignon argued that these should not be amputated, as even the smallest of fingers could 'gradually be strong enough to […] direct the activity in the prosthesis.'[63]

One example that illustrates how a child could experience the normalization process is the story of 'M,' a woman who spent parts of her childhood in the Eugenia Home. In 2011, she was interviewed in a radio documentary. M recalled the events that led to her toes being amputated somewhere between the ages of eight and ten. M's feet are attached near the hips. When using prosthetic legs, her toes bulged out underneath the fabric of her trousers. When V-jeans came into fashion, M decided to have her toes amputated: 'I wanted corduroys, because it looked so cool when people walked in them. And I remember the first pair I got from mum. Brown with pink pockets.' As an adult, however, M felt ambivalent about the pursuit of normalization. When asked how much hospitalization she considered necessary in her case, and how she felt about the surgeries she had received, she responded, 'I could claim that none of them was necessary, if I had been allowed to be the one I was. But since this was not the case, certain surgeries were important. It was the amputation […], the straightening of my wrist. But really, I have not been allowed to become the one I was born to be. […] Instead, I have a heap of scars on my body.'[64]

Another example of how normality was emphasized through the hope of technology is that of a girl born without arms. Her file stated, however, that her legs were 'completely normal.' In addition, she had normal sight and hearing, and was 'mentally well.' At age five, she had her prosthetic arms attached often, although she did not use them much. She was 'pretty irritable.' At age

61 'Avancerad behandling,' 25.

62 Board of Medicine, supporting data, 2.

63 Avignon, 'Den framtida vården,' 6.

64 Collmar, 'Det lagade barnet.'

six, she was equipped with advanced prosthetic arms. She attended preparatory class, a voluntary form of school offered to all Swedish children. There she mostly used her feet, although she 'carried boxes' with the prosthetics. She was well-adjusted and 'reasonable,' but 'lacking all spontaneity.' At home, she used her prosthetic arms less and less. The girl's way of using the prosthetic arm 'gives a stiff impression,' the counsellor noted.[65] The family was disappointed in the prosthetic technology: it was slow, although the maneuvering of the prosthetic arm worked from a technical point of view. It was believed that with time the girl could learn to tolerate the devices, as her own skills at steering improved. As she 'seemed exhausted,' use of the prosthetics was reduced to a minimum. One idea discussed was to provide a prosthetic arm designed to manage a single task, and to let her use it for this specific purpose, as it was observed that she felt 'free' while not using the prosthetics. At a later check-up, she was described as 'tense, exhausted, worried, and easily starts crying' when the prosthetics were 'failing.' The number of functions was drastically reduced to make her situation easier. A month later, she still had the arms attached often, but 'seldom' used them. She was reported as eager to 'oblige.'[66]

Like most thalidomide-affected children, this girl was attending a 'normal class' in primary school, 'blending in' well. She attended 'everything,' even ball games, and was never heard to say 'I can't.' Her teacher wrote that she was intellectually 'above average,' but was writing slowly. She only needed assistance at meals and when visiting the toilet. At age ten, she attended prosthetic training every week at the Eugenia Home, and had typewriting classes twice a week. She managed 'well' with her cosmetic hand. According to her file, the process of adjusting to the desired level of normality worked out well.[67] However, it came at the price of reducing her own mobility and restricting her ability to use her feet.

After a decade of struggling with artificial limbs, it was clear that they were causing conflicts for all involved, not least the children. Eventually, Karin Paulsson was assigned to evaluate how the children used their prosthetics. Paulsson found that the devices mostly hindered the children. This conclusion initially caused an uproar among both parents and engineers, but as Paulsson later stated in her own dissertation on the subject, it eventually led the rehabilitation group to look for alternative ways to cater for the needs of each child.[68]

65 National counsellor, personal dossier.
66 National counsellor, personal dossier.
67 National counsellor, personal dossier.
68 Yllner, *Bara en liten vit sömntablett*, 193–195; Paulsson, *'Dom säger,'* 75.

Prosthetic limbs, splints, medical care, medicine, training sessions, and practical aids were costly. Many of the orthopedic supplies were covered by general health insurance, but not all; neither were hearing or sight training sessions outside the rehabilitation facilities, personalized tools for eating, parents' journeys to the Eugenia Home, or their loss of income.[69] It became one of Juhlin's tasks to help the parents apply for additional coverage from their municipality or the county council. In other countries, people affected by thalidomide were excluded from the welfare system in order to avoid giving additional support to other groups with disabilities. This was the case in the United Kingdom, where the Government arranged a private fund to cater for their needs.[70] When Astra donated SEK 1 million and established a fund to complement public support for people affected by thalidomide in Sweden, it became common to apply to the fund for travel expenses, home alterations, parental courses involving expert lectures, individual support, and leisure activities.[71]

The society, however, wanted Astra to take full responsibility, as the company's donation would not compensate for the lifelong consequences that their children faced. The society retained the lawyer Henning Sjöström, and charges were filed in September 1965. A settlement was reached in October 1969, in which Astra agreed to pay lifelong, index-linked annual compensation to each child. The settlement meant that no criminal verdict was reached against Astra, but it offered a more economically favorable outcome for the children, according to Sjöström's own recollection of the case.[72]

The main argument from the society was, however, that full coverage of all medical care should be publicly financed. Minutes from a National Board of Medicine meeting in 1963 illustrates this standpoint. During the meeting, the chairman criticized differences in the county-level regulation of economic support for home care for children with disabilities, resulting in varying access to resources, depending on which region the families lived in.[73] However, already in November 1962 Juhlin had sent a survey to the county councils in which she referred to the need for economic support for home care, asking how each county handled this issue. In January 1963 the board of the coalition of county councils recommended that all counties provide the same amount

69 Board of Medicine, supporting data, 5.

70 Chisholm, *Life after the Scandal*, 111–12.

71 Juhlin, 'Neurosedynbarnens problem,' 3; Society for the Neurosedyn Affected to Astra Fund.

72 Nilsson and Sjöström, *Pillret som väckte världen*, 206–12.

73 Board of Medicine, minutes, September 5, 1963, 3.

of support for the care of children affected by thalidomide as was granted for other individuals with disabilities, and the measure was later put into effect.[74]

3 Rehabilitation with Dual Consequences

Inspired by a biopolitical perspective, this chapter has studied 'normalization' and rehabilitation of children affected by thalidomide in Sweden during the 1960s. As emphasized by Mika Ojakangas, the notion of biopower does not exclusively mean suppression; it also 'exerts a positive influence on life, endeavors to administer, optimize, and multiply it.'[75] These aspects of care and support resonate with fundamental features of the Swedish welfare state at the time: the welfare of each individual was a collective responsibility, and high-quality services should be provided equally to all citizens, regardless of income or status.[76] Applied to people affected by thalidomide, these principles resulted in efforts to optimize their lives based on the idea of normalization.

As we have seen, the management of the thalidomide scandal in the early 1960s was an efficient and far-reaching activity. One reason for its effectiveness was that the budget for health care and rehabilitation was considerably increased.[77] Another reason was that the enterprise was organized by the National Board of Medicine, resulting in centralized management and efficient implementation. A third reason was that the efforts of the Society for the Neurosedyn Affected and the rehabilitation program resulted in the reformulation of general welfare regulations to include care for people affected by thalidomide, unlike in, for instance, the United Kingdom. The new regulations, drawing on existing institutions and routines and covering the entire country, made this rapid organization possible.

However, the conflicts that arose from the role and function of prosthetic limbs in shaping normality is worth reflecting upon—particularly as the standards for altering the bodies of people affected by thalidomide have undergone significant changes since the early 1970s, as exemplified by M in the interview from 2011.

---

74 National counsellor, enqmries, 22; Board of Medicine, statement, 22. See also Björkman, 'Cost of Normalization.'

75 Ojakangas, 'Impossible Dialogue on Bio-Power,' 6.

76 Esping-Andersen, *Three Worlds of Welfare Capitalism*, 28; Aspalter, 'Worlds of Welfare Capitalism,' 9.

77 Swedish Ministry of Health and Social Affairs, *Bättre utbildning för handikappade*.

The Swedish welfare system stressed that the health and well-being of each individual was a collective responsibility. In the case of thalidomide, this responsibility also seems to have implicitly incorporated collective ideas about a 'standard body.' It was as if the welfare system was expected not only to provide efficient care and rehabilitation, but also to fulfill an implicit right to bodies that as closely as possible resembled 'normal' ones, with the help of technology.

At first, the experts at the National Board of Medicine, the rehabilitation institutions, and the Society for the Neurosedyn Affected seem to have agreed on and worked toward this implicit goal. As time passed and the children grew, it gradually became obvious that the prosthetic limbs did not live up to expectations. As the organization managing the prosthetic limbs reevaluated its work and changed its approach, the idea of normalization emerges as flexible, rather than fixed. The children's struggle with their prosthetic limbs, and the parents' complaints, eventually paved the way for investigating the functionality of the prosthetics.

The actions taken by parents, both individually and as represented by the society, shifted too. Initially they persistently requested more advanced and adequate prosthetic limbs, and were diligent in making the children practice. At the same time, they criticized the functionality of existing devices. It is clear that expectations placed on the technologies of normalization were initially shared by medical staff and parents, only to be adjusted later. For children, the situation was somewhat different. As we have seen in the example of the girl equipped with arm prosthetics, it is possible that it was the existing discourse around normalizing technologies that made her compliant, even when the artificial arms severely restricted her mobility. This phenomenon suggests that she had internalized ideas of a preferred, 'normal' body, which manifested in acts of self-governance. At the same time, although she was compliant on the surface, it was evident to the adults that she was on the brink of exhaustion, which, in its own way, constituted a silent protest. M, on the other hand, describes peer pressure during early adolescence as the motivating factor for a surgical, normalizing intervention. As I have shown, attempts at normalization for thalidomide-affected children had several consequences. These included newly organized means of both identifying who had been affected and categorizing the type and number of injuries, which, in turn, made it possible to grant individuals and families their rights to publicly financed medical care and rehabilitation. However, the same sorting procedure reproduced what was defined as a normal body and what was not. Ingunn Moser argues that although technology for people with disabilities is still often envisioned as a 'transformative power' that will enable individuals to become 'competent normal subjects,' the same technology instead contributes to the '(re)production of the asymmetries that they [...] seek to undo.' According to Moser, this is because the ideal of normalization, in which the technology is made to operate, continuously reenacts the dichotomy of 'abled and disabled, and normal and deviant.'[78] This holds true for people affected by thalidomide in 1960s Sweden.

As thalidomide-affected children became young adults, they assumed responsibility for the society from their parents. In a letter to the National Council for the Disabled, they described their plans for the future, among which was 'to live as independently as possible.'[79] In recent years, the society has, as part of its activities, run its own health project, focused on rehabilitation on members' own terms, financed by the Swedish Inheritance Fund.[80] In this way, old ideas about normalization have been replaced by the 'own normal' of people affected by thalidomide.

Bibliography

Anders, Abram. 'Foucault and "the Right to Life": From Technologies of Normalization to Societies of Control.' *Disability Studies Quarterly* 33, no. 3 (May 2013): https://dsq-sds.org/index.php/dsq/article/view/3340/3268.

Aspalter, Christian. 'Worlds of Welfare Capitalism: Examining Eight Different Models.' Research Center on Societal and Social Policy Research Paper Series 6 (2002).

'Avancerad behandling av neurosedynskadade barn i Västtyskland.' *Svensk vanföretidskrift* 40, no. 1 (January 1963): 25.

Avignon, Marcel d'. 'Den framtida vården av neurosedynskadade barn.' *Svensk vanföretidskrift* 40 no. 4 (April 1963): 4–6.

Avignon, Marcel d', Karin Hellgren, and Inga-Maj Juhlin. 'Thalidomidskadade barn, erfarenheter från Eugeniahemmet.' *Läkartidningen* 61 (1964): 2786–92.

Björkman, Jenny. *Vård för samhällets bästa: Tvångsvård av sjuka och missbrukare i Sverige 1850–1970*. Stockholm: Carlsson, 2001.

Björkman, Maria. 'The Cost of Normalization: The Thalidomide Affected and the Welfare State.' *Scandinavian Journal of History* 48, no. 3 (2023): 341–58.

Blue, Ruth. 'Adapting to Life as a Thalidomide Survivor,' from the Wellcome Collection project 'Voices of Thalidomide.' Accessed May 25, 2023. https://wellcomecollection.org/articles/YJEtbREAACIA4bQT.

78 Moser, 'Disability and the Promises of Technology,' 373.

79 Society for the Neurosedyn Affected to National Council for the Disabled.

80 Society for the Neurosedyn Affected, 'Vad gör FfdN?'

Ceccoli, Stephen. 'Divergent Paths to Drug Regulation in the United States and in the United Kingdom.' *Journal of Policy History* 12, no. 2 (2002): 135–69.

Chisholm, Christine. 'The Curious Case of Thalidomide and the Absent Eugenic Clause in Canada's Amended Abortion Law.' *Canadian Bulletin of Medical History* 33, no. 2 (Fall 2016): 493–516.

Chisholm, Christine. *Life after the Scandal: Thalidomide, Family, and Rehabilitation in Modern Canada, 1958–1990*. Ottawa: Carleton University, 2019.

Collmar, Lollo. 'Det lagade barnet.' Swedish Radio documentary, 2011. Transcript accessed November 24, 2019. https://sverigesradio.se/sida/artikel.aspx?programid=909&artikel=4807555.

Daemmrich, Arthur. 'A Tale of Two Experts: Thalidomide and Political Engagement in the United States and West Germany.' *Social History of Medicine* 15, no. 1 (April, 2002): 137–58.

Esping-Andersen, Gösta. *The Three Worlds of Welfare Capitalism*. Cambridge: Polity Press, 1990.

Grunewald, Karl. *Från idiot till medborgare: De utvecklingsstördas historia*. Stockholm: Gothia förlag, 2008.

Haegele, Justin Anthony, and Samuel Hodge. 'Disability Discourse: Overview and Critiques of the Medical and Social Models.' *Quest* 68, no. 2 (2016): 193–206.

Holme, Lotta. 'Disability, Identity and Ageing.' In *Ageing with Disability: A Lifecourse Perspective*, edited by Eva Jeppsson Grassman and Anna Whitaker, 35–53. Bristol: Bristol University Press, 2013.

Juhlin, Inga-Maj. 'Neurosedynbarnens problem—främst föräldrarnas problem.' *Socionomen* 8 (1963): 1–2.

Juhlin, Inga-Maj. *Rikskuratorn: Omhändertagandet av de neurosedynskadade barnen 1962–1970*. Stockholm: Carlsson, 2012.

Klausen, Susanne, and Julie Park. '"Are We Going to Stand By and Let These Children Come into the World?": The Impact of the "Thalidomide Disaster" in South Africa, 1960–1977.' *Journal of South Africa Studies* 41 (2015): 735–52.

Lalander, Nils. *Svenska miljöskandaler*. Stockholm: Sober, 1995.

Lennerhed, Lena. 'Sherri Finkbine Flew to Sweden: Abortion and Disability in the Early 1960s.' In *Abortion across Borders: Transnational Travel and Access to Abortion Services*, edited by Christabel Sethna and Gayle Davis, 25–45. Baltimore: Johns Hopkins University Press, 2019.

Lindqvist, Rafael. 'Swedish Disability Policies: Ideas, Values and Practices in a Historical Perspective.' In *The Routledge History of Disability*, edited by Roy Hanes, Ivan Brown, and Nancy E. Hansen, 216–30. London: Routledge, 2018.

Löwy, Ilana. *Imperfect Pregnancies: A History of Birth Defects and Prenatal Diagnosis*. Baltimore: Johns Hopkins University Press, 2017.

Lundmark, Lennart. *'Lappen är ombytlig, ostadig och obekväm–': Svenska statens samepolitik i rasismens tidevarv.* Bjurholm: Norrlands universitetsförlag, 2002.

McEnroe, Natasha. *Medicine: An Imperfect Science.* London: Scala Arts Publisher, 2020.

Moro, Adriana, and Noela Invernizzi. 'The Thalidomide Tragedy: The Struggle for Victims' Rights and Improved Pharmaceutical Regulation.' *História, Ciências, Saúde-Manguinhos* 24, no. 3 (July–September 2017): 603–22.

Moser, Ingunn. 'Disability and the Promises of Technology: Technology, Subjectivity and Embodiment within an Order of the Normal.' *Information, Communication & Society* 9, no. 3 (2006): 373–95.

Nilsson, Robert, and Henning Sjöström. *Pillret som väckte världen.* Stockholm: Sjöström & Sjöström, 1972.

Ojakangas, Mika. 'Impossible Dialogue on Bio-Power: Agamben and Foucault.' *Foucault Studies* 2 (May 2005): 5–28.

Parker, Clare. 'From Immorality to Public Health: Thalidomide and the Debate for Legal Abortion in Australia.' *Social History of Medicine* 25, no. 4 (October 2012): 863–80.

Paulsson, Karin. *'Dom säger att jag ser mer normal ut med benproteser': Om samhällskrav kontra barns behov.* Stockholm: Stockholms universitet, 1995.

Persson Bergvall, Inger, and Malena Sjöberg. *Åratal: Ur handikapphistorien.* Stockholm: Handikapphistoriska föreningen, 2012.

Quirke, Viviane. 'The Impact of Thalidomide on the British Pharmaceutical Industry: The Case of Imperial Chemical Industries.' In *Ways of Regulating: Therapeutic Agents between Plants, Shops and Consulting Rooms*, edited by Jean-Paul Gaudillière and Volker Hess, 137–52. Berlin: Max Planck Institute, 2008.

Roskies, Ethel. *Abnormality and Normality: The Mothering of Thalidomide Children.* Ithaca, NY: Cornell University Press, 1972.

Sewell, Claire. '"If One Member of the Family Is Disabled, the Family as a Whole Is Disabled": Thalidomide Children and the Emergence of the Family Carer in Britain, c. 1957–1978.' *Family & Community History* 18, no. 1 (2015): 37–52.

Society for the Neurosedyn Affected. 'Neurosedyn—vad var det som hände?' Accessed November 17, 2019. https://docplayer.se/115266742-Neurosedyn-vad-var-det-som-hande.html.

Society for the Neurosedyn Affected (website). 'Vad gör FfdN?' Accessed May 26, 2023. https://www.thalidomide.org/web/unnamned-thalidomide-1/.

Swedish Chancellor of Justice. Justitiekanslerns utlåtande angående neurosedynkatastrofen. Reg. no. 3195-02-90, April 30, 2003. https://www.jk.se/beslut-och-yttranden/2003/04/3195-02-90/.

Swedish Ministry of Health and Social Affairs. *Barnen som samhället svek: Åtgärder med anledning av övergrepp och allvarliga försummelser i samhällsvården.* SOU 2011:9. Stockholm: Fritze, 2011.

Swedish Ministry of Health and Social Affairs. *Bättre utbildning för handikappade: Förslag.* SOU 1969:35. Stockholm: Socialdepartementet, 1969.

Swedish Parliament. 'Nr 100. Kungl. Maj:ts proposition till riksdagen med förslag till lag angående ändrad lydelse av 1 och 4 §§ lagen den 17 juni 1938 (nr 318) om avbrytande av havandeskap; given Stockholms slott den 8 mars 1963.' In *Bihang till riksdagens protokoll 1963*. Collection 1, Vol. 10. *Kungl. Maj:ts propositioner nr 85–108*, 1–19. Stockholm: Riksdagen, 1963.

Tydén, Mattias. *Från politik till praktik: De svenska steriliseringslagarna 1935–1975*. Stockholm: Stockholms universitet, 2002.

Yllner, Nadja. *Bara en liten vit sömntablett: Historien om neurosedynkatastrofen*. Stockholm: Recito, 2007.

Archival Sources

Astra AB, to Swedish physicians, December 1961. F2:1, Documents concerning the Neurosedyn issue 1962–1964. NCN.

Board of Medicine. Memorandum on the care of the Neurosedyn children et cetera. F2:1, Documents concerning the Neurosedyn issue 1962–1964. NCN.

Board of Medicine. Minutes, September 5, 1963. F2:1, Documents concerning the Neurosedyn issue 1962–1964. NCN.

Board of Medicine. Statement on the Ombudsman's report on the Neurosedyn issue, referral. February 10, 1964. F2:1, Documents concerning the Neurosedyn issue 1962–1964. NCN.

Board of Medicine. Supplement to minutes, January 30, 1963. F2:1, Documents concerning the Neurosedyn issue 1962–1964. NCN.

Board of Medicine. Supporting data for the answer to the interpellation 'The care of children with neurosedyn-injury,' cost overview. F2:1, Documents concerning the Neurosedyn issue 1962–1964. NCN.

National counsellor. Enquiries about county council grants for N-injured children, November 1962. F2:1, Documents concerning the Neurosedyn issue 1962–1964. NCN.

National counsellor. Personal dossier. F1a:1–10, Neurosedyn-injured children 1959–1963. NCN.

Society for the Neurosedyn Affected, to Astra Fund, September 13, 1965. F4c:1, Society for the Neurosedyn Affected 1963–1972. NCN.

Society for the Neurosedyn Affected, to National Council for the Disabled, n.d. Statutes, register of members. F4c:1, Society for the Neurosedyn Affected 1963–1972. NCN.

Society for the Neurosedyn Affected, to Swedish Government Commission on Disability, November 11, 1966. F4c:1, Society for the Neurosedyn Affected 1963–1972. NCN.

CHAPTER 11

Unruly Bodies, Unruly Statistics: Thalidomide and the Birth of Reproductive Epidemiology in the Early 1960s

Francis Lee

In 1964 Sweden's National Board of Medicine decided to make permanent the Register of Congenital Malformations. This meant that from January 1, 1965, any congenital malformations were to be reported to the board's statistical department, and the newly formed Register of Congenital Malformations.[1] The aim of founding the register was that it would serve as an early warning system against fetal damages—whatever the source may be. The plan was that the register would be able to detect any increase in the number of infants born with congenital malformations, and any new patterns to these abnormalities.[2]

The decision to track congenital malformations in Sweden was, as in many other countries, a consequence of the thalidomide tragedy, in which almost six thousand infants were born with grave malformations globally.[3] The drug thalidomide was introduced in the late 1950s and was often prescribed for morning sickness in pregnant women. It was marketed in forty-six different countries under various names. In Sweden, thalidomide was introduced on the market in early 1959, and sold under the names Neurosedyn and Noxodyn. The birth defect epidemic caused by the drug consequently started in late 1959 in Sweden.[4]

This chapter deals with the events leading up to the foundation of the Register of Congenital Malformations, and the practical struggles to produce knowledge about unknown patterns of malformations through the statistical surveillance of birth defects. It investigates the tension between surveilling for unknown

1 Swedish Code of Statutes in the Field of Health and Sick Care, 'Kungliga Medicinalstyrelsens cirkulär.'

2 A note about the language of defects and malformations. In the chapter I use the words 'birth defects' and 'congenital malformations.' These words are both used in medical practice today, and I use them to reflect the medical language that I am trying to portray. See for instance Carachi and Doss, *Clinical Embryology*, which has the subtitle *An Atlas of Congenital Malformations*, and Singh, 'World Birth Defects Day.'

3 Lenz, 'Short History of Thalidomide Embryopathy'; Bergström et al., 'Talidomid-embryopati.' See also the chapter by Björkman in this volume.

4 Lenz, 'Short History of Thalidomide Embryopathy'; Bergström et al., 'Talidomid-embryopati.'

 | DOI:10.1163/9789004703759_013

abnormalities and standardized reporting, through the lens of the surveillance of congenital malformations. To do this, the chapter deals with the prehistory and the early days of the Register of Congenital Malformation and the challenges of using statistical methodologies for disease surveillance. The chapter seeks to analyze the practices of detecting unknown syndromes through the reporting of congenital malformations—which stands in contrast to medical practices of diagnosis using standardized categories of disease.

The aim of this chapter is to contribute to the history of Nordic epidemiology and disease surveillance. However, rather than focusing on epidemiological registry practices, such as linking records through unique identifiers, or the work of repurposing data from large-scale social and medical registries, this chapter approaches registry-based research from the point of view of the practices of classification.[5] It highlights how medical practitioners and statistical researchers struggled to standardize and bring under control that which belied the normal—their work to circumscribe, value, categorize, and track abnormalities in practice.

The structure of the chapter is as follows. First, it outlines some of the important events surrounding the thalidomide disaster in Sweden, identifying a number of key actors and events that preceded the foundation of the Register of Congenital Malformations. It contextualizes these events in relation to an international movement toward registries and control over pharmaceuticals. Second, it sketches a prehistory of the Register of Congenital Malformations and the main actors and debates leading up to its foundation, from the Tornblad Institute in Lund in southern Sweden, to the state inquiry into congenital malformation surveillance that was the forerunner to the register. Third, it delves into the practices of surveilling for unknown syndromes in a medical world obsessed with standardized paper technologies—and perhaps most importantly how the key actor, Bengt Källén, attempted to redesign the paper technologies of surveillance—to be able to sense the unknown in a world of knowns.

1 Thalidomide and the Emergence of Birth-Defect Surveillance

In the early 1960s thalidomide was found to cause grave birth defects.[6] The first signs of birth anomalies were discovered in West Germany, and the drug was recalled from the West German market in November 1961. However,

5 Bauer, 'From Administrative Infrastructure'; Bauer, 'Mining Data.'
6 Vargesson, 'Thalidomide-Induced Teratogenesis.'

thalidomide was still—even after the West German recall—sold on license outside Germany.[7] Nonetheless, owing to the mounting evidence of thalidomide's teratogenic effect on fetuses (i.e., that it causes congenital malformations), Swedish sales of the drug were halted a month later than in West Germany, on December 20, 1961.[8]

In the international medical literature, the first warning signals about thalidomide were sounded in the Lancet in 1961 and 1962 by William McBride and Widukind Lenz.[9] In Sweden, the Christian newspaper *Dagen* was the first to sound the public alarm in February 1962.[10] In March 1962, an article by A.-L. Bergström and coauthors, outlining the birth defects in Sweden, appeared in the Swedish medical journal *Svenska läkartidningen*.[11] Naturally, Swedish media headlines also reflected the fear of pharmaceutical damage to fetuses. For instance, in April 1962, a half page was devoted to the disaster. The page exclaimed, 'No pills—the fetus can be harmed!,' 'Fetal damage increased 300 times,' and 'Strong circumstantial evidence against thalidomide,' were published in the Swedish tabloid *Expressen*.[12] The fear of pharmaceutically induced malformations was palpable, and it contributed in many ways to the reshaping of how drugs were regulated, tested, and surveilled.[13]

Furthermore, in the wake of the thalidomide disaster, many countries set up registries for the reporting of birth defects. These were designed to be an early warning system for a new medically induced tragedy.[14] For instance, in Finland, a registry was founded in 1963.[15] In the United Kingdom a registry of malformations was set up in England and Wales in 1964.[16] In the United States,

7 Lennerhed, 'Kvinnan, aborten och teratologin.'

8 Swedish Chancellor of Justice, Justitiekanslerns utlåtande angående neurosedynkatastrofen.

9 Lenz, 'Short History of Thalidomide Embryopathy'; Lenz et al., 'Thalidomide and Congenital Abnormalities'; Mcbride, 'Thalidomide and Congenital Abnormalities.'

10 Lennerhed, 'Kvinnan, aborten och teratologin.'

11 Bergström et al., 'Talidomid-embryopati.'

12 Bernholm, 'Fosterskador ökade 300 gånger,' 7.

13 In the wake of the thalidomide tragedy a number of changes to pharmaceutical testing and malformation surveillance were instituted, aimed at preventing and detecting another pharmaceutical disaster. One important change was the reshaping of how drugs were tested and regulated, leading many countries to institute mandatory reporting of pharmaceutical studies to regulatory bodies. The famous three-phase randomized controlled trial (RCT) was born. Vargesson, 'Thalidomide-Induced Teratogenesis'; Olszynko-Gryn et al., 'Historical Argument for Regulatory Failure.'

14 International Centre for Birth Defects et al., *World Atlas of Birth Defects*.

15 Finnish Institute for Health and Welfare, 'Medfödda missbildningar.'

16 Misra, 'Evaluation'; Misra, Dattani, and Majeed, 'Congenital Anomaly Surveillance.'

the Center for Disease Control first started surveilling birth defects in 1967.[17] In Norway, the Medical Birth Registry was founded in 1967.[18] Consequently, the institution of Sweden's Register of Congenital Malformations in 1964 was part of an international movement to curtail pharmaceutical disaster by surveilling birth defects. The thalidomide tragedy thus left a lasting impression on the institutionalization of pharmaceutical safety procedures and the surveillance of birth defects.

2 The Welfare State and the Registration of the Population

However, the institutionalization of the Register of Congenital Malformations was not solely a reaction to the thalidomide tragedy. It was also situated in a period when the medical and epidemiological registration of the population in the Nordic countries boomed.[19] During this period many other registries were established across the region.[20] In Sweden, the Twin Register was established at the end of the 1950s, and the Patient Register was created in 1964.[21] As a part of this development, the reporting of deaths in Sweden was centralized to the Statistical Bureau in 1951.[22]

Thus, the development of the Register of Congenital Malformations can be understood in the context of 'long traditions of social engineering [... and] politics that became associated with the "Scandinavian" welfare states' as well as the establishment and growth of register-based research and epidemiology in the Nordic countries and elsewhere. Susanne Bauer has argued that this mode of medical investigation has been key in the rise of a specific 'Nordic style' of epidemiology based on the constant collection of data about the population, where personal identification numbers also became important.[23]

In sum, the Register of Congenital Malformations was part of an international movement toward surveillance of birth defects following the thalidomide disaster, participated in a long Nordic tradition of registering the

---

17 Edmonds et al., 'Congenital Malformations Surveillance.'

18 Bjerkedal, 'Protection of Privacy.'

19 This tradition of registering statistics about the population dates back to the 1700s in Sweden. See also Bondestam's chapter in this volume.

20 Bauer, 'From Administrative Infrastructure.'

21 Lichtenstein et al., 'Swedish Twin Registry'; National Board of Health and Welfare. 'Historik om patientregistret.'

22 Johansson, *Dödsorsaksstatistik*.

23 Bauer, 'From Administrative Infrastructure.'

population, and contributed to an international push to standardize the classification of disease. Consequently, the foundation of the register can be situated in a broader shift toward what David Armstrong has dubbed 'surveillance medicine,' in which population-based studies were used to delineate the normal standard of, for instance, children's development, as well as to define abnormalities and identify risk factors in individuals.[24]

3 The Prehistory: Comparative Embryology, Bengt Källén, and the Tornblad Institute

The surveillance of congenital malformations in Sweden was intimately intertwined with the work of embryologist and epidemiologist Bengt Källén. Through his work, Källén would develop into the most important actor for the surveillance of congenital malformations in Sweden. Källén was to become long-time director of the Tornblad Institute in Lund, where the Register of Congenital Malformations was eventually located. He was also instrumental in the work leading up to the foundation of the register as well as sometimes its sole custodian.[25]

The Tornblad Institute was founded by the anatomy professor Ivar Broman as an institute of comparative embryology in 1934. Broman was an avid collector of embryos and fetuses, and the macabre jars of fetuses were until recently available at the institute.[26] In the early 1950s Källén wrote his dissertation on comparative embryology at the Tornblad Institute, which led him to take an early interest in the abnormalities of fetal developments.[27] He would later describe the register as linked to his previous work on comparative embryology as well as his interest in fetal abnormalities and 'monsters.'[28]

Thus, in the early 1960s, when the thalidomide disaster became apparent, Källén and the Tornblad Institute seemed well positioned for taking up the teratogenic challenge that had been laid down by McBride and Lenz—and in the Swedish context by Bergström and coauthors—when they sounded the alarm about thalidomide in 1961 and 1962 in the Lancet.

24 Armstrong, 'Rise of Surveillance Medicine'; Rose, 'Psychological Complex.'
25 Källén, *Tornblad Institute in Lund*, chap. 7.
26 Källén, *Tornblad Institute in Lund*; Jülich, 'Historier kring Tornbladinstitutet.'
27 Källén, *Tornblad Institute in Lund*, chap. 7.
28 Källén, *Tornblad Institute in Lund*, chap. 1.

4 The Teratogenic Effect of Drugs and the Foundation of the Register of Congenital Malformations

Before the Register of Congenital Malformations was founded, malformations had been collated, reported, and analyzed annually in Sweden.[29] In the wake of the thalidomide disaster this approach was increasingly understood to be unsatisfactory as an early warning system for drug-induced medical disasters. For instance, Bergström and coauthors suggested, in their article on thalidomide embryopathy from March 1962, that 'a continuous, central registration and analysis of certain malformations' could become an important means of understanding the causes of malformations.[30]

During the spring of 1962 surveillance of malformations and drug consumption commenced on a trial basis. On February 26, 1962, the Register of Congenital Malformations instructed all maternity wards to send in monthly reports, between March 1 and May 31, of any congenital malformations as well as all mothers' consumption of sleeping aids during the first half of pregnancy. These monthly reports led to the discovery of widespread consumption of sleeping aids on the part of the pregnant women. On May 29 the board instructed the maternity wards to continue reporting any congenital malformations, as well as the drug consumption of mothers with malformed infants. They thus narrowed the scope of reporting for drug consumption, from all mothers to only those who had given birth to malformed infants.[31] The board deemed surveillance to be of importance, but the exact methods were still being worked out.

In addition, on April 1, 1962, the National Board of Medicine decided to start an inquiry into the teratogenic effect of drugs. The board gave pediatrician Jan Winberg—who was also one of Bergström's coauthors on the March 1962 article that sounded the alarm about thalidomide in the journal *Svenska läkartidningen*—the task of investigating.[32] Winberg's inquiry was dubbed Utredningen angående sambandet mellan läkemedel och fosterskador (the Inquiry into the Relationship between Pharmaceuticals and Congenital Malformations). Its remit was broader than thalidomide, and aimed to openly investigate any links between drugs and congenital malformations.

In 1963, the sore of thalidomide was still raw, and owing to findings in Winberg's ongoing inquiry, two other drugs, Postafen and Postadoxin (based

29 Källén and Winberg, 'Erfarenheter av kontinuerlig registrering,' 1943–44.

30 Bergström et al., 'Talidomid-embryopati,' 1021.

31 Winberg, 'Utredning: IV.'

32 Swedish Chancellor of Justice, Justitiekanslerns utlåtande angående neurosedynkatastrofen.

on the compound meclizine), received a warning label from the National Board of Medicine: 'not for pregnant women.' The Postafen warning label became a topic of debate between Winberg and Källén—who would both lay the groundwork for the Register of Congenital Malformations—in the journal *Svenska läkartidningen*. The point of contention was how to handle the preliminary results from Winberg's studies of the teratogenic effect of drugs. Winberg defended the application of the warning label on the basis of his preliminary investigation, while Källén argued that it was a premature, even incorrect decision, not based in the statistical evidence.[33] However, the use of statistics concerning abnormalities in medical regulation was not an easy task, and it was impossible for the National Board of Medicine to make any conclusive decisions about Postafen or Postadoxin on the basis of the Winberg study.[34]

Thus, at an early stage, the challenges of bringing unruly bodies and malformations under statistical surveillance were debated and acknowledged by two of the most important actors in the surveillance of congenital malformations in Sweden, Källén and Winberg. Questions about drawing conclusions from uncertain medical statistics would follow Källén throughout his career, and he would become a prolific writer about the pitfalls and methodologies of statistical epidemiology. However, both Källén and Winberg's early work on congenital malformations would help pave the way for a central register of congenital malformations.

The report from Winberg's inquiry was eventually published in five parts in *Svenska läkartidningen* in 1964. In it he lamented the state of the yearly reporting of malformations, and he identified multiple challenges with this approach to the statistical surveillance of malformation—for instance, uncertain and imprecise classifications according to the *International Classification of Diseases*, as well as overreporting of very common and 'meaningless' malformations. Just as in the 1962 article that he coauthored with Bergström, he argued that 'the current form of reporting and registration of malformations is unsatisfactory.'[35]

Before Winberg's inquiry concluded, the National Board of Medicine decided to explore the feasibility of the national monthly registration of congenital malformations starting in April 1964.[36] The board gave the task of running the trial to Källén and Winberg; it entailed mandatory reporting

33 Källén, Sjövall, and Ursing, 'Läkemedel och fosterskador—en replik.'

34 Winberg, 'Utredning: v.'

35 Winberg, 'Utredning: i & ii'; Winberg, 'Utredning: iii'; Winberg, 'Utredning: iv'; Winberg, 'Utredning: v.'

36 Lennerhed, 'Kvinnan, aborten och teratologin'; Källén, *Tornblad Institute in Lund*.

from women's clinics and maternity wards that had a pediatric consultant.[37] In January 1965 this new form of registration was made permanent, and the Register of Congenital Malformations was born, requiring 60 percent of Sweden's births to be reported.[38] Hopes for the new registry were high, and Källén, its first head, argued that the thalidomide tragedy would have been detected in only five months if this new type of reporting and statistical surveillance had been in effect.[39]

5 Classifying Malformations at the Bedside: Unruly Bodies, Unruly Professionals

Before the Register of Congenital Malformations was instituted, the foundation for the statistical classification of birth defects was the well-known *International Statistical Classification of Diseases, Injuries and Causes of Death* (ICD). The ICD was, and still is, the internationally accepted standard for classifying disease, and was used for statistical purposes. In Sweden during this time, two versions of the ICD were in use in medical classification. Both were based on the seventh version of the ICD, which was ratified by the World Health Organization in Geneva in 1955. The first Swedish version was printed in 1957, and the second in 1965.

In the Swedish ICD from 1957 congenital malformations are classified in chapter XIV. The classification spans two pages, from '750 *Monstra*'[40] to unspecified malformations that are not classified elsewhere: '759 *Maleformationes congenitae aliae s. Non definitae, alibi non classificatae*.' The newer version of the ICD broke down the categories of malformations further, specifying each in more detail. For example, the old category 750 *Monstra* is divided into several new ones: '750,00 *Acrania*,' '750,10 *Monstrum* (*of duplex type*),' '750,20 *Monstrum* (of undeveloped body shape—usually of the type where the head transitions directly to the trunk),' '750,99 *Monstrum aliud et* UNS' (where 'UNS' stands for unspecified). The monsters of the early modern period are thus subdivided, and other categories are developed to bring the abnormal infant into statistical and medical nomenclature.[41]

37 Källén, *Tornblad Institute in Lund*, chap. 7.

38 Källén and Winberg, 'Erfarenheter av kontinuerlig registrering av missbildningar,' 1943–44.

39 Källén and Winberg, 'Swedish Register of Congenital Malformations.'

40 Which includes 'Monstrum simplex: Acephalus, anencephalus, macrocephalus, etc. Monstrum duplex: Acardius, ischiopagus, thoracopagus, etc. Epignatus. Monstrum UNS.'

41 For monsters, see Bondestam's chapter in this volume.

However, the practices of producing medical statistics often have to contend with a multitude of practical challenges. Constant work is needed to produce medical and epidemiological statistics—and this work is not only of mathematical or statistical nature.[42] Birth defect registration grappled with a multitude of unruly bodies and professionals. A constant stream of local practices were translated into records, statistics—hopefully giving a clear sign when something is amiss—the goal being to avert a new thalidomide disaster.

To open up a window into the unruly realities of birth defect surveillance, the archive from Winberg's inquiry provides unique insights into the practical realities of the making of medical statistics in hospitals. This archive comprises thirty-six boxes of material, of which sixteen contain copies of medical records from births of children with congenital malformations. The medical records are drawn from all over the country and stem from small rural hospitals to large central university hospitals. They document the childbirth itself, as well as descriptions of the infants with congenital malformations and their treatment. The records provide rich details concerning how physicians struggled to bring the abnormal under standardized control in the late 1950s and early 1960s.[43]

The medical records were written on standardized forms, which are mostly unique for each hospital, printed at the local printers, or in some cases bought from a central printer, such as the large Swedish office supply depot ESSELTE. The records range from short handwritten and mostly illegible forms documenting a birth and some type of malformation, to meticulously typed and documented case histories spanning twenty or more pages, including charts for temperature, weight, Rh factor, and infant feeding as well as statements from specialists in radiology, urology, or endocrinology. In some hospitals the records were stamped with '*Partus Normalis* 660a' or a scribbled note on the record which says 'Y20,0' both of which are ICD codes for normal childbirth.

The malformations documented in the records range from genital abnormalities to hip subluxations (instabilities of the hip) and everything in between. Latin and Swedish diagnoses are both used to describe the infants: *Micrognathia, Syndactylia, Sista benigna, Medfödd näsanomali*. At the larger hospitals, and sometimes at the smaller ones, ICD codes are added to the diagnoses: *Monstrum* with the ICD code Y38,6; *Melfarmatio crane* Y20,0 (deformed infant and normal birth); *Hydrocephalus* 752 Y38,7 (giving two different ICD codes for hydrocephalus); *Mongolismus* 759.3 (mongoloid with an ICD code in another category); *Syndaktilia pedis dx* 759.1 (ICD for *Maleformationes cutis*); *Luxatio cong*. 758.0

42 Bowker and Star, *Sorting Things Out*.

43 Records of Winberg's inquiry are available at NBM-AB.

(in the same ICD category); *Klumpfot* 758,6 (ICD for Other skeletal and joint malformations); and so on. Different versions of ICD codes are used, as are different languages. The 'Other' category is used with some frequency.

Sometimes the diagnosis is discussed in the record. The case histories can range from a couple of terse sentences to long accounts spanning several years of treatment. For example, in one record from Karlskoga Hospital, the infant is described in an emotional register: 'The child has miserable congenital malformations, partly ugly clubfeet, partly similar malformations in the wrists and partly very stiff joints in general.'[44] The language of the record betrays the physician's feelings toward the newborn child in terms of their 'miserable,' 'ugly,' and 'stiff' state—without commenting on the ICD code. Another record, from the Women's Clinic of Malmö Municipal Hospital, uses clinical language to describe and diagnose the infant, and notes the ICD codes of the diagnosis: 'A cyst-like growth under the tongue. Ref. to ear clin. Diagnosis: *Cysta sublinqnisinales* 759,3.'[45]

The variations in the material point to the monumental task of standardizing medical information: different hospitals, different physicians, different secretaries, and different affinities with the codes of the ICD. Each record reflects the knowledge, practices, and different levels of commitment to standardizing medical knowledge at a particular hospital. The work of creating statistical medical knowledge thus starts at the patient's bedside—and reflects different local commitments to standardized medical knowledge and the statistics of fetal malformations.

Furthermore, the unruliness of diagnosing infant bodies is brought out time and time again in the records. Jotted annotations, question marks in the margins of the diagnosis, and uncertain and interpretative language constantly appear. The uncertainty of diagnosing congenital abnormalities is vividly reflected. For example, the struggle to know whether a child is born with congenital hip subluxations is tied to interpreting X-ray images, as well as keeping an infant still at the moment of exposure:

> with outstretched and inwardly rotated legs you can possibly get an impression of the left femur being slightly lower laterally than the right. One of the images unfortunately not completely [unreadable] as the child moved at the moment of exposure. There is no certain basis for congenital hip dislocation, but cannot be ruled out either.[46]

44 Record from Karlskoga Hospital.

45 Record from Women's Clinic of Malmö.

46 Follow-up assessment record.

Here, the bodily and material realities of the diagnosis of infants, as well as the difficulty of determining the normal range of the infant's form are brought to the fore. What is the normal configuration of an infant body? What could be said to be a normal configuration of the infant's hips? Physicians struggled to make diagnoses and pin down the heterogeneity of the human body. Another example concerns hip dislocations: 'Definite signs of dislocation do not exist, but a certain suspicion does exist that the l. femur is both pushed up and laterally dislocated.'[47] The language of these records reflects the constant efforts of medical staff and the difficulty of pinning down the human body on the diagnostic grid of the ICD. Physicians brandished the language of uncertainty: 'possibly,' 'relatively,' 'suspicion,' 'uncertain,' 'impression,' 'cannot be ruled out.'

What we can discern in these records is the difficult work of standardizing abnormality in practice. First, the classification of malformations relates to a multiplicity of infrastructures: partly the local standards that are articulated in the preprinted medical forms, partly the different translations of the ICD-7 in use in Sweden at the time. Second, the records reveal different traces of the practices of classification: the difficulty of making a certain diagnosis at the bedside, different commitments to the nationwide standardized statistical classification, but also the strong tendency toward normalizing mothers and infants. Each localized practice leaving traces in the forms, notes, language, and classifications.

The next step in the statistical surveillance of congenital malformations was to coerce these multiplicities into a statistical norm for malformations. This brings us to the practices of producing a constant statistical surveillance of congenital malformations. How did Källén intend to detect and stop the next thalidomide disaster using the Register of Congenital Malformations?

6 Surveilling Unruly Malformations: Problems in Practice

Transforming the multiplicities of congenital malformations into statistical surveillance was, and still is, a monumental challenge. How do you bring the abnormal under statistical control? Källén, as outlined above, was a driving force for this surveillance effort in Sweden. He published numerous texts on the classification of malformations. And he worked tirelessly to use the unruly medical data to produce statistics. The challenges that Källén identified in surveilling congenital malformations were many.

47 Record from the Central Hospital in Kalmar, Maternity Ward.

One challenge was that the very definition of malformation is multifarious and indefinite. Källén describes the border between an 'anatomical variation' and a malformation as uncertain, which in turn affects how classification is done in practice. Different research materials define the same diagnoses differently. Some are treated as a malformation, while others are not:

> The definition of malformation is fluid. The boundary against anatomical variations is often uncertain. Some materials have included anatomical variations, that are excluded in other materials. This often pertains to comparatively insignificant defects with relatively high frequency, which can completely skew the statistics. A clear definition of what has been registered as a malformation in a specific study is required, if the frequency numbers are to have any value.[48]

The challenge that Källén identifies thus points back to the practices of classification in different studies. His argument is that the interpretation of what a malformation is in local practices, and in specific investigations, will create completely different statistical understandings of malformations. In an interview in which Källén reflected on the early years of the Register of Congenital Malformations, he discussed the impossibility of classifying malformations using the grid defined in the ICD. The range of variation in congenital malformations constantly broke the standardized reporting formats of the ICD. The classes and diagnoses of the ICD were much too coarse to be useful for capturing the multifariousness and variability of medical malformations.[49]

Källén also ties the problem of standardized reporting of malformations to diagnostic practices and technologies, as well as the professional training and role of the diagnosing physician. In a textbook on teratology from 1967 he reflects on how classification procedures and practices vary:

> The diagnosis of a malformation can vary in exactness between different investigators. [...] In standardized reporting there is a larger risk that malformations are omitted. Experience shows that even easily observed malformations, for example cleft lip and grave defects of extremities are underreported. The precision of the diagnosis will also be dependent on whether autopsy is performed, if different exams (e.g. X-ray) have been performed, and whether the exam is performed by a pediatrician or pathologist or by nonspecialist physicians, midwives etc.[50]

48 Källén, *Teratologi*, 31.
49 Källén, interview with the author.
50 Källén, *Teratologi*, 31.

Here Källén gets close to how bedside practices reshape medical statistics and medical data. He brings up how easily observed malformations are not reported, and how certain malformations are not observable without specific forms of infrastructure and examination, such as X-rays. He also mentions that the training and experience of different professional groups skew statistics. In sum, he ties the statistical surveillance of congenital malformations to the varying classification practices of bedside reporting.

A further challenge that Källén brings up, in relation to reducing the explosive growth of medical archives in Sweden, is the impossibility of summarizing records without foreclosing the possibility of historical studies of congenital malformations. For instance, in a journal article he argues against archival deselection or even summarizing medical records to save space, since the knowledge and interests of the diagnosing physician will shape what the summary will contain, precluding future investigators from reclassifying the material:

> It is clear that the continued growth of the record archives must be slowed. Many different technical solutions can be discussed. An imminent possibility is to create record summaries, which are archived, while the record itself is destroyed after an appropriate time. Of course, such a record summary can also be stored in appropriate memory, e.g. a database. I would strongly advise against this possibility. The summary will reflect the summarizing person's knowledge and interests—it is impossible to predict what will be interesting in the future. [...] When writing the summary, some information is suppressed, which the summarizing physician deems to be uninteresting, leading to a nonrandom selection.[51]

The problem of summarizing medical records, according to Källén, is again tied to the practices of medical classification. Any summarizing of information will, according to Källén, reflect the current knowledge and interests of the person that summarizes the information. He also points to the impossibility of knowing what information could become interesting in the future. According to Källén, the original record—the messy, unruly documentation of the diagnosing medical personnel—needs to be retained in order to surveil congenital malformations. He ties this challenge back to the thalidomide tragedy, and how yearly summaries of birth defects were not sufficient to identify the relevant malformations among other more common ones:

51 Källén, 'Medicinsk-genetiska synpunkter på journalgallring,' 33.

> A concrete example of this is that, when the thalidomide injuries in neonates began to occur, it was not possible to distinguish these extremely specific and previously exceptionally unusual injuries from a number of other and common malformations of the extremities that were not related to thalidomide in the current summaries (annual reports).[52]

Again, Källén emphasized how the knowledge and interests of the person making the summary were not targeted enough to be able to perceive the change in statistical malformation patterns during the thalidomide disaster. The specific forms of malformations that the thalidomide disaster created were not possible to discern from the usual pattern of malformations. The existing standardized statistical classifications were not precise enough to be able to see the unexpected new patterns of malformation that emerged after the thalidomide disaster.

7 The Material Practices of Congenital Surveillance: Breaking Free from the ICD

In his constant attempts to solve the challenges of the surveillance of congenital malformations, Källén developed several methods for dealing with unruly and unclassifiable abnormalities, and the varying knowledge of the diagnosing personnel. For Källén the transformation of malformations into surveillance was a sustained effort. He struggled tirelessly to surveil congenital malformations as he attempted to create and run an early warning system that would protect against another thalidomide tragedy.

One attempt to solve the matter of imprecise reporting was specifically designed reporting cards that the National Board of Medicine distributed to all hospitals in Sweden. Information about congenital malformations was supposed to be recorded on these cards at the bedside of the patient. The cards showed a diagram of an infant, on which the physician was instructed to mark the location of the malformation on the back of the card, and to describe it verbally as clearly as possible. These reporting cards were then to be sent to the Register of Congenital Malformations, to be coded for the purposes of statistical surveillance. The cards were printed on thick, stiff paper, to make it easier for physicians to jot down their diagnosis at the bedside. But according to Källén these forms were also intended to create friction for the medical secretaries

52 Källén, 'Medicinsk-genetiska synpunkter på journalgallring,' 33.

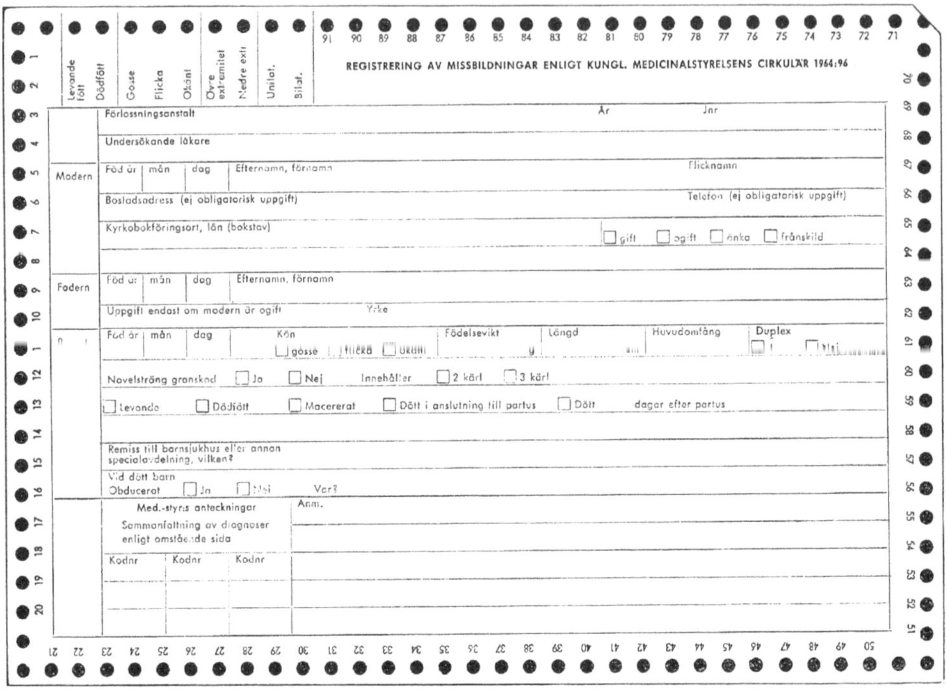

REGISTRERING AV MISSBILDNINGAR ENLIGT KUNGL. MEDICINALSTYRELSENS CIRKULÄR 1964:96

Levande fött | Dödfött | Gosse | Flicka | Okänt | Övre extremitet | Nedre extr | Unilat. | Bilat.

Förlossningsanstalt — År — Jnr

Undersökande läkare

Modern: Föd år | mån | dag | Efternamn, förnamn — Flicknamn

Bostadsadress (ej obligatorisk uppgift) — Telefon (ej obligatorisk uppgift)

Kyrkobokföringsort, län (bokstav) — ☐ gift ☐ ogift ☐ änka ☐ frånskild

Fadern: Föd år | mån | dag | Efternamn, förnamn

Uppgift endast om modern är ogift — Yrke

Föd år | mån | dag | Kön ☐ gosse ☐ flicka ☐ okänt | Födelsevikt g | Längd | Huvudomfång | Duplex

Navelsträng granskad ☐ Ja ☐ Nej — Innehåller ☐ 2 kärl ☐ 3 kärl

☐ Levande ☐ Dödfött ☐ Macererat ☐ Dött i anslutning till partus ☐ Dött dagar efter partus

Remiss till barnsjukhus eller annan specialavdelning, vilken?

Vid dött barn Obducerat ☐ Ja ☐ Nej — Var?

Med.-styr:s anteckningar — Sammanfattning av diagnoser enligt omstående sida — Anm.

Kodnr | Kodnr | Kodnr

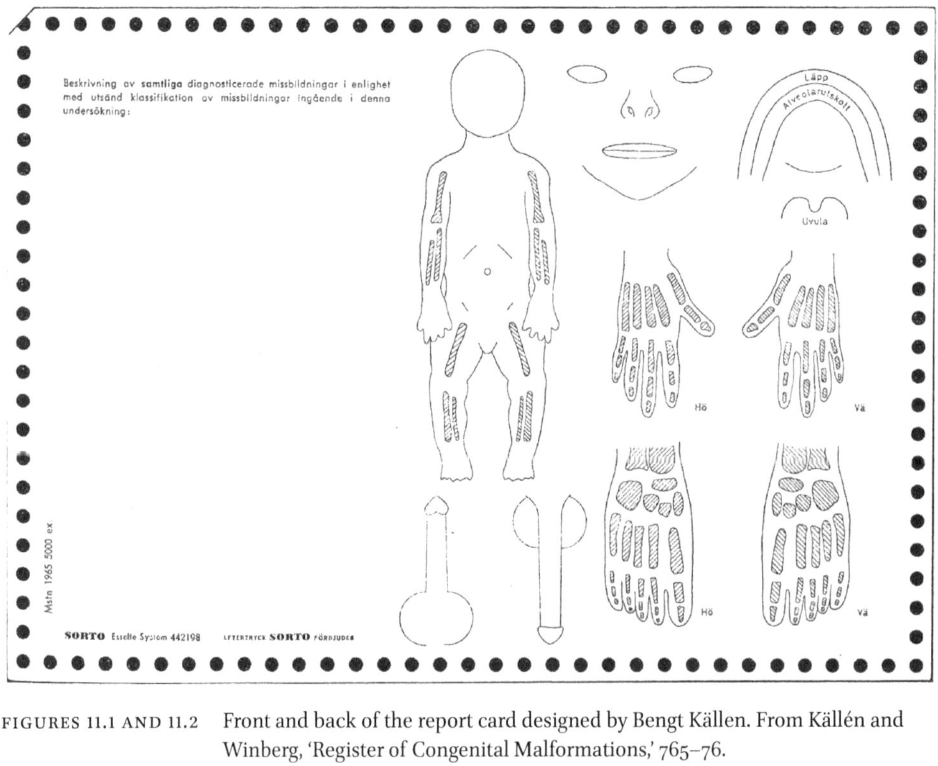

FIGURES 11.1 AND 11.2 Front and back of the report card designed by Bengt Källen. From Källén and Winberg, 'Register of Congenital Malformations,' 765–76.

who often typed the diagnoses on the forms. The stiff cards were purposefully difficult to get into the typewriter. By employing the cards' materiality, Källén wanted to entice hospital workers to collect the information directly from the source, while local physicians sometimes preferred to delegate the reporting work to a medical secretary.[53]

By requiring the reports to conform to this system, Källén hoped to bypass the coarse grid of the ICD diagnosis, as well as the shaping influence of the interests and knowledge of the diagnosing physicians. The report card purposefully asked for a bodily location and description of the malformation. Källén's hope was that his system would allow the reporting of *unknown* anomalies—the abnormalities that did not fit into the established grid of medical diagnosis. By doing this he attempted to keep alive the unruliness of congenital malformations, and allow for the unknown and unruly to be reported.

However, regardless of the reporting cards, Källén faced the same challenge as the diagnosing physicians: to categorize and classify the malformations for statistical analysis. What is a normal bodily malformation? What is the same malformation? What is a new abnormality? What is an unknown anomaly—perhaps caused by a new teratogenic pharmaceutical?

To classify the constant stream of reporting cards Källén argued that the crude grid of the ICD was not enough. Källén therefore created his own bespoke coding scheme, which was adapted to the latest data-processing technologies. He argued that the advantage of his system was the flexibility that it afforded in adding categories, when new malformations were discovered—for each newly discovered malformation, Källén himself could create a new category.[54]

The person translating the constant stream of report cards into statistical codes was Källén himself. He traveled regularly from his workplace in Lund, in the south of Sweden, to the National Board of Medicine in Stockholm to harvest new report cards, classify them, and enter them into the statistical analysis. By organizing the statistical classification of malformations in this manner, Källén attempted to address the many and difficult challenges that he had identified in surveilling congenital malformations. Using the report cards and his own code list, Källén attempted to solve several problems of standardizing the abnormal: he retained some of the unruliness of the bodily descriptions in the report cards, not immediately discarding description for classification; he attempted to make a finer grid of classifications in his own code list, circumventing the coarseness and inflexibility of the ICD; and by carrying out the coding alone, he tried to reduce the variations that resulted from

53 Källén, interview with the author.
54 Källén, interview with the author.

2

1XXXX	*missbildning i CNS*	*CNS malformation*
11XXX	slutningsmissbildning CNS	neural tube defect
11100	anencefali (akrani)	anencephaly
11210	myelomeningocele anterior	anterior MMC
11220	myelomeningocele posterior	spina bifida aperta
11300	encephalocele	encephalocele
11400	spina bifida utan myelomeningocele	spina bifida without MMC
11500	dermal sinus motsvarande spina bifida	dermal sinus at spina bifida
11600	defectus capilliti eller ländrygg	defectus capilliti or lumbar
12000	mikrocefali	microcephaly
13000	hydrocefali	hydrocephaly
14100	hydranencefali	hydranencephaly
14200	porencephali, hjärncystor	porencephaly, cerebral cysts
15000	holoprosencephali, arrhinencefali	holoprosencephaly
16XXX	övriga CNS-missbildningar	other CNS malformations
16100	Möbius syndrom	Moebius syndrome
16110	centronukleär myopati	centronuclear myopathy
16210	cerebellär hypoplasi	cerebellar hypoplasia
16220	övrig cerebellär missbildning	other cerebellar malformation
16310	pakygyri i cerebrala cortex	pakygyria of cerebral cortex
16320	mikropolygyri i cerebrala cortex	micropolygyria, cerebral cortex
16330	övrig missbildning i cerebrala cortex	other cerebral cortex malform.
16400	agenesi av corpus callosum	agenesis of corpus callosum
16401	AV fistel corpus callosum	AV fistula in corpus callosum
16402	dysgenesi av corpus callosum	dysgenesis of corpus callosum
1650x	facialispares	facial paresis
16600	diastematomyeli	diastematomyelia
16700	makrocefali	macrocephaly
16800	cebocefali (=15000)	cebocephaly (=15000)
16900	diverse hjärnmissbildningar	other brain malformations
16901	Dandy Walker cysta	Dandy Walker cyst
16902	aplasi av occipitalloben	occipital lobe aplasia
16990	oklar ryggmärgsmissbildning	unclear spinal cord malform.
16991	del av ryggmärg saknas	part of spinal cord missing
2XXXX	*missbildningar i sinnesorgan*	*sensory organ malformations*
21XXX	*ögonmissbildningar*	*eye malformations*
21100	cyklopi	cyclopia
21101	pseudocyklopi (tättsittande ögon)	pseudocyclopia
2121x	anoftalmi	anophthalmia
2122x	mikroftalmi	microphthalmia
2123x	kryptoftalmi	cryptophthalmia
213XX	slutningsdefekter av ögonen	eye closure defect
21311	iriscolobom	coloboma of iris
21312	retinacolobom	coloboma of retina
21313	linscolobom (=2151X)	coloboma of lens (=2151X)
21314	komplicerat colobom	complicated coloboma
21315	excentrisk pupill	excentric pupilla
21316	colobom av palpebrae	coloboma of eye lid
2132x	mikroftalmi med cysta	microphthalmia with cyst
2140x	aniridi	aniridia
2151x	coloboma lentis	coloboma lentis
2152x	afaki	aphakia
2153x	linsektopi	lens ectopia

FIGURE 11.3 A page from Bengt Källén's list of malformations. Courtesy of Bengt Källén

the different knowledges and interests of various professional groups.[55] It was Källén's know-how and experience that became the standard.

8 Statistical Surveillance and the Challenge of the Unknown

Medical statistics concerning malformations in the 1960s as well as today are based on unruly practices of classification and standardization of bodies that constantly break our grids of understanding. In statistical disease surveillance, the properties of any new disease are unknown—it is impossible to know what to be on the lookout for. What are the symptoms of a new thalidomide tragedy? What is a warning signal that a new pandemic flu has emerged? How do we know whether a new hemorrhagic fever is making its first cases known? In patient records—in the unruly diagnostic practices of different physicians, hospitals, or professions—might lurk the unknown disaster or disease.

In one publication, Källén argued that he would have been able to detect the thalidomide tragedy statistically only five months after its first cases were reported.[56] But that argument was of course made in hindsight, when the symptoms of the syndrome were already well known. He knew what to look for, and could therefore group the familiar malformations together in a recognized configuration.

In grappling with these challenges at the Register of Congenital Malformations, Källén devised a number of devices to help him detect, delineate, and act on new and unknown diseases. First, the reporting cards, where he attempted to entice medical personnel to report on symptoms and observed defects rather than ready-made diagnoses. Second, his bespoke and potentially infinite list of classifications was made to accommodate any new malformations. Both these tools put Källén's knowledge and experience at the center of the surveillance of congenital malformations. He thus attempted to make himself the central hub for detecting any new unknown disease. If a new malformation started to rear its head, Källén, using the report cards and his own list of malformation codes, hoped to be able to discern this new development through statistical comparison.

What Källén did in the setup of the Register of Congenital Malformations was to organize the classification and counting of malformations in a center of calculation, thus attempting to control how malformations were classified and

55 Källén, interview with the author.

56 Källén and Winberg, 'Swedish Register of Congenital Malformations.'

counted in the statistical surveillance.[57] However, the reporting of the cases and the filling in of the forms—and thus the first decision to count a specific biological variation as a malformation—were still delegated to the local hospitals. These decisions, sometimes made at the bedside by the reporting physician, and sometimes by medical secretaries, remained outside Källén's control, creating challenges in terms of the validity of the statistical inferences.

9 Sketching the History of the Register of Congenital Malformations

This chapter has sketched the history and material practices of birth defect surveillance in Sweden in the late 1950s and early 1960s. In doing this, it has first outlined the history, actors, and institutional work involved in setting up the Register of Congenital Malformations. It has situated the register in an international context, at the advent of medical regulation and surveillance, linking this development to the emergence of a Nordic style of epidemiology, based in the registration of the population.[58] Second, the chapter delves into the challenges and material practices of birth defect surveillance, especially those that abnormalities pose for medical-statistical surveillance. In this, it outlines how the unruliness of congenital malformations leads to a number of material practices that attempt to make them amenable to statistical surveillance.

In tracing the history of the Register of Congenital Malformations, this chapter brings to the fore certain challenges involved in the production of standardized medical knowledge. It highlights the difficulty of classifying congenital malformations in practice, the problems that arise in handling congenital malformations through standardized means, such as the ICD, and the struggles of medical practitioners to fit congenital malformations into the existing grid of medical classification. The multiplicity of congenital malformations constantly breaks out of the boundaries of medical standardization.

But perhaps more importantly, the chapter also brings to light the tensions between the unknown emerging syndrome and the known and standardized diagnosis in the surveillance of congenital malformations—and perhaps in medical surveillance for the unknown more broadly. According to Källén, the sensing infrastructure of medicine was steeped in physicians' judgment and previous knowledge as well as in the historically sedimented codes of the ICD—making it difficult to make room for and detect the unknown and emerging syndrome. This state of affairs spurred Källén to

57 Latour, *Science in Action.*
58 Bauer, 'From Administrative Infrastructure.'

centralize classification and judgment to his office—creating a center of classification and calculation—and to invent a bespoke and seemingly infinitely customizable classification system to break out of the sedimented and ready-made knowledge infrastructures of the medical system. His purpose was to invent an infrastructure for registry-based statistical surveillance—to make it possible to detect the unknown. In a sense he was trying to break away from—he resisted and reinvented—the existing paper technologies of classification (the ICD and preprinted diagnostic forms). He made his own bespoke paper-based infrastructure, attempting to remove physicians' judgments from the edges of this network, to form a controlled, one-man center of classification and calculation.[59]

One lesson here is about the tension between surveillance infrastructures—paper technologies of medicine—and the unruly and unknown syndrome. The chapter exemplifies how classification infrastructures and practices simplify, hide, split apart, or sometimes even do violence to the things they classify.[60] However, another lesson is about the tension between the already-known and classified and the emerging and unknown in surveillance medicine; it points to the infrastructural tensions between the ready-made and the bespoke, between the sedimented and the floating, and between nosology and unknown syndromes. The paper technologies of medicine create well-worn paths of classification that are difficult to break out of.

Bibliography

Armstrong, David. 'The Rise of Surveillance Medicine.' *Sociology of Health & Illness* 17, no. 3 (June 1, 1995): 393–404.

Bauer, Susanne. 'From Administrative Infrastructure to Biomedical Resource: Danish Population Registries, the "Scandinavian Laboratory," and the "Epidemiologist's Dream."' *Science in Context* 27, no. 2 (June 2014): 187–213.

Bauer, Susanne. 'Mining Data, Gathering Variables and Recombining Information: The Flexible Architecture of Epidemiological Studies.' *Studies in History and Philosophy of Science Part C: Studies in History and Philosophy of Biological and Biomedical Sciences* 39, no. 4 (December 2008): 415–28.

Bergström, A.-L., L. Nilsson, B. Pettersson, L. Söderling, L. Victorin, and J. Winberg. 'Talidomid-embryopati.' *Svenska läkartidningen* 59, no. 13 (1962): 1012–22.

59 Hess and Mendelsohn, 'Case and Series'; Hess, 'Paper Machine'; Mak and Bultman, 'Identity in Forms.' On centers of calculation, see Latour, *Science in Action*.

60 Bowker and Star, *Sorting Things Out*.

Bernholm, Bernt. 'Fosterskador ökade 300 gånger: Starka indicier mot neurosedyn.' *Expressen*, April 30, 1962.

Bjerkedal, Tor. 'Protection of Privacy against Protection of Health.' *Acta Obstetricia et Gynecologica Scandinavica* 79, no. 6 (June 2000): 520–22.

Bowker, Geoffrey C., and Susan Leigh Star. *Sorting Things Out: Classification and Its Consequences*. Cambridge, MA: MIT Press, 1999.

Carachi, Robert, and Sameh Helmi Edward Doss, eds. *Clinical Embryology: An Atlas of Congenital Malformations*. Cham: Springer International, 2019.

Edmonds, Larry D., Peter M. Layde, Levy M. James, J. William Flynt, J. David Erickson, and P. Oakley Godfrey. 'Congenital Malformations Surveillance: Two American Systems.' *International Journal of Epidemiology* 10, no. 3 (1981): 247–52.

Finnish Institute for Health and Welfare. 'Medfödda missbildningar.' September 4, 2020. https://thl.fi/sv/web/thlfi-sv/statistik/information-om-statistiken/kvalitetsbeskrivningar/missbildningar.

Hess, Volker. 'A Paper Machine of Clinical Research in the Early Twentieth Century.' *Isis* 109, no. 3 (September 1, 2018): 473–93.

Hess, Volker, and J. Andrew Mendelsohn. 'Case and Series: Medical Knowledge and Paper Technology, 1600–1900.' *History of Science* 48, no. 3–4 (September 2010): 287–314.

International Centre for Birth Defects, EUROCAT, World Health Organization, and Human Genetics Programme. *World Atlas of Birth Defects*. Geneva: Human Genetics Programme, Management of Noncommunicable Diseases, World Health Organization, 2003.

Johansson, Lars Age. *Dödsorsaksstatistik: Historik, produktionsmetoder och tillförlitlighet*. Stockholm: Socialstyrelsen, 2010.

Jülich, Solveig. 'Historier kring Tornbladinstitutet.' In *Embryologiska rum: Tornbladinstitutets samling av foster från människor och djur*, by Malin Thomas Nilsson and Solveig Jülich, 151–268. Göteborg: Makadam, 2022.

Källén, Bengt. Interview with the author. October 2018.

Källén, Bengt. 'Medicinsk-genetiska synpunkter på journalgallring.' *Arkiv, Samhälle och Forskning*, no. 21 (1979): 29–33.

Källén, Bengt. *Teratologi: Läran om missbildningar*. Stockholm: Almqvist & Wiksell, 1967.

Källén, Bengt. *The Tornblad Institute in Lund: From Comparative Embryology to Reproduction Epidemiology*. Lund: Royal Physiographic Society of Lund, 2014.

Källén, Bengt, Alf Sjövall, and Ingrid Ursing. 'Läkemedel och fosterskador—en replik.' *Svenska läkartidningen* 60 (1963): 1700–1703.

Källén, Bengt, and Jan Winberg. 'Erfarenheter av kontinuerlig registrering av missbildningar.' *Läkartidningen* 63, no. 20 (1966): 1941–51.

Källén, Bengt, and Jan Winberg. 'A Swedish Register of Congenital Malformations: Experience with Continuous Registration during 2 Years with Special Reference to Multiple Malformations.' *Pediatrics* 41, no. 4 (1968): 765–76.

Latour, Bruno. *Science in Action*. Cambridge, MA: Harvard University Press, 1987.

Lennerhed, Lena. 'Kvinnan, aborten och teratologin.' *Lychnos* (2015): 141–63.

Lenz, Widukind. 'A Short History of Thalidomide Embryopathy.' *Teratology* 38, no. 3 (1988): 203–15.

Lenz, Widukind, R. A. Pfeiffer, W. Kosenow, and D. J. Hayman. 'Thalidomide and Congenital Abnormalities.' *Lancet* 279, no. 7219 (January 6, 1962): 45–46.

Lichtenstein, Paul, Patrick F. Sullivan, Sven Cnattingius, Margaret Gatz, Sofie Johansson, Eva Carlström, Camilla Björk, et al. 'The Swedish Twin Registry in the Third Millennium: An Update.' *Twin Research and Human Genetics* 9, no. 6 (December 1, 2006): 875–82.

Mak, Geertje, and Saskia Bultman. 'Identity in Forms: Paper Technologies in Dutch Anthropometric Practices around 1900.' *International Journal for History, Culture and Modernity* 7, no. 1 (November 2, 2019): 64–109.

Mcbride, William G. 'Thalidomide and Congenital Abnormalities.' *Lancet* 278, no. 7216 (December 16, 1961): 1358.

Misra, T. 'Evaluation of the National Congenital Anomaly System in England and Wales.' *Archives of Disease in Childhood—Fetal and Neonatal Edition* 90, no. 5 (September 1, 2005): F368–73.

Misra, T., N. Dattani, and A. Majeed. 'Congenital Anomaly Surveillance in England and Wales.' *Public Health* 120, no. 3 (March 1, 2006): 256–64.

National Board of Health and Welfare. 'Historik om patientregistret.' Socialstyrelsen, January 30, 2019. https://www.socialstyrelsen.se/statistik-och-data/register/alla-register/patientregistret/historik/.

Olszynko-Gryn, Jesse, Eira Bjørvik, Merle Weßel, Solveig Jülich, and Cyrille Jean. 'A Historical Argument for Regulatory Failure in the Case of Primodos and Other Hormone Pregnancy Tests.' *Reproductive Biomedicine & Society Online* 6 (August 2018): 34–44.

Rose, Nikolas. 'The Psychological Complex: Mental Measurement and Social Administration.' *Ideology & Consciousness* 5 (1979): 5–68.

Singh, Poonam Khetrapal. 'World Birth Defects Day: Many Birth Defects, One Voice.' Accessed 15 August, 2023. https://www.who.int/southeastasia/news/detail/02-03-2023-world-birth-defects-day-many-birth-defects-one-voice.

Swedish Chancellor of Justice. Justitiekanslerns utlåtande angående neurosedynkatastrofen. Reg. no. 3195-02-90, April 30, 2003. https://www.jk.se/beslut-och-yttranden/2003/04/3195-02-90/.

Swedish Code of Statutes in the Field of Health and Sick Care. 'Kungliga Medicinalstyrelsens cirkulär angående rapportering av nyfödda med missbildning den

18 december 1964.' In *Samling av författningar och cirkulär m.m. angående medicinalväsendet.* MF 1964:96. Stockholm: Kungl. Medicinalstyrelsen, 1965.

Vargesson, Neil. 'Thalidomide-Induced Teratogenesis: History and Mechanisms.' *Birth Defects Research* 105, no. 2 (June 2015): 140–56.

Winberg, Jan. 'Utredning rörande det eventuella sambandet mellan fosterskador och läkemedel: Del I & II.' *Svenska läkartidningen* 61, no. 10 (1964): 718–41.

Winberg, Jan. 'Utredning rörande det eventuella sambandet mellan fosterskador och läkemedel: Del III.' *Svenska läkartidningen* 61, no. 11 (1964): 814–31.

Winberg, Jan. 'Utredning rörande det eventuella sambandet mellan fosterskador och läkemedel: Del IV.' *Svenska läkartidningen* 61, no. 12 (1964): 890–902.

Winberg, Jan. 'Utredning rörande det eventuella sambandet mellan fosterskador och läkemedel: Del V.' *Svenska läkartidningen* 61, no. 13 (1964): 980–87.

Archival Sources

Follow-up assessment record from the Maternity Ward at the Central Hospital in Kalmar, 1961, no. 281. Inquiry into the Relationship between Pharmaceuticals and Congenital Malformations. F54:1 (1962). NBM-AB.

Record from the Central Hospital in Kalmar, Maternity Ward, 1961, no. 215. Inquiry into the Relationship between Pharmaceuticals and Congenital Malformations. F54:1 (1962). NBM-AB.

Record from Karlskoga Hospital, no. 486/59. Inquiry into the Relationship between Pharmaceuticals and Congenital Malformations. F54:1 (1962). NBM-AB.

Record from Women's Clinic of Malmö Municipal Hospital, no. 2960/56. Inquiry into the Relationship between Pharmaceuticals and Congenital Malformations. F54:2 (1962). NBM-AB.

CHAPTER 12

Navigating between Risk Discourses: On the Early Adoption and Development of Obstetrical Ultrasound Imaging in Lund, ca. 1960–1980

Annika Berg

The first mention of ultrasound as a method for fetal diagnostics in the Swedish media occurred in January 1951. It appeared at the end of a somewhat sensational newspaper story about a Devonshire radio engineer who, in cooperation with a Polish priest and physicist, had constructed a kind of machine called a 'nodal indicator.' It was said that the machine had been conceived to help farmers distinguish between hen and rooster embryos, and that it worked by projecting the reflection of electrical waves onto a television-like screen. By chance, the engineer had discovered that when pregnant women walked into his shop, fetuses older than three months could be 'seen' on the screen 'in the form of a small circle, bigger for male fetuses, smaller for female ones.' Swedish engineers and gynecologists who were interviewed in the article dismissed the Englishman's claims. The gynecologist Gunnar af Geijerstam also questioned the ethics of revealing the sex of a child-to-be before birth. However, although dismissing the possibility of using radio waves for fetal diagnostics, the engineer Anders Djurberg conjectured that ultrasound could possibly be used for that purpose.[1]

In the following decade, ultrasound visualization *was* developed as a method for fetal diagnostics, mainly in Glasgow. The obstetrician Ian Donald, professor of midwifery at the University of Glasgow, and the engineer Thomas (Tom) Brown at Kelvin & Hughes Ltd. were pivotal in this development.[2] But Swedes were early adopters. The first researcher to transfer the Glaswegian technology into a new clinical environment was Bertil Sundén, a gynecologist based at Lund Hospital (closely associated with Lund University). In 1964 Sundén defended a two-hundred-page doctoral thesis on the uses of ultrasound for obstetrical and gynecological diagnostics, the first MD on diagnostic ultrasound outside the University of Glasgow.[3] In 2013, ninety-year-old Sundén

1 'Engelsk radioman avslöjar fosters kön.'

2 Nicolson and Fleming, *Imaging and Imagining the Fetus*.

3 Sundén, 'On the Diagnostic Value'; cf. Nicolson and Fleming, *Imaging and Imagining the Fetus*, 161–62.

 | DOI:10.1163/9789004703759_014

was given the unusual and prestigious award of being named professor by the Swedish Government for his pioneering work in diagnostic ultrasound.[4]

From our present standpoint, where ultrasound diagnostics is generally perceived as a harmless routine procedure, we might suppose that its establishment was an uncontroversial matter. However, in its historical context it was not necessarily so. This chapter explores some of the circumstances that allowed the adoption and experimental development of ultrasound diagnostics in Lund. Among them were direct cooperation with Glasgow, a preexisting interest in diagnostic technologies—and access to women undergoing abortion. But I also argue that ways of discussing *risk* were crucial for the early adoption and helpful in the establishment of ultrasound as a routine procedure for prenatal diagnostics in Sweden. Drawing on the key actor Bertil Sundén's applications for research funding, his doctoral thesis and scientific articles, I show how the use of ultrasound for diagnostic purposes was gradually legitimized by navigating between several different risk discourses.

While it may be forcefully argued that today we live in a 'risk society' of previously unimaginable proportions,[5] more or less modern ways of thinking about risk may be traced back several hundred years. Originally, 'risk' could refer to the probability of positive as well as negative outcomes; however, with time it has come to be exclusively associated with the latter. When used with greater precision, the concept of risk points at something more specific than uncertainty, implying that the probability of damage is somewhat calculable. Often too, the concept of risk is associated with man-made hazards rather than natural disasters. Medical innovation—understood as the process of introducing a new medical technology or drug—typically entails debates about risk and the weighing of benefits against dangers, which may or may not result in the new method's acceptance.[6] As Deborah Lupton points out, risk discourse may—despite its neutral demeanor—serve a number of rhetorical functions.[7]

In this study, when tracing and differentiating between risk discourses, I have looked out for discussions—outright or implicit—about potential damage or otherwise negative outcomes in relation to ultrasound: that is, negative outcomes that could be avoided by using diagnostic ultrasound (encompassing, as Ilana Löwy has put it, the establishment of prenatal ultrasound as a technology of risk management), but also those that might result from ultrasound itself, as

4 Ståhl, 'Bertil Sundén.'
5 Cf. Beck, *Risk Society*.
6 Schlich, 'Risk and Medical Innovation,' 1–17; see also, e.g., Wolf, *Cesarean Section*.
7 Lupton, 'Risk as Moral Danger,' 425–35.

potentially dangerous.[8] I have also attended to silences, considering what they may mean under different circumstances.

Anthropological and sociological studies of diagnostic ultrasound have mainly focused on its connection to 'the public fetus,' as Barbara Duden and others have conceptualized the nearly explosive spread of fetal images in popular media and elsewhere, and the ways in which this mediatization in turn has affected our views on fetuses, life, and personhood.[9] Fewer studies have dealt with the socio-technological development of ultrasound from a historical perspective.[10] And those who have, have generally touched rather briefly on the question of risk evaluations in this process. In their detailed book *Imaging and Imagining the Fetus*, Malcolm Nicolson and John Fleming dedicate minor passages to risks connected with the technology itself and the ways in which they were considered by Ian Donald and others in the early days of ultrasound visualization.[11] Ann Oakley also touched on the safety question—including Donald's take on it—in the part of her critical 1984 study on the history of antenatal care, *The Captured Womb*, that was dedicated to Ian Donald's experiments.[12] So, it should be noted, did Bertil Sundén himself, in a 2012 volume where a range of medical specialists looked back at Lund as a frontline environment in the development of ultrasound technologies, and where Sundén's visualization of a twin pregnancy in 1962 was highlighted as a world premiere.[13]

Besides shedding new light on the Swedish part of the history of ultrasound imaging, this chapter adds to earlier research by focusing more specifically on risk evaluations in the process of developing ultrasound as a technology for fetal imaging. It also argues that these considerations should be put into a historical context where ultrasound was not primarily conceptualized as an imaging technique, let alone a technique for imaging fetuses, but as a broadly applicable phenomenon, which was perceived as both promising and frightening.

First, I discuss why Lund provided fertile ground for the development of ultrasound imaging; then I consider the risk discourses that had to be reckoned with by the end of the 1950s. After that I follow Sundén through the 1960s and 1970s to see how he navigated between prevalent and emerging risk discourses,

---

8 Cf. Löwy, *Tangled Diagnoses*.

9 Duden, *Disembodying Women*; Petchesky, 'Fetal Images,' 263–92; Dijck, *Transparent Body*, chap. 6; Taylor, *Public Life*; Roberts, *Visualised Foetus*; Lupton, *Social Worlds of the Unborn*, chap. 2.

10 Cf. Löwy, *Imperfect Pregnancies*, 10.

11 Nicolson and Fleming, *Imaging and Imagining the Fetus*, 115–17, 130–31, 220–26. See also Tansey and Christie, *Looking at the Unborn*, 65–69.

12 Oakley, *Captured Womb*, 155–71.

13 See Eklöf, Lindström, and Persson, *Ultrasound in Clinical Diagnosis*, and especially Marčál and Sundén, 'Development of Ultrasound,'; Westling, 'Ultrasound in Lund.'

and weighed costs against benefits before different audiences. I conclude the study around 1980, when ultrasound was established as a mainstream technology for prenatal diagnostics.

1 Facilitating Factors

A number of coinciding factors may be seen to have paved the way for the appropriation, experimental use, and development of obstetric and gynecological ultrasound imaging in Lund. To begin with, the physicist Hellmuth Hertz and the cardiologist Inge Edler had used ultrasound technology to produce the world's first echocardiogram in 1953, and kept on developing the technology.[14] Also in Lund, the neurosurgeon Lars Leksell had experimented with different industrial flaw detectors to diagnose intracranial complications after skull injury.[15] Bertil Sundén, then a junior gynecologist, borrowed a flaw detector from Leksell to make ultrasound measurements of pregnant wombs.[16]

Sundén was also lucky that his interest in diagnostic technologies coincided with that of Alf Sjövall, who was professor in obstetrics and gynecology and chief consultant at the women's clinic at Lund Hospital, where Sundén was based. Sjövall was a pioneer in diagnostic laparoscopy, a method to visualize the inside of the pelvis or abdomen by inserting an optical device—a laparoscope—through a small cut in the abdominal wall.[17] Sjövall was the one who had prompted Sundén to approach Leksell in the first place. Later on, he would provide a link to Glasgow, which was crucial in the establishment of the women's clinic in Lund as a center for the development of ultrasound as an imaging technology. For while the Krautkrämer echoscope that Sundén borrowed from Leksell could produce one-dimensional measurements and diagrams, in Glasgow Tom Brown and Ian Donald were experimenting with a machine that made it possible to produce two-dimensional pictures of abdominal tumors and, potentially, fetuses, by way of ultrasound technology. Two-dimensional ultrasound imaging had been conceptualized in the early 1950s, but Brown's ingenuity took the technology to a new, and clinically promising, level. So when Donald visited Lund for a week in the late 1950s, aiming to study

14 On Hertz and Edler, see, e.g., Persson, Eskilsson, and Lundström, 'Development of Echocardiography in Sweden.'

15 Leksell, 'Echo-Encephalography'; 'Ekolodning i hjärnan kan påvisa blödning'; Nicolson and Fleming, *Imaging and Imagining the Fetus*, 29–31; Lunsford, 'Lars Leksell.'

16 Sundén, grant application, December 29, 1959.

17 Flam, 'Laparoskopi inom gynekologin,' 3396; Nicolson and Fleming, *Imaging and Imagining the Fetus*, 157. Protocols from the Lund University Hospital board show Sjövall's continuous support to Sundén in, e.g., applications for prolonged postings at his clinic.

the laparoscopic technique developed by Sjövall, Sundén received an invitation to visit Donald's clinic at the Western Infirmary in Glasgow. In 1959, Sundén went to Britain in order to learn more about ultrasound imaging, financed by grants from the Swedish Medical Research Council and Lund Medical Society.[18] Returning to Sweden, he was granted more money from the research council and was able to dedicate much of his time at the women's clinic to developing the technique further. Later on, in his 1964 doctoral thesis, Sundén would thank his 'chief' Sjövall for his 'stimulating interest' in the investigation and for 'invaluable help and advice.' (Donald and Hertz, who would also act as first and second opponents at the public defense, were acknowledged for 'inestimable' help and 'invaluable discussions,' respectively. Leksell got thanks for 'valuable help.')[19]

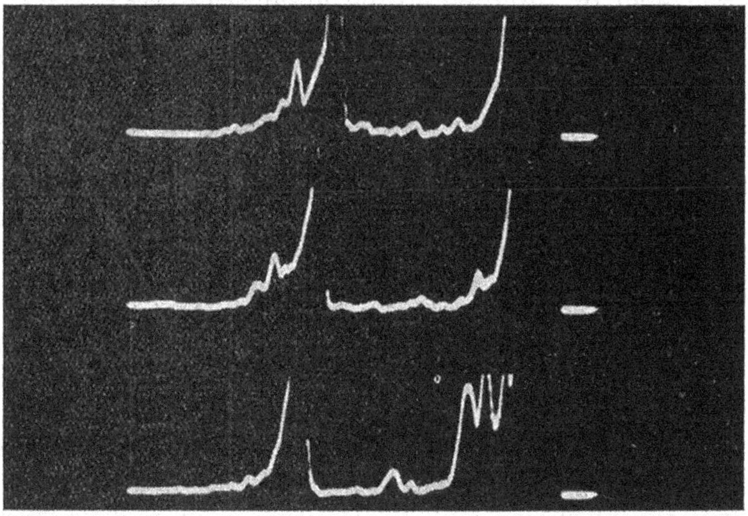

Fig. 3. Ekogram från en graviditet i mens III.

FIGURE 12.1 Bertil Sundén's first ultrasound examinations were made with a kind of apparatus that was normally used for industrial flaw detection. As illustrated and explained by Sundén in his 1960 article in *Svenska läkartidningen,* this kind of machinery could only produce one-dimensional representations. This particular illustration shows an echogram of a third-month pregnancy. From Sundén, 'Ultraljudsdiagnostik i obstetrik och gynekologi,' 774.

18 Sundén, 'Ultraljudsdiagnostik,' 782; Marčál and Sundén, 'Development of Ultrasound,' 50–51; various documents in F1:231, MRC. Cf. Donald, MacVicar, and Brown, 'Investigation of Abdominal Masses'; Nicolson and Fleming, *Imaging and Imagining the Fetus*, 119–43, 157.

19 Sundén, 'On the Diagnostic Value,' 178. Cf. Marčál and Sundén, 'Development of Ultrasound,' 52–54.

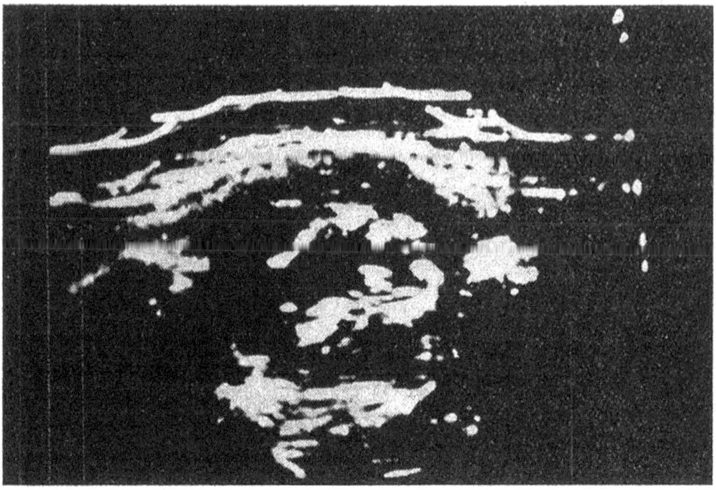

Fig. 8. Transversell bild av normal graviditet i mens IV.

FIGURE 12.2 By combining ultrasound echoes from a number of different angles, the new type of apparatus could produce pictures that showed a cross-section of the abdomen. This illustration, also from Sundén's *Svenska läkartidningen* article showed a transversal image of a normal, fourth-month pregnancy. From Sundén, 'Ultraljudsdiagnostik i obstetrik och gynekologi,' 780.

The development of ultrasound visualization techniques in Lund was thus enabled by a preexisting, general openness to new technology; a specific interest in ultrasound technologies; and the subsequent transfer of an even more specific—in fact, as we shall see, custom-made for Sundén—technology for ultrasound visualization.

But it was also helped by Swedish legislation. Like many of the other examples of fetal research discussed in this book, Sundén's experiments benefited from the comparatively liberal abortion law that had been in force in Sweden since the late 1930s, allowing abortions on medical, humanitarian, eugenic, and, since 1946, socio-medical indications. Researchers also benefited from access to a specific clinical environment, where women who had been granted abortion under the conditions of the law were at hand as research subjects.[20] In Glasgow, investigative ultrasound examinations were carried out on women waiting for either gynecological surgery or childbirth—not abortions.[21]

20 Cf. Sjövall, 'Operationsteknik vid havandeskapsavbrytande.'

21 Tansey and Christie, *Looking at the Unborn*, 46–47.

2 1950s Risk Discourses

That the development of ultrasound imaging was perceived as worthwhile to prioritize in the late 1950s and early 1960s may be connected to a specific risk discourse that was centered on X-rays. In the 1930s and 1940s, obstetricians had started, albeit occasionally, to employ X-rays for detection of major malformations, or for estimating of the age of a pregnancy. It could also be used to indicate sex, on the assumption that bone structures showed earlier in a female fetus. Obstetrical use of X-rays increased in the 1950s. However, so did the worries.[22] After Alice Stewart's first study on likely connections between childhood leukemia and prenatal X-ray exposure was published in *The Lancet* in 1956, the potential dangers of X-ray radiation could not be neglected (although a number of obstetricians were initially skeptical of Stewart's conclusions). And of course, there was also a more general apprehension toward ionizing radiation after the bombings of Hiroshima and Nagasaki.[23]

During this period, several technologies for fetal diagnostics were under development. From the 1950s, hemolytic disease of the newborn could be prevented through amniocentesis and measurement of bilirubin levels. Amniocentesis, although still a risky procedure, could also be used to confidently determine the sex of a fetus, and thereby—from about 1960—help to predict the occurrence of hemophilia. A new method for chromosome staining, also developed in Lund thanks to the liberal Swedish abortion law, led to the late-1950s identification of Down syndrome as a chromosomal condition and the growth of cytogenetics.[24] Laparoscopy could detect both extra- and intrauterine pregnancies.[25] But ultrasound stood out in that it was perceived to enable visualization of structures inside the body without any invasive procedures, and also without the obvious dangers of ionizing radiation. This, of course, made the technology attractive for researchers and clinicians as well as for financiers.

However, there was also a risk discourse that centered on ultrasound itself. This too had to be reckoned with. The descriptions of ultrasound technology in Swedish media in the 1930s and 1940s had often been alarmist. Ultrasound was typically described as a 'death ray of sound waves,' which could be used in

22 Löwy, *Imperfect Pregnancies*, 43–44.

23 Stewart et al., 'Preliminary Communication,' 447; Dry, 'Population as Patient.' Ian Donald was among the sceptics; see Nicolson and Fleming, *Imaging and Imagining the Fetus*, 85, 99–100. For a Swedish discussion on X-rays and fetal damage, see *Nordisk medicin* 59, no. 25 (1958), a special issue on ionizing radiation and radiation damage.

24 Löwy, *Imperfect Pregnancies*, 40–49.

25 Samuelsson and Sjövall, 'Laparoscopy in Suspected Ectopic Pregnancy.'

warfare as a 'secret, but humane and effective weapon.'[26] More constructive ways of using ultrasound were presented too.[27] Still, the promise consisted in harnessing a potentially lethal technology for productive purposes. In newspapers and popular media, narratives of the deadly properties of ultrasound lived on well into the 1950s, not least in connection with medical applications. Thus, new inventions that built on ultrasound technology were often presented with a caveat.[28] These alarms were not merely a popular-media phenomenon. That ultrasound examinations might result in damage, and especially fetal damage, was also a cause of continuous concern for Ian Donald and the other British pioneers, and, as we will see, for Sundén.[29]

3 Evaluating Risk as an Early-Career Researcher

I will now look more closely into the ways in which Bertil Sundén and people around him weighed costs and benefits in relation to ultrasound technology, and the ways in which these considerations transformed over time.

When Sundén applied for his first travel grant to go to Glasgow and study the new technology, his main argument was that it was able to create 'beautiful,' 'X-ray like' pictures, which could help to solve 'differential-diagnostic problems within obstetrics and gynecology.' In some respects, the technology even provided more information than X-rays. He also argued that it was a quick method that caused no discomfort for the 'patient' and, importantly, that 'no damaging effects had been observed.'[30] Sundén attached letters of recommendation from Alf Sjövall and Lars Leksell to his application, and also got a positive statement from a Gothenburg professor, Per Bergman. The professors emphasized that the method was not dangerous, or rather—significantly—that Sundén had described it as nondangerous.[31]

In the autumn of 1959, Sundén spent a few weeks with Donald at the gynecological ward of the Western Infirmary in Glasgow, learning and practicing the

26 'Dödad "dödsstråle."' See also, e.g., Holmberg, 'Ljudet som inte hörs'; 'Ljud som dödar'; '"Rent luckförsvar räcker ej."' For more on this topic, see Berg, 'Rays of Death.'

27 Berg, '"Det vita ljudet."'

28 See, e.g., Peter [pseud.], 'Ohörbart ljud botar magsår'; 'Dr Lindströms metod är "revolutionerande."'

29 Tansey and Christie, *Looking at the Unborn*, 65–69. Cf. Nicolson and Fleming, *Imaging and Imagining the Fetus*, 115–17, 130–31, 220–26.

30 Sundén, grant application, May 21, 1959.

31 Leksell and Sjövall to the Medical Research Council; Bergman to the Medical Research Council.

new technique, and also visited the engineers at Kelvin & Hughes.[32] Shortly after returning to Sweden, Sundén applied for more than SEK 45,000 (equivalent to two years' wages for a junior physician at the time) from the Medical Research Council for the purchase of his own custom-made ultrasound apparatus for two-dimensional visualization and differential diagnostics. A key argument in this application was the absence of danger, and the possibility of avoiding ionizing radiation. Sundén also described the technique as quick and harmless—at the (undefined) frequencies and exposure times used for diagnostic purposes. Implicitly here, Sundén not only distinguished between dangerous X-rays and nondangerous ultrasound, but also made a distinction between diagnostic (safe) and therapeutic uses of ultrasound.[33] His descriptions thus engaged with two different discourses of risk. This time another professor, the physiologist Torsten Teorell, gave Sundén his approval, with reference to Sundén's own description of the method as completely harmless at the frequencies and intensities used.[34]

In a scientific paper attached to the application and published a few months later in the Swedish medical journal *Svenska läkartidningen*, Sundén explained the technology in an instructive manner. He also wrote more explicitly about phenomena that could indicate potential risks, such as energy absorption and cavitation, and named them as potentially dangerous. At the same time though, he mentioned several studies that indicated that diagnostic ultrasound was harmless. He was also careful to contrast his diagnostic methods against earlier, and in his own view rather 'uncritical,' uses of ultrasound for therapeutic purposes, where energy absorption and heat production were actually the goal. However, he did not clarify what frequencies, amplitudes, or exposure times would ensure safety; nor did he draw any clear line between diagnostic and therapeutic frequencies or intensities. In his own previous experiments, he had used frequencies of two megahertz, which was within the spectrum employed for detection of flaws in metal structures.[35]

In describing these earlier experiments, using Leksell's apparatus, Sundén was careful to note that they had been conducted on women who would later undergo legal abortions.[36] In the application proper, Sundén did not mention that his 'patients' were women whose fetuses would soon be aborted. Instead,

32 Sundén, grant application, December 29, 1959; Sundén, 'Ultraljudsdiagnostik' (manuscript). See also Nicolson and Fleming, *Imaging and Imagining the Fetus*, 157; Tansey and Christie, *Looking at the Unborn*, 14; Marčál and Sundén, 'Development of Ultrasound.'

33 Sundén, grant application, December 29, 1959.

34 Teorell to the Medical Research Council, March 8, 1960.

35 Sundén, 'Ultraljudsdiagnostik' (manuscript); cf. Sundén, 'Ultraljudsdiagnostik.'

36 Sundén, 'Ultraljudsdiagnostik' (manuscript), 5.

he highlighted the possibility of deciding whether an early pregnancy was 'fetal' or not as a matter of 'great importance' in order to prevent (spontaneous) abortions.[37] Sundén's highlighting the potential prevention of miscarriages was perhaps an attempt to steer away from the sensitive issue of induced abortion. Although access to women and fetuses in line for abortion may have been relatively uncontroversial in Lund at the time, Sundén had to consider that several of the influential obstetricians whose approval he needed—Ian Donald among them—were very restrictive in their views on abortion.[38] Sundén's own standpoint is hard to pinpoint from the material at hand, but in any case, he took advantage of the abortion law for his research purposes.

The comment in the manuscript—that experiments had only involved fetuses that would be aborted anyway—can also be read as an acknowledgment of diagnostic ultrasound as potentially hazardous. However, Sundén pointed out that the principal weakness of the technology available in Lund was that it lacked precision. The main problems were that it could only be used to examine rather simple kinds of tissue, could not reach very far into the body, and could only make one-dimensional measurements.[39] The Scottish machinery, on the other hand, opened a world of new possibilities.[40]

Sundén was granted the money he requested to purchase an ultrasound scanner.[41] Two years later, on March 30, 1962, the custom-made machinery was delivered from Glasgow to Lund.[42] The scanner—a major order for Kelvin & Hughes and its parent company, Smiths Industries Ltd.—was one of a kind, an attempt to combine the reliability of the 'doctor-proof' automatic scanner that Tom Brown had recently constructed for Donald with the versatility of a manual scanner. It was also the first scanner to be exported abroad, and the only one to be exported for several years. It was not until the second half of the 1960s that any kind of serial production of ultrasound scanners got underway.[43]

Tom Brown and the designer Dugald Cameron described the 'Sundén machine' as an attempt to make examinations as comfortable and unintimidating as possible for the patients.[44] Some physicians too showed concern for

37 Sundén, grant application, December 29, 1959.

38 On Donald's attitudes to abortion, see also Nicolson and Fleming, *Imaging and Imagining the Fetus*, 5, 238–47; cf. Donald, 'Abortion and the Obstetrician.'

39 Sundén, 'Ultraljudsdiagnostik' (manuscript), 6–9, quotation on 6.

40 Sundén, 'Ultraljudsdiagnostik,' 8–13.

41 Medical Research Council to Sundén, March 30, 1960.

42 Nicolson and Fleming, *Imaging and Imagining the Fetus*, 161.

43 Nicolson and Fleming, *Imaging and Imagining the Fetus*, chap. 7.

44 Tansey and Christie, *Looking at the Unborn*, 21–23, quotation on 21; cf. Nicolson and Fleming, *Imaging and Imagining the Fetus*, 160–61.

the women. One of Sundén's arguments in favor of the technology was that it caused 'no discomfort whatsoever' for the patient.[45] At a 1998 witness seminar, several of the British physicians also recalled considering the women's health and comfort. However, concern did not equal informed consent. In hindsight, James Willocks and John MacVicar, who assisted and collaborated with Donald in the 1950s and early 1960s, reflected that a modern-day ethical committee would never have let them get away with experimenting with industrial flaw detectors on women who were already in a crisis situation, waiting either for gynecological surgery or childbirth.[46] Similarly, in Sweden at that time, there were no ethical committees to approve or reject Sundén's experiments.[47]

Immediately after the machine was delivered and installed, Sundén set out to scan a great number of patients.[48] A year later, he applied for more money from the Medical Research Council to complete his studies. This time, the ultrasound risk discourse was more directly addressed. In particular, it was emphasized that in addition to clinical studies on pregnant women, experimental animal studies were made to address the question—suddenly presented as controversial—of potentially harmful effects of ultrasound on sensitive tissues such as ovaries and fetuses. For this purpose, Sundén needed to employ a laboratory assistant to take care of all the lab rats involved for half a year.[49] Evaluations of the application were positive, and especially so in regard to the animal studies, which were described as crucial.[50]

In May 1963, the Medical Research Council decided to grant Sundén SEK 5,000—a little less than the SEK 7,000 he had applied for. However, the rat part of the study—dedicated to exploring the method's safety—received full funding.[51] One year later, in spring 1964, Sundén applied for money to finish and publish his research, with largely the same motivation as the year before.[52] Torsten Teorell, who was once again consulted to evaluate the application, recommended that Sundén should receive the whole sum he had applied for. And he did so largely because of the importance of the animal studies in relation to the still-unsolved question of potential risks of tissue damage.[53]

45 Sundén, 'Ultraljudsdiagnostik,' 778.
46 Tansey and Christie, *Looking at the Unborn*, 46–47.
47 See Tinnerholm Ljungberg's chapter in this volume.
48 Nicolson and Fleming, *Imaging and Imagining the Fetus*, 161.
49 Sundén, grant application, March 11, 1963.
50 Ingelman-Sundberg to the Medical Research Council.
51 Medical Research Council to Bertil Sundén, May 6, 1963.
52 Sundén, grant application, March 12, 1964.
53 Teorell to the Medical Research Council, April 22, 1964.

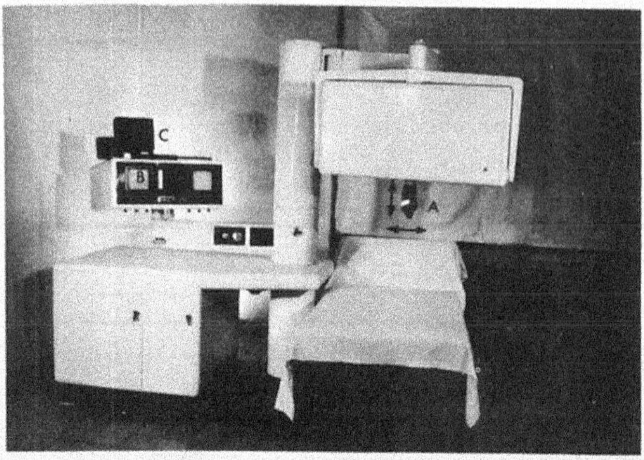

Fig 1 Ultrasonic scanning machine. For details see text

The crystal, which both generates the sound and receives the echoes, is enclosed in the probe (A in Fig 1). The ultrasound is pulsed and a frequency of 50 pulses per second is used. The mean value of the intensity received by the patient is 1 or $2mW/cm^2$ at the skin. The probe is attached to a stand above the patient's abdomen and can be moved vertically or horizontally and rocked ± 110°. Ultrasound examination is performed with the patient supine. To eliminate air bubbles, which reflect the sound, between the probe and the skin, a thin film of olive oil is applied as a contact medium. The probe is moved either longitudinally from the costal arch down to the symphysis pubis or transversely from one flank to the other (Fig 2). The movements of the probe are carried out by hand. The probe is rocked during the longitudinal and transverse movement so that the ultrasound strikes inter-

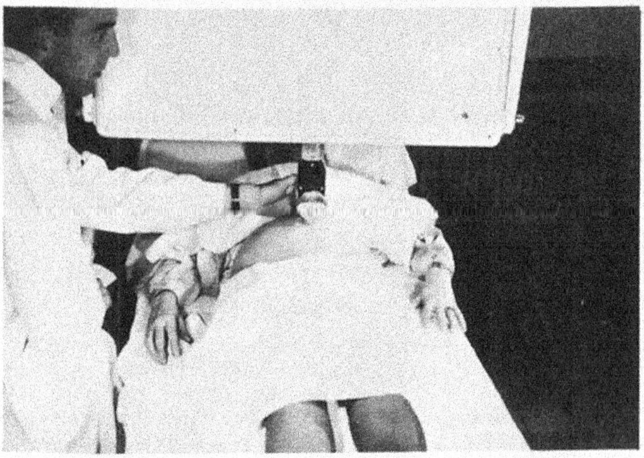

Fig 2 Transverse scanning

FIGURE 12.3
The apparatus that was delivered exclusively to Bertil Sundén in Lund was designed to be both versatile and 'doctor-proof.' As Sundén described it in his 1967 article in *Ultrasonics*, its use caused 'no discomfort' for the patient. From Sundén, 'Obstetric Diagnosis with Ultrasound,' 67.

What can be noticed here is that as the project progressed, Sundén became more willing to admit that the question of risk was still open. In part this was likely due to the very specific historical circumstance that the thalidomide scandal had unfolded in the years between Sundén's second and third applications to the Medical Research Council, raising awareness of medical risks more generally.[54] However, as we have seen, there was also a preexisting discourse on the more specific risks of ultrasound that Sundén must have been aware of from the start. Arguably, for Sundén personally, a balancing act had to be made between, on the one hand, highlighting the harmlessness of the method, and on the other hand, highlighting the importance of securing that harmlessness. And this balancing act had to be continued throughout the research process. The tipping of the balance one way or the other was likely dependent on external circumstances—but also on the stage of the research and the precise purposes of the funding applications. When there was still a long way to go and Sundén was unsure of getting any funding at all, any risks inherent in the new technology would have been hazardous to mention. But as he approached the conclusion of the study, it actually became an advantage for him to show that he had taken the question of risk seriously.

4 Risk Discourses and Risk Analysis in Sundén's Doctoral Thesis

In Sundén's 1964 doctoral thesis, 'On the Diagnostic Value of Ultrasound in Obstetrics and Gynaecology,' a thirty-five page-long chapter was dedicated to 'the biological effects of ultrasound'—or rather, implicitly, biological *risks* that might be connected with the technology. After a review of previous research, from which he concluded that *high*-intensity ultrasound could damage living tissue, largely through heating, Sundén went on to describe his rat experiments. In order to mimic clinical diagnostic examinations on women, he had applied ultrasound at relatively low intensity to groups of albino rats. He had also used pulsed ultrasound in order to avoid unnecessary exposure, and an examination technique where 'the crystal' (referring to the piezoelectric ultrasound generator) was continuously moved along and across the rat's abdomen. In comparison with the unirradiated rats in his control groups, Sundén concluded that rats exposed to low-intensity, pulsed ultrasound exhibited no changes in behavior or appetite, no histological or functional changes in their ovaries or pregnant uteruses, and no higher percentage of stillborn or

54 Cf. Brynner and Stephens, *Dark Remedy*, 1–59; Sjöström and Nilsson, *Thalidomide*, 131–36; Björkman's chapter in this volume.

deformed offspring. Ultrasound did not provoke abortion, intrauterine death, or premature birth, and had not affected the subsequent fertility of either the irradiated rats or their offspring.[55] After describing his animal experiments in detail and concluding that no harmful effects had been observed from them, Sundén added in a subparagraph that he had also used the scanner to diagnostically examine more than four hundred women since 1962, and that none of them had reported any discomfort; neither had any adverse effects been observed. Sundén referred to this as 'clinical experience' that helped confirming the safety of the method (although the human examinations had in fact started before the animal experiments).[56]

The rest of the thesis was dedicated to descriptions of different applications of the technique as a 'method of investigation in obstetrics and gynaecology' that had been tried and developed by Sundén himself.[57] The different chapters dealt with the diagnosis of, for example, twin pregnancies, molar pregnancies, excessive amniotic fluid, 'monsters,' and, on the gynecological side, various tumors. The choice to dedicate a whole chapter to 'monsters' was apparently made during his work on the thesis, and may be seen as a reflection of the new risk discourse on fetal malformations that had been triggered by the thalidomide scandal.[58] Also, in identifying fetal malformations by way of ultrasound, Sundén indeed broke new ground internationally.[59] Before him, Donald had identified hydrocephalus in the third semester, but otherwise it was not until real-time scanning in the 1970s that the diagnosis of malformations took off.[60]

55 Intensities used were 1–2 milliwatts/square cm; frequencies of ultrasound 1.5 or 2.5 MHz, and frequency of pulses 25 per second. Each rat was examined for 3 minutes. Sundén, 'On the Diagnostic Value,' 46–80. Cf. Nicolson and Fleming, *Imaging and Imagining the Fetus*, 115–17, on Donald's early considerations about safety, including some animal experiments.

56 Sundén, 'On the Diagnostic Value,' 79–80. The animal experiments were carried out August 1962–January 1964 (67). I have not been able to trace any firsthand accounts from the women who underwent those experimental examinations.

57 Sundén, 'On the Diagnostic Value,' 81–173.

58 'Monstra' was the first category of congenital malformations listed in the 1957 Swedish version of the *International Classification of Diseases*, still in use when Sundén published his thesis. See Lee's chapter in this volume.

59 In 1998, Stuart Campbell reminisced that Sundén, 'in the early 1960s,' was probably the first to record anencephaly by way of ultrasound, several years ahead of Campbell himself (in early 1970s London). Tansey and Christie, *Looking at the Unborn*, 54–55. Cf. also Nicolson and Fleming, *Imaging and Imagining the Fetus*, 214. What Sundén actually claimed to have visualized was three cases of acrania (a condition often associated with anencephaly). This too was a first. Sundén, 'On the Diagnostic Value,' 121–23.

60 Nicolson and Fleming, *Imaging and Imagining the Fetus*, 214–15; Tansey and Christie, *Looking at the Unborn*, 55.

In the end, after summarizing his own results, Sundén confidently concluded that the safety of the method had been 'demonstrated beyond doubt, not only in this investigation but also in the investigations of others.'[61] Thus, at the point of finishing his MD, Sundén was very assertive in his claims about the safety of diagnostic ultrasound—however, this assertiveness was still dependent on a thoroughly described risk analysis.

5 Establishing Unambiguous Harmlessness

In media of the mid- and late 1960s, ultrasound prevailed as a strong symbol of modernity and progress, especially in relation to industrial and construction work. Measuring and imaging techniques for brain and heart diagnostics were mentioned from time to time, and, occasionally, the possibility of visualizing fetuses as well. In October 1967, an article in the leading daily newspaper *Dagens Nyheter* reported on an 'explosive development' in medical electronics, including the development of 'ultrasound instruments for determining fetal life within the uterus.'[62] However, if there was one innovation relating to diagnostic ultrasound that got publicity, it was not fetal imaging but Hellmuth Hertz's invention of the inkjet printer, which was originally conceived to make his and Inge Edler's work with cardiac ultrasound more effective.[63]

Popular descriptions of ultrasound as potentially dangerous became rare in the late 1960s, and Sundén's texts followed a similar trajectory. In the years that followed the publication of his doctoral thesis, he published several articles in which he presented diagnostic ultrasound more and more unambiguously as a simple-to-use, reliable method that was comfortable for the patient and harmless in comparison with X-rays. An article in *Ultrasonics* in 1967 largely repeated the main findings in the obstetrical part of the doctoral thesis, illustrated with state-of-the-art ultrasound images. Risks were only mentioned indirectly, in the declaration that the ultrasound scanner could be used with three different intensities, but that Sundén had only used the two lower ones when examining pregnant uteruses. When discussing the potential use of ultrasound for localizing the placenta, Sundén noted that his series of rat experiments had 'failed to demonstrate any harmful effects on ovaries, pregnancy or young.' In the rest of the article, where more established ways of using ultrasound were discussed,

61 Sundén, 'On the Diagnostic Value,' 177.

62 Karsberg, '"Explosionsutveckling" i medicinsk elektronik.'

63 See, e.g., Karsberg, 'Ny fotokopiering spar silver'; 'Dagens namn.'

the only risks that were mentioned were those that could be *avoided* by the use of ultrasound.[64]

In the years that followed, Sundén worked on developing the method for the examination of human placentas.[65] In the article 'Ultrasonic Placentography,' published in *Acta Obstetricia et Gynecologica Scandinavica* in 1969, Sundén compared ultrasound with X-rays and concluded by stating that ultrasonic placentography was 'highly reliable' and 'safe to child and mother.'[66] 'Placentography by Ultrasound' was published in the same journal in 1970. It dealt with the same subject as the previous article, but in more detail. It was also even more assertive in launching ultrasound as an easy, reliable, and harmless method, ending with the statement that 'the ultrasound examination does not cause the patient any discomfort whatsoever, and the method is in no way harmful to mother or child.'[67] Notably, in both these articles, published in 1969 and 1970, Sundén wrote about 'the mother and child' as the objects of examination. This choice of language indicates the coming of a new era in that the method, apparently, was intended for examining women whose pregnancies were meant to result in a child—that is, for clinical use.

In the ten years since Sundén's first trip to Glasgow, his descriptions of the technology had evolved from something promising and probably harmless in comparison with X-rays, to something that had to be carefully tested for safety, and finally into something that could quite confidently be launched as non-dangerous. Throughout the process, his descriptions had mirrored different risk narratives that, apparently, always had to be taken into consideration, but at the same time not exaggerated—not to other researchers, let alone people who could help to fund his experiments.

6 Continuing Anxieties

In a 1970 article in *The Lancet*, an international group of researchers, including Sundén and Donald, focused specifically on addressing the safety of diagnostic

64 Sundén, 'Obstetric Diagnosis with Ultrasound,' 67–71, quotation on 71.

65 Sundén's publications on placentography were preceded by publications by Ken Gottesfeld (in 1966) and by Ian Donald and Usama Abdulla (in 1968); however, Sundén had localized the placenta in his earlier article 'Obstetric Diagnosis with Ultrasound' too. Donald and Abdulla were arguably the first to actually visualize the placenta. Tansey and Christie, *Looking at the Unborn*, 11, 29–30, 54. Cf. Donald and Abdulla, 'Placentography by Sonar'; Taylor et al., 'Ultrasonic Placentography.'

66 Sundén, 'Ultrasonic Placentography,' 161.

67 Sundén, 'Placentography by Ultrasound.'

ultrasound in obstetrics.[68] Nicolson and Fleming describe this publication as an answer to 'a certain generalized anxiety about the biological effects of ultrasound,' especially in the United States, where rumors spread that Canadian scientists had reared a giant chicken, standing more than one meter tall, after treating fertilized eggs with ultrasound.[69] In the *Lancet* article, the obstetricians established—albeit with the caveat that 'our findings do not prove conclusively the safety of diagnostic ultrasound in pregnancy'—that ultrasound examinations of 1,114 'apparently normal pregnant women' at three different clinics (in Brooklyn, Glasgow, and Lund) had not resulted in a higher incidence of fetal abnormality than in the general population.[70]

If the leading researchers had reached some kind of consensus on the probable harmlessness of diagnostic ultrasound in obstetrics by 1970, ultrasound retained an ambiguous aura in the press.[71] Occasionally the question of potential danger was re-triggered by scientific claims as well. A South African study in the early 1970s indicated chromosomal damage from ultrasound, and stirred commotion among obstetricians as well as the press and general public. However, the results of the study were soon refuted, even by the authors themselves.[72]

7 A Discourse of Risk Management

The question of safety was never fully resolved.[73] Still today, authorities typically state that ultrasound equipment should only be handled by trained and experienced personnel, in doses 'as low as reasonably achievable' and only when medically motivated. Special warnings are also issued to counteract a growing 'keepsake' industry.[74] Nevertheless, it seems that over the course of the 1970s, it became less and less important for researchers to address safety

68 Hellman et al., 'Safety of Diagnostic Ultrasound.'

69 Nicolson and Fleming, *Imaging and Imagining the Fetus*, 221.

70 Hellman et al., 'Safety of Diagnostic Ultrasound,' 1133.

71 See, e.g., 'Tårgas, epilepsi senaste vapnen rädda gisslan.'

72 Tansey and Christie, *Looking at the Unborn*, 65–67; Nicolson and Fleming, *Imaging and Imagining the Fetus*, 222–24; Lele, 'Revue,' 312–13. Cf. Macintosh and Davey, 'Chromosome Aberrations,' 92–93.

73 Nicolson and Fleming, *Imaging and Imagining the Fetus*, 224–26.

74 Cf., e.g., American Institute of Ultrasound in Medicine, 'As Low as Reasonably Achievable'; Kollman et al., 'EFSUMB Clinical Safety Statement'; US Food and Drug Administration, 'Ultrasound Imaging'; Swedish Radiation Safety Authority, 'Ultraljudsundersökning vid graviditet.'

in their writings. Toward the end of the 1970s, it appears that the harmlessness of the diagnostic use of ultrasound within obstetrics and gynecology had been established as a fact to the extent that potential dangers did not even have to be mentioned in scientific articles. This development can be associated to yet another risk discourse. Notably, it went hand in hand with the establishment of ultrasound and other methods for prenatal diagnosis as technologies of risk *management*, as historian Ilana Löwy has put it. As the resolution of ultrasound images increased, ultrasonography could be more effectively used to detect fetal malformations. Thanks to its power to determine the age of a pregnancy, it enabled the use of serum markers to indicate neural tube defects and, later on, Down syndrome. Ultrasound could also be used to minimize the risks associated with other methods for prenatal diagnosis, such as amniocentesis.[75] Also, it should be added, the mid-1970s saw the introduction of real-time ultrasound scanning, which provided moving high-resolution pictures, and was easier to use.[76] Together, these developments further facilitated the framing of ultrasound as a means of risk reduction rather than a risk in itself.

This framing is clearly mirrored in Sundén's publications. In a 1977 article in *Läkartidningen*, Sundén—who was now a senior consultant, still based at the women's clinic in Lund—made a detailed overview of the rapid development of diagnostic ultrasound on pregnant women in the last twenty years. He wrote about the development of the technology, as well as the growing numbers of women examined annually, just adding a short note on the lack of evidence for any damaging effects at the very end of the text.[77] And in the article 'Diagnostic Ultrasound in Threatened Abortion and Suspected Ectopic Pregnancy,' published by Sundén and three other researchers in *Acta Obstetricia et Gynecologica Scandinavica* 1980, fetal diagnostic ultrasound was exclusively discussed as a means of risk reduction and prognosis, and an 'excellent' one at that, with no mention whatsoever of even improbable risks related to the method itself.[78]

75 Löwy, *Tangled Diagnoses*, 8–15. Cf. Nicolson and Fleming, *Imaging and Imagining the Fetus*, 214–15.

76 Tansey and Christie, *Looking at the Unborn*, 39–42; Nicolson and Fleming, *Imaging and Imagining the Fetus*, 229–33. Routine ultrasound screening of pregnant women was for the first time—arguably worldwide—introduced in 1973 at Malmö Municipal Hospital, which was closely connected with Lund University. Marčál and Sundén, 'Development of Ultrasound,' 54–55; Grennert, Persson, and Gennser, 'Benefits of Ultrasonic Screening.'

77 Sundén, 'Obstetrisk ultraljudsdiagnostik.'

78 Jörgensen et al., 'Diagnostic Ultrasound.'

8 Conclusion

In this chapter, I have shown how the early adoption and development of ultrasound imaging in Lund was enabled by a number of coinciding factors. A precondition was that the key actor, Bertil Sundén, could get access to women who were scheduled to have abortions for 'safe' experiments at the women's clinic at Lund Hospital. Significantly, Sundén was not alone in his interest in new diagnostic technologies at Lund University and Lund Hospital; colleagues such as Alf Sjövall, Hellmuth Hertz, and Lars Leksell helped pave the way for his experiments and contributed to a culture that was willing to embrace new technologies. Sjövall also provided a crucial link to Ian Donald in Glasgow, where the technology of ultrasound imaging was first developed. Crucially too, Sundén managed to secure the money needed for a rather costly technological transfer.

However, these early adoptions, as well as the further development and establishment of obstetric ultrasound imaging in Sweden, were also dependent on Sundén's ability to navigate between different discourses of risk. One was a preexisting discourse on the dangers of X-rays and other kinds of ionizing radiation. Another was attached to ultrasound itself. As Sundén's research moved on, he also had to deal with a more general discourse on medical risks, triggered by the thalidomide scandal in the early 1960s and, later on, a discourse on ultrasound and other means of prenatal diagnosis as methods for risk management. Sometimes, successful navigation meant steering away from risk narratives, and sometimes, taking advantage of them—until, at the brink of the 1980s, diagnostic ultrasound imaging was ready to be launched and marketed to mothers-to-be as a routine and harmless prenatal procedure.[79]

Bibliography

American Institute of Ultrasound in Medicine. 'As Low as Reasonably Achievable (ALARA) Principle.' Last modified May 19, 2020. https://www.aium.org/resources/official-statements/view/as-low-as-reasonably-achievable-(alara)-principle.

Beck, Ulrich. *Risk Society: Towards a New Modernity*. London: Sage, 1992.

Berg, Annika. '"Det vita ljudet": Ultraljud som synestetisk teknologi.' In *Sinnen i arbete*, edited by Daniel Normark and Ingemar Pettersson. Lund: Arkiv förlag, 2024.

79 Also cf. Lele, 'Revue,' 318–19.

Berg, Annika. 'Rays of Death and Visions of Life: Ultrasound Narratives, Risk Evaluations, and Prenatal Imaging.' *Technology and Culture* 65, no. 3 (2024): 933–65.

Brynner, Rock, and Trent Stephens. *Dark Remedy: The Impact of Thalidomide and Its Revival as a Vital Medicine*. New York: Basic Books, 2001.

'Dagens namn: Hellmuth Hertz, idéspruta med bläckspruta.' *Dagens Nyheter*, April 15, 1970.

Dijck, José van. *The Transparent Body: A Cultural Analysis of Medical Imaging*. Seattle: University of Washington Press, 2004.

'Dödad "dödsstråle."' *Dagens Nyheter*, September 13, 1940.

Donald, Ian. 'Abortion and the Obstetrician.' *The Lancet* 297, no. 7711 (1971): 1233.

Donald, I., and U. Abdulla. 'Placentography by Sonar.' *Journal of Obstetrics and Gynaecology of the British Commonwealth* 75, no. 10 (1968): 993–1006.

Donald, Ian, J. MacVicar, and T. G. Brown. 'Investigation of Abdominal Masses by Pulsed Ultrasound.' *The Lancet* 271, no. 7032 (1958): 1188–95.

'Dr Lindströms metod är "revolutionerande."' *Svenska Dagbladet*, September 2, 1953.

Dry, Sarah. 'The Population as Patient: Alice Stewart and the Controversy over Low-Level Radiation in the 1950s.' In *The Risks of Medical Innovation: Risk Perception and Assessment in Historical Context*, edited by Thomas Schlich and Ulrich Tröhler, 108–22. London and New York: Routledge, 2006.

Duden, Barbara. *Disembodying Women: Perspectives on Pregnancy and the Unborn*. Cambridge, MA: Harvard University Press, 1993.

Eklöf, Bo, Kjell Lindström, and Stig Persson, eds. *Ultrasound in Clinical Diagnosis: From Pioneering Developments in Lund to Global Application in Medicine*. Oxford: Oxford University Press, 2012.

'Ekolodning i hjärnan kan påvisa blödning.' *Dagens Nyheter*, July 5, 1957.

'Engelsk radioman avslöjar fosters kön med ny apparat.' *Dagens Nyheter*, January 4, 1951.

Flam, Folke. 'Laparoskopi inom gynekologin: För- och nackdelar, vilket väger tyngst?' *Läkartidningen* 94, no. 40 (1997): 3496–500.

Grennert, Lars, Per-Håkan Persson, and Gerhard Gennser. 'Benefits of Ultrasonic Screening of a Pregnant Population.' *Acta Obstetricia et Gynecologica Scandinavica* 57, suppl. 78 (1978): 5–14.

Hellman, Louis M., Gillian M. Duffus, Ian Donald, and Bertil Sundén. 'Safety of Diagnostic Ultrasound in Obstetrics.' *The Lancet* 295, no. 7657 (1970): 1133–35.

Holmberg, Carl Bertil. 'Ljudet som inte hörs.' *Svenska Dagbladet*, February 6, 1938.

Jörgensen, Connie, Johannes Skjaerris, Bertil Sundén, and Anders Åberg. 'Diagnostic Ultrasound in Threatened Abortion and Suspected Ectopic Pregnancy.' *Acta Obstetricia et Gynecologica Scandinavica* 59, no. 3 (1980): 233–35.

Karsberg, Arne. '"Explosionsutveckling" i medicinsk elektronik.' *Dagens Nyheter*, October 18, 1967.

Karsberg, Arne. 'Ny fotokopiering spar silver.' *Dagens Nyheter*, June 7, 1969.

Kollman, Christian, Klaus-Vitold Jenderka, Carmel M. Moran, Ferdinando Draghi, J. F. Jimenez Diaz, and Ragnar Sande. 'EFSUMB Clinical Safety Statement for Diagnostic Ultrasound—(2019 revision).' *Ultraschall in der Medizin* 41, no. 4 (2020): 387–89.

Leksell, Lars. 'Echo-Encephalography: I. Detection of Intracranial Complications Following Head Injury.' *Acta Chirurgica Scandinavica* 110, no. 4 (1955): 301–15.

Lele, Padmakar P. 'Revue: Safety and Potential Hazards in the Current Applications of Ultrasound in Obstetrics and Gynecology.' *Ultrasound in Medicine & Biology* 5, no. 4 (1979): 307–20.

'Ljud som dödar, nytt vapen i USA.' *Svenska Dagbladet*, December 2, 1947.

Löwy, Ilana. *Imperfect Pregnancies: A History of Birth Defects and Prenatal Diagnosis*. Baltimore: Johns Hopkins University Press, 2017.

Löwy, Ilana. *Tangled Diagnoses: Prenatal Diagnosis, Women, and Risk*. Chicago: University of Chicago Press, 2018.

Lunsford, L. Dade. 'Lars Leksell: Notes at the Side of a Raconteur.' *Stereotactic and Functional Neurosurgery* 67, no. 3–4 (1996–97): 153–68.

Lupton, Deborah. 'Risk as Moral Danger: The Social and Political Functions of Risk Discourse in Public Health.' *International Journal of Health Services* 23, no. 3 (1993): 425–35.

Lupton, Deborah. *The Social Worlds of the Unborn*. Basingstoke: Palgrave Macmillan, 2013.

Macintosh, I. J. C., and D. A. Davey. 'Chromosome Aberrations Induced by an Ultrasonic Fetal Pulse Detector.' *British Medical Journal* 4, no. 5727 (1970): 92–93.

Marčál, Karel, and Bertil Sundén. 'The Development of Ultrasound in Obstetrics and Gynecology in Sweden.' In *Ultrasound in Clinical Diagnosis: From Pioneering Developments in Lund to Global Application in Medicine*, edited by Bo Eklöf, Kjell Lindström, and Stig Persson, 50–62. Oxford: Oxford University Press, 2012.

Nicolson, Malcolm, and John E. E. Fleming. *Imaging and Imagining the Fetus: The Development of Obstetric Ultrasound*. Baltimore: Johns Hopkins University Press, 2013.

Nordisk medicin 59, no. 5 (1958): 827–88. [Special issue on ionizing radiation and radiation damage.]

Oakley, Ann. *The Captured Womb: A History of the Medical Care of Pregnant Women*. Oxford: Blackwell, 1984.

Persson, Stig, Jan Eskilsson, and Nils-Rune Lundström. 'The Development of Echocardiography in Sweden.' In *Ultrasound in Clinical Diagnosis: From Pioneering Developments in Lund to Global Application in Medicine*, edited by Bo Eklöf, Kjell Lindström, and Stig Persson, 8–20. Oxford: Oxford University Press, 2012.

Petchesky, Rosalind Pollack. 'Fetal Images: The Power of Visual Culture in the Politics of Reproduction.' *Feminist Studies* 13, no. 2 (1987): 263–92.

Peter [pseud.]. 'Ohörbart ljud botar magsår, gör Eau de Vie till Martell.' *Svenska Dagbladet*, May 28, 1950.

'"Rent luckförsvar räcker ej": Marktrupper härdigast mot stormakt, tror "radiomajoren" såsom överste.' *Dagens Nyheter*, January 7, 1948.

Roberts, Julie. *The Visualised Foetus: A Cultural and Political Analysis of Ultrasound Imagery*. London: Routledge, 2012.

Samuelsson, Stig, and Alf Sjövall. 'Laparoscopy in Suspected Ectopic Pregnancy.' *Acta Obstetricia et Gynecologica Scandinavica* 51, no. 1 (1972): 31–35.

Schlich, Thomas. 'Risk and Medical Innovation: A Historical Perspective.' In *The Risks of Medical Innovation: Risk Perception and Assessment in Historical Context*, edited by Thomas Schlich and Ulrich Tröhler, 1–17. London and New York: Routledge, 2006.

Sjöström, Henning, and Robert Nilsson. *Thalidomide and the Power of the Drug Companies*. Harmondsworth: Penguin Books, 1972.

Sjövall, Alf. 'Operationsteknik vid havandeskapsavbrytande.' *Svenska läkartidningen* 45, no. 16 (1948): 753–57.

Ståhl, Katrin. 'Bertil Sundén tilldelas Professors namn av regeringen.' Published October 24, 2013. https://www.lu.se/artikel/bertil-sunden-tilldelas-professors-namn-av-regeringen.

Stewart, Alice, Josefine Webb, Dawn Giles, and David Hewitt. 'Preliminary Communication: Malignant Disease in Childhood and Diagnostic Irradiation In Utero.' *The Lancet* 268, no. 6940 (1956): 447.

Sundén, Bertil. 'Obstetric Diagnosis with Ultrasound.' *Ultrasonics* 5, no. 2 (1967): 67–71.

Sundén, Bertil. 'Obstetrisk ultraljudsdiagnostik.' *Läkartidningen* 74, no. 6 (1977): 431–33.

Sundén, Bertil. 'On the Diagnostic Value of Ultrasound in Obstetrics and Gynaecology.' *Acta Obstetricia et Gynecologica Scandinavica* 43, suppl. 6 (1964): 1–191.

Sundén, Bertil. 'Placentography by Ultrasound.' *Acta Obstetricia et Gynecologica Scandinavica* 49, no. 2 (1970): 179–84.

Sundén, Bertil. 'Ultraljudsdiagnostik i obstetrik och gynekologi.' *Svenska läkartidningen* 57, no. 11 (1960): 769–82.

Sundén, Bertil. 'Ultrasonic Placentography.' *Acta Obstetricia et Gynecologica Scandinavica* 48, suppl. 3 (1969): 161–63.

Swedish Radiation Safety Authority. 'Ultraljudsundersökning vid graviditet.' Last modified February 14, 2018. https://www.stralsakerhetsmyndigheten.se/omraden/stralning-i-varden/berattigande-och-optimering/ultraljudsundersokning-vid-graviditet/.

Tansey, E. M., and D. A. Christie, eds. *Looking at the Unborn: Historical Aspects of Obstetric Ultrasound; A Witness Seminar Held at the Wellcome Institute for the History of Medicine, London, on 10 March 1998*. London: Wellcome Trust, 2000.

'Tårgas, epilepsi senaste vapnen rädda gisslan.' *Dagens Nyheter*, August 28, 1973.

Taylor, E. S., J. H. Holmes, H. E. Thompson, and K. R. Gottesfeld. 'Ultrasonic Placentography: A New Method for Placental Localization.' *American Journal of Obstetrics and Gynecology* 96, no. 4 (1966): 538–47.

Taylor, Janelle S. *The Public Life of the Fetal Sonogram: Technology, Consumption, and the Politics of Reproduction*. New Brunswick, NJ, and London: Rutgers University Press, 2008.

US Food and Drug Administration. 'Ultrasound Imaging.' Last modified January 12, 2024. www.fda.gov/radiation-emitting-products/medical-imaging/ultrasound-imaging.

Westling, Håkan. 'Ultrasound in Lund: Three World Premieres.' In *Ultrasound in Clinical Diagnosis: From Pioneering Developments in Lund to Global Application in Medicine*, edited by Bo Eklöf, Kjell Lindström, and Stig Persson, 1–7. Oxford: Oxford University Press, 2012.

Wolf, Jaqueline H. *Cesarean Section: An American History of Risk, Technology and Consequence*. Baltimore: Johns Hopkins University Press, 2018.

Archival Sources

Bergman, Per. Written statement to the Medical Research Council, August 11, 1959. F1:231, Application documents, 1955–1965. MRC.

Ingelman-Sundberg, Axel. Written statement to the Swedish Medical Research Council, April 8, 1963. F1:231, Application documents, 1955–1965. MRC.

Leksell, Lars, and Alf Sjövall to the Medical Research Council. Recommendation letter, May 21, 1959. F1:231, Application documents, 1955–1965. MRC.

Medical Research Council to Bertil Sundén. Decision letter, March 30, 1960. F1:231, Application documents, 1955–1965. MRC.

Medical Research Council to Bertil Sundén. Decision letter, May 6, 1963. F1:231, Application documents, 1955–1965. MRC.

Protocols of the Lund University Hospital board. A1A:57–66, Protocols 1958–1964. LUH.

Sundén, Bertil. Grant application to the Medical Research Council. May 21, 1959. F1:231, Application documents, 1955–1965. MRC.

Sundén, Bertil. Grant application to the Medical Research Council. December 29, 1959. F1:231, Application documents, 1955–1965. MRC.

Sundén, Bertil. 'Ultraljudsdiagnostik i obstetrik och gynekologi.' Article manuscript attached to grant application, December 29, 1959. F1:231, Application documents, 1955–1965. MRC.

Sundén, Bertil. Grant application to the Medical Research Council. March 11, 1963. F1:231, Application documents, 1955–1965. MRC.

Sundén, Bertil. Grant application to the Medical Research Council, March 12, 1964. F1:231, Application documents, 1955–1965. MRC.

Teorell, Torsten. Written statement to the Medical Research Council, March 8, 1960. F1:231, Application documents, 1955–1965. MRC.

Teorell, Torsten. Written statement to the Medical Research Council, April 22, 1964. F1:231, Application documents, 1955–1965. MRC.

CHAPTER 13

Visual Wonders and Shocks: Images of Human Fetuses in Television Programs on Abortion and Fetal Research, 1969–1988

Elisabet Björklund

The 1960s are often described as the beginning of a new visual culture of the fetus in the Western world. With the publication of Swedish photographer Lennart Nilsson's images of human embryos and fetuses in the American *Life* magazine and the best-selling book *Ett barn blir till* (*A Child Is Born*) in 1965, as well as the breakthrough of ultrasound in maternity care during subsequent decades, images of fetuses increasingly became part of the public sphere.[1] In the late 1980s and early 1990s, feminist scholars started to use the concept of 'the public fetus' to describe this growing production of images of the unborn and their dissemination in the media and elsewhere. They regarded this development critically because of its potential negative consequences for women's reproductive rights. For instance, fetal images—not least the ones by Nilsson—were widely mobilized in anti-abortion campaigns.[2]

However, this historiography has also been criticized, particularly by scholars demonstrating that visualizations of embryos and fetuses have a much longer history.[3] Moreover, it has been argued that discussions of 'the public fetus' have largely focused on the United States, without accounting for other cultural contexts. For instance, Nilsson's images have a complex history in Sweden. While they have mostly been associated with progressive sex education, Solveig Jülich has shown that they were used in Swedish anti-abortion campaigns before they were published in *A Child Is Born* and achieved their international breakthrough. Hence, the meanings of the images have shifted greatly depending on their historical and cultural context.[4]

1 See, e.g., Lupton, *Social Worlds of the Unborn*, 33–51. For an analysis of the production of Lennart Nilsson's *A Child Is Born*, see Jülich, 'Making of a Best-Selling Book.'

2 For a historiographic overview and discussion of this research, see Jülich and Björklund, 'Public Fetus.'

3 Hopwood, 'Producing Development'; Hopwood, *Haeckel's Embryos*; Dubow, *Ourselves Unborn*; Björklund and Jülich, *Rethinking the Public Fetus*.

4 Jülich, 'Picturing Abortion Opposition'; Jülich, 'Fetal Photography.' For more on Nilsson's images in school sex-education films, see Björklund, *Most Delicate Subject*, chap. 5, esp. 283–84.

 | DOI:10.1163/9789004703759_015

This chapter provides further nuances to these discussions by exploring the uses and reception of images of fetuses in a specific medium and historical framework: Swedish television programs on abortion and fetal research in the period from the late 1960s to the late 1980s. This was a time of change within politics, medicine, and the media. Swedish abortion legislation was hotly debated in the early 1960s, which sparked a process that eventually led to the introduction of abortion on demand in 1975.[5] Alongside this development, the related and controversial issue of fetal research received attention through various media debates and investigations.[6] Moreover, the media landscape was transformed as television was introduced in the late 1950s and rapidly grew in popularity. Drawing on previous research on fetal imagery during this time period, I explore how the sensitive issue of research on human fetuses was brought into the public realm through television and how the medium's visual character was handled in these programs.

More specifically, I am interested in how these depictions related to larger shifts in media representations of human fetuses. Scholars who have examined the visual culture of the fetus during the second half of the twentieth century have demonstrated how two contrasting ways of depicting human fetuses became dominant during this era. On the one hand, the fetus was represented as alive through photographs like those in American science writer Geraldine Lux Flanagan's pregnancy guide *The First Nine Months of Life* (1962) and Nilsson's images. On the other, the fetus was depicted as dead, through so-called 'war pictures'—gruesome images of aborted fetuses that the US anti-abortion movement began to distribute in the wake of *Roe v. Wade* (1973).[7] While the former type of image has been analyzed as using an aesthetic that creates a sense of wonder in the spectator and making the fetus symbolically represent 'life,' the latter can be understood as having the opposite aim: to show a particular dead or dying fetus and thereby create feelings of shock, disgust, and sadness in the viewer.[8] It has been argued that these

For a discussion of Nilsson's images in Franco's Spain, see Santesmases, 'Public Fetus in Franco's Spain.'

5 Swärd, *Varför Sverige fick fri abort*; Lennerhed, *Frihet att njuta*, 141–45; Lennerhed, 'Sherri Finkbine's Choice.'

6 Jülich, 'Fosterexperimentens produktiva hemlighet.'

7 Morgan, *Icons of Life*; Gorney, *Articles of Faith*, 99–106; Hughes, 'Burning Birth Certificates,' 553. Representations of fetuses as beautiful, living babies did exist earlier. Rose Holz has analyzed the widespread series of sculptures called *The Birth Series*, which depicted the fetus in this way in the late 1930s. See Holz, 'Biological Bodies, Unfettered Imaginations.'

8 Franklin, Lury, and Stacey, *Global Nature, Global Culture*, 33–36; Stormer, 'Looking in Wonder'; Hughes, 'Burning Birth Certificates.'

opposing representational strategies have left little room for seeing the fetus in other ways. Lynn Morgan claims that the efforts of anti-abortion groups in the United States to equate dead fetuses with abortion have created a polarized divide between depictions of human fetuses as either 'icons of life' or 'specters of death,' giving rise to a taboo around dead fetuses.[9] 'According to this ideology,' she writes, 'there are only two kinds of fetuses: "good" ones that represent life, beauty, innocence, and our collective well-being, and "bad" ones that are unattractive, morally polluting, ethically suspect, and make us squeamish.'[10]

By paying attention to these different ways of representing fetuses in Swedish television and the discussions they provoked, this chapter demonstrates that representations clearly showing the fetus as dead or dying were increasingly problematized in Sweden following the 1960s. This is similar to the development that Morgan discusses in the United States, but there are also important differences between the two contexts. I argue that at a time when 'the political attack on abortion rights moved further into the terrain of mass culture and imagery' in the United States, with films like *The Silent Scream* (Dabner, 1984) airing on major US television networks, as discussed by Rosalind Petchesky,[11] mainstream Swedish media denounced explicit depictions of dead fetuses. Furthermore, I claim that this distancing was connected with a growing tendency to associate this type of imagery precisely with US anti-abortion activism. Not only did Nilsson's images travel across borders during this era, but images from the US media also circulated in Sweden. However, in the discussions around these images, one can note how the Swedish images were generally understood as 'good' and the American ones as 'bad.' Hence, the chapter contributes to international research emphasizing the need to study the circulation of images across different media and national contexts, and to understand anti-abortion activism as a transnational phenomenon.[12]

The material used in this chapter was located through searches in the database of the broadcasting company Swedish Television, while the most relevant programs found through these searches were made available by the National Library of Sweden. While searches using very general key words (like 'fetus' and 'abortion') were initially made to obtain an overview of the material, I eventually chose to focus on a number of documentary programs in which research

9 Morgan, *Icons of Life*, 29–31, 228.

10 Morgan, *Icons of Life*, 232.

11 Petchesky, 'Fetal Images,' 263. For a detailed account of the 'public fetus' in the United States, see Hopwood, 'Visual Strategies.'

12 Hopwood, *Haeckel's Embryos*; Slattery, 'Building a "World Coalition for Life"'; Kuźma-Markowska and Kelly, 'Anti-abortion Activism in Poland.'

on human fetuses is a clear topic. They include medical documentaries and programs on societal issues as well as some news programs.

In the first section of this chapter, I briefly introduce the context of Swedish television, early medical television programs, and images of human fetuses in 1960s audiovisual media. The second section provides an analysis of the use of fetal images in a controversial television program on abortion broadcast in 1969. This is followed by a section discussing fetal imagery in television and in Swedish visual culture in the 1970s and 1980s more broadly. The last section offers an analysis of fetal images in three programs on fetal research made in the 1980s.

1 Early Swedish Television, Medical Programs, and Fetal Imagery

During the period studied here, television was a medium with huge impact in both Europe and the United States, which is explained by its wide reach but still limited number of channels.[13] This was clearly the case in the Swedish context, as there was only one television channel between 1956, when regular broadcasts began, and 1969, and only two in the period until the late 1980s. Television's spread was also rapid in Sweden, surpassed only by the United States. By the late 1960s, 83 percent of Swedish households owned a television set.[14] In the 1970s, television reached almost everyone.[15] This makes it a crucial medium to study when discussing visual culture from the 1960s onward.

But it is also important to highlight the specificity of different national media contexts. Television in Sweden was a public service institution, modeled on the British Broadcasting Corporation (BBC), meaning that it had goals and ideals connected to education, democracy, and independence.[16] This, of course, influenced how controversial issues such as abortion and fetal research could be handled. Moreover, Swedish television underwent important transformations during its first three decades. Not only did it change aesthetically (with, for example, black and white being replaced by color during the 1970s), but it also can be seen to have shifted in perspective, with the more paternalistic mode that characterized its early years giving way to an increased focus on social critique in the late 1960s and early 1970s.[17] Toward the end of the

13 von Hodenberg, *Television's Moment*, 75.
14 Höijer, *Det hörde vi allihop!*, 198.
15 Höijer, *Det hörde vi allihop!*, 216.
16 Weibull, 'New Media,' 41–45.
17 Furhammar, 'From Affluence to Poverty.'

1980s, cable and satellite television posed increasing competition, ultimately breaking the monopoly held by the public service company.[18] Nevertheless, the two public service channels remained the most popular until the early 1990s.[19]

Medical topics became part of television programming relatively early and reached audiences through a variety of formats. Among them were various types of medical documentaries, educational programs with different physicians in the spotlight, and more critical journalistic reports. The visual character of television was exploited at an early stage, not least by many programs showing explicit scenes of surgical procedures. Programs visualizing births were also relatively common. For instance, a program on how children take their first breath after being born, coproduced with the BBC, was shown as early as 1961. Scenes like these were not confined to television, however. The relationship between television and other media, especially the press, was close, and images frequently traveled between them. Upcoming television programs were announced in the magazine *Röster i radio-tv* (Voices in radio-TV), where pictures from the programs were often printed in articles to raise interest, and newspapers and the tabloid press treated television programs as news to report on. Hence, spectacular medical images from television programs could often be seen in various other media as well.[20]

But images also traveled the other way—from printed media to moving images. As discussed above, photographic images of fetuses were spreading during this period, and Nilsson's images from *A Child Is Born* were reused in many other media forms, among them film and television.[21] The most well-known example is the film *Så börjar livet* (*The Beginning of Life: A Documentary*), which narrated the course of fertilization and fetal development until birth and was based almost entirely on these images. The film was aired on Swedish television in 1965 and was distributed internationally.[22] Nilsson's pictures also appeared in a school television program called *Så kom du till* (How you were made), broadcast in 1966, and in the films *Barnet* (The child, Håkan Cronsioe, 1967) and *Ett barn blir till* (A child is born, Thomas Hellberg, 1974), which were distributed to Swedish schools.[23] Through television, moving images of biological processes thus became a familiar phenomenon in the 1960s and 1970s, and the medium was, furthermore, one among many in which

---

18 Furhammar, *Sex, såpor och svenska krusbär*, 20–21.

19 Höijer, *Det hörde vi allihop!*, 262–63.

20 See Björklund, 'Medicinens och televisionens ögonblick.'

21 Jülich, 'Fetal Photography,' 130–33.

22 For a discussion of this film, see Jülich, 'Televising Inner Space.' See also Hopwood, 'Visual Strategies.'

23 Björklund, *Most Delicate Subject*, 281–87.

images of fetuses were disseminated. To my knowledge, however, television seldom displayed fetal images in connection with abortion until the late 1960s.

2 1969—Abortion on Television

On the evening of October 15, 1969, a program titled *Abort: Fakta och synpunkter om avbrytande av havandeskap* (Abortion: Facts and opinions about terminating pregnancy) was broadcast on Sweden's only television channel, causing widespread controversy.[24] The program presented information about the Abortion Act and the procedures for having a legal abortion through voice-over, staged scenes of a woman applying for abortion, and interviews with medical doctors and social workers, but also included explicit and authentic scenes demonstrating different abortion methods. The scene perceived as the most upsetting showed an abdominal hysterotomy, an abortion method used in the second trimester, in which a fetus of seventeen to eighteen weeks was aborted through 'small cesarean section' and displayed in close-up after being put in a metal kidney dish. This scene was furthermore closely linked with a sequence in which the delicate issue of research on human fetuses was discussed. Before the broadcast, newspapers had warned sensitive viewers, but the program nevertheless triggered strong reactions.[25]

This program is significant for two main reasons: First, because of its explicit depiction of a fetus being aborted in the mainstream media. This was not the first time an abortion had been shown in moving images in Sweden. In 1952, there was a minor scandal when an uncensored medical film of an abortion was screened at a public debate on the abortion issue in the city of Uppsala. However, only around 250 people had been present at the meeting, a very small audience compared with the number of television viewers on an ordinary evening in the late 1960s.[26] Abortion had also been represented on television. Various shows, from news and debate programs to TV-theater plays, had dealt with the controversial issue since the late 1950s.[27] A real abortion procedure had also been shown. In 1966, almost exactly three years before *Abort*, *Ronden* had aired an episode in which an abortion through dilation and curettage was demonstrated.[28] This depiction was, however, not very explicit.

---

24 *Abort.*

25 Steen, 'TV varnar'; Gadd, 'Abort-chock.'

26 Jülich, 'Picturing Abortion Opposition,' 288–89.

27 Björklund, 'Waiting for Abortion.'

28 *Ronden.*

The physician was filmed in a medium shot from the side with the camera placed so that only the patient's leg in the gynecological chair was slightly visible to the right in the frame, and only glimpses of the fetal parts could be seen as they were quickly removed and put away off-screen. In contrast to these examples, *Abort* was both widely seen and very graphic.

Second, *Abort* appeared at a critical point in time. In the early 1960s, a substantial debate on abortion had started in the Swedish media, as liberal and social democratic youth and student organizations began to question the existing Abortion Act. A governmental abortion committee was commissioned in 1965 and was expected to present its conclusions during the fall of 1969, which was the reason for making the program at this particular point, although the committee's report was delayed until 1971.[29] Moreover, research on living fetuses had been the subject of debate for some time, and a report to the Parliamentary Ombudsman had recently been made to investigate the issue.[30] When *Abort* was broadcast, it was thus part of an ongoing media discussion of abortion and fetal knowledge production.

The program begins and ends with an image of a fetus in close-up, as a heartbeat is heard on the soundtrack, putting the fetus at the center of concern. Although the origins of this image are not stated, it reminds the viewer of Lennart Nilsson's images of fetuses. Moreover, the heartbeat clearly constructs a connection between the image and a conception of life. It is not clear whether the heartbeat is supposed to be that of the fetus or the pregnant woman. If understood as the heartbeat of the fetus, it is slower than normal and must be understood symbolically rather than realistically. If interpreted as the heartbeat of the pregnant woman, on the other hand, the viewer is positioned as sharing the perspective of the fetus. In both cases, the heartbeat clearly represents the fetus as alive, by ascribing to it either a beating heart or the sense of hearing.

The inclusion and repetition of this scene create a sharp contrast to the other fetal representation in the program—the one of the fetus aborted through hysterotomy. While the image in the beginning of the program symbolizes life in general, the other images represent a particular dying fetus. The circumstances of the abortion are never revealed, and the scene is not placed within a fictional narrative, but the context of the images renders the fetus concrete rather than abstract—we have seen it being lifted from the uterus in the amniotic sac and placed in a dish. In contrast to the other fetal image, it is clear that this fetus has been aborted. The cinematography itself supports this—camera

29 Steen, 'TV varnar'; Swedish Ministry of Justice, *Rätten till abort*.

30 Jülich, 'Fosterexperimentens produktiva hemlighet,' 27–32.

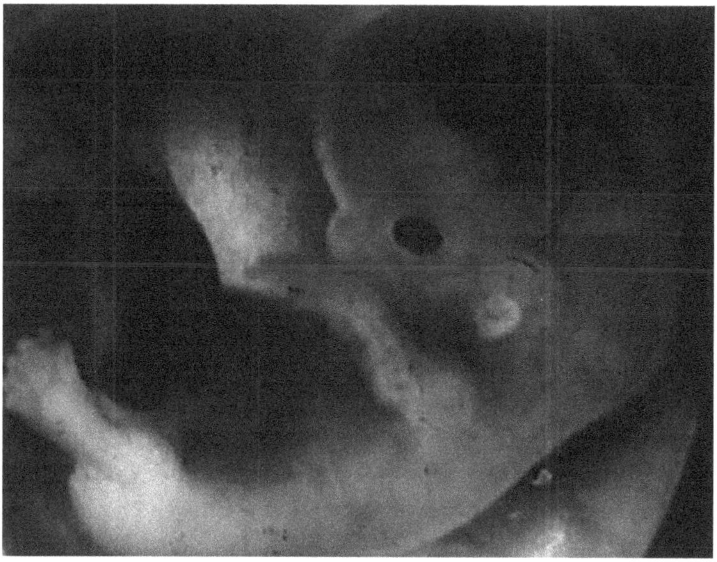

FIGURE 13.1 The fetus accompanied by the sound of a beating heart in the beginning of the controversial television program *Abort* broadcasted in 1969.

movements changing the framing and the use of a zoom lens make the viewer aware that the camera is present at the surgery. The sterile environment further contributes to the impact of the scene. The fetus at the beginning and end of the program is shown in close-up, filling the whole frame, thus creating the impression that it is embedded in the uterus. In stark contrast, the images of the aborted fetus show it being handled by gloved hands and put into a metal container.

The structure of the program is also significant. In contrast to the other abortion methods demonstrated—vacuum aspiration, dilation and curettage, and saline injection—the hysterotomy is placed at the end of the program, thus becoming its dramaturgical climax.[31] This is followed by a sequence in which first gynecologist Irma Wright and then pediatrician Olov Celander are interviewed about the issue of abortions mistakenly performed too late (after

31 In dilation and curettage, the cervix is dilated, and the physician then uses various instruments to evacuate the uterus. From the early 1960s, this method was gradually replaced by the new technique of vacuum aspiration, in which a tube connected to a suction pump is used for the evacuation instead. In saline injection, which was also a new method during this era but used for later abortions, saline is injected into the uterus, causing a miscarriage. See Ramsey, *Swedish Abortion Pill*, 49–50; Swedish Ministry of Justice, *Rätten till abort*, 39–40, 44–47.

week twenty-four). The doctors describe the very rare situation in which the length of the pregnancy has been miscalculated and the aborted fetus shows signs that it might survive outside the womb, and how the doctors in those cases have tried to save its life, but never succeeded. In this sequence, images of a premature child in an incubator are also displayed as Celander describes the small chances that a child born extremely early will survive (10 percent of the children born at week twenty-eight, he says) and the problems that arise for those who do. This is followed by a sequence about fetal research. Here, Professor Astrid Fagraeus and Sven Erik Svehag from the National Bacteriological Laboratory talk about different uses of fetal tissue and organs—such as diagnosis of virological and immunological diseases, hormone and vaccine research, and the production of serums used in organ transplantations—followed by neurologist Olof Gilland, who addresses whether or not aborted fetuses feel pain. Gilland's conclusion is that there is no certainty around the issue of when pain develops, but that in his opinion a fetus should have the same rights as any person as long as it is alive. Gilland's voice forms a sound bridge as images of the fetus in the kidney dish are intercut with the interview. The structuring of these three sequences, together with the editing choices, creates a suggestive chain of associations connecting the thought of fetuses being used for scientific purposes while still alive and possibly in pain with the emotional effects evoked by the images of an actual abortion and of a small premature child.

While this reading interprets the program as critical of abortion, the contemporary reception was actually divided. The program was described in the press as a 'shock' for viewers, and adjectives such as 'horrible,' 'nasty,' 'deterrent,' and 'repulsive' were used about the images.[32] Some reviewers, on the other hand, found the program to be balanced and expressed positive opinions about it.[33] This view was also shared by a number of executives at the broadcasting enterprise Swedish Radio. When the program was discussed at a meeting with the manager, three out of four people who shared their opinions stated that they found it neutral and nuanced.[34] Several commentators in the press, however, interpreted it as critical of abortion, and three representatives of the feminist organization Grupp 8 also reported it to the Radio Committee for being biased. The committee did not share this interpretation.[35]

32 Gadd, 'Abort-chock'; Öhlander, 'Så upplevde'; Ramsby, 'En chock för TV-tittarna'; Sten, 'Bilderna i går.'

33 Jolanta, 'Balanserat om abort.'

34 Minutes from the manager's program meeting.

35 Steen, 'TV varnar'; Bolinder, Svanberg, and Åkerstedt, report to Radionämnden; Radionämnden to Bolinder, Svanberg, and Åkerstedt. The Radio Committee was a

EXPRESSEN ★ Torsdagen den 16 oktober 1969 7

Bilden av ett 18 veckor gammalt foster — placerat i en rondskål

EN CHOCK FÖR TV-TITTARNA

Av ÅGE RAMSBY

TV:s abortprogram blev ett skrämselprogram. Bilden som chockade ser ni här intill — fostret i rondskålen. En 18 veckor gammal människa . . .

Bilden av fostret som togs ur livmoderhålan var den mest dramatiska sekvensen i TV-filmen.

Under några korta sekunder, när fostret lyftes ut och placerades i rondskålen, syntes det tydligt hur det andades.

De två forskarna, professor Astrid Fagreus och laborator Sven-Eric Svehag, Statens bakteriologiska laboratorium, är oroliga i dag:

Risk för missförstånd

— Risken för att TV-publiken missförstod oss är stor, säger professor Fagreus. Vi var inte heller så väl förberedda.

— Frågan om fostret känner smärta kom som en fullständig överraskning. Sånt är jag inte expert på.

— Värst är om folk tror att vi använder levande foster för experiment. Så är det inte.

— Men vi behöver fostervävnaden så tidigt som möjligt. Fostren får inte ha varit döda i mer än någon timme.

— Det är rätt i så måtto att fostren kan vara levande när de tas ut genom ett kejsarsnittingrepp.

Det var en lurig fråga professor Fagreus fick om levande foster. Den löd ordagrant så här:

Forskning på levande foster?

— Känner ni till om man bedriver någon ytterligare forskning här i landet på levande foster?

Professor Fagreus svarade ordagrant så här:

— Ja, den hormonala förstås och sen har vi den neurologiska.

Det vill säga, det är under fosterlivet som nervceller utbildas, och sen ett viktigt forskningsområde är ju vilka ämnen som passerar genom moderkakan från modern till fostret och tvärtom . . .

Laborator Svehag om fosterorgan:

— Vi har mycket svårt att få tag i tillräckligt med organ från mänskliga foster — det är väldigt ont om dem.

— Vi har en så svår situation att vi måste söka oss till andra djurslag, apa företrädesvis, för att se om vi kan ersätta den mänskliga vävnaden med apvävnad. I vissa fall går det i andra inte alls . . .

Nu vädjar forskarna om att ingen ska missförstå dem. Professor Fagreus:

— Det är ont om fostervävnad i dag, men det beror på att man numera i större utsträckning använder en annan abortteknik, nämligen koksaltsinsprutning i stället för genom kejsarsnitt!

— Jag trodde inte jag behövde gå in på aborttekniken. Jag fann det självklart som bakgrund till att det är ont om fostervävnad.

— Ingen ska tro att vi nu önskar flera aborter bara för att få mer fostervävnad.

— Personligen uppfattade jag programmet i sin helhet som en väckarklocka för alla dem som håller på med abortärenden.

— Bilden av det aborterade fostret i rondskålen hade nog en våldsam effekt på många tittare. En ytterst kärv information.

"Vi känner oss som mördare!"

GÖTEBORG (Expressen). — Vi känner oss som mördare efter TV-programmet. Så ringde och berättade uppskakade kvinnor efter TV-programmet i går kväll. Sveriges Radio fick efter sändningen flera samtal från upprörda kvinnor som någon gång själva upplevt en abort och nu via TV fick uppleva alla fruktansvärda kval igen. Karl-Axel Jansson, informationschef på Sveriges Radio i Göteborg:

— Det var nog tur att vi informerade tittarna om programmets innehåll i förväg.

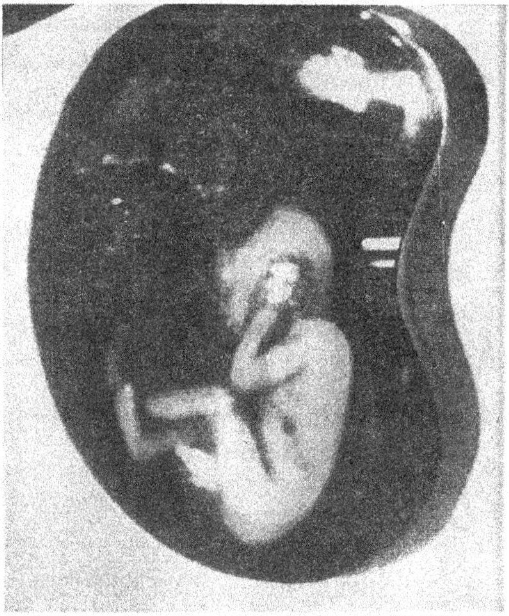

Ett 18-veckors foster i en rondskål. Kvinnan som opererades var flerbarnsmor. Det fanns risk för att hon inte skulle klara av ett nytt havandeskap, berättar docent Göran Rybo vid Sahlgrenska sjukhuset i Göteborg. Det var han som gjorde aborten. Kvinnan är i 40-årsåldern. Hon gav själv sitt medgivande till TV-producenten Birgitta Bergman att filma aborten.

Bilderna i går de ruskigaste jag sett i TV

Hemming Sten

Bilderna i TV:s abortprogram var otäcka och frånstötande och helt meningslösa — om de inte visades i avskräckande syfte.

Hela programmet verkade över huvud taget tillkommet för att injaga skräck och varnagel: se här så ruskiga, motbjudande ingreppen är.

Bilderna av det levande, fullgångna fostret var kanske det värsta jag sett i den vägen i TV — och då spelar det ändå mindre roll vad jag och andra blödiga personer tycker, jämfört med den effekt sådana bilder har på kvinnor som kan komma i den situationen att de måste söka abort.

För dem kan resultatet bli förödande. När stunden kommer vågar de inte söka abort, eftersom de är uppskrämda och avskräckta.

Och det var väl inte meningen med programmet?

Eller var det?

Var fanns allt det positiva som ligger till grund för vår allt liberalare abortlagstiftning? Den frihetstanke som ligger bakom, det ansvar som lagen lägger på individen; i hög grad är det vi själva som ska bestämma när vi vill sätta barn till världen.

FIGURE 13.2 The program *Abort* received strong reactions in the press due to its explicit depictions of abortion. In this report in *Expressen*, the controversial shot of the fetus in the kidney dish was reproduced and described as 'a shock to TV viewers' in the headline. From Ramsby, 'En chock för TV-tittarna.' Courtesy of *Expressen*.

Arguing that the program was neutral might have been a way to express support for an anti-abortion standpoint, as commentators who were openly critical of abortion praised the program. 'Trying scenes from operations illustrated eloquently how the Swedish industry of death operates,' a blurb on the front page of the Christian newspaper *Dagen* stated two days after the broadcast, next to a picture of the small hands of a twelve-week fetus, reproduced from Flanagan's *The First Nine Months of Life*, which had been published in Swedish in 1963.[36] Inside the paper, an article by editor Olof Djurfeldt appeared under the headline 'I protest,' expressing the anger that the program had triggered in him.[37]

It is revealing that the fetus in the kidney dish received the most attention in the press, not the fetus with the sound of a beating heart. For instance, a front-page headline in *Dagen* cited a question by prosecutor Dagmar Heurlin: 'What happened to the little one in the kidney dish?'[38] Although the aim of this question was to argue that information about the handling of aborted fetuses in general should be made public, it is still notable that Heurlin used the explicitly aborted fetus in this rhetoric. The different fetuses in the program clearly represented diametrical opposites: universal life and concrete death.

3 Fetal Images and Abortion in Swedish Visual Culture of the 1970s and 1980s

Even though the images in *Abort* were much questioned, images from abortions were not banned from television following this program. Some programs from the 1970s also depict abortion operations. For instance, a 1973 documentary about family planning in India showed sterilizations and an abortion in the seventh week, including a close-up of the embryo.[39] To my knowledge, however, no program showed late abortions.

During the 1970s and 1980s, the practice of displaying aborted fetuses was increasingly associated with anti-abortion activists and groups.[40] In 1974,

governmental agency between 1936 and 1994, which had the task of ensuring that radio and television companies in Sweden followed the Radio Act and the agreements made with the state.

36 'TV-programmet om abortfrågan.' Flanagan, *Livets första 9 månader*.

37 Djurfeldt, 'Jag protesterar.'

38 P. Ö., 'Dagmar Heurlin frågar överåklagaren.'

39 *Den röda triangeln*.

40 This section discusses some of the same material that I analyze more thoroughly in 'Contested Pictures of Persuasion.'

the newspaper *Aftonbladet* reported that Irma Wright—one of the doctors who had appeared in *Abort*—had planned to show a real aborted fetus in a discussion of abortion on the popular debate program *Kvällsöppet*. Wright had carried the fetus in a plastic bag in her handbag and showed it to host Per Grevér before the broadcast; Grevér, however, had made her promise not to display it on the program. Wright's plan was described as an effort to shock viewers, but she defended herself, stating that she did not aim to shock, and that a fetus in itself could not be offensive. 'Is it really more shocking to carry a fetus around than to kill it?' she asked rhetorically in a written statement.[41]

That same year, Wright also wrote an article about the event in *Läkartidningen* (a journal for physicians) and in a journal called *Operation Sverige* (Operation Sweden).[42] The latter was published by a morally conservative Christian movement with the same name that had been started in 1968. The organization was opposed to abortion and the Social Democratic government of Olof Palme, and many of the writers in the magazine had connections with Swedish right-wing extremist or Nazi movements.[43] The front page of the issue with Wright's article stated that the Palme government 'allowed 30,000 living human fetuses to be murdered each year,' next to an image of a pile of dead fetuses in a black plastic bag. This image originated from material distributed by US anti-abortion activists John C. and Barbara Willke and is thus an early example of how American anti-abortion imagery started to appear in Sweden.[44] In the parliamentary debate preceding the vote on the new Abortion Act in 1974, one of the Social Democratic members of Parliament referred to the front page of *Operation Sverige* and also mentioned that an image of a fetus had been sent anonymously to members of Parliament, as examples of what he called the 'fascist methods' adopted by opponents of the proposal.[45]

By the end of 1980, a number of television broadcasts dedicated attention to a new anti-abortion group called Rätt till liv (Right to Life) and its campaign 'Ja till livet' (Yes to Life). This organization, started in 1979, had published several brochures and other types of material with explicit images of aborted fetuses, among them a brochure with a translated supplement written by the

41 Therner, 'Kvinnlig läkare.' In 1980, large color photographs of this fetus were, however, published in a Sunday supplement to the newspaper *Göteborgs-Posten*. See 'Många blir inte äldre', and Teghammar, 'Nu blir det strid.'

42 Wright, 'Abortdebatten i TV'; Wright, 'TV förbjöd visning av människofoster!'

43 Nilsson, *Överklass, nazism och högerextremism*, 209–33.

44 'Regeringen Palme'; Gorney, *Articles of Faith*, 105–6.

45 Swedish Parliament, 'Förslag till abortlag, m.m.' 101–2.

Willkes.[46] In a religious news program called *Mellan himmel och jord* (Between heaven and earth), examples from this material were shown, raising the issue of whether this method could properly be considered Christian.[47] Rätt till liv also published a Swedish translation of the Willkes' book *Handbook on Abortion* in 1980 and produced a film called *Ja till livet* (Kvist & Wahl, 1981) with the small company Cymbal Film.[48] While a scene showing an abortion through vacuum aspiration was included in this film, it did not, however, contain any 'war pictures.' Instead, Nilsson's photographs play a central part, as the young protagonist, who has gone through an abortion, is overwhelmed by guilt when seeing the pictures in *A Child Is Born* and starts to seek the 'truth' of her abortion. In December of 1980, the team behind the film was interviewed in an episode of the television program *Magasinet* (The magazine)—a program on societal issues—focusing on abortion, and scenes from the shooting of the film as well as clips from the final production were shown.[49]

In 1985, *Magasinet* drew attention to the issue again. It presented the group Rätt till liv and their use of visual material such as slides and, in a longer feature, reported on the anti-abortion movement in the United States, incorporating clips from the US film *The Silent Scream*.[50] Ever since its launch, this notorious anti-abortion film, in which former abortionist Dr. Bernard N. Nathanson guides the viewer through the video screening of an abortion as seen through an ultrasound scan, has been harshly criticized for its 'visual distortions and verbal fraud.'[51] This was also the case in Sweden. After the feature, a studio debate followed between social welfare officer Ingrid Olsson; gynecologist Karl-Gösta Nygren, from the National Board of Health and Welfare; Peder Teglund, from Rätt till liv; and feminist Margareta Garpe, who had recently written the screenplay for a movie with an abortion theme—*Sally och friheten* (*Sally and Freedom*, Lindblom, 1981). The only one who was positive toward *The Silent Scream* was Teglund; the rest were deeply critical toward it. Among other things, Nygren stated that he found the film completely untrue, that he was tremendously upset, and that he had tried to stop Swedish Television from showing clips. The general rejection of the film can also be seen in the press. Announcing the program in *Aftonbladet*, Lars Bjelf wrote about the 'hysterical opposition against abortion in USA' and called *The Silent Scream* a 'propaganda

46 Djurfeldt et al., *Rätt till liv?* See also Andersson and Rätt till liv, Borås, *Argument i abortfrågan*.

47 *Mellan himmel och jord*.

48 Willke and Willke, *Handbok om abort*.

49 *Magasinet*, 1980.

50 *Magasinet*, 1985.

51 Petchesky, 'Fetal Images,' 267.

film.'[52] The newspaper *Expressen* also wrote that even Alf Svensson—leader of the Christian Democratic Unity, a political party—rejected the film, although he supported showing images of fetal development in schools.[53] *The Silent Scream*, however, continued to circulate among anti-abortion groups in Sweden at least until the 1990s.[54]

4 Fetal Research in Television of the 1980s

When *Abort* was aired in 1969, it provided fuel for an ongoing debate about fetal research, which resulted in a number of investigations aimed at clarifying whether experiments were conducted on living human fetuses in Sweden. In the mid-1970s, the National Board of Health and Welfare concluded that the stories circulating about such experiments were groundless, and the debates died down after 1975.[55] In the 1980s, however, fetal research again came into the public eye through a number of television programs.

The first, an episode of *Magasinet* aired in 1982, deals with the use of human and animal fetal tissue in beauty treatments in Europe as well as in Swedish and international medical research.[56] The program is made in the style of investigative journalism, with a reporter seeking to expose secrets, but the information presented about the research is quite vague and to some extent built on rumors or secondary sources, resulting in a rather sensationalist tone. The program attracted major headlines in the press, especially highlighting a few scenes from the beauty clinic La Prairie in Switzerland (allegedly visited by celebrities and top politicians like Charlie Chaplin and Ronald Reagan), where fetuses from sheep were used in various rejuvenation treatments.[57] The program also includes a studio discussion of Swedish fetal research in the 1960s and 1970s and an interview with medical doctor Agneta Philipson, who was indicted for grave robbing in the United States in the 1970s—charges which were later dismissed—following her studies on aborted fetuses to examine the effect of antibiotics during pregnancy.[58]

52 Bjelf, 'Hysteriskt abortmotstånd i USA.' See also Mollberger, 'Skräckpropaganda.'

53 Schönstedt, 'Tittarstorm efter TV-film om aborter.'

54 Persson, '"Ni ljuger om aborter, Maranata!"'; advertisement for Maranata meetings; Seidal, 'Skakande ultraljudsfilm om abort'; Oscarsson, '"Det tysta skriket."'

55 Jülich, 'Fosterexperimentens produktiva hemlighet.'

56 *Magasinet*, 1982.

57 Larsson, 'Dunderkuren'; Persson, 'Smuggel av djupfrysta foster.'

58 See Dubow, *Ourselves Unborn*, 67–75, and the introduction in this volume.

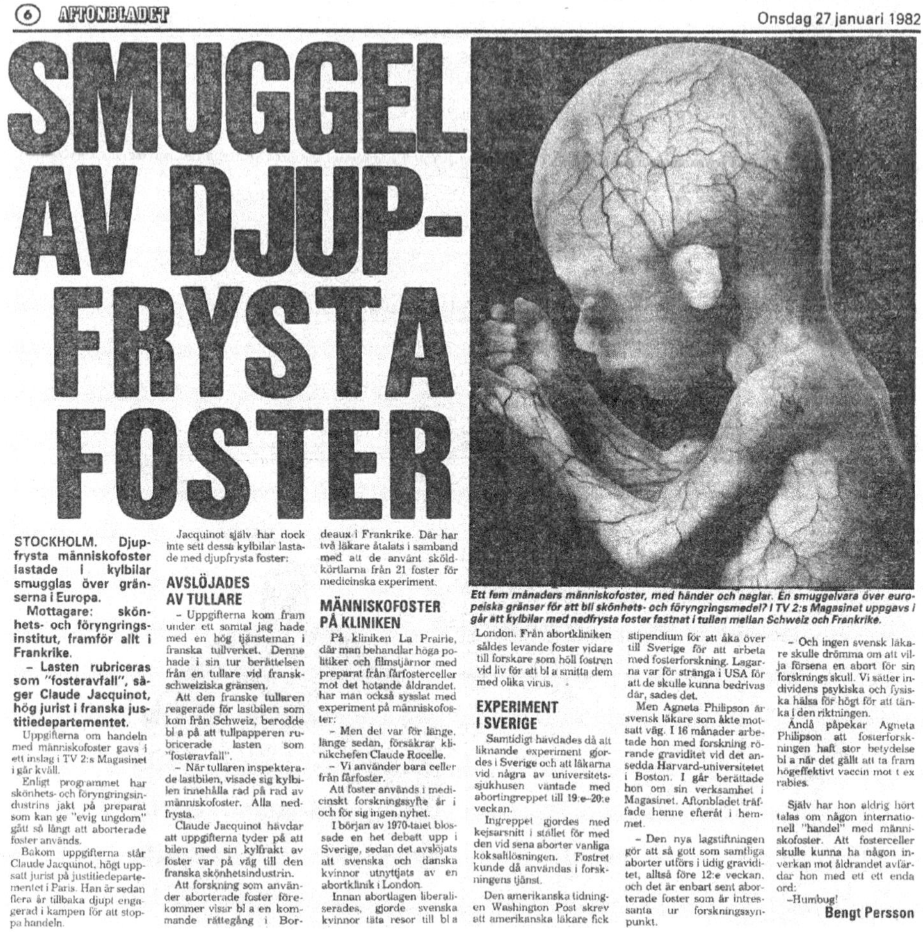

6 AFTONBLADET Onsdag 27 januari 1982

SMUGGEL AV DJUPFRYSTA FOSTER

Ett fem månaders människofoster, med händer och naglar. En smuggelvara över europeiska gränser för att bli skönhets- och föryngringsmedel? I TV 2:s Magasinet uppgavs i går att kylbilar med nedfrysta foster fastnat i tullen mellan Schweiz och Frankrike.

STOCKHOLM. Djupfrysta människofoster lastade i kylbilar smugglas över gränserna i Europa.

Mottagare: skönhets- och föryngringsinstitut, framför allt i Frankrike.

– Lasten rubriceras som "fosteravfall", säger Claude Jacquinot, hög jurist i franska justitiedepartementet.

Uppgifterna om handeln med människofoster gavs i ett inslag i TV 2:s Magasinet i går kväll.

Enligt programmet har skönhets- och föryngringsindustrins jakt på preparat som kan ge "evig ungdom" gått så långt att aborterade foster används.

Bakom uppgifterna står Claude Jacquinot, högt uppsatt jurist på justitiedepartementet i Paris. Han är sedan flera år tillbaka djupt engagerad i kampen för att stoppa handeln.

Jacquinot själv har dock inte sett dessa kylbilar lastade med djupfrysta foster:

AVSLÖJADES AV TULLARE

– Uppgifterna kom fram under ett samtal jag hade med en hög tjänsteman i franska tullverket. Denne hade i sin tur berättelsen från en tullare vid fransk-schweiziska gränsen.

Att den franske tullaren reagerade för lastbilen som kom från Schweiz, berodde bl a på att tullpapperen rubricerade lasten som "fosteravfall".

– När tullaren inspekterade lastbilen, visade sig kylbilen innehålla rad på rad av människofoster. Alla nedfrysta.

Claude Jacquinot hävdar att uppgifterna tyder på att bilen med sin kylfrakt av foster var på väg till den franska skönhetsindustrin.

Att forskning som använder aborterade foster förekommer visar bl a en kommande rättegång i Bordeaux i Frankrike. Där har två läkare åtalats i samband med att de använt sköldkörtlarna från 21 foster för medicinska experiment.

MÄNNISKOFOSTER PÅ KLINIKEN

På kliniken La Prairie, där man behandlar höga politiker och filmstjärnor med preparat från fårfosterceller mot det hotande åldrandet, har man också sysslat med experiment på människofoster:

– Men det var för länge, länge sedan, försäkrar klinikchefen Claude Rocelle.

– Vi använder bara celler från fårfoster.

Att foster används i medicinskt forskningssyfte är i och för sig ingen nyhet.

I början av 1970-talet blossade en het debatt upp i Sverige, sedan det avslöjats att svenska och danska kvinnor utnyttjats av en abortklinik i London.

Innan abortlagen liberaliserades, gjorde svenska kvinnor täta resor till bl a London. Från abortkliniken såldes levande foster vidare till forskare som höll fostren vid liv för att bl a smitta dem med olika virus.

EXPERIMENT I SVERIGE

Samtidigt hävdades då att liknande experiment gjordes i Sverige och att läkarna vid några av universitetssjukhusen väntade med abortingreppet till 19:e–20:e veckan.

Ingreppet gjordes med kejsarsnitt i stället för med den vid sena aborter vanliga koksaltlösningen. Fostret kunde då användas i forskningens tjänst.

Den amerikanska tidningen Washington Post skrev att amerikanska läkare fick stipendium för att åka över till Sverige för att arbeta med fosterforskning. Lagarna var för stränga i USA för att de skulle kunna bedrivas där, sades det.

Men Agneta Philipson är svensk läkare som åkte motsatt väg. I 16 månader arbetade hon med forskning rörande graviditet vid det ansedda Harvard-universitetet i Boston. I går berättade hon om sin verksamhet i Magasinet. Aftonbladet träffade henne efteråt i hemmet.

– Den nya lagstiftningen gör att så gott som samtliga aborter utförs i tidig graviditet, alltså före 12:e veckan, och det är enbart sent aborterade foster som är intressanta ur forskningssynpunkt.

– Och ingen svensk läkare skulle drömma om att vilja försena en abort för sin forsknings skull. Vi sätter individens psykiska och fysiska hälsa för högt för att tänka i den riktningen.

Ändå påpekar Agneta Philipson att fosterforskningen haft stor betydelse bl a när det gällt att ta fram högeffektivt vaccin mot t ex rabies.

Själv har hon aldrig hört talas om någon internationell "handel" med människofoster. Att fosterceller skulle kunna ha någon inverkan mot åldrandet avfärdar hon med ett ett enda ord:

–Humbug!

Bengt Persson

FIGURE 13.3 A 1982 newspaper report on the television program *Magasinet* with the headline 'Smuggling of frozen fetuses.' The picture by Lennart Nilsson featured here does not depict one of the frozen fetuses referred to in the article. It was published without credit and originally appeared in a different context in the newspaper twenty years earlier (Bergengren, 'Den osedda människan'). From Persson, 'Smuggel av djupfrysta foster.' Courtesy of *Aftonbladet* and Lennart Nilsson Photography/SPL.

The program does not include any explicit images of abortions; instead, the fetus is represented through a clip from Nilsson's television film *The Beginning of Life: A Documentary*. This footage appears early in the program, after an interview with French lawyer Claude Jacquinot, who tells reporter Catrin Jacobs how he discovered a transnational traffic in human fetuses. Images from Nilsson's film are then shown as Jacobs says in voice-over, 'The World Health Organization sets the border of independent life to week 22 and at least 500 grams. This is how a human looks at that age in the pictures of Lennart

Nilsson. Here, but no further, the light is green. As long as no price is put on the head of the fetus. No money can change hands.' It is also stated that a research team in Bordeaux had used twenty-one fetuses to cure a patient with diabetes. 'They are prosecuted now—thanks to indignant people—but ironically not for the fetal experiments as such, only for how they obtained the fetuses.' After this, Jacquinot continues to explain that fetuses are aborted with cesarean section and then kept alive in order to be used in research. A research team in Bordeaux has even managed to keep fetuses alive for three years, he states.

Nilsson's images and the reference to Nilsson made by the voice-over trigger the viewer to interpret the images as representing life—*The Beginning of Life* demonstrates fetal development, and the images used in the film were by this time well-known, to say the least. Using clips from this film—and not just a number of still images—also adds a layer to the construction of meaning, as *The Beginning of Life* has an extraordinary soundtrack by composer Karl-Birger Blomdahl, which in this context contributes to a sense that the fetus is endangered. Phrases like 'as long as no price is put on the head of the fetus' also link the practice of obtaining fetuses for research to hunting and killing, and the reference to 'indignant people' indicates the type of feelings that the program itself is meant to evoke.

While the feature in *Magasinet* mainly reported on European research, Swedish fetal research again came into focus in the late 1980s. In this period, research was carried out on the possibility of transplanting cells from fetuses to treat a variety of conditions. In Uppsala, insulin-producing cells from human fetuses had been transplanted to patients with diabetes, and in Lund a research group was working on transplanting brain cells from fetuses to patients with Parkinson's disease.[59] Here, I highlight two programs reporting on this research which display radically different strategies for showing fetal imagery.

The first is a program called *Livsviktigt* (Vital), which was aired in February 1988.[60] The program does not show any images of human fetuses or operation on humans, but instead includes numerous scenes with images of animal fetuses and detailed demonstrations of operations on animals. For instance, the program opens with a close-up of an aborted pig fetus as the topic of the program is introduced by a voice-over. Very early in the program, there is also a scene from a pig farm in which a sow is slaughtered and the pig fetuses are taken out and put in a cooler for transportation to a lab. After a short interview with the pig farmer, a scene shows how a researcher at the lab takes out one of the pig fetuses and starts cutting it up to extract the pancreas.

59 Swedish Ministry of Health and Social Affairs, *Aborterade foster, m.m.*, 33–37.

60 *Livsviktigt*.

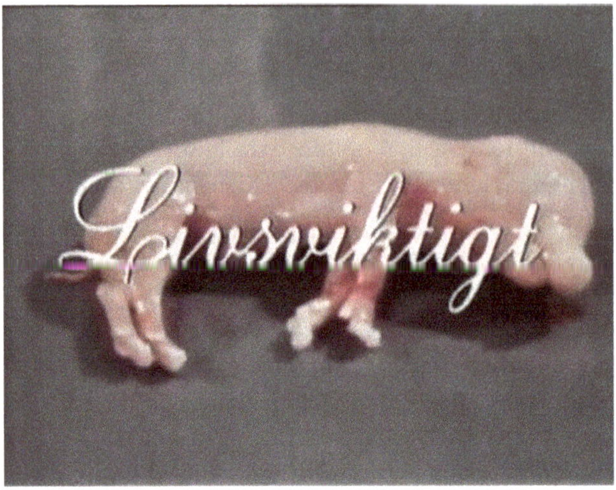

FIGURE 13.4
A pig fetus shown in the beginning of the television program *Livsviktigt* broadcast in 1988.

The use of human fetuses in research is never displayed in this program, probably in order to avoid the problematic meanings and controversies that such images could set off. However, the visual absence of the fetus can have other effects. It can create the feeling that images of human fetuses are taboo and that an unwatchable 'truth' is being hidden. It can also provoke mental images of the fetus among spectators. Even though a large part of the program concerns research on animals, the question of human fetal research constantly looms in the background. Consequently, when a doctoral student states in an interview that 'just like any person who would see an aborted [human] fetus, I can sometimes find it a bit disgusting,' the viewer is prompted to imagine this sight, perhaps by mentally replacing the program's explicit and numerous images of animal fetuses with subjective visualizations of human fetuses. Another such moment is created at the end of the program, when the reporter presses Anders Björklund, a professor of histology at Lund University, to specify what it is that is problematic about using human fetuses in research. After repeatedly trying to avoid the question, Björklund finally states that an abortion should never be connected to a certain purpose. It is not unreasonable to presume that, having seen the graphic images of a pig being slaughtered in order to obtain its fetuses at the beginning of the program, viewers hearing this comment might experience unpleasant visions of women being forced to have abortions.

The second program that I wish to highlight is an episode of *Mellan himmel och jord* aired in December of 1988.[61] Here, the opposite strategy is used as

61 *Mellan himmel och jord.* The use of human fetuses in research on Parkinson's disease was discussed in other programs as well. The science program *Vetenskap* (Science) introduced

images from an actual abortion are shown. This program raises the ethical issues of fetal research, and two medical doctors in Gothenburg are interviewed—one who is against fetal research and one who is supportive of it. The fetal images are central. The program starts as the camera pans over a number of pictures in frames, including a fetal image, meant to hint at the topics addressed by the program. Even though one such image has thus already been shown, presenter Siewert Öholm warns sensitive viewers about upcoming images when later presenting the feature. The images had also been announced in the press. The editorial secretary noted when interviewed that to his knowledge, 'images like these have never before been shown on Swedish television.'[62] While a voice-over explains how vacuum aspiration is done—'the fetus is torn apart and ends up in a glass container with the mucous membrane and placenta'—images are shown of the instruments followed by a bloody mass on top of some sort of filter. A person with a green mask is seen separating the fetal parts from the mass, and the image briefly freezes in an extreme close-up of the mass, in which it is possible to see an arm with a hand and a round part that is possibly a head. Despite these pictures, the program did not meet with much discussion in the mainstream press. One of the few who did comment on it was journalist Åsa Moberg, who quite tellingly noted that the use of fetal images degraded the 'admirably sober tone' of Swedish religious discussion on the abortion issue to an 'American slaughterhouse standard.'[63]

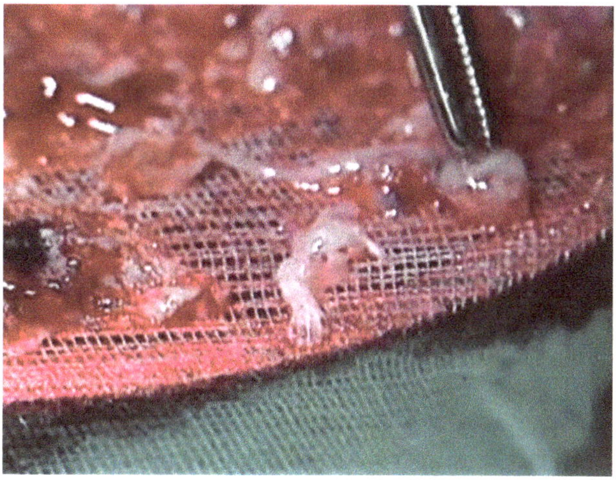

FIGURE 13.5
A picture showing how fetal parts are collected after a vacuum aspiration abortion in the television program *Mellan himmel och jord* broadcast in 1988.

the topic in October the same year, but was—like *Livsviktigt*—careful with showing fetal images. In this program, there is only a brief display of one of Lennart Nilsson's pictures.

62 'Religiöst TV-magasin.'

63 Moberg, 'Dystra herrar.'

5 Conclusion

This chapter has explored fetal images in television programs on abortion and fetal research aired in Sweden between 1969 and 1988. In 1969, the program *Abort* featured lengthy and detailed images of actual abortions, including close-ups of an aborted fetus, which triggered reactions of shock and stirred up widespread debate. This program displays two different representations of fetuses: the fetus as a symbol of life in general and the particular, aborted, dead or dying fetus. But while the program in itself is an example of how fetal images were made public in a new way in the 1960s, its display of aborted fetuses explicitly represented as dead or dying was exceptional in the mainstream media. Perhaps as a consequence of reactions to this program, Swedish television rarely showed images of explicitly aborted fetuses in the 1970s and 1980. And when it did, these images were presented in a framework associating the practice mainly with US anti-abortion campaigns and minor Christian activist groups like Rätt till liv. It is telling that, among the programs discussed here, the only one reporting on fetal research in the 1980s that did include images from an abortion was the religious news program *Mellan himmel och jord*. The other two employed different strategies: using only the familiar images of Lennart Nilsson or completely avoiding images of human fetuses. However, while not seen as shocking, these strategies can have other effects. By connoting 'life,' the Nilsson sequence in *Magasinet* is used to create associations with threatened life, while the absence of human fetuses in *Livsviktigt* might—intentionally or not—function to stir up disturbing mental images.

Consequently, this chapter demonstrates that in the first three decades of television in Sweden, Swedish media representations of abortion and fetuses developed in a different direction from those in the United States. It thus provides a new perspective on the history of 'the public fetus,' which has mostly been examined in the US context. However, while differences between Swedish and US media are expected, this chapter also adds contradictions and nuances to this picture. In the period studied, fetal images circulated nationally and transnationally. Nilsson's images were widespread in Sweden in various sex education materials, but were also used by the anti-abortion movement, both in Sweden and in the United States. At the same time, anti-abortion groups in Sweden adopted US strategies and used US material. But while the use of Nilsson's images and similar ones in the television programs that I have studied were seldom criticized or even commented on, explicit pictures of abortions were generally denounced. As Moberg's comment on *Mellan himmel och jord* indicates, in the 1980s an association had also developed between this type of imagery and American anti-abortion activism. Hence, to return to Morgan's discussion of the divide between 'good' and 'bad' fetuses referred to in the beginning of this chapter, one interpretation could be that in the Swedish media there was also a line created between Sweden, and its 'good' fetuses portrayed by Lennart Nilsson, and the United States, where 'bad' pictures of fetuses were disseminated. This perceived difference, however, overlooks the fact that the Nilsson images were also of aborted fetuses and that Swedish television had shown explicit images of abortion already in the 1960s, before the strategy of using 'war pictures' had emerged among US anti-abortion activists.

Bibliography

'Abortprotester av KDU i Östersund.' *Dagen*, October 23, 1969.

Advertisement for Maranata meetings. *Dagens Nyheter*, June 15, 1985.

Andersson, Jonas, and Rätt till liv, Borås, eds. *Argument i abortfrågan*. Järfälla: Salt & Ljus, 1980.

Bergengren, Kurt. 'Den osedda människan.' *Aftonbladet*, April 2, 1961.

Bjelf, Lars. 'Hysteriskt abortmotstånd i USA.' *Aftonbladet*, March 14, 1985.

Björklund, Elisabet. 'Contested Pictures of Persuasion: American Images of Foetuses in Swedish Antiabortion Campaigns of the 1970s and 1980s.' In *Nordic Media Histories of Propaganda and Persuasion*, edited by Fredrik Norén, Emil Stjernholm, and C. Claire Thomson, 97–116. Cham: Palgrave Macmillan, 2023.

Björklund, Elisabet. 'Medicinens och televisionens ögonblick: Om det medicinska magasinet *Ronden* (1966–1978).' In *Medicinjournalistikens efterkrigstida historia i Sverige: Aktörer, arenor och ideal ca. 1945–2020*, edited by Jonatan Samuelsson (under review).

Björklund, Elisabet. *The Most Delicate Subject: A History of Sex Education Films in Sweden*. Lund: Lund University, 2012.

Björklund, Elisabet. 'Waiting for Abortion: Narratives of Passing Time, Decision-Making, and Late Abortions in Swedish TV Theater of the Late 1960s and Early 1970s.' *Body Politics: Zeitschrift für Körpergeschichte* 8, no. 12 (2020): 108–34.

Björklund, Elisabet, and Solveig Jülich, eds. *Rethinking the Public Fetus: Historical Perspectives on the Visual Culture of Pregnancy*. Rochester, NY: University of Rochester Press, 2024.

Djurfeldt, Olof. 'Jag protesterar.' *Dagen*, October 17, 1969.

Djurfeldt, Olof, Ingrid Pejrud, Eskil Albertsson, Stefan Swärd, and Tommy Lindén, eds. *Rätt till liv?* Järfälla: Salt & Ljus, [1980]. [Brochure in the Lund University Library collection of printed ephemera]

Dubow, Sara. *Ourselves Unborn: A History of the Fetus in Modern America*. New York: Oxford University Press, 2011.

Edström, Bror. 'Abort är mord!' *Dagen*, October 23, 1969.

Flanagan, Geraldine Lux. *Livets första 9 månader*. Stockholm: Forum, 1963.

Franklin, Sarah, Celia Lury, and Jackie Stacey. *Global Nature, Global Culture*. London, Thousand Oaks, CA, and New Delhi: Sage, 2000.

Furhammar, Leif. 'From Affluence to Poverty: The Early Swedish TV Documentary.' In *A History of Swedish Broadcasting: Communicative Ethos, Genres and Institutional Change*, edited by Monika Djerf-Pierre and Mats Ekström, 241–59. Gothenburg: Nordicom, 2013.

Furhammar, Leif. *Sex, såpor och svenska krusbär: Television i konkurrens*. Stockholm: Ekerlids förlag, 2006.

Gadd, Pia. 'Abort-chock i TV i kväll.' *Expressen*, October 15, 1969.

Gorney, Cynthia. *Articles of Faith: A Frontline History of the Abortion Wars*. New York: Simon & Schuster, 1998.

Hodenberg, Christina von. *Television's Moment: Sitcom Audiences and the Sixties Cultural Revolution*. New York and Oxford: Berghahn Books, 2017.

Höijer, Birgitta. *Det hörde vi allihop! Etermedierna och publiken under 1900-talet*. Stockholm: Prisma, 1998.

Holz, Rose. 'Biological Bodies, Unfettered Imaginations: The 1939 Dickinson-Belskie *Birth Series* Sculptures and the Unexpected Origins of Modern Antiabortion Imagery.' In Björklund and Jülich, *Rethinking the Public Fetus*, 94–118.

Hopwood, Nick. *Haeckel's Embryos: Images, Evolution, and Fraud*. Chicago: University of Chicago Press, 2015.

Hopwood, Nick. 'Producing Development: The Anatomy of Human Embryos and the Norms of Wilhelm His.' *Bulletin of the History of Medicine* 74, no. 1 (2000): 29–79.

Hopwood, Nick. 'Visual Strategies of Antiabortion Activism and Their Feminist Critique: The Public Fetus in the United States.' In Björklund and Jülich, *Rethinking the Public Fetus*, 193–224.

Hughes, Richard L. 'Burning Birth Certificates and Atomic Tupperware Parties: Creating the Antiabortion Movement in the Shadow of the Vietnam War.' *Historian* 68, no. 3 (2006): 541–58.

Jolanta. 'Balanserat om abort.' *Svenska Dagbladet*, October 16, 1969.

Jülich, Solveig. 'Fetal Photography in the Age of Cool Media.' In *History of Participatory Media: Politics and Publics, 1750–2000*, edited by Anders Ekström, Solveig Jülich, Frans Lundgren, and Per Wisselgren, 125–41. New York: Routledge, 2011.

Jülich, Solveig. 'Fosterexperimentens produktiva hemlighet: Medicinsk forskning och vita lögner i 1960- och 1970-talets Sverige.' *Lychnos* (2018): 10–49.

Jülich, Solveig. 'The Making of a Best-Selling Book on Reproduction: Lennart Nilsson's *A Child Is Born*.' *Bulletin of the History of Medicine* 89, no. 3 (2015): 491–525.

Jülich, Solveig. 'Picturing Abortion Opposition in Sweden: Lennart Nilsson's Early Photographs of Embryos and Fetuses.' *Social History of Medicine* 31, no. 2 (2018): 278–307.

Jülich, Solveig. 'Televising Inner Space: Lennart Nilsson's Early Medical Documentaries on the Interior of the Human Body.' In *Representational Machines: Photography and the Production of Space*, edited by Anna Dahlgren, Dan Petersson, and Nina Lager Vestberg, 149–70. Aarhus: Aarhus University Press, 2013.

Jülich, Solveig, and Elisabet Björklund, 'The Public Fetus: A Traveling Concept.' In Björklund and Jülich, *Rethinking the Public Fetus*, 289–309.

'KDU: Fria aborter det fria samhällets bankruttförklaring.' *Dagen*, October 21, 1969.

Kuźma-Markowska, Sylwia, and Laura Kelly. 'Anti-abortion Activism in Poland and the Republic of Ireland, c. 1970s–1990s.' *Journal of Religious History* 46, no. 3 (2022): 526–51.

Larsson, Ann-Hjördis. 'Dunderkuren som ska göra Reagan ung igen.' *Expressen*, January 26, 1982.

Lennerhed, Lena. *Frihet att njuta: Sexualdebatten i Sverige på 1960-talet*. Stockholm: Norstedts, 1994.

Lennerhed, Lena. 'Sherri Finkbine's Choice: Abortion, Sex-Liberalism and Feminism in Sweden in the 1960s and 1970s.' *Women's History Magazine* 73 (2013): 13–18.

Lupton, Deborah. *The Social Worlds of the Unborn*. Basingstoke: Palgrave Macmillan, 2013.

Moberg, Åsa. 'Dystra herrar.' *Aftonbladet*, December 19, 1988.

Mollberger, Bertil. 'Skräckpropaganda.' *Dagens Nyheter*, March 15, 1985.

Morgan, Lynn M. *Icons of Life: A Cultural History of Human Embryos*. Berkeley: University of California Press, 2009.

'Många blir inte äldre än såhär.' *G-P nu*, Sunday supplement to *Göteborgs-Posten*, November 9, 1980.

Nilsson, Karl N. Alvar. *Överklass, nazism och högerextremism 1945–1995*. Stockholm: Carlssons, 1998.

Öhlander, Karin. 'Så upplevde en kvinna som genomgått två legala aborter TV:s chockprogram: Jag har inte sovit i natt.' *Expressen*, October 16, 1969.

Oscarsson, Mikael. '"Det tysta skriket" sågs av 1.5 miljoner: Mediaexplosion.' *Ja till livet-nytt*, no. 2 (1997): 2.

Persson, Bengt. 'Smuggel av djupfrysta foster.' *Aftonbladet*, January 27, 1982.

Persson, Magnus. '"Ni ljuger om aborter, Maranata!"' *Dagens Nyheter*, March 26, 1985.

Petchesky, Rosalind Pollack. 'Fetal Images: The Power of Visual Culture in the Politics of Reproduction.' *Feminist Studies* 13, no. 2 (1987): 263–92.

P. Ö. 'Dagmar Heurlin frågar överåklagaren: Vad hände med den lille i rondskålen?' *Dagen*, October 24, 1969.

Ramsby, Åge. 'En chock för TV-tittarna.' *Expressen*, October 16, 1969.

Ramsey, Morag. *The Swedish Abortion Pill: Co-producing Medical Abortion and Values, ca. 1965–1992*. Uppsala: Uppsala University, 2021.

'Regeringen Palme tillåter att cirka 30. 000 levande människofoster mördas per år!' *Operation Sverige*, no. 5–6 (1974): front page.

'Religiöst TV-magasin visar bilder från en abort.' *Svenska Dagbladet*, December 18, 1988.

Santesmases, María Jesús. 'The Public Fetus in Franco's Spain: Women, Doctors, and Feminists in the Circulation of Pregnancy Images.' In Björklund and Jülich, *Rethinking the Public Fetus*, 171–192.

Schönstedt, Tommy. 'Tittarstorm efter TV-film om aborter.' *Expressen*, March 15, 1985.

Seidal, Tomas. 'Skakande ultraljudsfilm om abort.' *Ja till livet-nytt*, no. 4–5 (1995), 4.

Slattery, Kathryn. 'Building a "World Coalition for Life": Abortion, Population Control and Transnational Pro-life Networks, 1960–1990.' PhD diss., University of New South Wales, 2010.

Steen, Kjell-Åke. 'TV varnar känsliga tittare för abortprogrammet i kväll.' *Aftonbladet*, October 15, 1969.

Sten, Hemming. 'Bilderna i går de ruskigaste jag sett i TV.' *Expressen*, October 16, 1969.

Stormer, Nathan. 'Looking in Wonder: Prenatal Sublimity and the Commonplace "Life."' *Signs* 33, no. 3 (2008): 647–73.

Swedish Ministry of Health and Social Affairs. *Aborterade foster, m.m.: Betänkande.* SOU 1991:42. Stockholm: Allmänna förlaget, 1991.

Swedish Ministry of Justice. *Rätten till abort.* SOU 1971:58. Stockholm: Justitiedepartementet, 1971.

Swedish Parliament. 'Förslag till abortlag, m.m.' In *Riksdagens protokoll*, no. 93, 3–131. Stockholm: Riksdagen, 1974.

Swärd, Stefan. *Varför Sverige fick fri abort: Ett studium av en policyprocess.* Stockholm: Stockholms universitet, 1983.

Teghammar, Karin. 'Nu blir det strid om fria aborterna.' *G-P nu*, Sunday supplement to *Göteborgs-Posten*, November 9, 1980.

Therner, Bengt. 'Kvinnlig läkare som är emot abort försökte chocka tv-tittarna.' *Aftonbladet*, April 2, 1974.

'TV-programmet om abortfrågan.' *Dagen*, October 17, 1969.

Weibull, Lennart. 'New Media between Technology and Content: The Introduction of Radio and Television in Sweden.' In *A History of Swedish Broadcasting: Communicative Ethos, Genres, and Institutional Change*, edited by Monika Djerf-Pierre and Mats Ekström, 31–54. Gothenburg: Nordicom, 2013.

Willke, John C., and Barbara Willke. *Handbok om abort.* Translated by Ingrid Pejrud. 1971. Järfälla: Salt & Ljus, 1980.

Wright, Irma. 'Abortdebatten i TV.' *Läkartidningen* 71, no. 17 (1974): 1717.

Wright, Irma. 'TV förbjöd visning av människofoster!' *Operation Sverige*, no. 5–6 (1974): 4–5.

Film and Television Productions

Abort: Fakta och synpunkter om avbrytande av havandeskap. Aired on October 15, 1969. Sweden: Sveriges Radio Göteborg.

Dabner, Jack. *The Silent Scream.* United States: American Portrait Films, 1984.

Den röda triangeln: Om familjeplanering i Indien. Aired on March 18, 1973, on TV2. Sweden: Sveriges Radio.

Kvist, Karin, and Lars Gunnar Wahl. *Ja till livet.* Sweden: Cymbal Film, 1981.

Lindblom, Gunnel. *Sally och friheten.* Sweden: Cinematograph/Svenska filminstitutet/Sandrews, 1981.

Livsviktigt. Aired on February 23, 1988, on TV2. Sweden: Sveriges Television Malmö.

Mellan himmel och jord. Aired on November 23, 1980, on TV1. Sweden: Sveriges Television.

Mellan himmel och jord. Aired on December 18, 1988, on TV2. Sweden: Sveriges Television.

Magasinet. Aired on December 9, 1980, on TV2. Sweden: Sveriges Television.

Magasinet. Aired on January 26, 1982, on TV2. Sweden: Sveriges Television.

Magasinet. Aired on March 14, 1985, on TV2. Sweden: Sveriges Television.

Ronden. Aired on October 18, 1966, on TV2. Sweden: Sveriges Radio.

Så börjar livet. Aired on December 29, 1965. Sweden: Sol-film.

Vetenskap: Nytt liv i hjärnan. Aired on October 3, 1988, on TV1. Sweden: Sveriges Television.

Archival Sources

Bolinder, Birgitta, Birgitta Svanberg, and Åsa Åkerstedt. Report to the Radio Committee. April 24, 1970. A12 F3:4, 106/70, SRA.

Minutes from the manager's program meeting, October 24, 1969. A04 A6A:4, SRA.

The Radio Committee, to Birgitta Bolinder, Birgitta Svanberg, and Åsa Åkerstedt. Copy. Appendix to minutes nr 54, June 30, 1970. A12 F3:4, 106/70, SRA.

CHAPTER 14

The Moral Landscape of Prenatal Diagnosis

Anna Tunlid

In 1984, the Swedish Government appointed a commission of inquiry to examine issues related to the protection of the fetus and the ethical and legal questions surrounding prenatal diagnosis. The backdrop was a broad political and public debate concerning the moral status of the fetus, particularly in relation to emerging reproductive and genetic technologies, as well as the societal, political, and moral consequences of prenatal diagnosis. At this point in time there were no specific guidelines or legislation that regulated the practice of prenatal diagnosis in Sweden, with the exception of the 1974 Abortion Act, which defined the conditions for abortion if a woman decided to terminate a pregnancy. Apart from that, the practice of prenatal diagnosis was ruled by general medical praxis.

The call for regulation touched on a number of critical issues: feminists' long-term struggles for abortion and reproductive rights; the status and rights that were ascribed to the fetus by various groups, from medical experts to Christian communities; and the disability movement's opinion that selective abortions of impaired fetuses might negatively affect attitudes toward people with disabilities.[1] In addition, the long history of eugenics cast a shadow over the issue, although the context of prenatal diagnosis differed in many ways from eugenic practices of the early 1900s.[2] The practice and regulation of prenatal diagnosis was therefore a complex configuration of medical technologies, cultural values, social norms, and legal cultures. Being the result of historical, social, and political processes, such configurations are particular to individual countries.

Regardless of how these configurations have changed in specific contexts, the introduction of prenatal diagnostics in the 1970s altered perceptions of both the fetus and the pregnant woman. This diagnostic method was originally developed to help women in so-called risk groups make informed decisions about whether to terminate a pregnancy if the fetus was found to have

1 There are several studies on prenatal diagnosis; see, e.g., Rapp, *Testing Women, Testing the Fetus*; Löwy, *Imperfect Pregnancies*; Löwy, *Tangled Diagnoses*.

2 Whether there is a link between early twentieth-century eugenics and later reproductive genetics, including prenatal diagnosis, is controversial. See, e.g., Bashford, 'Epilogue'; Paul, 'Reflections on the Historiography.'

 | DOI:10.1163/9789004703759_016

abnormalities. However, the close links between prenatal diagnosis and selective abortion meant that the technology was controversial from the outset and gave rise to heated debates. According to medical historian Ilana Löwy, selective abortion of impaired fetuses has been the main focus of the public debate on prenatal diagnosis since its introduction.[3]

The technology also had a decisive impact on individual pregnant women. Those women considering prenatal diagnosis faced a series of difficult deliberations and decisions and became, in the words of anthropologist Rayna Rapp, 'moral pioneers.'[4] However, the increasingly advanced biomedical methods for identifying fetal characteristics also led to a very different discussion over the possibility of curing the fetus while still *in utero*. Although the potential to do so has historically been very limited, this hope helped to promote the view of the fetus as a patient with its own rights and interests.[5] Contributing to this increased attention on the fetus was also the emphasis on its vulnerability to drugs, alcohol, and toxic substances in the environment, and thus its need for protection, in some cases even against the pregnant woman and her behavior.[6]

The view of the fetus as a patient with potential rights or as a vulnerable body had profound consequences for the pregnant woman and her experience of pregnancy. The biomedical discourse defined both the fetal and the pregnant body, giving them meaning and regulating them. In this process, the pregnant woman and the fetus were increasingly recognized as two separate individuals with, at times, conflicting interests and rights. However, as historian Sara Dubow has reminded us, we should not exaggerate the importance of technology in understanding the changing significance attributed to the fetus; we must also examine the social values and political circumstances that have shaped various discourses on the fetus.[7] While the conceptions of the fetus and the pregnant woman had implications for reproductive rights and policy more broadly, they also formed the backdrop to the discussion of prenatal diagnosis.

This chapter deals with the 1984 investigation concerning regulation of prenatal diagnosis in Sweden and the various arguments posed for or against such regulation, including whether there should be any changes in the legislation of late-term abortions. The investigation was a so-called governmental commission, a political institution with a long tradition in Sweden. Being appointed

3 Löwy, *Imperfect Pregnancies*, 7.

4 Rapp, *Testing Women, Testing the Fetus*, 306–11.

5 For a critical discussion of fetal surgery and reproductive politics, see Casper, *Making of the Unborn Patient*.

6 Lupton, *Social Worlds of the Unborn*, 92–112.

7 Dubow, *Ourselves Unborn*, 3.

by the Government but formally independent, the task of commissions is to produce policy-relevant knowledge for political decisions.[8] The governmental commission that was assigned to address issues concerning the protection of the fetus and prenatal diagnosis published two official reports: an interim report in 1987, on social and legal measures in cases of women's drug abuse during pregnancy, and a final report in 1989, concerning the potential regulation of prenatal diagnosis and late-term abortions. This chapter mainly deals with the final report, focusing in particular on how issues concerning prenatal diagnosis were discussed in relation to women's reproductive rights, the moral rights of the fetus, and human dignity. Besides the commission's report, the referral opinions issued by consulting bodies will be analyzed, as well as the government bill about prenatal diagnosis and late abortion that was submitted to Parliament in 1995.

Using the spatial metaphor of a 'moral landscape,' I will explore how various actors—the commission, the numerous consulting bodies, and the Government—tried to negotiate their position on a controversial issue that was shaped by novel medical technologies and the critical questions that these technologies engendered. The moral landscape in which these negotiations took place could be likened to a topography of values and practices intersected by various pathways, created by the actors as they tried to navigate these complex issues.[9] By analyzing the positions taken by various actors, I will demonstrate how their paths were guided not only by abstract bioethical principles—although those were present—but also by their efforts to negotiate and reconcile the sometimes conflicting values and practices of prenatal diagnosis. During these negotiations, the moral landscape was constantly transformed as new positions were shaped and reshaped. The image of finding one's way in a moral landscape thus draws attention to the temporal and multifaceted process of creating moral positions.

After briefly surveying the 1974 Abortion Act and the introduction of prenatal diagnosis within the Swedish healthcare system, the chapter deals with emerging public discussions on the issue. This is followed by an analysis of the commission's reports as well as the various referral opinions and the final governmental bill. The last section discusses the changing moral landscape of prenatal diagnosis, arguing that although the practice raised questions about the moral status of the fetus and human dignity, the official regulation

8 Wisselgren, 'Reforming the Science-Policy Boundary.'

9 Helgason and Palsson, 'Contested Commodities'; Koch and Svendsen, 'Negotiating Moral Value.'

defended women's reproductive rights, while other views and values were relegated to the margins.

1 Development of Prenatal Diagnosis and the 1974 Abortion Act

The development of prenatal diagnosis was based on the innovation of several biomedical technologies: the improvement of amniocentesis, the study of human chromosomes, the description of biochemical markers of fetal anomalies in maternal blood, and the invention of obstetric ultrasound.[10] A crucial step was taken at Lund University in Sweden in 1956, when the cytogeneticists Albert Levan and Joe Hin Tjio suggested that the number of human chromosomes was forty-six, not forty-eight, which was the previously accepted view.[11] The number was soon confirmed, which paved the way for extensive studies of chromosomal anomalies. Another technology with strong links to Swedish biomedical research was obstetric ultrasound, which the gynecologist Bertil Sundén started to develop in the late 1950s.[12] The development of both technologies benefited from the 1938 Abortion Act, which allowed abortion under certain circumstances. Moreover, close links between biomedical research and clinical practice facilitated the introduction of these technologies within Swedish healthcare.

By using the new technologies, or a combination of them, it was possible to detect chromosomal abnormalities, genetic diseases, and structural anomalies of the fetus. These technologies developed rapidly, and new ones evolved, thereby increasing the number of conditions that could be diagnosed antenatally. Their introduction in obstetric care took place at the same time as Lennart Nilsson's images of the fetus began to circulate in his best-selling book *Ett barn blir till* (*A Child Is Born*, 1965).[13] While Nilsson's aestheticized images of the fetus were produced to display 'the miracle of life,' the emergent technologies formed the basis of what Löwy has called the 'biomedical fetus'—that is, a conception of the fetus shaped by new medical technologies.[14]

In Sweden, the clinical practice of prenatal diagnosis was introduced in early 1970. It soon became associated with amniocentesis, although several

10 Löwy, *Imperfect Pregnancies*, 2.

11 de Chadarevian, 'Chromosome Photography.'

12 See Berg's chapter in this volume.

13 Nilsson, Ingelman-Sundberg, and Wirsén, *Ett barn blir till*. The first American edition was published in 1966 by Delacorte Press and the first British edition in 1967 by Allen Lane/Penguin Press. For a discussion of the book, see Jülich, 'Making of a Best-Selling Book.'

14 Löwy, *Tangled Diagnoses*, 16.

other tests were also used. In 1972, ninety amniocenteses were performed in Sweden, and three years later the number had risen to more than six hundred per year.[15] During these early years, prenatal diagnosis was almost exclusively discussed among medical geneticists and other medical specialists. For them, the tests became valuable tools in genetic counselling for parents who were considered to belong to 'risk families'—that is, families with a known history of genetic disease. Another group was women who already had a child with genetic disease or chromosome abnormalities, and a third was women aged thirty-five or older. If a pregnant woman belonged to any of these categories, she could be offered prenatal testing.[16]

The medical experts had several arguments for performing prenatal testing. The tests could prevent abortion of a healthy fetus when the pregnant woman was afraid of having (another) impaired child. They could also be used to decide whether to abort an impaired fetus, thereby preventing the expected child from suffering and easing the burden on the afflicted family. A third argument was that the tests could be used to calm anxious prospective mothers in those cases where there was no obvious medical risk to the fetus. In addition to the medical and psychological arguments, economic reasons were put forward: prenatal diagnosis, followed by abortion of impaired fetuses, could decrease public spending on medical care for the disabled.[17] Although the medical experts carefully pointed out that it was women who decided whether to take the test or have an abortion, the economic argument introduced a societal interest in prenatal diagnosis. This train of thought was not unique to Sweden; in several countries an explicit link was drawn between prenatal diagnosis and economic benefits to society in the 1970s.[18]

The development of prenatal diagnosis occurred at the same time as Sweden adopted new, liberal abortion legislation that guaranteed women's right to make their own decisions about abortion, albeit with some restrictions. The former legislation, the 1938 Abortion Act, was very restrictive and had only legalized abortions on specific indications. However, in 1963 the law was amended to also allow abortion in cases where there was a risk of serious fetal impairment. The reason for this reform was the birth defects caused by the tranquillizer thalidomide, which provoked considerable debate in Sweden.[19]

15 Lindsten and Beckman, *Klinisk genetik*, 40.

16 Björkman and Tunlid, 'Establishment of Genetic Counselling,' 356–57.

17 Björkman and Tunlid, 'Establishment of Genetic Counselling,' 356–60.

18 E.g., Nemec and Moser, 'Counselling, Risk and Prevention,' 381–84; Stern, *Telling Genes*, 161–64.

19 Lennerhed, 'No Backlash'; Lennerhed, *Kvinnotrubbel*, chap. 5. See also Björkman's chapter in this volume.

As Leslie Reagan has pointed out, in the United States both thalidomide and outbreaks of German measles produced a new image of abortions as respectable and responsible, before the procedure was decriminalized nationwide in 1973.[20] In Sweden, too, attention to the fetal impairment caused by thalidomide led to a greater understanding of women seeking abortions for this reason. However, the woman still had to apply for permission from authorities to have an abortion.

In contrast, the 1974 Abortion Act stated that until the eighteenth week of pregnancy, the choice to have an abortion was entirely up to the woman. After the eighteenth week, permission could only be given by the National Board of Health and Welfare. These 'late abortions' were only allowed in cases with severe indications and as long as the fetus was not 'viable.' In this context, viability meant the ability of the fetus to survive and develop outside the woman's body. When the 1974 Abortion Act was introduced, this was considered to occur at the twenty-fourth week of pregnancy if advanced neonatal care was provided. The time limit for late-term abortions was set at twenty-two weeks to provide a sufficient margin of safety for a viable fetus.[21]

A fundamental notion in the new abortion legislation was that the fetus was considered part of the woman's body in early pregnancy and that the fetus's right to life increased gradually during its development. This was expressed in the eighteen-week limit on the woman's right to make her own decision and in the ban on abortions of viable fetuses (abortion after this threshold was only permitted if the woman's life was in danger). Fetal rights were only briefly mentioned in the report by the governmental commission, *Rätten till abort* (The right to abortion), which preceded the legislation. However, the subsequent government bill discussed it to some extent.[22] Here it was concluded that the eighteen-week limit was reasonable, considering fetal viability but also with respect to the psychological strain of late abortions.[23] The disputed issue in the late 1970s was whether selective abortions—before or after the eighteenth week—differed from other abortions and if they had to be regulated in any specific way. These discussions concerned the issue of fetal rights but also societal attitudes toward people with disabilities and opened up new pathways in the moral landscape.

---

20 Reagan, *Dangerous Pregnancies*.

21 Swedish Parliament, 'Nr 70. Kungl. Maj:ts proposition.' The viability concept was also included in the US Supreme Court decision *Roe v. Wade*. On this, see Lupton, *Social Worlds of the Unborn*, 28.

22 Swedish Ministry of Justice, *Rätten till abort*. See also the reservation by the conservative member of Parliament Astrid Kristensson, concerning legal protection of the fetus.

23 Swedish Parliament, 'Nr 70. Kungl. Maj:ts proposition.'

2 A Changing Moral Landscape

The public debate concerning prenatal diagnosis was initiated in the late 1970s by people in close contact with those living with disabilities. While physicians usually pointed out that the main reason for prenatal diagnosis was to reduce the future suffering of children and to ease the burden on afflicted families, critical voices argued that the ultimate reason was to reduce public spending on health care and support for people living with disabilities. Some voices even warned that prenatal diagnosis could lead to eugenic tendencies.[24] According to this view, prenatal diagnosis with a subsequent abortion posed a threat to human dignity, especially for people with disabilities, and risked increasing discriminatory attitudes toward this group. The critique sparked a wider debate about the ethical principles of prenatal diagnosis and possible regulation.[25]

In parallel, the issue of fetal rights emerged from two partly overlapping developments. One concerned abortion in general, specifically the 1974 Abortion Act, which according to its critics did not take sufficient account of the moral and legal status of the fetus.[26] The other was more intimately linked to the development of prenatal diagnosis, claiming that these diagnostic tools had demonstrated beyond doubt that the fetus was a unique individual. Moreover, rapid technological development made it likely that in the near future it would be possible not only to diagnose diseases in the fetus but also to treat them. The fetus could thus be considered as a potential patient, which raised the issue of its legal status. This view was held by the physician Gustav Giertz, chairman of the Ethical Committee of the Swedish Society of Medicine, among others. According to Giertz, a paradoxical situation had arisen: 'A physician can theoretically be held liable if he does not initiate the treatment required by the fetus's condition—but the pregnant woman is legally entitled to abortion of the same fetus.'[27] The increasing interest in 'the unborn child' (this notion was repeatedly used) became clear in a symposium organized by the Ethical Committee with the title 'Who Takes Responsibility for the Unborn?,' which covered a broad range of topics related to the fetus—such as pregnant women's smoking and drug abuse, chemical exposure in work environments, and future opportunities for fetal therapy.[28] According to the Ethical Committee,

24 E.g., 'Fostertest.'

25 Swedish National Association for People with Intellectual Disability to MHSA. The association suggested a governmental commission about prenatal diagnosis with representation from the disability organizations.

26 E.g., Swedish Parliament, 'Motion 1980/81:376.'

27 Karlsson, '"Det ofödda barnets rätt."'

28 Karlsson, 'Vem svarar för den ofödde?'

'the fetus [was] a developing individual, whose interests [had] to be taken into account,' and its legal status should be further analyzed.[29]

On several occasions in the late 1970s and early 1980s, issues about abortions, prenatal diagnosis, and fetal rights were also brought up in the Swedish Parliament.[30] Although the political majority stood behind the main principle of the 1974 Abortion Act, recurring discussions about the legal and moral status of the fetus influenced the debate in a way that could ultimately affect women's reproductive autonomy.[31] This became clear in a report by the National Board of Health and Welfare concerning prenatal diagnosis.[32] One of several questions that the board raised was whether there were grounds for introducing special rules for abortions in weeks fourteen to eighteen, implying an obligation to inform the authorities when abortions were performed because of fetal impairments. This suggestion would violate the woman's legal right to have an abortion without giving any reason. The board's concern was that in the future, more and more congenital disorders would be possible to detect before the eighteenth week of pregnancy, meaning that these abortions would be performed without the authorities' approval. As a consequence, society would lose the ability to surveil the development. Another concern was that an increasing number of less serious impairments could be diagnosed, leading to 'quality control' of the fetus and devaluation of people with disabilities. The board thus asked whether the woman herself should have the right to decide on abortions motivated by fetal traits. Although the board did not suggest any changes to the 1974 Abortion Act, questions like these linked the issue of prenatal diagnosis to, on the one hand, the situation of people with disabilities and, on the other, to women's reproductive rights.[33]

In a few years, the moral landscape of prenatal diagnosis had thus changed, as the status of the fetus and the situation of people with disabilities came under increasing scrutiny. The emerging landscape included a complex tangle of values and interests, and it became the task of the 1984 commission of inquiry to propose how prenatal diagnosis and late-term abortions should be regulated.

---

29 Swedish Society of Medicine's Ethics Delegation, 'Stärk skyddet för det ofödda barnet!'

30 E.g., Swedish Parliament, 'Nr 14. Socialutskottets betänkande.'

31 The concept of reproductive autonomy began to appear in the context of the fight for more liberal abortion legislation in the United States in the 1960s. For a brief history of the concept, see Johnston and Zacharias, 'Future of Reproductive Autonomy.'

32 National Board of Health and Welfare, *Fosterdiagnostik*.

33 For a discussion about the intersections of disability and reproductive rights from a European perspective, see Herzog, *Unlearning Eugenics*.

3 The Commission of the Unborn Child

The assignment was given to Tor Sverne, who was assisted by a committee made up of members of Parliament and experts on medicine, psychology, and theology. Sverne had a background as a lawyer and was deeply engaged in issues concerning children's rights.[34] On several occasions in the early 1980s, he had discussed whether it was time to also protect the unborn child.[35] The commission, which adopted the name Utredningen om det ofödda barnet (The Commission of the Unborn Child), had two tasks: first, to consider situations when a pregnant woman did not realize the risk of her behavior for the expected child, primarily concerning the use of alcohol and tobacco but also drug abuse; and second, to investigate 'the principled and ethical issues that prenatal diagnosis actualized and to analyze the problems associated with possible legislation.'[36]

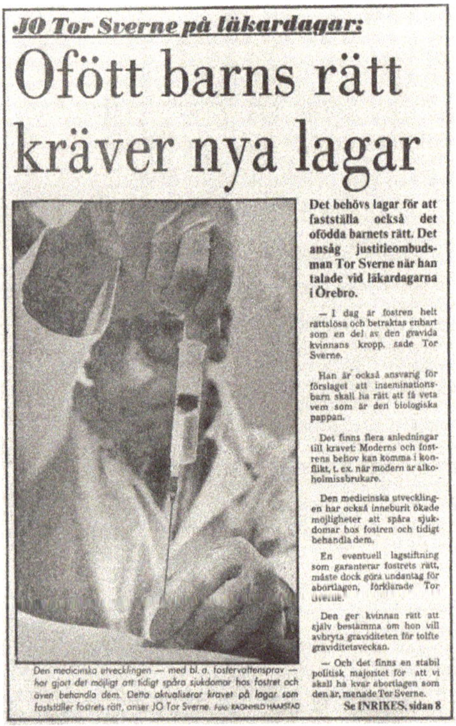

JO Tor Sverne på läkardagar:

Ofött barns rätt kräver nya lagar

Det behövs lagar för att fastställa också det ofödda barnets rätt. Det ansåg justitieombudsman Tor Sverne när han talade vid läkardagarna i Örebro.

— I dag är fostren helt rättslösa och betraktas enbart som en del av den gravida kvinnans kropp, sade Tor Sverne.

Han är också ansvarig för förslaget att inseminationsbarn skall ha rätt att få veta vem som är den biologiska pappan.

Det finns flera anledningar till kravet: Moderns och fostrens behov kan komma i konflikt, t. ex. när modern är alkoholmissbrukare.

Den medicinska utvecklingen har också inneburit ökade möjligheter att spåra sjukdomar hos fostren och tidigt behandla dem.

En eventuell lagstiftning som garanterar fostrets rätt, måste dock göra undantag för abortlagen, förklarade Tor Sverne.

Den ger kvinnan rätt att själv bestämma om hon vill avbryta graviditeten för tolfte graviditetsveckan.

— Och det finns en stabil politisk majoritet för att vi skall ha kvar abortlagen som den är, menade Tor Sverne.

Se INRIKES, sidan 8

Den medicinska utvecklingen — med bl. a. fostervattensprov — har gjort det möjligt att tidigt spåra sjukdomar hos fostret och även behandla dem. Detta aktualiserar kravet på lagar som fastställer fostrets rätt, anser JO Tor Sverne. Foto: RAGNHILD HAARSTAD

FIGURE 14.1
In this article from 1984, Tor Sverne who was chair of The Commission of the Unborn Child stated that the fetus currently had no rights and was considered only a part of the pregnant woman's body. However, medical developments, including amniocentesis, had demonstrated the need for new laws to establish the rights of the unborn child. From 'Ofött barns rätt kräver nya lagar.' Courtesy of *Svenska Dagbladet*

34 E.g., as chairman of the governmental commission 'Om barnens rätt' (On children's rights) during the 1970s.

35 Ewerlöf, Röst Andréasson, and Sverne, *Barnets bästa*, 119–120. See also Swedish Parliament, 'Nr 4. Sammanfattning av hearing.'

36 Swedish Ministry of Justice, *Den gravida kvinnan*, 19.

The commission's first report, *Skydd för det väntade barnet* (Protection of the expected child), which dealt with issues related to drug abuse, argued that the fetus was a developing human life that had to be protected. In the words of the commission, 'the mother and the prospective child are two individuals that are both worthy of protection. Their interests may coincide but may also conflict.'[37] By this statement, the commission chose a path in the moral landscape that departed from the notion that the fetus was part of the woman's body. This view became fundamental to the commission's deliberations. However, regarding the use of alcohol, tobacco, and drugs, the commission claimed that in most cases there was no conflict between the pregnant woman and the fetus since in principle, all women wanted to have a healthy child.[38] Therefore, most women adapted their way of life and reduced their use of alcohol and other drugs during pregnancy. Increased information about the risks of using these substances during pregnancy was sufficient. In cases of more severe drug problems, the commission suggested outreach measures and voluntary treatment but no coercive actions. Thus, while efforts to protect the fetus permeated the report, measures aimed at the pregnant woman were limited.

The notion of the pregnant woman and the fetus as two individuals worthy of protection was further developed in the commission's second report, *Den gravida kvinnan och fostret—två individer: Om fosterdiagnostik; Om sena aborter* (The pregnant woman and the fetus—two individuals: On prenatal diagnosis; On late-term abortions). In this report, the commission stressed that the status of the fetus had changed since the 1974 Abortion Act. One reason was the development of prenatal diagnosis; another was the changing perception of children and their rights, which, according to the commission, naturally drew attention to the rights of the unborn child.[39] Central to the commission's deliberations on fetal rights was an ethical perspective called *en humanistisk människosyn* (a humanistic perspective on human beings), emphasizing human dignity, the inviolability of life, and personal integrity. According to the commission, every human being was a goal in itself. This view contrasted with a technocratic perspective, which would regard human beings as objects that could be manipulated.[40] Concerning the disputed issue of when the fetus should be recognized as a person and granted human dignity, the commission

37 Swedish Ministry of Justice, *Skydd för det väntade barnet*, 69.

38 Swedish Ministry of Justice, *Skydd för det väntade barnet*, 42.

39 Swedish Ministry of Justice, *Den gravida kvinnan*, 80.

40 Swedish Ministry of Justice, *Den gravida kvinnan*, 75. 'En humanistisk människosyn' is a central concept in Swedish discussions on medical ethics. Hermerén, 'Det svårfångade människovärdet.'

argued that there was a distinction between 'life as a possibility' and 'life as developed.'[41] Life as a possibility started with conception, and this life had to be protected as far as possible (e.g., from harmful substances) but was not inviolable. Human personhood, on the other hand, developed gradually.[42] Therefore, the legal protection of the fetus should increase as its development progressed.

While the fetus did not have the status of a person in its early development, according to the commission it still had legitimate interests. In principle, the commission argued, the fetus had the right to develop and be born; this was in the fetus's interest even if it was diagnosed with some impairment, the only exception being when serious damage placed it at risk of dying during or shortly after birth. On the other hand, the commission continued, it was in the interest of the woman to have the right to make decisions on prenatal diagnosis and selective abortions based on her specific situation. Personal integrity and autonomy were important parts of human dignity. The ethical conflict then, the commission argued, was between the fetus's human dignity and value, regardless of health and functioning, and the woman's autonomy, particularly how she assessed her ability to care for a child with disabilities. The balance of interests between the woman and the fetus was, according to the commission, 'difficult and delicate,' yet it was obvious that in certain situations the interest of one had to take precedence over the other.[43] In early pregnancy, the commission argued, the interest of the woman outweighed that of the fetus, while the interest of the fetus became increasingly significant as fetal development progressed. Thus, despite viewing the fetus as an individual, in practice the commission followed the current abortion legislation, in which the woman had the right to make her own decision in early pregnancy, while the fetus's interest—that is, its right to life—took over in late pregnancy.

Although the commission argued that the fetus's interests were subordinated to the woman's in early pregnancy, it seemed deeply concerned about the development of prenatal diagnosis, especially in light of the rapid scientific advancement and the possibility of diagnosing a greater number of anomalies. In its view, selective abortions posed a threat to human dignity and the principle of equal value of all human beings. Trying to detect every possible deviation of the fetus, the commission emphasized, was unethical and could lead to the pursuit of perfection, causing elitist attitudes toward human life.

---

41 Swedish Ministry of Justice, *Den gravida kvinnan*, 77.

42 On the contested status of the unborn, see Lupton, *Social Worlds of the Unborn*, 13–19.

43 Swedish Ministry of Justice, *Den gravida kvinnan*, 78.

The concerns of the disability movement were 'very understandable.'[44] Therefore, society had to be informed about the scientific development of prenatal diagnosis as well as its clinical use and, if necessary, regulate its applications.

The commission's rather skeptical attitude toward prenatal diagnosis was reflected in its deliberations about guidelines and regulations. Basically, prenatal diagnosis should only be used for monitoring pregnancy or detecting serious diseases or conditions of the fetus. General fetal screening was dismissed since it might be regarded as a routine attempt to detect abnormalities. However, the commission also defended women's reproductive rights by emphasizing their entitlement to full information about prenatal diagnosis as well as the complete test results. It also proposed that the current indications for prenatal diagnosis, based on specific risk groups, should be discarded. The woman herself, in discussion with her physician, should decide whether she wanted to undergo prenatal diagnosis.[45] Regarding late-term abortions, the commission argued that the safety margin for a viable fetus was sufficient, and there was no need to lower the eighteen-week limit for unrestricted abortion.

The commission's deliberations demonstrate the difficulties of reconciling a restrictive approach to prenatal diagnosis with a defense of women's autonomy, and in the end, the commission did not propose any specific legislation related to prenatal diagnosis.[46] One reason may have been that it did not have the mandate to propose any major changes to the 1974 Abortion Act. However, its thorough discussions about fetal rights and human dignity changed the topography of the moral landscape. Women's reproductive rights were now situated close, on the one hand, to notions of fetal rights and, on the other hand, to critiques from the disability rights movement. In discussing prenatal diagnosis and selective abortions, all actors had to navigate between these positions. This became clear in the report's referral opinions from consulting bodies. Several authorities and organizations responded to the report, developing various positions in the moral landscape.[47]

---

44 Swedish Ministry of Justice, *Den gravida kvinnan*, 81.

45 This procedure followed a basic principle in Swedish health care: ultimately it was the physician who decided whether a treatment was medically justified.

46 Only minor adjustments of the 1974 Abortion Act were suggested.

47 Forty-five referral responses were made by authorities, political organizations, and various interest groups. It should be noted that the term 'fetus' was used throughout these responses, and no distinction was made between 'embryo' and 'fetus,' presumably because the opinions concerned fetal diagnosis.

4 Navigating the Moral Landscape

The commission's premise that the pregnant woman and the fetus were two individuals was questioned by several consulting bodies who argued that it was contradictory to regard the fetus as an individual and yet not give it full protection throughout pregnancy. However, as these critics noted, such a view would have undermined the foundations of the current abortion legislation. Others agreed with the commission's statement, drawing the conclusion that fetal rights had to be respected. This was the opinion of a joint statement by several Christian churches, including the Swedish State Church, which had been one of the sharpest critics of the proposal for liberal abortion legislation in the early 1970s.[48] Taking a critical approach to the current law, which, according to the churches, did not take into account the fetus's rights in early pregnancy, the statement expressed deep concerns that prenatal diagnosis could lead to selective abortions. The fetus, they argued, had human dignity from conception; human dignity was inherent in human existence and was not dependent on the level of development, or on any human characteristics or functions. The 'unborn child was a specific human life and as such an individual with human interests and with the right of life and development.'[49] This view, the statement emphasized, was consistent with Christian belief and tradition but could also be supported by biomedical developments that had demonstrated that the fetus was an independent individual. Therefore, to be able to examine and, in the future, even treat the fetus and still not give it legal protection was ethically untenable. While abortions in general posed a threat to the inviolability of life, selective abortions risked undermining the equal value of all human beings. However, maintaining these principles was a matter for society as a whole. Denouncing the tendency to individualize the ethical conflict of selective abortions with its existential and social dimensions, the churches' statement emphasized societies' responsibility to support those taking care of children with disabilities. Selective abortions, they concluded, were an emergency measure that should only be used in particularly vulnerable situations.[50] Framed by a general critique of abortion, this path in the moral landscape thus turned toward protecting fetal rights, while women's reproductive autonomy was challenged.

48 Joint statement of opinion to MHSA. On the Swedish State Church's opinion of the proposal for new abortion legislation, see Swedish Ministry of Justice, *Abortfrågan*, 96–108.

49 Joint statement of opinion to MHSA.

50 Joint statement of opinion to MHSA.

Taking a somewhat different route, a large segment of the disability movement also expressed deep concerns about prenatal diagnosis, particularly selective abortions. This position was not primarily based on the protection of fetal rights but on worries that selective abortion might threaten the principle of the equal value of all people and negatively affect societal attitudes toward people with disabilities. This would be a setback for the disability community in Sweden, whose situation had started to improve during the 1960s and 1970s, through government policy focusing on normalization and integration.[51]

However, prenatal diagnosis was a complex issue, and the disability movement was not entirely unanimous in its views; how to value this medical technology had been a thorny issue within the movement for several years. When the technology was introduced in the 1970s, many were cautiously positive. As the Swedish Disability Rights Federation, one of the largest associations, initially argued, prenatal diagnosis was a means to prevent disabilities.[52] When the debate evolved, and the moral landscape changed, this perspective seemed increasingly untenable to many members. The movement tried to find new pathways, navigating between respectful attitudes toward those who thought prenatal diagnosis and selective abortions could be justified in specific situations, and those who stressed that abortions of impaired fetuses undermined human dignity.

Central to all disability organizations' reactions to the commission's report was the equal value of all human beings. Prenatal diagnosis should not be used to screen out people with disabilities. Instead, it was society's responsibility to provide the necessary conditions so that all people, regardless of characteristics or functioning, could live a good life.[53] The argument that selective abortions could prevent suffering was dismissed. Loss of functioning was not suffering in itself; it was exclusion from society and the lack of equality that caused suffering.[54] However, as the Disability Rights Federation carefully pointed out, the strict view of prenatal diagnosis did not mean condemning women who saw abortion of an impaired fetus as the only solution to a difficult situation. What they demanded was that society take its responsibility, defend the equal value of all people, and support families living with children with disabilities.[55] This

51 Lindqvist, 'Swedish Disability Policy.'

52 Gustafson, *Fosterdiagnostik*, 66.

53 See, e.g., National Association of the Disabled, statement of opinion to MHSA; National Association of the Neurologically Disabled, statement of opinion to MHSA; National Council for the Disabled, statement of opinion to MHSA; Swedish Disability Rights Federation, statement of opinion to MHSA.

54 National Association of the Disabled, statement of opinion to MHSA.

55 Swedish Disability Rights Federation, statement of opinion to MHSA.

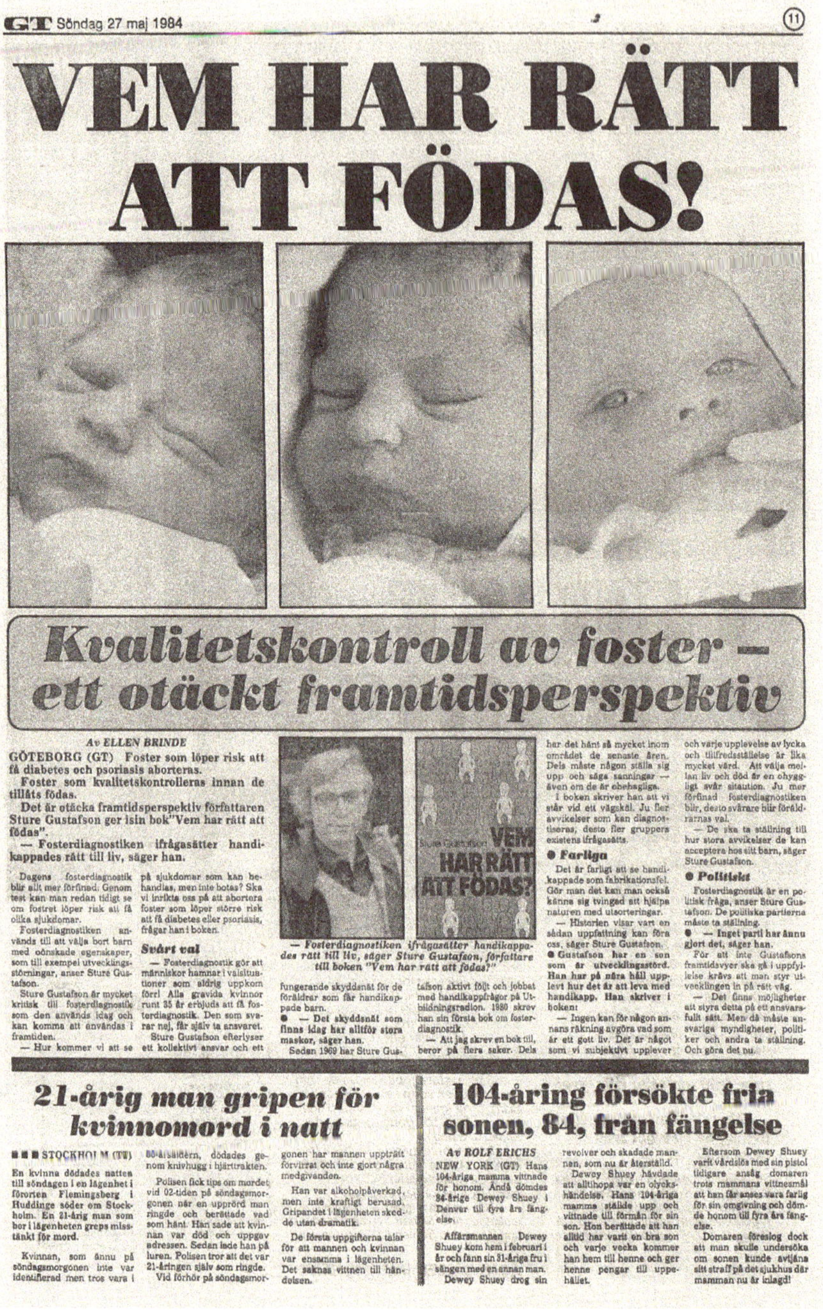

GT Söndag 27 maj 1984 11

VEM HAR RÄTT ATT FÖDAS!

Kvalitetskontroll av foster – ett otäckt framtidsperspektiv

Av ELLEN BRINDE

GÖTEBORG (GT) Foster som löper risk att få diabetes och psoriasis aborteras.

Foster som kvalitetskontrolleras innan de tillåts födas.

Det är otäcka framtidsperspektiv författaren Sture Gustafson ger i sin bok "Vem har rätt att födas".

— Fosterdiagnostiken ifrågasätter handikappades rätt till liv, säger han.

Dagens fosterdiagnostik blir allt mer förfinad. Genom test kan man redan tidigt se om fostret löper risk att få olika sjukdomar.

Fosterdiagnostiken används till att välja bort barn med oönskade egenskaper, som till exempel utvecklingsstörningar, anser Sture Gustafson.

Sture Gustafson är mycket kritisk till fosterdiagnostik som den används idag och kan komma att användas i framtiden.

— Hur kommer vi att se på sjukdomar som kan behandlas, men inte botas? Ska vi inrikta oss på att abortera foster som löper större risk att få diabetes eller psoriasis, frågar han i boken.

Svårt val

— Fosterdiagnostik gör att människor hamnar i valsituationer som aldrig uppkom förr! Alla gravida kvinnor runt 35 år erbjuds att få fosterdiagnostik. Den som svarar nej, får själv ta ansvaret.

Sture Gustafson efterlyser ett kollektivt ansvar och ett fungerande skyddsnät för de föräldrar som får handikappade barn.

● **— Det skyddsnät som finns idag har alltför stora maskor, säger han.**

Sedan 1969 har Sture Gustafson aktivt följt och jobbat med handikappfrågor på Utbildningsradion. 1980 skrev han sin första bok om fosterdiagnostik.

— Att jag skrev en bok till, beror på flera saker. Dels har det hänt så mycket inom området de senaste åren. Dels måste någon ställa sig upp och säga sanningar — även om de är obehagliga.

I boken skriver han att vi står vid ett vägskäl. Ju fler avvikelser som kan diagnostiseras, desto fler gruppers existens ifrågasätts.

● Farliga

Det är farligt att se handikappade som fabrikationsfel. Gör man det kan man också känna sig tvingad att hjälpa naturen med utsorteringar.

— Historien visar vart en sådan uppfattning kan föra oss, säger Sture Gustafson.

● Gustafson har en son som är utvecklingsstörd. Han har på nära håll upplevt hur det är att leva med handikapp. Han skriver i boken:

— Ingen kan för någon annans räkning avgöra vad som är ett gott liv. Det är något som vi subjektivt upplever och varje upplevelse av lycka och tillfredsställelse är lika mycket värd. Att välja mellan liv och död är en ohyggligt svår sitaution. Ju mer förfinad fosterdiagnostiken blir, desto svårare blir föräldrarnas val.

— De ska ta ställning till hur stora avvikelser de kan acceptera hos sitt barn, säger Sture Gustafson.

● Politiskt

Fosterdiagnostik är en politisk fråga, anser Sture Gustafson. De politiska partierna måste ta ställning.

● **— Inget parti har ännu gjort det, säger han.**

För att inte Gustafsons framtidsvyer ska gå i uppfyllelse krävs att man styr utvecklingen in på rätt väg.

— Det finns möjligheter att styra detta på ett ansvarsfullt sätt. Men då måste ansvariga myndigheter, politiker och andra ta ställning. Och göra det nu.

— Fosterdiagnostiken ifrågasätter handikappades rätt till liv, säger Sture Gustafson, författare till boken "Vem har rätt att födas?"

21-årig man gripen för kvinnomord i natt

■■■ STOCKHOLM (TT)

En kvinna dödades natten till söndagen i en lägenhet i förorten Flemingsberg i Huddinge söder om Stockholm. En 21-årig man som bor i lägenheten greps misstänkt för mord.

Kvinnan, som ännu på söndagsmorgonen inte var identifierad men tros vara i 80-årsåldern, dödades genom knivhugg i hjärttrakten.

Polisen fick tips om mordet vid 02-tiden på söndagsmorgonen när en upprörd man ringde och berättade vad som hänt. Han sade att kvinnan var död och uppgav adressen. Sedan lade han på luren. Polisen tror att det var 21-åringen själv som ringde.

Vid förhör på söndagsmorgonen har mannen uppträtt förvirrat och inte gjort några medgivanden.

Han var alkoholpåverkad, men inte kraftigt berusad. Gripandet i lägenheten skedde utan dramatik.

De första uppgifterna talar för att mannen och kvinnan var ensamma i lägenheten. Det saknas vittnen till händelsen.

104-åring försökte fria sonen, 84, från fängelse

Av ROLF ERICHS

NEW YORK (GT) Hans 104-åriga mamma vittnade för honom. Ändå dömdes 84-årige Dewey Shuey i Denver till fyra års fängelse.

Affärsmannen Dewey Shuey kom hem i februari i år och fann sin 81-åriga fru i sängen med en annan man.

Dewey Shuey drog sin revolver och skadade mannen, som nu är återställd.

Dewey Shuey hävdade att alltihopa var en olyckshändelse. Hans 104-åriga mamma ställde upp och vittnade till förmån för sin son. Hon berättade att han alltid har varit en bra son och varje vecka kommer han hem till henne och ger henne pengar till uppehället.

Eftersom Dewey Shuey varit vårdslös med sin pistol tidigare ansåg domaren trots mammans vittnesmål att han får anses vara farlig för sin omgivning och dömde honom till fyra års fängelse.

Domaren föreslog dock att man skulle undersöka om sonen kunde avtjäna sitt straff på det sjukhus där mamman nu är inlagd!

FIGURE 14.2 Journalist Sture Gustafson, author of the book *Vem har rätt att födas*? (Who has the right to be born?), was a prominent voice in the debate on prenatal diagnosis in the early 1980s. Gustafson argued that developments in prenatal diagnosis called into question the right to life of people with disabilities. From Brinde, 'Vem har rätt att födas?' Courtesy of *Expressen*

responsibility included providing women with information about all aspects of prenatal diagnosis but also what it meant to live with disability. Otherwise, an informed and free decision was not possible. Insufficient information, indirect recommendations, and prejudices about living with disabilities threatened women's autonomy.[56] In this way, many of the disability organizations also defended a woman's right to make her own decision. However, others explicitly argued for stricter regulations of prenatal diagnosis.[57]

A third path in the moral landscape more explicitly defended women's rights. Referring to the 1974 Abortion Act, actors in this position argued that the woman's interest took precedence over fetal interests in early pregnancy and that women were competent to make difficult decisions about prenatal diagnosis and selective abortions.[58] Ascribing the fetus moral status as an individual, with the right to protection that this status implied, was criticized. As the Swedish Society of Medicine emphasized, this would mean that abortion could not be defended at all. Instead, the fetus should be considered as a potential individual, whose interest in some cases had to be subordinated to the woman's (or parents') situation.[59] Nowhere did the Society of Medicine argue that the fetus might be a patient, which was one of the issues that Giertz, the former chairman of the society's Ethics Committee, had brought up as an argument for changing the moral status of the fetus. One reason might have been that the possibility of providing treatment to the fetus had proved very limited.[60] Instead, the Society of Medicine deplored the moral debates about prenatal diagnosis and selective abortion, as they had caused families to refrain from 'a medically well-motivated examination.'[61] In the same spirit, one of the women's organizations pointed out that discussions about the 'inviolability of life,' which tended to be brought up in relation to the moral status of the fetus, too often led to 'a violation of the woman's integrity and autonomy, which is unjustifiable.'[62]

At the same time, these referral opinions carefully pointed out that prenatal diagnosis and selective abortions did not mean any downgrading of people

---

56 Swedish Disability Rights Federation, statement of opinion to MHSA.

57 E.g., National Association of the Neurologically Disabled, statement of opinion to MHSA, and National Council for the Disabled, statement of opinion to MHSA.

58 E.g., Fredrika Bremer Association, statement of opinion to MHSA; and Swedish Association for Sexuality Education, statement of opinion to MHSA.

59 Swedish Society of Medicine, statement of opinion to MHSA. See also Karolinska Institute, statement of opinion to MHSA.

60 Cf. Swedish Ministry of Justice, *Den gravida kvinnan*, 26.

61 Swedish Society of Medicine, statement of opinion to MHSA.

62 Fredrika Bremer Association, statement of opinion to MHSA.

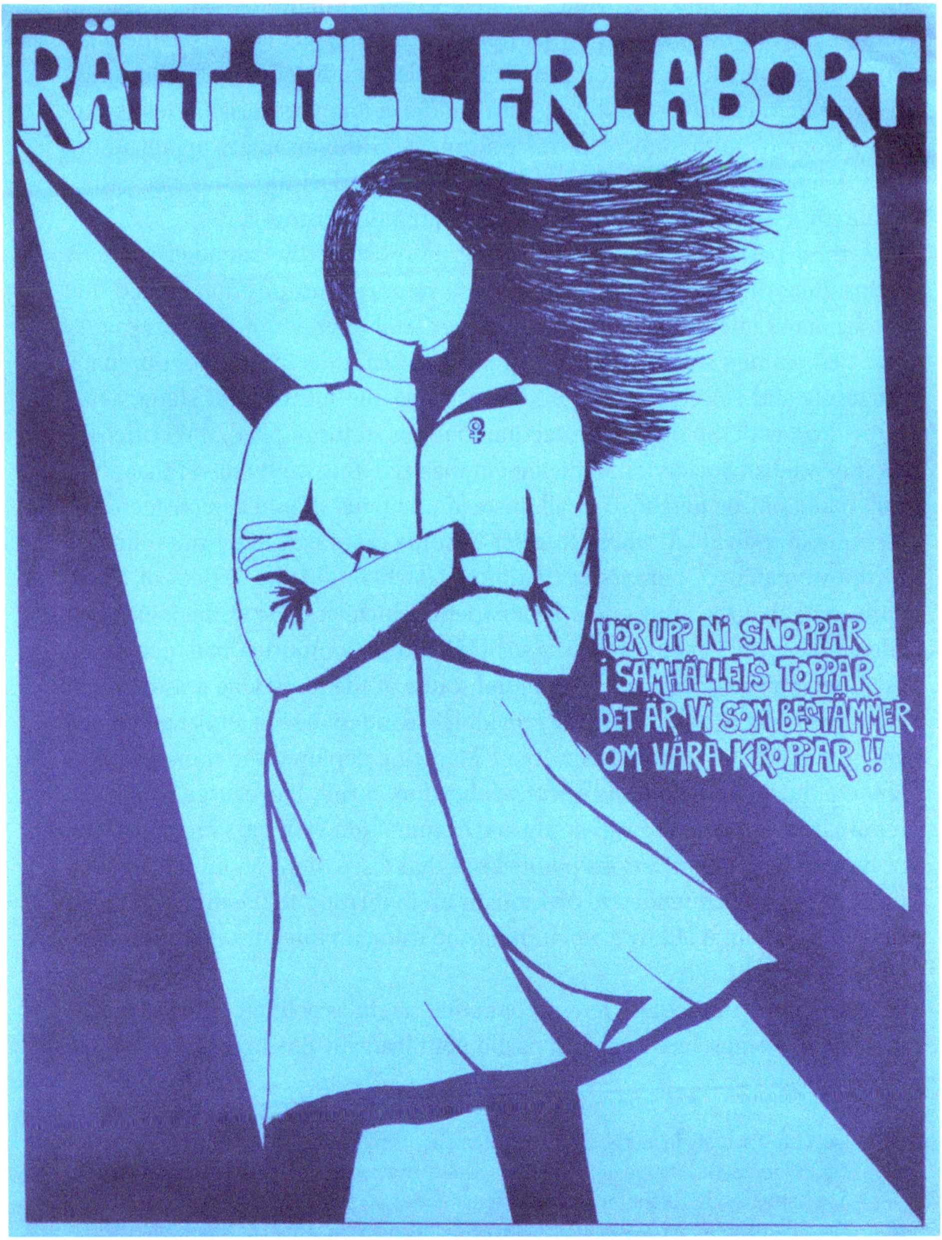
RÄTT TILL FRI ABORT
HÖR UPP NI SNOPPAR
I SAMHÄLLETS TOPPAR
DET ÄR VI SOM BESTÄMMER
OM VÅRA KROPPAR !!

FIGURE 14.3 Probably from the 1970s, this poster proclaims the 'Right to free abortion' (*Rätt till fri abort*). Women's right to decide on abortion was well established in Sweden and the regulation of prenatal diagnosis and selective abortions was, according to the women's movement, a restriction of this right. The text at the right-side reads: 'Listen up you dicks at the top of society; we are the ones who decide about our bodies!!' Unknown artist. KvinnSam, Gothenburg University Library.

with disabilities.[63] It was important to make a distinction between the individual motives and society's goals. For the woman, the motives concerned her specific situation, while society's goal must be to support all people, including those living with disabilities.[64] It was even argued that decisions about selective abortions could actually be based on certain traits of the fetus and the expected child's quality of life, and not only on the family's situation. This had to be accepted since selective abortions were allowed. However, the individual valuation had to be distinguished from that of society, which must not even be suspected of calling into question the equal worth of all human beings.[65] The objections of the disability movement were thus met by two arguments: that it was possible to distinguish between individual choices and societal norms, and that society had to provide support to people living with disabilities. The previous argument that prenatal diagnosis could be justified from an economic point of view, which was initially posed by medical experts, was no longer suggested, either by actors taking this path in the moral landscape or by anyone else.

Several years after the commission's report and the consultation process, the Government submitted a bill to Parliament about prenatal diagnosis and abortion.[66] Although the fetus's right to protection during its development was recognized, the Government clearly defended women's reproductive rights: No matter how difficult the decision on prenatal diagnosis was, no one was better suited to make it than the woman herself, in consultation with her physician. Therefore, no regulation of prenatal diagnosis was suggested. Access to adequate knowledge about the medical examination and the implications of the tests, as well as information about society's support for people with disabilities, was, however, a prerequisite for an informed choice. According to the Government, 'information and knowledge was one of the central issues of prenatal diagnosis.'[67] The bill was approved by Parliament, and ten years after the appointment of the Commission of the Unborn Child, Sweden ended up with a decision that no special legislation on prenatal diagnosis and selective abortion was needed.[68] Prenatal diagnosis thus became inseparably linked to

63 Swedish Society of Medicine, statement of opinion to MHSA.

64 Swedish Medical Association, statement of opinion to MHSA; and National Board of Health and Welfare's advisory board for ethical issues, statement of opinion to MHSA.

65 National Board of Health and Welfare's advisory board for ethical issues, statement of opinion to MHSA.

66 Swedish Parliament, 'Nr 142. Fosterdiagnostik och abort.'

67 Swedish Parliament, 'Nr 142. Fosterdiagnostik och abort,' 22–23.

68 Only minor changes to the 1974 Abortion Act were made—for example, that the woman should be offered a meeting with a counsellor before and after the termination of a pregnancy if she so desired.

the liberal abortion legislation of 1974 and the emphasis on a woman's individual choice. It should be noted that this choice was always situated and dependent on the individual woman's circumstances as well as the social, political, and cultural context.[69]

5 Discussion

Parliament's decision marked the end of a debate on prenatal diagnosis that had been going on for almost two decades. During this time, the moral landscape underwent various changes as new arguments and positions developed, while others were abandoned or downplayed. In the end, the political decision demonstrated that the main path was to defend women's reproductive autonomy, while the notion that life was inviolable from conception did not receive much support.

Although the regulation of prenatal diagnosis did not primarily concern abortion legislation, there were obvious overlaps, and the balance between the interests of the fetus and the woman that had been established by the 1974 Abortion Act also shaped the view of prenatal diagnosis. This outcome points to the strong political support for liberal abortion legislation in Sweden, particularly with regard to women's reproductive autonomy.[70] The Swedish anti-abortion movement never gained the scope and political influence that it did in the United States, where political conflicts over abortion-related issues have always been intense.[71]

Another sign of broad support for women's reproductive autonomy was that the Church of Sweden (until 2000, the Swedish State Church), along with several other churches in Sweden, gradually accepted the right to abortion, arguing that although the 'the unborn life' had human dignity and should be protected, there was no room to change the abortion legislation and no alternative to women's autonomy.[72] The churches' influence on the issue of abortion was arguably diminishing in Sweden, which is often considered as one of the most secularized countries in the world.[73] Nevertheless, their recognition of the

69 For a discussion of liberal abortion legislation as well as decisions about development, prenatal diagnosis, and reproduction in other European countries, see, e.g., Löwy, *Tangled Diagnoses*, chap. 3 on France; and Doetz, 'Healthy, Happy, Rational' on the GDR.

70 See Lennerhed, 'No Backlash.' For a brief discussion about Swedish anti-abortion activists, see Björklund's chapter in this volume.

71 Linders, 'Victory and Beyond'; Lennerhed, 'No Backlash.'

72 Kumlien, *'Kristet synsätt på abort?*, 41–43.

73 Zuckerman, 'Why Are Danes and Swedes.'

right to abortion may be taken as a sign that women's reproductive rights had gained acceptance in wide circles.

As this chapter has demonstrated, the debate on prenatal diagnosis also concerned the practice's consequences for people with disabilities, with the differences of opinion centered on whether prenatal diagnosis and selective abortions expressed negative and discriminatory attitudes toward people with disabilities, a view that has been called the expressivist argument.[74] Some actors addressed this dilemma by distinguishing between individual choice and societal norms and values. In this way, support for women's reproductive autonomy and a respectful view of persons with disabilities could be reconciled. However, this approach was not convincing to the disability movement, whose members felt that prenatal diagnosis risked undermining essential social values and ultimately society's support for persons with disabilities. This argument was important when these public debates emerged in Sweden, and it was further developed in referral opinions to the commission's report. However, the government bill mentioned it only briefly, focusing instead on the conflict of interest between the woman and the fetus. The tension between women's reproductive autonomy and the potential devaluing of people with disabilities thus remained and has continued to be addressed in relation to new reproductive biotechnologies.[75]

Several of the arguments in the Swedish debate on prenatal diagnosis and selective abortions show similarities with corresponding debates in other countries, although the emphasis and focus have varied.[76] Common features included socioeconomic arguments in the early debates, the perception that prenatal diagnosis and selective abortion were tools to prevent suffering, and the reactions of the disability movement. The increased focus on the fetus and its potential rights has also attracted much attention, as have, of course, the pregnant woman, her experiences of pregnancy, and her reproductive rights. However, the Swedish investigation and subsequent responses provide a vivid picture of how the different aspects were weighed against each other in a specific historical situation.

Finally, it should be noted that prenatal diagnosis formed part of a larger moral landscape of developing genetic and reproductive technologies such as preimplantation diagnostics, as well as medical research involving fertilized

---

74 See, e.g., Parens and Asch, *Prenatal Testing and Disability Rights*; Hofmann, "'You Are Inferior!'"

75 See, e.g., Hofmann, "'You Are Inferior!'"

76 See, e.g., Löwy, *Tangled Diagnoses*; Lupton, *Social Worlds of the Unborn*; Stern, *Telling Genes*, chap. 7.

eggs, embryos, and fetuses. Within these contexts, embryos and fetuses were conceptualized and valued from various standpoints, for example, as entities at the beginning of human life, as collections of cells, or as precious resources for understanding and treating diseases. The view of the fetus has thus continued to be dependent on broader scientific, political, and moral values.

Bibliography

Bashford, Alison. 'Epilogue.' In *The Oxford Handbook of the History of Eugenics*, edited by Alison Bashford and Philippa Levine, 539–58. New York: Oxford University Press, 2010.

Björkman, Maria, and Anna Tunlid. 'The Establishment of Genetic Counselling in Sweden: 1940–1980.' In *History of Human Genetics: Aspects of Its Development and Global Perspectives*, edited by Heike I. Petermann, Peter S. Harper, and Susanne Doetz, 339–66. Cham: Springer International, 2017.

Brinde, Ellen. 'Vem har rätt att födas?' *Göteborgs-Tidningen*, May 27, 1984.

Casper, Monica J. *The Making of the Unborn Patient: A Social Anatomy of Fetal Surgery.* New Brunswick, NJ: Rutgers University Press, 1998.

de Chadarevian, Soraya. 'Chromosome Photography and the Human Karyotype.' *Historical Studies in the Natural Sciences* 45 (2015): 115–46.

Doetz, Susanne. 'Healthy, Happy, Rational: Reflections on Genetic Counselling in the GDR.' *Medical Humanities* 49, no. 2 (2023): 236–47.

Dubow, Sara. *Ourselves Unborn: A History of the Fetus in Modern America.* New York: Oxford University Press, 2011.

Ewerlöf, Göran, Barbro Röst Andréasson, and Tor Sverne. *Barnets bästa: Om föräldrars och samhällets ansvar.* Stockholm: Liber Förlag, 1982.

'Fostertest: Rätt eller plikt?' *Dagens Nyheter*, June 18, 1980.

Gustafson, Sture. *Fosterdiagnostik—för vem?* Stockholm: LT:s förlag, 1980.

Gustafson, Sture. *Vem har rätt att födas? En bok om människosyn och fosterdiagnostik.* Stockholm: LT:s förlag, 1984.

Helgason, Agnar, and Gísli Pálsson. 'Contested Commodities: The Moral Landscape of Modernist Regimes.' *Journal of the Royal Anthropological Institute* 3 (1997): 451–71.

Hermerén, Göran. 'Det svårfångade människovärdet.' In *Det svårfångade människovärdet: En debattskrift*, 61–99. Etiska vägmärken 4. Stockholm: Statens Medicinsk-etiska råd, 1991.

Herzog, Dagmar. *Unlearning Eugenics: Sexuality, Reproduction, and Disability in Post-Nazi Europe.* Madison: University of Wisconsin Press, 2018.

Hofmann, Bjørn. '"You Are Inferior!" Revisiting the Expressivist Argument.' *Bioethics* 31 (2017): 505–14.

Johnston, Josephine, and Rachel L. Zacharias. 'The Future of Reproductive Autonomy.' *Hastings Center Report* 47 (2017): S6–S11.

Jülich, Solveig. 'The Making of a Best-Selling Book on Reproduction: Lennart Nilsson's *A Child Is Born*.' *Bulletin of the History of Medicine* 89, no. 3 (2015): 491–526.

Karlsson, Yngve. '"Det ofödda barnets rätt" etisk nyckelfråga som får ny aktualitet genom fosterdiagnostiken.' *Läkartidningen* 77 (1980): 1266–68.

Karlsson, Yngve. 'Vem svarar för den ofödde?' *Läkartidningen* 37 (1981): 3131–36.

Koch, Lene, and Mette N. Svendsen. 'Negotiating Moral Value: A Story of Danish Research Monkeys and Their Humans.' *Science, Technology, & Human Values* 40 (2015): 368–88.

Kumlien, Mats. *Finns det ett kristet synsätt på abort?* Uppsala Faculty of Law, Working Paper 2012:2. Uppsala: Uppsala universitet, 2012.

Lennerhed, Lena. *Kvinnotrubbel: Abort i Sverige 1938–1974*. Möklinta: Gidlunds, 2017.

Lennerhed, Lena. 'No Backlash for Swedish Women? The Right to Abortion on Demand, 1975–2000.' *Journal of Modern European History* 17, no. 3 (2019): 326–36.

Linders, Annulla. 'Victory and Beyond: A Historical Comparative Analysis of the Outcomes of the Abortion Movements in Sweden and the United States.' *Sociological Forum* 19 (2004): 371–404.

Lindqvist, Rafael. 'Swedish Disability Policy: From Universal Welfare to Civil Rights?' *European Journal of Social Security* 2 (2000): 399–418.

Lindsten, Jan, and Lars Beckman. *Klinisk genetik: Supplement till Medicinsk service.* Stockholm: Socialstyrelsen 1976.

Löwy, Ilana. *Imperfect Pregnancies: A History of Birth Defects and Prenatal Diagnosis.* Baltimore: Johns Hopkins University Press, 2017.

Löwy, Ilana. *Tangled Diagnoses: Prenatal Diagnosis, Women and Risk.* Chicago: University of Chicago Press, 2018.

Lupton, Deborah. *The Social Worlds of the Unborn.* Basingstoke: Palgrave Macmillan, 2013.

National Board of Health and Welfare. *Fosterdiagnostik: Rapport från en av Socialstyrelsen tillsatt expertgrupp.* Stockholm: Socialstyrelsen, 1982.

Nemec, Birgit, and Gabriele Moser. 'Counselling, Risk and Prevention in Human Genetic Early Diagnosis in the Federal Republic of Germany.' In *History of Human Genetics: Aspects of Its Development and Global Perspectives,* edited by Heike I. Petermann, Peter S. Harper, and Susanne Doetz, 367–92. Cham: Springer International, 2017.

Nilsson, Lennart, Axel Ingelman-Sundberg, and Claes Wirsén. *Ett barn blir till: En bildskildring av de nio månaderna före födelsen; En praktisk rådgivare för den blivande mamman.* Stockholm: Bonnier, 1965.

'Ofött barns rätt kräver nya lagar.' *Svenska Dagbladet,* April 10, 1984.

Parens, Erik, and Adrienne Asch, eds. *Prenatal Testing and Disability Rights.* Baltimore: Georgetown University Press, 2000.

Paul, Diane B. 'Reflections on the Historiography of American Eugenics: Trends, Fractures, Tensions.' *Journal of the History of Biology* 49 (2016): 641–58.

Rapp, Rayna. *Testing Women, Testing the Fetus*. New York: Routledge, 1999.

Reagan, Leslie J. *Dangerous Pregnancies: Mothers, Disabilities, and Abortion in Modern America*. Berkeley: University of California Press, 2010.

Stern, Alexandra Minna. *Telling Genes: The Story of Genetic Counselling in America*. Baltimore: Johns Hopkins University Press, 2012.

Swedish Ministry of Justice. *Abortfrågan: Remissyttranden över 1965 års abortkommittés betänkande Rätten till abort (SOU 1971:58)*. SOU 1972:39. Stockholm: Justitiedepartementet, 1972.

Swedish Ministry of Justice. *Den gravida kvinnan och fostret—två individer: Om fosterdiagnostik; Om sena aborter*. SOU 1989:51. Stockholm: Justitiedepartementet, 1989.

Swedish Ministry of Justice. *Rätten till abort*. SOU 1971:58. Stockholm: Justitiedepartementet, 1971.

Swedish Ministry of Justice. *Skydd för det väntade barnet. 1. Åtgärder vid missbruk m.m. under graviditet*. SOU 1987:11. Stockholm: Justitiedepartementet, 1987.

Swedish Parliament. 'Nr 14. Socialutskottets betänkande om lagstiftning till skydd för ofödda m. m.' In *Riksdagens protokoll*. Collection 12, Vol. E9. *Socialutskottets betänkanden och yttranden nr 1–56*, 1–37. Stockholm: Riksdagen, 1981–82.

Swedish Parliament. 'Nr 4. Sammanfattning av hearing 1984-09-04. Bilaga till Socialutskottets betänkande om vissa medicinsk-etiska frågor.' In *Riksdagens protokoll*. Collection 12, Vol. E9. *Socialutskottets betänkanden och yttranden*, 28–49. Stockholm: Riksdagen, 1984–85.

Swedish Parliament. 'Nr 70. Kungl. Maj:ts proposition med förslag till abortlag m.m.; given den 8 mars.' In *Riksdagens protokoll*. Collection 1, Vol. B9. *Kungl. Maj:ts propositioner nr 51–76*, 1–123. Stockholm: Riksdagen, 1974.

Swedish Parliament. 'Nr 142. Fosterdiagnostik och abort.' In *Riksdagens protokoll*. Collection 1, Vol. B21. *Regeringens propositioner nr 130–149*, 1–82. Stockholm: Riksdagen, 1994–95.

Swedish Parliament. 'Motion 1980/81:376 av Mårten Werner och Gunnar Oskarson om tilläggsdirektiv till 1980 års abortkommitté.' In *Riksdagens protokoll*. Collection 3, Vol. D2. *Motioner nr 180–520*, 13–14. Stockholm: Riksdagen, 1980–81.

Swedish Society of Medicine's Ethics Delegation. 'Stärk skyddet för det ofödda barnet!' *Läkartidningen* 37 (1981): 3139–41.

Wisselgren, Per. 'Reforming the Science-Policy Boundary: The Myrdals and the Swedish Tradition of Governmental Commissions.' In *Academics and Public Intellectuals*, edited by Sven Eliaeson and Ragnvald Kalleberg, 173–95. Newcastle: Cambridge Scholars, 2008.

Zuckerman, Phil. 'Why Are Danes and Swedes So Irreligious?' *Nordic Journal of Religion and Society* 22 (2009): 55–69.

Archival Sources

Rätt till fri abort. Poster, n.d. The Archive of the Woman's House in Stockholm. B68:13. KvinnSam. Gothenburg University Library.

Fredrika Bremer Association. Statement of opinion to MHSA, April 26, 1990. E1A:2583. MHSA.

Joint statement from the Catholic Bishops' Office, the Swedish Ecumenical Board, the Bishops' Meeting of the Church of Sweden, the Swedish Council of Free Churches with the main agreement of the Central Board of the Church of Sweden. Statement of opinion MHSA, May 10, 1990. E1A:2583. MHSA.

Karolinska Institute. Statement of opinion to MHSA, May 4, 1990. E1A:2583. MHSA.

National Association of the Disabled. Statement of opinion to MHSA, April 4, 1990. E1A:2583. MHSA.

National Association of the Neurologically Disabled. Statement of opinion to MHSA, April 20, 1990. E1A:2583. MHSA.

National Board of Health and Welfare's advisory board for ethical issues. Statement of opinion to MHSA, March 30, 1990. E1A:2583. MHSA.

National Council for the Disabled. Statement of opinion to MHSA, April 18, 1990. E1A:2583. MHSA.

Swedish Association for Sexuality Education. Statement of opinion to MHSA, August 28, 1990. E1A:2583. MHSA.

Swedish Disability Rights Federation. Statement of opinion to MHSA, April 25, 1990. E1A:2583. MHSA.

Swedish Medical Association. Statement of opinion to MHSA, April 23, 1990. E1A:2583. MHSA.

Swedish National Association for People with Intellectual Disability to MHSA, December 21, 1983. Vol. 1, 'Commission of the Unborn Child.' NAS, Stockholm.

Swedish Society of Medicine. Statement of opinion to MHSA, May 8, 1990. E1A:2583. MHSA.

EPILOGUE

Controversy and Fetal Research: The Swedish Case

Solveig Jülich

In her seminal study on the development of the reproductive sciences in the United States, Adele Clarke asked, 'What makes a line of scientific work morally controversial?' Using an interactionist arena model, she understood controversies as the collision of different perspectives or 'social worlds' of actors participating in a certain area. In the broader arena of US reproduction during the twentieth century, interest groups consisted of not only professionals working in biology, medicine, and agriculture but also family planning advocates, religious groups, feminists, pharmaceutical companies, research funding organizations, and others. Clarke highlighted several realms of controversy around the reproductive sciences as well as scientists' strategies for managing their controversial status and gaining access to research funding. Importantly, she emphasized that although some controversies can be 'black boxed,' rendering them invisible, such closures are rarely definitive.[1]

The present volume has contributed fresh insights on the reproductive arena by focusing on fetal knowledge production within a Swedish historical context. We have adopted a broad scope of inquiry, highlighting the activities of embryologists, obstetricians, endocrinologists, and other categories of actors as well as crucial religious, legal, political, and visual aspects involved in the uses and handling of fetuses, stillborn, reproductive organs, and pregnant bodies. In addition, addressing a significantly longer period than Clarke did in her study, the authors have brought to light conflicted concepts, values, and practices involved in fetal knowledge production in Sweden.

In this epilogue, I address the issue of public controversy around the scientific uses of fetal material in the latter part of the twentieth century. Drawing on the chapters that deal with this theme, I return to the overarching questions raised in the introduction: Which specific interests were involved in postwar fetal research in Sweden? What strategies were developed to manage controversy? In addition, I ask to what extent fetal research has become a controversial part of Swedish medical history. In order to suggest answers to these questions, I engage with controversy studies as well as perspectives from

1 Clarke, 'Controversy,' quotation on p. 18; Clarke, *Disciplining Reproduction*, chap. 8.

 | DOI:10.1163/9789004703759_017

ignorance studies. As others have discussed, controversy around reproductive biomedicine can be linked to diverse and sometimes competing forms of ignorance production related to, for instance, risky innovations tested on women's bodies. Yet ignorance production does not always have to be strategically planned.[2] With respect to public controversies, the term may also draw attention to what is left out, unspoken, or cast into oblivion. In conclusion, I claim that postwar human fetal research involved many facets of public controversy, including 'uncontroversy,' 'tamed controversy,' and 'selective controversy.'[3]

According to Duncan Wilson, a new genre of '"social unease" literature' has emerged in both popular and academic domains that narrates the histories of tissue cultures in various national contexts. He dwells particularly on the 2010 best-seller *The Immortal Life of Henrietta Lacks*, in which author Rebecca Skloot drew attention to the lack of patient consent or any thought of ownership concerning the use of Lacks's biopsy for research.[4] Criticism, he states, has also been applied more widely to the establishment of non-consented human tissue cultures in the United States during the mid-twentieth century, portraying these as 'tissues with a troubled past.'[5] Wilson claims that these assumptions are unfair and inaccurate. Detailing the history of 'tissue culture in twentieth-century Britain,' he argues that the practices involved in obtaining and using human tissues were seen by both professionals and the public as 'unproblematic.' No secrecy was involved. Newspapers were enthusiastic over tissues and raised no concerns over their use for research. Moreover, Wilson argues that demands for informed consent 'often emanated from the scientists

2 In Jülich and Dussauge's chapter the notion of the 'strategic production of ignorance' was introduced to emphasize how actors created and disseminated specific sorts of information about the polio vaccine while witholding or downplaying others, such as the risky abortion operations that were a source of material for the vaccine's production. On ignorance production about teratogenic risks, see Nemec and Olszynko-Gryn, 'Duogynon Controversy and Ignorance Production.' Varieties of ignorance are discussed in Smithson, 'Afterword,' 387–90.

3 Following Jülich and Dussauge in this volume, I use 'uncontroversy' to describe how, for various reasons, public controversy does not break out even if a subject is sensitive or contains controversial elements. I speak of 'tamed controversy' to refer to a public debate in which some actors construct controversy around a topic and others exert authority to prevent its development into full-fledged controversy. The term 'selective controversy' is used to highlight how diverse conditions, including past controversies, affect which topics are rendered controversial. Even though these terms have emerged in relation to examining Swedish postwar fetal research, I believe that they may have a more general relevance.

4 Wilson, 'Troubled Past?,' 248–50.

5 Wilson mentions the *Nature* editorial 'Culture of Consent,' but not Meredith Wadman's historical article 'Medical Research,' on the creation of cell line WI-38 from an aborted fetus in Sweden, in the same issue. It is unclear how he positions Landecker's *Culturing Life* in relation to this '"social unease" literature.'

themselves.' He thinks that his more 'balanced' history can 'benefit present debates on the biomedical uses of human tissue.'[6]

According to Wilson, the '"social unease" literature' builds on a false dichotomy between science and its publics and runs the risk of deepening the public mistrust toward science and medicine. Instead, he stresses the importance of redefining tissue cultures as '*sites of engagement*, where scientific and popular interests converge.' In many ways this approach recalls the interactionist arena model that Clarke developed in *Disciplining Reproduction*.[7] It also has affinities with current studies of scientific controversies within the field of science and technology studies (STS). There is no longer an assumption of clear boundaries around expertise. Controversies involving science, medicine, health, and technology are examined in a wide array of settings today, including the media, social movements, and the state. This development has also directed attention toward the role of audiences for specific controversies.[8] More recently, controversy studies and ignorance studies have been brought together, providing a fertile ground for multidisciplinary dialogue and exchange.[9] However, this is not the approach that Wilson takes.

As a historian, one might find it easy to sympathize with Wilson's criticism of obsolete morals as well as his call for more balanced accounts of tissue cultures that can contribute relevant perspectives to contemporary public debates. However, the research presented in this volume highlights weaknesses in his own historical analysis of controversy. I will shortly return to the development of the Swedish polio vaccine and to perfusion studies of aborted fetuses at the Karolinska Institute (KI) to nuance his claim that 'the scientific collection of tissue for research was widely viewed as unproblematic for much of the twentieth century.'[10] But before discussing controversy in this context, we need to recognize the central participants. The next section probes the hopes and interests involved in making Sweden a powerful actor in the international field of reproductive research in the postwar period.

---

6 Wilson, 'Troubled Past?,' 250; Wilson, *Tissue Culture*, 54–55, 67–68.

7 Wilson echoes Clarke's discussion when stating that controversy surrounding the scientific use of tissues arises when the social worlds of interdependent actors come into conflict. Similarly, he holds that views on specific issues can differ within as well as overlap between social worlds, and that the process or outcome of specific controversies can 're-shape the terms of engagement and the status of tissue itself.' He prefers, then, to think in terms of 'the ongoing formation of hybrid sciences-and-publics,' rather than drawing a line between science and public. Wilson, *Tissue Culture*, 92, 122–23.

8 Pinch, 'Scientific Controversies,' 284–85.

9 Topçu and Maffi, 'Rethinking Ignorance Production,' 218.

10 Wilson, *Tissue Culture*, 92.

1 A Great Power of Sorts

'There Sweden is a great power,' boasted a 1965 Swedish newspaper article, in reference to the Hormone Laboratory at the Karolinska Hospital in Stockholm. A photograph showed a group of male guest researchers from Austria, Canada, France, West Germany, Ireland, Italy, and the United States with the director of the laboratory, Egon Diczfalusy, in the middle at the back. The reporter went on to list several more countries that were represented at the Karolinska Hospital and the KI through guest researchers affiliated to other departments and units. Apart from the Soviet Union, China, and East Germany, few were missing. He urged readers to reflect on the extraordinary achievements and enormous international publicity that the researchers' presence in Sweden entailed: 'Perhaps it gives us a legitimate reason to think for a few moments that a small nation high up in the north has been able to build hospitals and medical research institutions that the world outside is curious about.' Above all, the reporter contended, the Hormone Laboratory, with its dynamic research milieu, had attracted attention from international experts.[11]

It was not uncommon to label Sweden a great power of sorts at the time. During the Cold War some argued that Swedish internationalism should earn it the title of 'the moral superpower,' in harsh competition with, among others, Canada, Norway, and the Netherlands. What distinguished Sweden from these other countries was its nonaligned security doctrine ('neutrality'), which, according to its supporters, created an ideal position between the Soviet Union and the United States, enabling it to pursue an independent strand of foreign policy. One important area where Sweden was said to be a pioneer and international role model was family planning programs in developing countries. To its critics, the self-proclaimed title of moral superpower was an expression of the Social Democratic Party's monopoly on governmental power in Sweden from the 1930s onward. In reality, it was neither neutral, moral, nor a superpower.[12]

More recently, historians have claimed that this idea of Sweden as a moral superpower was not an invention of Social Democratic postwar foreign aid but rather an expression of a political culture that can be traced back to the emergent state idealism of the nineteenth century and even further, to early modern 'Protestant ideas about the duty and responsibility of a Christian person.'[13]

11 Öhquist, 'Där är Sverige stormakt.'

12 For an analysis that sides with the critics, see Nilsson, *Den moraliska stormakten*; Dahl, 'Sweden.'

13 Åselius, *Vietnamkriget*, 82. For a similar argument, see Berggren and Trädgårdh, *Är svensken människa?*

As others have pointed out, both of these variants of Swedish exceptionalism are too simplistic. According to an extensive historical analysis of Swedish foreign aid after the Second World War, national self-interest was always interwoven with altruism, solidarity, and collaboration.[14]

This problematization of Swedish exceptionalism is relevant for the overarching argument of this volume. Reproductive and population research, as demonstrated in several chapters, was considered an important element in Sweden's foreign-aid policy, especially after the Swedish International Development Cooperation Agency (Sida) had been established in 1965.[15] This was part of a broader Swedish ambition to be a leading actor in international development aid and family planning programs after World War II. Norway had similar aspirations.[16] Swedish as well as Danish, Finnish, and Norwegian medical researchers were sponsored by US funding agencies.[17]

Moreover, there is historical evidence suggesting that the use of aborted fetuses for research and vaccine development was not unique to Sweden in the Nordic region during the postwar period. For instance, in Norway 'embryos' (or rather fetuses) that had been 'evacuated per vaginam' were employed for the making of tissue cultures for polio vaccine at the Kaptein Wilhelm Wilhelmsen og Frues bakteriologiske institutt at Rikshospitalet in Oslo in the mid-1950s.[18] In Copenhagen a Laboratory for Fetal Research was set up in the 1960s with support from the Association for the Aid of Crippled Children in New York.[19] The US National Commission for the Protection of Human Subjects of Biomedical and Behavioral Research described studies of fetal physiology in Finland, including those in which the head of the fetuses had been cut off and the brains perfused with glucose and other substances. The British Peel Report, on the other hand, mentioned only Swedish contributions.[20] More historical work is needed to determine the scope and duration of these human fetal research activities in other Nordic countries.[21]

---

14 Here I follow the discussion in Berg, Lundberg, and Tydén, *En svindlande uppgift*, 270–72. See also Bengtsson, 'Swedish *Sonderweg* in Question,' and Ekengren and Götz, 'One Per Cent Country.'

15 See also Brodén Gyberg, *Aiding Science.*

16 Berg, Lundberg, and Tydén, *En svindlande uppgift*; Engh, 'Conscience of the World?'

17 Engh, 'Rockefeller Foundation'; Ramsey, *Swedish Abortion Pill*, 58–60.

18 See, e.g., Lahelle, 'Multiplication of Poliomyelitis,' 436.

19 This laboratory and its head, the pediatrician Henning Andersen, are acknowledged, for instance, in Zachariae, 'Histamine and Mast Cells,' 63.

20 National Commission for the Protection of Human Subjects of Biomedical and Behavioral Research, *Research on the Fetus*, 13–14; United Kingdom Department of Health and Social Security, *The Use of Fetuses*, 13.

21 For a starting place, see Jülich, 'Rise and Fall.'

All the same, the Swedish context stands out for its strong state and government support for fetal research, the expanded infrastructure for supplying aborted fetal material, and the strategic ignorance production involved in this scientific enterprise. The Swedish Medical Research Council, a state agency, actively promoted fetal research and encouraged the international exchange and collaboration of researchers in order to strengthen medical science in Sweden. American governmental and private funding agencies, for their part, took advantage of Sweden's permissive attitude to launch research that was difficult to pursue in the United States. The Swedish Government emphasized reproductive research as a tool in the nation's mission to help solve the global overpopulation crisis. As demonstrated in Ramsey's chapter this also included changing the legislation to allow for clinical trials on pregnant women to test the abortion pill. Information about fetal research was not altogether secret but, as discussed in more detail below, public knowledge was controlled and restricted in various ways.

As we have argued in this volume, because of certain conditions, the most important being its abortion legislation, Sweden did acquire a unique position within the transnational field of fetal research in the postwar period. It was not a coincidence that in 1965 the Hormone Laboratory at the Karolinska Hospital could be described as a space where Sweden was a 'great power.' Certainly, this perception aligned with national rhetoric used by medical researchers. In retrospect, Diczfalusy self-confidently spoke of the 'fetoplacental empire' that arose during the 'merry post-war period' in Sweden thanks to access to aborted fetuses and US funding.[22]

But more significant is the large number of official documents that, as showcased by chapters in this book, rehearsed the view that aborted fetuses were a national resource that other countries lacked. It would thus be an unfortunate waste not to use the material to improve reproductive health conditions both nationally and globally—producing polio vaccine to save the health and lives of citizens, developing the abortion pill to make abortion safer and more widely accessible, exploring the potential of obstetrical ultrasound to create a less risky method for prenatal diagnosis, and testing dangerous pharmaceuticals to protect future beings. At the same time, such claims can be understood as a strategy to gain legitimacy for controversial research and to counter criticism from divergent audiences.[23]

Thus, many powerful actors were allied through their common interest in developing fetal knowledge as well as through their claims to provide new or

22 Diczfalusy, 'My Life with the Fetal-Placental,' 29.

23 Cf. Clarke, *Disciplining Reproduction*, 255.

improved means of controlling reproduction, including termination of pregnancy and testing for fetal anomalies. Yet, these actors were not always in agreement. As shown in this book, physicians were critical of the Abortion Act, in particular after the 1946 socio-medical amendment. A majority of gynecologists and obstetricians were in opposition, sometimes even refusing to perform abortion operations. They actively participated in public debates revolving around abortion legislation and risky abortion methods. Religious voices were also heard in these discussions, whereas women's movements usually supported the current legislation and did not demand abortion on demand until around 1970. But even if abortion was a controversial topic in the 1950s and 1960s, did anyone really object to using aborted fetuses for research and vaccine development? As we recall, Duncan Wilson claimed that, in the British case, no secrecy was involved and that both professional and popular media wholly endorsed the project.

2 Uncontroversy

As described by Jülich and Dussauge in this volume, Swedish virologists set out to produce a specific version of the polio vaccine in the early 1950s. The international vaccine race was on, and different vaccines against polio had already been developed in the United States by Jonas Salk and Albert Sabin. Sven Gard and the other virologists at the National Bacteriological Laboratory (NBL) were nonetheless confident that Sweden could take a lead thanks to their unique access to fetal material from legal abortions. However, when the infrastructure for supplying aborted fetuses failed, the production apparatus had to be reorganized in order to adapt to monkey tissues, which in turn delayed the launch of mass vaccinations.

We found no social worlds in collision when reading Swedish newspapers and popular magazines from the 1950s. Most reports on the production of the polio vaccine were neutral or positive, some even enthusiastic. Abortion as a source of fetal tissues was mentioned several times, and no explicit criticism was expressed. Nevertheless, there were voices of discontent in the press, concerning not only the delay of the vaccine but also the lack of information from the Government and NBL. Several journalists indicated that secrecy had been imposed by the Ministry of the Interior and expressed doubts about the freedom of the press.

Scientific and professional journals, in contrast, raised concerns with the media. In a paper first presented at the Scandinavian Congress of Pathology and Bacteriology in Denmark in 1955, Gard addressed the problem of sharing

17

FROM INSTITUTIONEN FÖR VIRUSFORSKNING, KAROLINSKA INSTITUTET, STOCKHOLM

ACTIVE IMMUNIZATION AGAINST POLIOMYELITIS

By

S. Gard

There is scarcely any other virus problem which is of so great current interest as the one of active immunization against poliomyelitis. However, during recent months the discussion on vaccination seems to have been led astray. The professional discussion has taken place behind closed doors, and only a few selected experts have been allowed to participate. The only open debate, the one carried on in the daily press, threatens to become politically tinged. It seems to me that it is high time to find a sounder, more dignified and matter-of-fact form for the discussion of this important problem.

As you know, the British maintain that scientific discoveries and results of scientific research should not be presented to the general public until they have been critically analyzed and assessed by the experts. A strict observation of this rule satisfies the sense of propriety but it also serves a purpose beyond that. The press, radio and television are capable of creating public opinion from one day to the next. A sensational discovery within the field of medicine is something which concerns all human beings; it is an item of news of great interest to the public and is treated accordingly. A distorted or one-sided presentation of such news may cause great harm.

These remarks are truisms, but it seems as if even old truths must be repeated now and again. The manner in which the results of the American vaccine field trial of 1954 were made public should be a matter of great concern. By the use of a complicated code system, by allocating various partial tasks to a great number of different laboratories, and thus concentrating the possibilities of analyzing and evaluating the results on one hand, attempts were made to prevent the dissemination of premature and incomplete information. This whole gigantic experiment was staged as a perfect thriller. Gradually the excitement was screwed up to a climax in the last scene of the last act, and the solution was presented in a grandiose finale with the press, radio and television in the stalls. According to the reports, 500 specially selected scientists were invited to be present, but these acted only as extras, as an effectful background. The message was aimed over their heads direct to the public.

FIGURE 15.1 First page of Sven Gard's paper on vaccination reveals three different national strategies in handling relationships between science, the media, and the public. From Gard, 'Active Immunization against Poliomyelitis,' 17. Courtesy of John Wiley and Sons.

the results of polio vaccination, and of scientific research more generally, with the public (see figure 15.1). In Sweden, he stated, the 'professional discussion has taken place behind closed doors,' with the participation of only a few select experts. On the other hand, 'the only open debate,' carried out in the newspapers, 'threatens to become politically tinged.' According to him, the press, radio, and television had great influence over the public, and there was always a risk that news of scientific discoveries might become harmfully distorted.[24]

Gard's discussion is interesting for several reasons. First, it constructs a divide between experts and the public, stressing that the media can create public ignorance through misleading information. This perspective is more closely aligned with a conventional view of linear science communication than with Wilson's conception of tissue cultures as a 'site of engagement' between science and the public. Second, Gard's report on professional discussions behind 'closed doors,' in tension with politically charged 'open debate,' confirms that there were indeed strategies to exclude the media and to restrict public knowledge about vaccine production. We sense no complete consensus among members of the public about the polio vaccine, and it seems plausible that information could have been missing or difficult to interpret (for instance, because it was presented in a scientific idiom). In other words, controversy presupposes not only public interest but also public awareness of an event or action. In this case, although the production of the Swedish polio vaccine in the 1950s was linked to the controversial abortion issue, it never sparked a public controversy; thus, uncontroversy resulted.

Third, Gard's discussion suggests that there existed various national styles of communicating about science to the media and the public. Without revealing any details about the Swedish approach, he emphasized his preference for the British model of presenting scientific research only after it had been examined and evaluated by experts. As a counterexample, he referred to the manner in which the 1954 mass vaccination trials in the United States were made public: 'This whole gigantic experiment was staged as a perfect thriller.' The media played the leading role, and the scientists only acted as extras when the solution was presented in a finale, suggesting that polio no longer represented a problem because the vaccine worked. In light of the Cutter Incident, in which many people were paralyzed and some even died, this appeared to Gard as a grave misinterpretation.[25]

In sum, the case of the Swedish polio vaccine demonstrates a significantly more complex view of the role of human tissue cultures in the 1950s than

24 Gard, 'Active Immunization against Poliomyelitis,' 17–18.

25 Gard, 17–18.

that conveyed by Wilson in his discussion about the British and US contexts. From one perspective, the production of a new vaccine against polio was a huge scientific success, and public knowledge about the importance of vaccination increased. Yet, from another perspective, scientists' distrust of the public and the media meant that they withheld or restricted information about the aborted fetuses that were the source of the polio vaccine, thereby creating ignorance. Relationships between science and its publics played out in different ways in different countries, but Sweden, which had staked its success on the availability of fetal tissues, chose the politics of half-open (or half-closed) doors, producing uncontroversy. In the 1960s this politics changed, as the media revealed scientific experiments on living human fetuses, but rather than full-fledged controversy we find controversy tamed by the medical and governmental actors involved. But first, it is interesting to note how the 'thalidomide scandal,' which arose during the same period, was both subject to attempts at information control and itself used to tame the controversy over human fetal experimentation.

3 Tamed Controversy

In 1962, newspapers in Sweden and other countries reported that the drug thalidomide could cause fetal damage. Maria Björkman and Francis Lee demonstrate in their respective chapters how the Swedish welfare state responded to this alarming information and the unfolding tragedy, including an amending abortion legislation, changing drug regulations, and establishing a national register of congenital malformations. During the early phase, the National Board of Medicine decided to halt the sale of thalidomide, but refrained from warning the public. The press reportedly complied with this decision and agreed not to cover the topic until a fuller picture was available. However, the Christian newspaper *Dagen* disregarded the medical authorities, and once the news was out, the other media acted accordingly. The National Board of Medicine maintained that it had followed protocols and had not published the matter to avoid causing distress to pregnant women.

In light of the events surrounding the Swedish polio vaccine, the handling of the thalidomide tragedy seems less remarkable. Measures were taken to restrict the flow of sensitive information to the public, which was perceived to be in need of guidance. However, it should be acknowledged that the welfare state also sought to assume responsibility in various ways. As discussed by Björkman, children affected by thalidomide received publicly financed medical care, and an ambitious rehabilitation program was launched in order to improve their lives. Yet, new conflicts arose over the functionality and role of prosthetics in shaping normal, abled bodies.

Following the thalidomide tragedy, medical experts and researchers began to justify the use of aborted fetuses in research to gain crucial knowledge about the harmful effects of drugs during the vulnerable period of gestation. However, scientific studies on fetuses from abortions had already been conducted since the end of the Second World War. In the 1950s, this research primarily focused on improving the understanding of how the human fetus contributes to its own physiological development in the uterus. Practical benefits were of secondary importance.[26]

Like the virologists at the NBL, Swedish reproductive scientists did not conduct their research in complete secrecy. Throughout the 1950s, they received grants from various funding agencies for studies involving human fetal tissues, which sometimes received attention in the newspapers. The researchers reported on their activities in international scientific publications and shared their results with colleagues at conferences and seminars. Yet the research was not altogether open. The Medical Research Council requested that grant recipients maintain a low profile and limit public transparency. For this reason, it is difficult to grasp how people would have responded to information about the human fetal research taking place at several university clinics and laboratories.[27] What we do know, through Jülich and Dussauge's chapter in this book, is that the abortion method used to obtain intact fetuses suitable for the research, the so-called small cesarean section, was publicly disputed.

As discussed in the introduction and by Tinnerholm Ljungberg in this volume, controversy started to emerge in the early 1960s, when the media reported on Diczfalusy's success in getting US funding for the perfusion studies at the KI. This reporting led to a debate between concerned parliamentary members and the minister of justice, but no further action was taken. Increasing numbers of actors became involved, including journalists, religious groups, and disability organizations. Investigations were initiated, and knowledge about the experiments became more publicly available. After 1975, when the new Abortion Act was introduced, the debate came to an end.

At the center of the controversy was the status of the fetus. In the 1960 parliamentary debate, the minister of justice, following the National Board of Medicine, claimed that the fetuses used as research objects were fully comparable to organs, tissues, and cells removed during surgery and then kept alive so that their functions could be studied. They were 'nonviable' and in

26 Jülich, 'Pusseltävlingar för de ofödda,' 433.

27 Jülich, 'Fosterexperimentens produktiva hemlighet,' 16.

legal terms stillborn. For others, this was not an acceptable parallel. A pastor and Liberal party member maintained that if the abortion operation was performed twenty weeks after conception, it was a question of experimenting not on 'tissues' but instead on a 'fetus' or even a 'child.' Neither did he accept that the fetuses were 'nonviable,' since they had been registered as showing cardiac activity, breathing, and reflex movements—signs of life that obligated the civil registry to report a fetus. He moreover implied that women undergoing abortions should be asked for their consent to use the aborted fetus for research.[28]

Following this parliamentary debate, the established definition put forward by medical actors was that aborted fetuses used for perfusion studies were comparable to tissue cultures. It was common to remind audiences about the role that human fetal tissues had played in the development of the successful Swedish polio vaccine. This comparison highlighted not only the good and legitimate cause of the research but also implied that the fetal material was dead. Critics, on the other hand, refuted this notion of the research object as a mere assemblage of bodily tissues. They maintained that the fetuses in these experiments were 'alive.' This polarization in the debate over the status of the fetus continued over the years. A parliamentary investigation published in 1974 concluded that no experimentation on living fetuses had been conducted and that the conditions for research on viable fetuses had in any case been eliminated by the new Abortion Act.

It is illustrative to compare this episode to Duncan Wilson's historical account of this period. As mentioned earlier, he holds that no controversy around human tissue culture emerged in Britain or the United States in the 1960s. However, by defining 'tissue culture' as 'a blanket term that covers the culture of cells and whole organs, known as "cell culture" and "organ culture" respectively,' he adopts the view of the winning side of the historical controversy.[29] In other words, he overlooks the fact that the debate revolved around the very definition of the object of fetal research. Sweden was hardly the only country where terminology was an issue and medical actors strived to control discourse. In fact, as Tinnerholm Ljungberg recounts in her chapter, the British Peel Advisory Group made a substantial effort to categorize fetal material as comparable to a tumor or any other unwanted body part.

It is uncertain what effects the Swedish controversy had on ethical regulations. Some of the critical participants strived to establish a link between Swedish fetal research and Nazi medical experiments. Another recurrent point of reference in the 1960s was British physician Maurice Pappworth's widely

28 This is discussed in Jülich, 21–22.

29 Wilson, *Tissue Culture*, 125n5.

discussed report on unethical experiments with human subjects. But unlike Pappworth's writings, which fueled international change in research ethics, the controversy in Sweden never escalated into a scandal, and no one was ever convicted of or blamed for unlawful or unethical professional behavior.[30]

As Tinnerholm Ljungberg has demonstrated, the first research ethics committee at the Karolinska Hospital was inaugurated because of demands from the US National Institutes of Health but had no practical effect on fetal research. Later on, the British Peel Report seems to have affected Swedish parliamentary debates on the need to expand the system of research ethics committees and also to include laymen, which generally meant politicians. But no evidence suggests that it was the scientists themselves who developed ethical guidelines, out of their own concern or in response to criticism. Quite the contrary; theirs was a plea to protect free science from public interference and control.

The conflict over fetal experimentation can perhaps best be described as a 'tamed controversy.' It was more transparent and open than those emerging in the 1950s, but boundaries between the science and the public were still maintained and guarded. The media continued to be portrayed as sensationalistic and a source of popular ignorance. In various ways the information provided by medical researchers and authorities was still restricted. Even if controversy broke out, the experiments at its core were never fully disclosed, followed by silence and historiographic oblivion.

4 Selective Controversy

As we learn from controversy studies, disputes that are settled or closed can be reopened.[31] Interestingly, this has not been the case with the strands of medical research discussed here. Since 1975, postwar fetal research has been largely absent from public debates in Sweden. No controversy or scandal has emerged around the use of lung tissues from aborted fetuses for developing the Swedish polio vaccine.[32] The 'live fetus experiments' at the KI have not made the headlines or gone viral. The link between the development of the

30 On associations with Nazi experiments, see Jülich, 'Fosterexperimentens produktiva hemlighet,' 22. The Swedish reception of Pappworth's report is discussed in Jülich, 'Rise and Fall.'

31 Pinch, 'Scientific Controversies.'

32 For instance, Wadman's work on the 'Swedish source' of the cell line WI-38 has not been discussed at all in a Swedish context. See Wadman, *Vaccine Race*, chap. 6.

analysis of chromosomal anomalies and access to material from legal abortions has mostly gone unnoticed. Neither have voices condemned the testing of abortion pills and obstetric ultrasound technology on women granted abortion. Certainly, other controversial topics have emerged—for instance, around IVF and embryonic stem cell research—but the historical legacy of postwar fetal research has not been discussed in the Swedish media or in academic publications.[33]

The work of ignoring or forgetting the history of fetal experiments may have involved a complex set of motives. One important reason is probably the fact that the legality of abortion has not been the subject of major political controversy in Sweden since the introduction of abortion on demand in 1975. As discussed by Björklund and Tunlid in this volume, the anti-abortion movement in Sweden never gained the scale and political influence of its counterpart in the United States, where conflicts over abortion-related issues have been heated and indeed continue to be so.[34] The Church of Sweden, along with several free churches, accepted the right to abortion, indicating broad support for women's reproductive autonomy. Tellingly, Lennart Nilsson's fetal photographs have largely been used for sex education in a Swedish context, whereas in the United States they were appropriated early on for anti-abortion campaigns.[35]

Instead, public debates have focused on other parts of Swedish medical history. From the early 1980s historical collections of human remains and their association with nineteenth- and early twentieth-century racial science has been a recurrent theme. The outcry started with an article in a daily newspaper alerting readers that an attic in the Anatomy Department at Lund University housed a cranial collection that had presumably been assembled in an unethical way. Soon afterward, similar collections in Stockholm and Uppsala were reported on. During the 1990s new research on the history of race biology and eugenics became available, which led to the so-called sterilization debate in 1997, when Sweden's 'dark history' made the headlines in both national and foreign newspapers.[36] Here abortion was seen as an important issue—not the legislation as such, but rather its historical link to involuntary and voluntary sterilizations. Many participants in this debate argued that the Social Democratic welfare state was responsible for the forced sterilization of 'inferior

33 Gunnarsson Payne, 'Reproducing the Legitimate Swedish Family'; Ideland, 'Stem Cells.'

34 For historical discussions about national legacies in shaping ethical controversies about embryo/fetal research, see also Banchoff, *Embryo Politics*, 14–19, and Wilson, *Tissue Cultures*, 95.

35 Jülich, 'Fetal Photography.'

36 Jülich, 'Historier kring Tornbladinstitutet.'

citizens,' especially intellectually disabled people, revealing connections to racial and Nazi ideologies.[37]

Historical researchers showed that this view was based on a number of misconceptions, including the portrayal of the Nordic countries, especially Sweden, as a unique case. Instead, they emphasized that political support for the sterilization policy was almost unanimous among all parties. A common pattern in these countries was the presence of influential medical professions, a strong belief in science, lack of resistance from the Catholic Church, and a heritage of earlier racial research. The largest category of sterilized people in Sweden was 'worn-out women,' who accepted sterilization as a condition for abortion. Yet even in the absence of direct coercion, it has not been possible to establish how voluntary these sterilizations really were.[38]

These media debates have lingered. In 2015 the obstetrical collection examined by Franzén in this volume was 'rediscovered' and framed as problematic cultural heritage. A journalist described the collection of women's pelves at the Museum of Medical History in Uppsala as part of a 'dark history' with strong links to race biology. He stressed that at least a third of the individuals to whom these bones belonged had descended from non-Swedish groups. He also emphasized that the former owner of the collection, Magnus Retzius, was the brother of Anders Retzius, 'the father of Swedish skull measurement.' However, until the publication of Franzén's research, not much was known about the history of this university collection.[39]

Embryological collections were also presented as part of this controversial history. Swedish Radio reported that human embryological specimens were still kept at many older secondary schools, where they had been used in biology classes. The journalists asked whether the fetuses in the Tornblad Collection at Lund University, discussed by Jülich in this volume, had been obtained in an ethical manner. Moreover, the editor of a magazine published by the Church of Sweden linked the Tornblad Institute to Auschwitz, stating that it was rooted in race biology that we know today led to one of humanity's darkest chapters. In 2017 the wet human fetal specimens were moved from the institute building to the Biological Museum of Lund University, where they were restored. The

37 For a useful review of the larger 1990s debate, see Liljeborg, 'En genomgång av 1997.'

38 The historical research on the Nordic countries was presented in Broberg and Roll-Hansen, *Eugenics and the Welfare State*. For a recent analysis, see Alaattinoğlu, *Grievance Formation, Rights and Remedies*, chap. 3.

39 For a discussion of this media report, see Franzén, *Kroppar i förvandling*, 13.

medical faculty's promise to return the Tornblad Collection to its former building has yet to be fulfilled.[40]

In other cases, these debates have led to the destruction of embryological specimens. In 2018, politicians on the Västra Götaland Region Council decided that all human remains at schools and museums within the region should be destroyed or 'reburied,' including the 'Siamese twins' that had been on display at the Gothenburg Natural History Museum. The argument was that the way the bodies had been acquired did not meet present standards of ethics and human rights. Museum professionals as well as researchers in archaeology, osteology, and history protested that the decision would make it impossible to create new historical knowledge about the collection, including histories about vulnerable individuals. Nevertheless, the 'Siamese twins,' despite their unknown identity or religious background, were cremated and the ashes buried in a Lutheran memorial grove.[41]

Looking back at the past decades, these debates about problematic medical heritage can be characterized as 'selective controversies' that constructed a history of racial science and the violation of human rights. They were selective in the sense that certain episodes and phenomena were foregrounded, framed, and dramatized in specific ways. They did not include the scientific uses of human fetuses in postwar Sweden, which has long enjoyed historical amnesia. Even so, many of the features that historians have highlighted as crucial conditions for establishing Swedish sterilization policy during the period between the world wars are relevant for understanding the rise of postwar fetal research, including a consensual political culture, strong faith in science, medicine, and technology, influential medical professions, and weak opposition from the church and religious groups.

5 Conclusion

Adele Clarke's study of controversy and the development of the reproductive sciences in the Unites States has been valuable in understanding the Swedish case. In Sweden, fetal research emerged as a new scientific field during the postwar period, largely because of the availability of legal abortions. Medical authorities, organizations, and researchers did not widely share information about or discuss this research. There were differing and critical voices among

40 Jülich, 'Historier kring Tornbladinstitutet,' 151–52, 260–61.
41 Jülich, 152, 267–68.

the public. However, these debates can only be partially described as a collision of social worlds. As demonstrated, controversy took many different forms.

First, I discussed 'uncontroversy' to highlight how the production of the Swedish polio vaccine in the 1950s, although linked to the controversial abortion issue, never sparked a public controversy. An important condition for this outcome was the secrecy imposed by the Government and medical experts. This analysis diverges from Duncan Wilson's history of tissue culture in Britain and the United States. According to him, the '"social unease" literature' has built a false dichotomy between science and its publics. Yet, we have to acknowledge that for various reasons historical actors have chosen to draw boundaries between science and the public. As shown here, medical experts manifested a paternalistic attitude toward people's capacity to understand and take a stance on difficult scientific matters.

Second, I described the perfusion studies of aborted fetuses in the 1960s and early 1970s as an instance of 'tamed controversy.' As with the thalidomide tragedy, it was evident that there were attempts to control and restrict the information to the public. Even if some non-medical actors publicly contested fetal experimentation, the topic never developed into a full-fledged controversy. The central question was whether the aborted fetus should be considered as an assemblage of nonviable tissues or whether it was alive and had human value. Medical experts did not agree with the definition of a living fetus, nor with the idea that permission must be obtained from the abortion patients whose terminated pregnancies the research relied upon. This standpoint became the established view, and after the introduction of the Abortion Act in 1975, the dispute came to an end.

Third, the notion of 'selective controversy' is helpful in understanding why postwar Swedish fetal research has not been discussed in Sweden after the disputes of the 1960s and 1970s. The subject was black boxed, to use a favorite term in controversy studies. Other aspects of Swedish medical history have been highlighted as controversial in past decades. Above all, public debates have linked involuntary sterilizations and obstetrical and embryological collections to race science and the violation of human rights. The selective nature of this controversy could be due to the relative consensus around the legality of abortion and reproductive rights. Other factors may also have contributed to the unwillingness to look back and discuss the past, not least the promotion of Sweden as a leading nation in medical science that contributes positively to the good of humanity.

According to the dominant historiography, human fetal research became controversial after the liberalization of abortion in the United States and Britain. But this story is ripe for revision in several respects. In Sweden, conflicts around abortion broke out much earlier, owing to a fairly liberal abortion law and experimentation on human fetuses. This point is significant not only for Swedish medical history but also for its transnational and international connections. Many countries viewed Sweden as a hospitable environment for human fetal research and supported it, but eventually the controversy they wished to avoid came home to roost. In sum, we need to have histories other than those of the major Atlantic democracies because they diversify and add complexity to the big picture.

This volume has highlighted the conflicting values and difficult balancing acts involved in fetal knowledge production during five hundred years of Swedish history. Postwar fetal research is notable for several reasons. A moral economy emerged in which the use of aborted fetuses and pregnant women scheduled for abortion was justified in terms of the benefits to science, the nation, and humanity. Those who were responsible for authorizing, supporting, and conducting this research navigated a stormy sea. On the one hand, they achieved new scientific knowledge that helped to combat epidemic disease and, in some ways, improved reproductive health and rights for women. On the other, in an attempt to avoid controversy, they produced and maintained public ignorance about the necessary conditions for developing this knowledge.

Bibliography

Alaattinoğlu, Daniela. *Grievance Formation, Rights and Remedies: Involuntary Sterilisation and Castration in the Nordics, 1930s–2020s*. Cambridge: Cambridge University Press 2023.

Åselius, Gunnar. *Vietnamkriget och de svenska diplomaterna 1954–1975*. Stockholm: Dialogos, 2019.

Banchoff, Thomas. *Embryo Politics: Ethics and Policy in Atlantic Democracies*. Ithaca, NY: Cornell University Press, 2011.

Bengtsson, Erik. 'The Swedish *Sonderweg* in Question: Democratization and Inequality in Comparative Perspective, *c*. 1750–1920.' *Past and Present*, no. 244 (August 2019): 123–61.

Berg, Annika, Urban Lundberg, and Mattias Tydén. *En svindlande uppgift: Sverige och biståndet 1945–1975*. Stockholm: Ordfront, 2021.

Berggren, Henrik, and Lars Trädgårdh. *Är svensken människa? Gemenskap och oberoende i det moderna Sverige*. Stockholm: Norstedts, 2006.

Broberg, Gunnar, and Nils Roll-Hansen, eds. *Eugenics and the Welfare State: Sterilization Policy in Denmark, Sweden, Norway, and Finland*. East Lansing: Michigan State University Press, 1996.

Brodén Gyberg, Veronica. *Aiding Science: Swedish Research Aid Policy 1973–2008*. Linköping: Linköpings universitet, 2013.

Clarke, Adele E. 'Controversy and the Development of Reproductive Sciences.' *Social Problems* 37, no. 1 (1990): 18–37.

Clarke, Adele E. *Disciplining Reproduction: Modernity, American Life Sciences, and 'the Problems of Sex.'* Berkeley: University of California Press, 1998.

'A Culture of Consent.' *Nature* 498 (June 26, 2013): 407.

Dahl, Ann-Sofie. 'Sweden: Once a Moral Superpower, Always a Moral Superpower?' *International Journal* 61, no. 4 (2006): 895–907.

Dahl, Ann-Sofie. *See also* Nilsson, Ann-Sofie.

Diczfalusy, Egon R. 'My Life with the Fetal-Placental Unit.' *American Journal of Obstetrics and Gynecology* 193, no. 6 (2005): 2025–29.

Ekengren, Ann-Marie, and Norbert Götz. 'The One Per Cent Country: Sweden's Internalisation of the Aid Norm.' In *Saints and Sinners: Official Development Aid and Its Dynamics in a Historical and Comparative Perspective*, edited by Thorsten Borring Olesen, Helge Pharo, and Kristian Paaskesen, 21–49. Oslo: Akademika forlag, 2013.

Engh, Sunniva. 'The Conscience of the World? Swedish and Norwegian Provision of Development Aid.' *Itinerario* 33, no. 2 (2009): 65–82.

Engh, Sunniva. 'The Rockefeller Foundation, Scandinavian Aid Agencies and the "Population Explosion."' In *American Foundations and the European Welfare States*, edited by Klaus Petersen, John Stewart, and Michael Kuur Sørensen, 181–202. Odense: Syddansk Universitetsforlag, 2013.

Franzén, Helena. *Kroppar i förvandling: Obstetriska och embryologiska samlingar vid Uppsala universitet, ca 1830–1930*. Uppsala: Uppsala universitet, 2022.

Gard, Sven. 'Active Immunization against Poliomyelitis.' In *Transactions of the Eleventh Scandinavian Congress of Pathology and Bacteriology: Aarhus, June 20th–22nd 1955*, 17–26. *Acta pathologica et microbiologica Scandinavica*. Supplement 111. Copenhagen: E. Munksgaard, 1956.

Gunnarsson Payne, Jenny. 'Reproducing the Legitimate Swedish Family: Kinship Grammars in the Context of Assisted Reproductive Technologies.' *Jahrbuch für Europäische Ethnologie* 16/17 (2023): 139–62.

Idеland, Malin. 'Stem Cells between Ethics and Entrepreneurship: How a Contested Bio-Object Became 'Normal.' *Studies in Media and Communication* 2, no. 2 (2014): 82–92.

Jülich, Solveig. 'Fetal Photography in the Age of Cool Media.' In *History of Participatory Media: Politics and Publics, 1750–2000*, edited by Anders Ekström, Solveig Jülich, Frans Lundgren, and Per Wisselgren, 125–41. New York: Routledge, 2011.

Jülich, Solveig. 'Fosterexperimentens produktiva hemlighet: Medicinsk forskning och vita lögner i 1960-och 1970-talets Sverige.' *Lychnos* (2018): 10–49.

Jülich, Solveig. 'Historier kring Tornbladinstitutet.' In *Embryologiska rum: Tornbladinstitutets samling av foster från människor och djur*, by Thomas Nilsson and Solveig Jülich, 151–268. Göteborg: Makadam, 2022.

Jülich, Solveig. 'Pusseltävlingar för de ofödda: *Expressens* insamling till prenatal forskning 1957–1990.' *Historisk tidskrift* 143, no. 3 (2023): 409–43.

Jülich, Solveig. 'The Rise and Fall of the Fetoplacental Empire: Human Fetal Research in Sweden, ca. 1950–1975.' Unpublished manuscript.

Lahelle, Oskar. 'Multiplication of Poliomyelitis and Echo Viruses in Tissue Cultures Prepared from Human Amniotic Membranes.' *Acta Pathologica et Microbiologica Scandinavica* 40, no. 5 (1957): 436–44.

Landecker, Hannah. *Culturing Life: How Cells Became Technologies*. Cambridge, MA: Harvard University Press, 2007.

Liljeborg, Olov. 'En genomgång av 1997 års tvångssteriliseringsdebatt i svensk dagspress.' Levande historia, 2009. Accessed January 26, 2024. https://www.levandehistoria.se/.

National Commission for the Protection of Human Subjects of Biomedical and Behavioral Research. *Research on the Fetus: Report and Recommendations*. US Department of Health, Education and Welfare, Publication No. (OS) 76–127. Washington, DC: Government Printing Office, 1975.

Nemec, Birgit, and Jesse Olszynko-Gryn. 'The Duogynon Controversy and Ignorance Production in Post-Thalidomide West Germany.' *Reproductive Biomedicine & Society Online* 14 (2022): 75–87.

Nilsson, Ann-Sofie. *Den moraliska stormakten: En studie av socialdemokratins internationella aktivism*. Stockholm: Timbro, 1991.

Nilsson, Ann-Sofie. *See also* Dahl, Ann-Sofie.

Öhquist, Nils. 'Där är Sverige stormakt: Läkare från hela världen forskar i Sverige.' *Aftonbladet*, April 10, 1965.

Pinch, Trevor. 'Scientific Controversies.' In *International Encyclopedia of the Social and Behavioral Sciences*. 2nd ed. Edited by James D. Wright. Vol. 21. Amsterdam: Elsevier, 2015.

Ramsey, Morag. *The Swedish Abortion Pill: Co-producing Medical Abortion and Values, ca. 1965–1992*. Uppsala: Uppsala University, 2021.

Skloot, Rebecca. *The Immortal Life of Henrietta Lacks*. New York: Crown, 2010.

Smithson, Michael. 'Afterword: Ignorance Studies; Interdisciplinary, Multidisciplinary, and Transdisciplinary.' In *Routledge International Handbook of Ignorance Studies*, edited by Matthias Gross and Linsey McGoey, 385–99. Abingdon: Routledge, 2015.

Topçu, Sezin, and Irène Maffi. 'Rethinking Ignorance Production in the Field of Reproductive Biomedicine: An Introduction.' *Reproductive Biomedicine & Society Online* 14 (2022): 216–21.

United Kingdom Department of Health and Social Security. *The Use of Fetuses and Fetal Material for Research: Report of the Advisory Group*. London: HMSO, 1972.

Wadman, Meredith. 'Medical Research: Cell Division.' *Nature* 498 (June 26, 2013): 422–46.

Wadman, Meredith. *The Vaccine Race: Science, Politics, and the Human Costs of Defeating Disease*. New York: Viking, 2016.

Wilson, Duncan. *Tissue Culture in Science and Society: The Public Life of a Biological Technique in Twentieth Century Britain*. Basingstoke: Palgrave Macmillan, 2011.

Wilson, Duncan. 'A Troubled Past? Reassessing Ethics in the History of Tissue Culture.' *Health Care Analysis* 24, no. 3 (2016): 246–59.

Zachariae, Hugh. 'Histamine and Mast Cells in Human Fetal Skin.' *Proceedings of the Society for Experimental Biology and Medicine* 117 (October 1964): 63–65.

Glossary

Bishops' Meeting of the Church of Sweden Svenska kyrkans biskopsmöte
Catholic Bishops' Office Katolska biskopsämbetet
Center Party Centerpartiet
Central Bacteriological Laboratory of Stockholm City Bakteriologiska centrallaboratoriet i Stockholm
Central Board of the Church of Sweden Svenska kyrkans centralstyrelse
Central Hospital in Kalmar Kalmar lasarett
Christian Democratic Unity (Christian Democrats) Kristen Demokratisk Samling (today Kristdemokraterna)
Church of Sweden Svenska kyrkan
Church Law of 1686 1686 års kyrkolag
Civil Code of 1734 1734 års lag
College of Health Sundhetscollegium
committe report, parliamentary utskottsbetänkande, riksdagen
Conservative Party, Moderate Party Högerpartiet (today Moderaterna)
Eugenia Home Eugeniahemmet
Finnish Institute for Health and Welfare Institutet för hälsa och välfärd, Finland
First Chamber of the Parliament Första kammaren i riksdagen
Fredrika Bremer Association Fredrika-Bremer-Förbundet
Geatish Society Göthiska förbundet
Gothenburg Natural History Museum Göteborgs naturhistoriska museum
Gothenburg University Göteborgs universitet
government bill proposition från regeringen
Hagströmer Library of the Karolinska Institute Hagströmerbiblioteket
Helsingborg's Maternity Hospital Helsingborgs Barnbördshus
Infanticide Act of 1778 Barnamordsplakatet
interpellation (written question put to a minister) interpellation
Karlskoga Hospital Karlskoga lasarett
Karolinska Hospital Karolinska sjukhuset
Karolinska Institute Karolinska Institutet
King in Council, Royal Majesty Kunglig Majestät, Kungl. Maj:t (until 1974)
Liberal People's Party (Liberals) Folkpartiet (today Liberalerna)
Lund University Lunds universitet
Lund (University) Hospital Lunds lasarett, Lunds universitetssjukhus
Malmö Municipal Hospital Malmö Allmänna Sjukhus
Medical Research Council Medicinska forskningsrådet
motion (proposal to the Parliament by one or several MP:s) motion

Museum of Drawings in Laholm Teckningsmuseet i Laholm
Museum of Medical History in Uppsala Medicinhistoriska museet i Uppsala
Museum of Work in Norrköping Arbetets museum, Norrköping
National Association of the Disabled De handikappades riksförbund
National Association of the Neurologically Disabled Neurologiskt handikappades riksförbund
National Bacteriological Laboratory Statens bakteriologiska laboratorium
National Board of Health and Welfare Socialstyrelsen
National Board of Health and Welfare's advisory board for ethical issues Socialstyrelsens rådgivande nämnd för etiska frågor
National Board of Medicine Medicinalstyrelsen
National Council for the Disabled Statens handikappråd
National Counsellor for the Neurosedyn issue Rikskuratorn för neurosedynfrågan
National News Agency Tidningarnas Telegrambyrå
National Organization against Polio Riksföreningen mot polio
National Pharmaceutical Laboratory Statens farmaceutiska laboratorium
Nordic Museum Nordiska museet
Office for Tabulation Tabellverket
Parliamentary Committee on Education Utbildningsutskottet, riksdagen
Parliamentary Ombudsman justitieombudsmannen
Radio Committee Radionämnden
research ethics committees forskningsetiska kommittéer
Royal Institute of Technology Kungliga Tekniska högskolan
Royal Swedish Academy of Sciences Kungl. Vetenskapsakademien
Sabbatsberg Hospital Sabbatsbergs sjukhus
Sahlgrenska University Hospital Sahlgrenska universitetssjukhuset
Scandinavian Association of Naturalists Nordiska Naturforskare-Sällskapet
Second Chamber of the Parliament Andra kammaren i riksdagen
Social Democratic Party Socialdemokraterna
Society for the Neurosedyn Affected Föreningen för de Neurosedynskadade
Society of German Natural Scientists and Physicians Gesellschaft Deutscher Naturforscher und Ärzte
South Swedish Society for the History of Medicine Sydsvenska medicinhistoriska sällskapet
State Institute for Race Biology Statens institut för rasbiologi
Statistics Sweden Statistikmyndigheten, Statistiska centralbyrån
Stockholm City Council Stockholms stadsfullmäktige
Stockholm City Hospital Directorate Stockholms stads sjukvårdsstyrelse
Swedish Association for Sexuality Education Riksförbundet för sexuell upplysning (RFSU)

Swedish Chancellor of Justice Justitiekanslerämbetet
Swedish Code of Statutes Svensk författningssamling
Swedish Code of Statutes in the Field of Health and Sick Care Medicinalförfattningar
Swedish Council of Free Churches Sveriges frikyrkoråd
Swedish Disability Rights Federation Handikappförbundens Centralkommitté
Swedish Ecumenical Board Svenska ekumeniska nämnden
Swedish Ethical Review Authority Etikprövningsmyndigheten
Swedish Freedom of the Press Act (1766) Tryckfrihetsförordningen
Swedish Government regeringen (from 1975)
Swedish Government Commission on Disability Handikapputredningen
Swedish Government Commission Official Reports Statens offentliga utredningar (SOU)
Swedish International Development Cooperation Agency Styrelsen för internationellt utvecklingssamarbete (Sida)
Swedish Medical Association Sveriges Läkarförbund
Swedish Medical Journal *Svenska läkartidningen, Läkartidningen*
Swedish Midwives Journal *Jordemodern*
Swedish Ministry of Health and Social Affairs Socialdepartementet
Swedish Ministry of the Interior Inrikesdepartementet
Swedish Ministry of Justice Justitiedepartementet
Swedish National Association for People with Intellectual Disability Riksförbundet för utvecklingsstörda barn, ungdomar och vuxna
Swedish National Council on Medical Ethics Statens medicinsk-etiska råd (Smer)
Swedish Parliament riksdagen
Swedish Radiation Safety Authority Strålsäkerhetsmyndigheten
Swedish Radio Sveriges Radio
Swedish Register of Congenital Malformations Missbildningsregistret
Swedish Society of Biology Biologiska Föreningen
Swedish Society of Medicine Svenska läkaresällskapet
Swedish Society of Medicine's Ethics Delegation Svenska läkaresällskapets delegation för medicinsk etik
Swedish Society for Racial Hygiene Svenska sällskapet för rashygien
Swedish Television Sveriges Television
Tabulation Commission Tabellkommissionen
Tornblad Institute for Comparative Embryology, Lund University Tornbladinstitutet för komparativ embryologi, Lunds universitet
Twin Register Tvillingregistret
Uppsala University Uppsala universitet
Uppsala University Hospital Akademiska sjukhuset
Västra Götaland Region Council Västra Götalandsregionen

Selected Bibliography

The bibliography consists of secondary sources cited in the introduction, chapters, and the epilogue. The emphasis is on titles in English.

Åhrén, Eva. *Death, Modernity and the Body: Sweden 1870–1940*. Rochester, NY: University of Rochester Press, 2009.

Åhrén, Eva. 'Figuring Things Out: Visualizations in the Work of Anders and Gustaf Retzius, 1829–1921.' *Nuncius: Journal of the Material and Visual History of Science* 32, no. 1 (2017): 166–211.

Åhrén, Eva. 'Making Space for Specimens: The Museums of the Karolinska Institute, Stockholm.' In *Medical Museums: Past, Present, Future*, edited by Samuel J. M. M. Alberti and Elizabeth Hallam, 102–15. London: Royal College of Surgeons, 2013.

Al-Gailani, Salim, and Angela Davis. 'Introduction to "Transforming Pregnancy Since 1900."' *Studies in History and Philosophy of Biological and Biomedical Sciences* 47, Pt. B (September 2014): 229–32.

Alaattinoğlu, Daniela. *Grievance Formation, Rights and Remedies: Involuntary Sterilisation and Castration in the Nordics, 1930s–2020s*. Cambridge: Cambridge University Press 2023.

Alberti, Samuel J. M. M. *Morbid Curiosities: Medical Museums in Nineteenth-Century Britain.* Oxford: Oxford University Press, 2011.

Andersson, Jenny, and Mary Hilson. 'Images of Sweden and the Nordic Countries.' *Scandinavian Journal of History* 34, no. 3 (2009): 219–28.

Ariès, Philippe. *Centuries of Childhood*. London: Pimlico, 1996.

Armstrong, David. 'The Rise of Surveillance Medicine.' *Sociology of Health & Illness* 17, no. 3 (June 1, 1995): 393–404.

Axelsson, Per. 'The Cutter Incident and the Development of a Swedish Polio Vaccine, 1952–1957.' *Dynamis* 32, no. 2 (2012): 311–28.

Banchoff, Thomas. *Embryo Politics: Ethics and Policy in Atlantic Democracies*. Ithaca, NY: Cornell University Press, 2011.

Barton, H. Arnold. 'Scandinavianism, Fennomania, and the Crimean War.' *Journal of Baltic Studies* 36, no. 2 (2005): 131–56.

Bashford, Alison. *Global Populations: History, Geopolitics, and Life on Earth*. New York: Columbia University Press, 2013.

Bauer, Susanne. 'From Administrative Infrastructure to Biomedical Resource: Danish Population Registries, the "Scandinavian Laboratory," and the "Epidemiologist's Dream."' *Science in Context* 27, no. 2 (June 2014): 187–213.

Bauer, Susanne, and Ayo Wahlberg, eds. *Contested Categories: Life Sciences in Society*. Ashgate: Farnham, 2009.

Bengtsson, Erik. 'The Swedish *Sonderweg* in Question: Democratization and Inequality in Comparative Perspective, *c.* 1750–1920.' *Past and Present*, no. 244 (August 2019): 123–61.

Berg, Annika. 'Rays of Death and Visions of Life: Ultrasound Narratives, Risk Evaluations, and Prenatal Imaging.' *Technology and Culture* 65, no. 3 (2024): 933–65.

Berg, Annika. 'A Suitable Country: The Relationship between Sweden's Interwar Population Policy and Family Planning in Post-independence India.' *Berichte zur Wissenschaftsgeschichte* 33, no. 3 (2010): 297–320.

Berg, Annika, Urban Lundberg, and Mattias Tydén. *En svindlande uppgift: Sverige och biståndet 1945–1975*. Stockholm: Ordfront, 2021.

Björklund, Elisabet. 'Contested Pictures of Persuasion: American Images of Foetuses in Swedish Antiabortion Campaigns of the 1970s and 1980s.' In *Nordic Media Histories of Propaganda and Persuasion*, edited by Fredrik Norén, Emil Stjernholm, and C. Claire Thomson, 97–116. Cham: Palgrave Macmillan, 2023.

Björklund, Elisabet. *The Most Delicate Subject: A History of Sex Education Films in Sweden*. Lund: Lund University, 2012.

Björklund, Elisabet. 'Waiting for Abortion: Narratives of Passing Time, Decision-Making, and Late Abortions in Swedish TV Theater of the Late 1960s and Early 1970s.' *Body Politics: Zeitschrift für Körpergeschichte* 8, no. 12 (2020): 108–34.

Björklund, Elisabet, and Solveig Jülich, eds. *Rethinking the Public Fetus: Historical Perspectives on the Visual Culture of Pregnancy*. Rochester, NY: University of Rochester Press, 2024.

Björkman, Maria. 'The Cost of Normalization: The Thalidomide Affected and the Welfare State.' *Scandinavian Journal of History* 48, no. 3 (2023): 341–58.

Björkman, Maria, and Anna Tunlid. 'The Establishment of Genetic Counselling in Sweden: 1940–1980.' In *History of Human Genetics: Aspects of Its Development and Global Perspectives*, edited by Heike I. Petermann, Peter S. Harper, and Susanne Doetz, 339–66. Cham: Springer International, 2017.

Björkman, Maria, and Sven Widmalm. 'Selling Eugenics: The Case of Sweden.' *Notes and Records of the Royal Society of London* 64, no. 4 (2010): 379–400.

Bock von Wülfingen, Bettina, Christina Brandt, Susanne Lettow, and Florence Vienne, eds. 'Temporalities of Reproduction: Practices and Concepts from the Eighteenth to the Early Twenty-First Century.' Special issue, *History and Philosophy of the Life Sciences* 37, no. 1 (2015).

Bondestam, Maja, ed. *Exceptional Bodies in Early Modern Culture: Concepts of Monstrosity Before the Advent of the Normal*. Amsterdam: Amsterdam University Press, 2020.

Bondestam, Maja. *See also* Larsson, Maja.

Broberg, Gunnar, and Nils Roll-Hansen, eds. *Eugenics and the Welfare State: Sterilization Policy in Denmark, Sweden, Norway, and Finland*. East Lansing: Michigan State University Press, 1996.

Brodén Gyberg, Veronica. *Aiding Science: Swedish Research Aid Policy 1973–2008.* Linköping: Linköpings universitet, 2013.

Buklijas, Tatjana, and Nick Hopwood. *Making Visible Embryos* (online exhibition). 2008–10. Accessed May 6, 2023. http://www.hps.cam.ac.uk/visibleembryos/.

Buklijas, Tatjana, and Salim Al-Gailani. 'A Fetus in the World: Physiology, Epidemiology, and the Making of Fetal Origins of Adult Disease.' *History and Philosophy of the Life Sciences* 45, no. 44 (2023): 1–34.

Campbell, Patricia. 'Making Sense of the Abortion Pill: A Sociotechnical Analysis of RU486 in Canada.' *Health Sociology Review* 27, no. 2 (January 2018): 121–35.

Carlhed, Carina. 'The Rise of the Professional Field of Medicine in Sweden.' *Professions and Professionalism* 3, no. 2 (2013): 1–15.

Casper, Monica J. 'At the Margins of Humanity: Fetal Positions in Science and Medicine.' *Science, Technology & Human Values* 19, no. 3 (1994): 307–23.

Casper, Monica J. *The Making of the Unborn Patient: A Social Anatomy of Fetal Surgery.* New Brunswick, NJ: Rutgers University Press, 1998.

Cházaro, Laura. 'From Anatomical Collection to National Museum, ca 1895: How Skulls and Female Pelvises Began to Speak the Language of Mexican National History.' In *Beyond Alterity: Destabilizing the Indigenous Other in Mexico*, edited by Paula López Caballero and Adriana Acevedo-Rodrigo, 173–98. Tucson: University of Arizona Press, 2018.

Christoffersen-Deb, Astrid. 'Viability: A Cultural Calculus of Personhood at the Beginnings of Life.' *Medical Anthropology Quarterly* 26, no. 4 (2012): 575–94.

Claes, Tinne. '"By What Right Does the Scalpel Enter the Pauper's Corpse?" Dissections and Consent in Late Nineteenth-Century Belgium.' *Social History of Medicine* 31, no. 2 (2018): 258–77.

Clarke, Adele E. *Disciplining Reproduction: Modernity, American Life Sciences, and 'the Problems of Sex.'* Berkeley: University of California Press, 1998.

Clarke, Adele E. 'Research Materials and Reproductive Sciences in the United States, 1910–1940.' In *Physiology in the American Context 1850–1940*, edited by Gerald L. Geison, 323–50. Bethesda: American Physiological Society, 1987.

Clarke, Adele E. and Teresa Montini. 'The Many Faces of RU486: Tales of Situated Knowledges and Technological Contestations.' *Science, Technology & Human Values* 18, no. 11 (Winter 1993): 42–78.

Conklin, Alice L. *In the Museum of Man: Race, Anthropology, and Empire in France, 1850–1950*. Ithaca, NY: Cornell University Press, 2013.

Crawford, Catherine. 'Legalizing Medicine: Early Modern Legal Systems and the Growth of Medico-Legal Knowledge.' In *Legal Medicine in History*, edited by Michael Clark and Catherine Crawford, 89–116. Cambridge: Cambridge University Press, 1994.

Creager, Angela N. H., and Hannah Landecker. 'Technical Matters: Method, Knowledge, and Infrastructure in Twentieth-Century Life Science.' *Nature Methods* 6, no. 10 (2009): 701–5.

Cressy, David. 'Lamentable, Strange, and Wonderful: Headless Monsters in the English Revolution.' In *Monstrous Bodies/Political Monstrosities in Early Modern Europe*, edited by Laura Lunger Knoppers and Joan B. Landes, 40–63. Ithaca, NY: Cornell University Press, 2004.

Czarnowski, Gabriele, and Sabine Hildebrandt. 'Research on the Boundary between Life and Death: Coercive Experiments on Pregnant Women and their Fetuses during National Socialism.' In *From Clinic to Concentration Camp: Reassessing Nazi Medical and Racial Research, 1933–1945*, edited by Paul Weindling, 73–99. London: Routledge, 2017.

Daston, Lorraine, and Peter Galison. *Objectivity*. New York: Zone Books, 2007.

Daston, Lorraine, and Katharine Park. *Wonders and the Order of Nature, 1150–1750*. New York: Zone Books, 1998.

Davies, Douglas J. *Death, Ritual and Belief: The Rhetoric of Funerary Rites*. London and Washington, DC: Cassell, 1997.

Davis, Lennard J. *Enforcing Normalcy: Disability, Deafness, and the Body*. London: Verso, 1995.

de Chadarevian, Soraya. 'Chromosome Photography and the Human Karyotype.' *Historical Studies in the Natural Sciences* 45 (2015): 115–46.

de Chadarevian, Soraya. *Heredity under the Microscope: Chromosomes and the Study of the Human Genome*. Chicago: University of Chicago Press, 2020.

Dias, Nélia. 'The Visibility of Difference: Nineteenth-Century French Anthropological Collections.' In *The Politics of Display: Museums, Science, Culture*, edited by Sharon MacDonald, 36–52. London: Routledge, 1998.

Dijck, José van. *The Transparent Body: A Cultural Analysis of Medical Imaging*. Seattle: University of Washington Press, 2004.

Dittmar, Jenna M., and Mitchell Piers. 'From Cradle to Grave via the Dissection Room: The Role of Foetal and Infant Bodies in Anatomical Education from the Late 1700s to Early 1900s.' *Journal of Anatomy* 229 (2016): 713–22.

Doetz, Susanne. 'Healthy, Happy, Rational: Reflections on Genetic Counselling in the GDR.' *Medical Humanities* 49, no. 2 (2023): 236–47.

Dolan, Brian. 'Malthus's Political Economy of Health: The Critique of Scandinavia in the *Essay on Population*.' In *Malthus, Medicine and Morality: 'Malthusianism' after 1798*, edited by Brian Dolan, 9–32. Amsterdam: Rodopi, 2000.

Donaghy, Paige. 'Miscarriage, False Conceptions, and Other Lumps: Women's Pregnancy Loss in Seventeenth- and Eighteenth-Century England.' *Social History of Medicine* 34, no. 4 (2021): 1138–60.

Donaghy, Paige. 'The Secrets of the Placenta in European Anatomy and Midwifery, 1560–1700.' *Isis* 114, no. 2 (2023): 249–71.

Dron, Heather A. *Teratology Transformed: Uncertainty, Knowledge, and Conflict over Environmental Etiologies of Birth Defects in Midcentury America*. Diss. San Francisco: University of California, 2016.

Dry, Sarah. 'The Population as Patient: Alice Stewart and the Controversy over Low-Level Radiation in the 1950s.' In *The Risks of Medical Innovation: Risk Perception and Assessment in Historical Context*, edited by Thomas Schlich and Ulrich Tröhler, 108–22. London and New York: Routledge, 2006.

Dubow, Sara. *Ourselves Unborn: A History of the Fetus in Modern America*. New York: Oxford University Press, 2011.

Duden, Barbara. *Disembodying Women: Perspectives on Pregnancy and the Unborn*. Cambridge, MA: Harvard University Press, 1993.

Duden, Barbara. 'Quick with Child: An Experience That Has Lost Its Status.' *Technology in Society* 14, no. 3 (1994): 335–44.

Duden, Barbara, Jürgen Schlumbohm, and Patrice Veit, eds. *Geschichte des Ungeborenen: Zur Erfahrungs- und Wissenschaftgeschichte der Schwangerschaft, 17.–20. Jahrhundert*, Göttingen: Vandenhoeck and Ruprecht, 2002.

Dussauge, Isabelle, Claes-Fredrik Helgesson, and Francis Lee, eds. *Value Practices in the Life Sciences and Medicine*. Oxford: Oxford University Press, 2015.

Ekengren, Ann-Marie, and Norbert Götz. 'The One Per Cent Country: Sweden's Internalisation of the Aid Norm.' In *Saints and Sinners: Official Development Aid and Its Dynamics in a Historical and Comparative Perspective*, edited by Thorsten Borring Olesen, Helge Pharo, and Kristian Paaskesen, 21–49. Oslo: Akademika forlag, 2013.

Ekerwald, Hedvig. 'The Modernist Manifesto of Alva and Gunnar Myrdal: Modernization of Sweden in the Thirties and the Question of Sterilization.' *International Journal of Politics, Culture, and Society* 14, no. 3 (2001): 531–61.

Engh, Sunniva. 'The Conscience of the World? Swedish and Norwegian Provision of Development Aid.' *Itinerario* 33, no. 2 (2009): 65–82.

Engh, Sunniva. 'The Rockefeller Foundation, Scandinavian Aid Agencies and the "Population Explosion."' In *American Foundations and the European Welfare States*, edited by Klaus Petersen, John Stewart, and Michael Kuur Sørensen, 181–202. Odense: Syddansk Universitetsforlag, 2013.

Ericsson, Martin. 'What Happened to "Race" in Race Biology? The Swedish State Institute for Race Biology, 1936–1960.' *Scandinavian Journal of History* 46, no. 1 (2021): 125–48.

Evans, Jennifer, and Sara Read. '"Before Midnight She Had Miscarried": Women, Men, and Miscarriage in Early Modern England.' *Journal of Family History* 40, no. 1 (2015): 3–23.

Fabian, Ann. *The Skull Collectors: Race, Science, and America's Unburied Dead*. Chicago: University of Chicago Press, 2010.

Fannin, Maria. 'Making an "Embryological Vision of the World": Law, Maternity and the Kyoto Collection.' In *Reproductive Geographies: Bodies, Places and Politics*, edited by Marcia R. England, Maria Fannin, and Helen Hazen, 17–30. London: Routledge, 2018.

Fausto-Sterling, Anne. 'Gender, Race, and Nation: The Comparative Anatomy of "Hottentot" Women in Europe, 1815–1817.' In *Deviant Bodies: Critical Perspectives of Difference in Science and Popular Culture*, edited by Jennifer Terry and Jacqueline Urla, 19–48. Bloomington: Indiana University Press, 1995.

Foscati, Alessandra. '"Nonnatus Dictus Quod Caeso Defunctae Matris Utero Prodiit": Postmortem Caesarean Section in the Late Middle Ages and Early Modern Period.' *Social History of Medicine* 32, no. 3 (2019): 465–80.

Foucault, Michel. *Abnormal: Lectures at the Collège de France, 1974–1975*. Edited by Valerio Marchetti and Antonella Salomoni. Translated by Graham Burchell. London: Verso, 2003.

Foucault, Michel. 'The Politics of Health in the Eighteenth Century.' In *The Essential Foucault: Selections from Essential Works of Foucault, 1954–1984*, edited by Paul Rabinow and Nikolas Rose, 90–105. New York: New Press, 2003.

Franklin, Sarah. 'Rethinking Reproductive Politics in Times, and Time in UK Reproductive Politics: 1978–2008.' *Journal of the Royal Anthropological Institute* 20, no. 1 (2014): 109–25.

Franklin, Sarah, Celia Lury, and Jackie Stacey. *Global Nature, Global Culture*. London, Thousand Oaks, CA, and New Delhi: Sage, 2000.

Franzén, Helena. 'From Patient to Specimen and Back Again: Radical Surgeries and Pelvic Pathologies in the Museum Obstetricum.' *Lychnos* (2020): 33–57.

Franzén, Helena. '"The Precious Material": Obtaining Human Fetal Bodies for an Embryological Collection at Uppsala University ca. 1890–1930.' *Scandinavian Journal of History* 47, no. 2 (2022): 178–202.

Fur, Gunlög. 'Colonialism and Swedish History: Unthinkable Connections?' In *Scandinavian Colonialism and the Rise of Modernity: Small Time Agents in a Global Arena*, edited by Magdalena Naum and Jonas M. Nordin, 17–36. New York: Springer, 2013.

Gélis, Jacques. *Les enfants des limbes: Mort-néz et parents dans l'Europe chrétienne*. Paris: Louis Audibert, 2006.

Gorney, Cynthia. *Articles of Faith: A Frontline History of the Abortion Wars*. New York: Simon & Schuster, 1998.

Gottweis, Herbert, Brian Salter, and Catherine Waldby. *The Global Politics of Human Embryonic Stem Cell Science: Regenerative Medicine in Transition*. Basingstoke: Palgrave Macmillan, 2009.

Gowing, Laura. *Common Bodies: Women, Touch, and Power in Seventeenth-Century England*. New Haven, CT: Yale University Press, 2003.

Grant, Joanna. '"Those Parts Peculiar to Her Organization": Some Observations on the History of Pelvimetry, a Nearly Forgotten Obstetric Sub-speciality.' In *The Female Body in Medicine and Literature*, edited by Andrew Mangham and Greta Depledge, 135–47. Liverpool: Liverpool University Press, 2011.

Grell, Ole Peter. 'The Protestant Imperative of Christian Care and Neighborly Love.' In *Health Care and Poor Relief in Protestant Europe 1500–1700*, edited by Andrew Cunningham and Ole Peter Grell, 43–65. London: Routledge, 1997.

Guerrini, Anita. 'The Material Turn in the History of Life Science.' *Literature Compass* 13, no. 7 (2016): 469–80.

Gunnarsson Payne, Jenny. 'Reproducing the Legitimate Swedish Family: Kinship Grammars in the Context of Assisted Reproductive Technologies.' *Jahrbuch für Europäische Ethnologie* 16/17 (2023): 139–162.

Hagner, Michael. 'Enlightened Monsters.' In *The Sciences in Enlightened Europe*, edited by William Clark, Jan Golinski, and Simon Schaffer, 175–217. Chicago: University of Chicago Press, 1999.

Hall, Patrik. *The Social Construction of Nationalism: Sweden as an Example*. Lund: Lund University, 1998.

Hallam, Elizabeth. *Anatomy Museum: Death and the Body Displayed*. London: Reaktion Books, 2016.

Han, Sallie, Tracy K. Betsinger, and Amy B. Scott, eds. *The Anthropology of the Fetus: Biology, Culture, and Society*. New York: Berghahn Books, 2018.

Hedgecoe, Adam. '"A Form of Practical Machinery": The Origins of Research Ethics Committees in the UK, 1967–1972.' *Medical History* 53, no. 3 (2009): 331–50.

Hedlund, Maria. 'Democratic Expert Influence through Bioethical Advisory Commissions? The Case of PGD Legislation in Sweden.' In *Quality Issues in Clinical Genetic Services*, edited by Ulf Kristoffersson, J. J. Cassiman, and Jörg Schmidtke, 233–242. Dordrecht: Springer, 2010.

Hedlund, Maria. 'Ethicisation and Reliance on Ethics Expertise.' *Res Publica* (2023), https://doi.org/10.1007/s11158-023-09592-5

Helgason, Agnar, and Gisli Palsson. 'Contested Commodities: The Moral Landscape of Modernist Regimes.' *Journal of the Royal Anthropological Institute* 3 (1997): 451–71.

Hendriksen, Marieke. 'The Fate of the Beaded Babies: Forgotten Early Colonial Anatomy.' In *The Fate of Anatomical Collections*, edited by Rina Knoeff and Robert Zwijnenberg, 179–94. Farnham: Ashgate, 2015.

Herzog, Dagmar. *Unlearning Eugenics: Sexuality, Reproduction, and Disability in Post-Nazi Europe*. Madison: University of Wisconsin Press, 2018.

Hess, Volker, and J. Andrew Mendelsohn. 'Case and Series: Medical Knowledge and Paper Technology, 1600–1900.' *History of Science* 48, no. 3–4 (September 2010): 287–314.

Hilson, Mary. 'Denmark, Norway, and Sweden: Pan-Scandinavism and Nationalism.' In *What Is a Nation? Europe 1789–1914*, edited by Timothy Baycroft and Mark Hewitson, 192–209. Oxford: Oxford University Press, 2006.

Hopwood, Nick. *Embryos in Wax: Models from the Ziegler Studio*. Cambridge: Whipple Museum of the History of Science, 2002.

Hopwood, Nick. *Haeckel's Embryos: Images, Evolution, and Fraud.* Chicago: University of Chicago Press, 2015.

Hopwood, Nick. 'Plastic Publishing in Embryology.' In *Models: The Third Dimension of Science*, edited by Soraya de Chadarevian and Nick Hopwood, 170–206. Stanford, CA: Stanford University Press, 2004.

Hopwood, Nick. 'Producing Development: The Anatomy of Human Embryos and the Norms of Wilhelm His.' *Bulletin of the History of Medicine* 74, no. 1 (2000): 29–79.

Hopwood, Nick, Rebecca Flemming, and Lauren Kassel, eds. *Reproduction: Antiquity to the Present Day.* Cambridge: Cambridge University Press, 2018.

Hopwood, Nick, Peter Murray Jones, Lauren Kassell, and Jim Secord, eds. 'Communicating Reproduction.' Special issue, *Bulletin of the History of Medicine* 89, no. 3 (2015).

Hornuff, Daniel, and Heiner Fangerau, eds. *Visualisierung des Ungeborenen: Interdisziplinäre Perspektiven.* Paderborn: Brill/Fink, 2020.

Huet, Marie-Hélène. *Monstrous Imagination.* Cambridge, MA: Harvard University Press, 1993.

Hughes, Richard L. 'Burning Birth Certificates and Atomic Tupperware Parties: Creating the Antiabortion Movement in the Shadow of the Vietnam War.' *Historian* 68, no. 3 (2006): 541–58.

Hurlbut, Benjamin. *Experiments in Democracy: Human Embryo Research and the Politics of Bioethics.* New York: Columbia University Press, 2017.

Ideland, Malin. 'Stem Cells between Ethics and Entrepreneurship: How a Contested Bio-Object Became 'Normal.' *Studies in Media and Communication* 2, no. 2 (2014): 82–92.

Jackson, Mark. 'Suspicious Infant Deaths: The Statute of 1624 and Medical Evidence at Coroners' Inquests.' In *Legal Medicine in History*, edited by Michael Clark and Catherine Crawford, 64–86. Cambridge: Cambridge University Press, 1994.

Jacobs, Noortje. *Ethics by Committee: A History of Reasoning Together about Medicine, Science, Society, and the State.* Chicago: Chicago University Press, 2022.

Jacobs, Noortje, and Helena Tinnerholm Ljungberg, eds. 'How Ethics Travels: The International Development of Research Ethics Committees in the Late Twentieth Century.' Special issue, *European Journal for the History of Medicine and Health* 78, no. 2 (2021).

Jasanoff, Sheila. 'Making the Facts of Life.' In *Reframing Rights: Bioconstitutionalism in the Genetic Age*, edited by Sheila Jasanoff, 59–83. Cambridge, MA: MIT Press, 2011.

Joffe, Carole, and Tracy Weitz. 'Normalizing the Exceptional: Incorporating the "Abortion Pill" into Mainstream Medicine.' *Social Science & Medicine* 56, no. 12 (2003): 2353–66.

Johannisson, Karin. 'The People's Health: Public Health Policies in Sweden.' In *The History of Public Health and the Modern State*, edited by Dorothy Porter, 165–82. Amsterdam: Rodopi, 1994.

Jülich, Solveig. 'The Drama of the Fetoplacental Unit: Reimagining the Public Fetus of Lennart Nilsson.' In Björklund and Jülich, *Rethinking the Public Fetus*, 143–70.

Jülich, Solveig. 'Fetal Photography in the Age of Cool Media.' In *History of Participatory Media: Politics and Publics, 1750–2000*, edited by Anders Ekström, Solveig Jülich, Frans Lundgren, and Per Wisselgren, 125–41. New York: Routledge, 2011.

Jülich, Solveig. 'The Making of a Best-Selling Book on Reproduction: Lennart Nilsson's *A Child Is Born*.' *Bulletin of the History of Medicine* 89, no. 3 (2015): 491–525.

Jülich, Solveig. 'Picturing Abortion Opposition in Sweden: Lennart Nilsson's Early Photographs of Embryos and Fetuses.' *Social History of Medicine* 31, no. 2 (2018): 278–307.

Jülich, Solveig. 'Televising Inner Space: Lennart Nilsson's Early Medical Documentaries on the Interior of the Human Body.' In *Representational Machines: Photography and the Production of Space*, edited by Anna Dahlgren, Dan Petersson, and Nina Lager Vestberg, 149–70. Aarhus: Aarhus University Press, 2013.

Keller, Eve. 'Embryonic Individuals: The Rhetoric of Seventeenth-Century Embryology and the Construction of Early-Modern Identity.' *Eighteenth-Century Studies* 33, no. 3 (2000): 321–48.

Kent, Julie. *Regenerating Bodies: Tissue and Cell Therapies in the Twenty-First Century*. London and New York: Taylor and Francis, 2012.

Keupper Valle, Rosemary. 'The Cesarean Operation in Alta California during the Franciscan Mission Period (1769–1833).' *Bulletin of the History of Medicine* 48, no. 2 (1974): 265–75.

Kirejczyk, Marta. 'Parliamentary Cultures and Human Embryos: The Dutch and British Debates Compared.' *Social Studies of Science* 29, no. 6 (1999): 889–912.

Koch, Lene, and Mette N. Svendsen. 'Negotiating Moral Value: A Story of Danish Research Monkeys and Their Humans.' *Science, Technology, & Human Values* 40 (2015): 368–88.

Kosmin, Jennifer F. *Authority, Gender, and Midwifery in Early Modern Italy: Contested Deliveries*. London: Routledge, 2020.

Kosmin, Jennifer F. 'When the Fetus Becomes a Child: Some Reflections from the Long Eighteenth Century.' In *Medical Humanities: Perspectives from the Arts and the Social Sciences*, edited by Rinaldo F. Canalis, Massimo Ciavolella, and Valeria Finucci, 51–70. Berlin: De Gruyter, 2023.

Kuźma-Markowska, Sylwia, and Laura Kelly. 'Anti-abortion Activism in Poland and the Republic of Ireland, c. 1970s–1990s.' *Journal of Religious History* 46, no. 3 (2022): 526–51.

LaFleur, William. *Liquid Life: Abortion and Buddhism in Japan*. Princeton, NJ: Princeton University Press, 1992.

Landecker, Hannah. *Culturing Life: How Cells Became Technologies*. Cambridge, MA: Harvard University Press, 2007.

Larsson, Maja. 'From Frightening Beast to Primitive Stage: On the Normalization of the Monstrous Body in Swedish Medicine.' In *Body Claims*, edited by Janne Bromseth, Lisa Folkmarson Käll, and Katarina Mattsson, 26–57. Uppsala: Uppsala University, 2009.

Larsson, Maja. *See also* Bondestam, Maja.

Law, Jane Marie, and Vanessa R. Sasson, eds. *Imagining the Fetus: The Unborn in Myth, Religion and Culture*. Oxford: Oxford University Press, 2008.

Lee, Francis, Solveig Jülich, and Isa Dussauge. 'The Politics of Valuation: Value Disjunctures in Bioethics and Fetal Research During the Twentieth Century.' *Nordic Journal of Science and Technology Studies*, 12, no. 2 (2024): 5–17.

Lemke, Thomas. *Biopolitics: An Advanced Introduction*. New York: New York University Press, 2011.

Lennerhed, Lena. 'No Backlash for Swedish Women? The Right to Abortion on Demand, 1975–2000.' *Journal of Modern European History* 17, no. 3 (2019): 326–36.

Lennerhed, Lena. 'Sherri Finkbine's Choice: Abortion, Sex-Liberalism and Feminism in Sweden in the 1960s and 1970s.' *Women's History Magazine* 73 (2013): 13–18.

Lennerhed, Lena. 'Taking the Middle Way: Sex Education Debates in Sweden in the Early Twentieth Century.' In *Shaping Sexual Knowledge: A Cultural History of Sex Education in Twentieth Century Europe*, edited by Lutz Sauerteig and Roger Davidson, 55–70. London: Routledge, 2009.

Lennerhed, Lena. 'Troubled Women: Abortion and Psychiatry in Sweden in the 1940s and 1950s.' In *Transcending Borders: Abortion in the Past and Present*, edited by Shannon Stettner, Katrina Ackerman, Kristin Burnett, and Travis Hay, 89–100. Cham: Springer International, 2017.

Linders, Annulla. 'Victory and Beyond: A Historical Comparative Analysis of the Outcomes of the Abortion Movements in Sweden and the United States.' *Sociological Forum* 19 (2004): 371–404.

Lindqvist, Rafael. 'Swedish Disability Policy: From Universal Welfare to Civil Rights?' *European Journal of Social Security* 2 (2000): 399–418.

Littoz-Monnet, Annabelle. *Governing through Expertise: The Politics of Bioethics*. Cambridge: Cambridge University Press. 2020.

Løkke, Anne. 'Responsibility and Emotion: Parental, Governmental and Almighty Responses to Infant Death in Denmark in the Mid-eighteenth to the Mid-nineteenth Century.' In *Death, Emotion and Childhood in Premodern Europe*, edited by Katie Barclay, Kimberley Reynolds, and Ciara Rawnsley, 191–208. London: Palgrave Macmillan, 2016.

Löwy, Ilana. *Imperfect Pregnancies: A History of Birth Defects and Prenatal Diagnosis*. Baltimore: Johns Hopkins University Press, 2017.

Löwy, Ilana. *Tangled Diagnoses: Prenatal Diagnosis, Women, and Risk*. Chicago: University of Chicago Press, 2018.

Lundin, Per, and Niklas Stenlås. 'Technology, State Initiative, and National Myths in Cold War Sweden: An Introduction.' In *Science for Welfare and Warfare: Technology and State Initiative in Cold War Sweden*, edited by Per Lundin, Niklas Stenlås, and Johan Gribbe, 1–34. Sagamore Beach, MA: Science History Publications, 2010.

Lupton, Deborah. *The Social Worlds of the Unborn*. Basingstoke: Palgrave Macmillan, 2013.

MacDonald, Helen. 'Corpse Stories: Anatomy, Bodies and a Colonial World.' In *Bodies beyond Borders: Moving Anatomies, 1750–1950*, edited by Kaat Wils, Raf de Bont, and Sokhieng Au, 73–90. Leuven: Leuven University Press, 2017.

MacDonald, Helen. *Human Remains: Dissection and Its Histories*. New Haven, CT: Yale University Press, 2006.

Maehle, Andreas-Holger. *Contesting Medical Confidentiality: Origins of the Debate in the United States, Britain, and Germany*. Chicago: University of Chicago Press, 2016.

Maehle, Andreas-Holger. *Doctors, Honour, and the Law: Medical Ethics in Imperial Germany*. Basingstoke: Palgrave Macmillan, 2009.

Maienschein, Jane, Marie Glitz, and Garland E. Allen, eds. *Centennial History of the Carnegie Institution of Washington*. Vol. 2, *The Department of Embryology*. Cambridge: Cambridge University Press, 2004.

Marks, Lara. 'Human Guinea Pigs? The History of the Oral Contraceptive Clinical Trials.' *History and Technology* 14, no. 4 (1999): 263–88.

Martin, Emily. *The Woman in the Body: A Cultural Analysis of Reproduction*. Boston: Beacon Press, 1987.

Matthews, Kirstin R. W., and Daniel Moralí. 'National Human Embryo and Embryoid Research Policies: A Survey of 22 Top Research-Intensive Countries.' *Regenerative Medicine* 15, no. 7 (2020): 1905–17.

Maynard-Moody, Steven. *The Dilemma of the Fetus: Fetal Research, Medical Progress and Moral Politics*. New York: St. Martin's Press, 1995.

McClive, Cathy. 'Blood and Expertise: The Trials of the Female Medical Expert in the Ancien-Régime Courtroom.' *Bulletin of the History of Medicine* 82, no. 1 (2008): 86–108.

McClive, Cathy. 'The Hidden Truths of the Belly: The Uncertainties of Pregnancy in Early Modern Europe.' *Social History of Medicine* 15, no. 2 (2002): 209–27.

McLeary, Erin Hunter. 'Science in a Bottle: The Medical Museum in North America, 1860–1940.' PhD diss., University of Pennsylvania, 2001.

Morgan, Lynn M. *Icons of Life: A Cultural History of Human Embryos*. Berkeley: University of California Press, 2009.

Morgan, Lynn M. '"Properly Disposed of": A History of Embryo Disposal and the Changing Claims on Fetal Remains.' *Medical Anthropology* 21, no. 3–4 (2002): 247–74.

Morgan, Lynn M. 'When Does Life Begin? A Cross-Cultural Perspective on the Personhood of Fetuses and Young Children.' In *Talking about People: Readings in Contem-*

porary Cultural Anthropology, edited by William A. Haviland, Robert J. Gordon, and Luis A. Vivanco, 35–46. Boston, MA: McGraw-Hill, 2002.

Naum, Magdalena, and Jonas M. Nordin. 'Introduction: Situating Scandinavian Colonialism.' In *Scandinavian Colonialism and the Rise of Modernity: Small Time Agents in a Global Arena*, edited by Magdalena Naum and Jonas M. Nordin, 3–16. New York: Springer, 2013.

Nemec, Birgit, and Jesse Olszynko-Gryn. 'The Duogynon Controversy and Ignorance Production in Post-Thalidomide West Germany.' *Reproductive Biomedicine & Society Online* 14 (2022): 75–87.

Nemec, Birgit, and Gabriele Moser. 'Counselling, Risk and Prevention in Human Genetic Early Diagnosis in the Federal Republic of Germany.' In *History of Human Genetics: Aspects of Its Development and Global Perspectives*, edited by Heike I. Petermann, Peter S. Harper, and Susanne Doetz, 367–92. Cham: Springer International, 2017.

Nicolson, Malcolm, and John E. E. Fleming. *Imaging and Imagining the Fetus: The Development of Obstetric Ultrasound.* Baltimore: Johns Hopkins University Press, 2013.

Nordin, Jonas M., and Carl-Gösta Ojala. 'Collecting, Connecting, Constructing: Early Modern Commodification and Globalization of Sámi Material Culture.' *Journal of Material Culture* 23, no. 1 (2018): 58–82.

Nordlund, Christer. *Hormones of Life: Endocrinology, the Pharmaceutical Industry, and the Dream of a Remedy for Sterility, 1930–1970*. Sagamore Beach, MA: Science History Publications, 2011.

Nyhart, Lynn K. *Biology Takes Form: Animal Morphology and the German Universities, 1800–1900.* Chicago: University of Chicago Press, 1995.

Oakley, Ann. *The Captured Womb: A History of the Medical Care of Pregnant Women.* Oxford: Blackwell, 1984.

Olszynko-Gryn, Jesse, Eira Bjørvik, Merle Weßel, Solveig Jülich, and Cyrille Jean. 'A Historical Argument for Regulatory Failure in the Case of Primodos and Other Hormone Pregnancy Tests.' *Reproductive Biomedicine & Society Online* 6 (August 2018): 34–44.

Olszynko-Gryn, Jesse, and Caroline Rusterholz. 'Reproductive Politics in Twentieth-Century France and Britain.' *Medical History* 63, no. 2 (2019): 117–33.

Olszynko-Gryn, Jesse, Patrick Ellis, and Caithan Gainty, eds. 'Reproduction on Film.' Special issue, *British Journal for the History of Science* 50, no. 3 (September 2017).

Oudshoorn, Nelly. *Beyond the Natural Body: An Archeology of Sex Hormones.* London: Routledge, 1994.

Parens, Erik, and Adrienne Asch, eds. *Prenatal Testing and Disability Rights.* Baltimore: Georgetown University Press, 2000.

Park, Katherine. 'Birth and Death.' In *A Cultural History of the Human Body in the Medieval Age*, edited by Linda Kalof, 17–37. London: Bloomsbury Academic, 2010.

Park, Katherine. 'The Death of Isabella Della Volpe: Four Eyewitness Accounts of a Postmortem Caesarean Section in 1545.' *Bulletin of the History of Medicine* 82, no. 1 (2008): 169–87.

Park, Katharine. *Secrets of Women: Gender, Generation, and the Origins of Human Dissection*. New York: Zone Books, 2006.

Paul, Diane B. 'Reflections on the Historiography of American Eugenics: Trends, Fractures, Tensions.' *Journal of the History of Biology* 49 (2016): 641–58.

Paulsson Holmberg, Tove. 'Ambiguous and Transitional Bodies: Stillbirth in Stockholm, 1691–1724.' In *Exceptional Bodies in Early Modern Culture: Concepts of Monstrosity before the Advent of the Normal*, edited by Maja Bondestam, 163–84. Amsterdam: Amsterdam University Press, 2020.

Petchesky, Rosalind Pollack. 'Fetal Images: The Power of Visual Culture in the Politics of Reproduction.' *Feminist Studies* 13, no. 2 (1987): 263–92.

Pfeffer, Naomi, and Julie Kent. 'Framing Women, Framing Fetuses: How Britain Regulates Arrangements for the Collection and Use of Aborted Fetuses in Stem Cell Research and Therapies.' *BioSocieties* 2, no. 4 (2007): 429–47.

Pickstone, John V. *Ways of Knowing: A New History of Science, Technology, and Medicine*. Chicago: University of Chicago Press, 2001.

Pinch, Trevor. 'Scientific Controversies.' In *International Encyclopedia of the Social and Behavioral Sciences*. 2nd ed. Edited by James D. Wright. Vol. 21. Amsterdam: Elsevier, 2015.

Poort, Looneke, Tora Holmberg, and Malin Ideland. 'Bringing in the Controversy: Re-politicizing the De-politicized Strategy of Ethics Committees.' *Life Sciences, Society and Policy* 9, no. 11 (2013): https://doi.org/10.1186/2195-7819-9-11.

Prescott, Heather Munro. *The Morning After: A History of Emergency Contraception in the United States*. New Brunswick, NJ: Rutgers University Press, 2011.

Proctor, Robert N. 'Agnotology: A Missing Term.' In *Agnotology: The Making and Unmaking of Ignorance*, edited by Robert N. Proctor and Londa Schiebinger, 1–33. Stanford, CA: Stanford University Press, 2008.

Quirke, Viviane, and Jean-Paul Gaudillière. 'The Era of Biomedicine: Science, Medicine, and Public Health in Britain and France after the Second World War.' *Medical History* 52, no. 4 (2008): 441–52.

Ramsey, Morag. *The Swedish Abortion Pill: Co-producing Medical Abortion and Values, ca. 1965–1992*. Uppsala: Uppsala University, 2021.

Rapp, Rayna. *Testing Women, Testing the Fetus*. New York: Routledge, 1999.

Ray, Sara. 'From Monsters to Malformations: Anatomical Preparations as Objects of Evidence for a Developmental Paradigm of Embryology, 1770–1850.' *Journal of the History of Biology* 55, no. 1 (2022): 35–57.

Reagan, Leslie J. *Dangerous Pregnancies: Mothers, Disabilities, and Abortion in Modern America*. Berkeley: University of California Press, 2010.

Reagan, Leslie J. *When Abortion Was a Crime: Women, Medicine, and Law in the United States, 1867–1973*. Berkeley: University of California Press, 1997.

Reinarz, Jonathan. 'The Age of Museum Medicine: The Rise and Fall of the Medical Museum at Birmingham's School of Medicine.' *Social History of Medicine* 18, no. 3 (2005): 419–37.

Rich, Miriam. 'The Curse of Civilised Woman: Race, Gender and the Pain of Childbirth in Nineteenth-Century American Medicine.' *Gender and History* 28, no. 1 (2016): 57–76.

Roberts, Julie. *The Visualised Foetus: A Cultural and Political Analysis of Ultrasound Imagery*. London: Routledge, 2012.

Rocca, Julius. *Forging a Medical University: The Establishment of Sweden's Karolinska Institutet*. Stockholm: Karolinska Institutet University Press, 2006.

Roe, Shirley A. *Matter, Life, and Generation: 18th-Century Embryology and the Haller-Wolff Debate*. Cambridge: Cambridge University Press, 1981.

Roque, Ricardo. 'Stories, Skulls, and Colonial Collections.' *Configurations* 19 (2011): 1–23.

Rothman, David J. *Strangers at the Bedside: A History of How Law and Bioethics Transformed Medical Decision Making*. 1991. New Brunswick, NJ: AldineTransaction, 2003.

Ruberg, Willemijn. 'Travelling Knowledge and Forensic Medicine: Infanticide, Body and Mind in the Netherlands, 1811–1911.' *Medical History* 57, no. 3 (2013): 359–76.

Rusnock, Andrea A. *Vital Accounts: Quantifying Health and Population in Eighteenth-Century England and France*. New York: Cambridge University Press, 2002.

Schiebinger, Londa. *The Mind Has No Sex? Women in the Origins of Modern Science*. Cambridge, MA: Harvard University Press, 1989.

Schiebinger, Londa. *Nature's Body: Gender in the Making of Modern Science*. Boston: Beacon Press, 1993.

Schlich, Thomas. 'Risk and Medical Innovation: A Historical Perspective.' In *The Risks of Medical Innovation: Risk Perception and Assessment in Historical Context*, edited by Thomas Schlich and Ulrich Tröhler, 1–17. London and New York: Routledge, 2006.

Schoen, Johanna. *Abortion after* Roe. Chapel Hill: University of North Carolina Press, 2015.

Sheldon, Sally, Gayle Davis, Jane O'Neill, and Clare Parker. *The Abortion Act 1967: A Biography of a UK Law*. Cambridge: Cambridge University Press, 2022.

Skloot, Rebecca. *The Immortal Life of Henrietta Lacks*. New York: Crown, 2010.

Sköld, Peter. 'The Birth of Population Statistics in Sweden.' *History of the Family* 9, no. 1 (2004): 5–21.

Stark, Laura. *Behind Closed Doors: IRBs and the Making of Ethical Research*. Chicago: University of Chicago Press, 2012.

Stern, Alexandra Minna. *Telling Genes: The Story of Genetic Counselling in America*. Baltimore: Johns Hopkins University Press, 2012.

Stormer, Nathan. 'Looking in Wonder: Prenatal Sublimity and the Commonplace "Life."' *Signs* 33, no. 3 (2008): 647–73.

Svärd, Per-Anders, and Helena Tinnerholm Ljungberg. 'Fetal and Animal Research in Sweden: The Construction of Viable Lives in Regulatory Policy Debates, 1970–1980.' *Studies in History and Philosophy of Science, Part A* 89 (2021): 248–56.

Svendsen, Mette N., and Lene Koch. 'Unpacking the "Spare Embryo": Facilitating Stem Cell Research in a Moral Landscape.' *Social Studies of Science* 38, no. 1 (2008): 93–110.

Takala, Tuija, and Matti Häyry. 'Physicians Controlling Women's Reproductive Choices: The Slow Liberalization of Abortion Laws in Finland.' *Cambridge Quarterly of Healthcare Ethics* 32, no. 3 (2023): 391–96.

Taylor, Janelle S. *The Public Life of the Fetal Sonogram: Technology, Consumption, and the Politics of Reproduction*. New Brunswick, NJ, and London: Rutgers University Press, 2008.

Tinnerholm Ljungberg, Helena. 'Regulating Research: The Origins and Institutionalization of Research Ethics Committees in Sweden.' *European Journal for the History of Medicine and Health* 78, no. 2 (2021): 267–86.

Topçu, Sezin, and Irène Maffi. 'Rethinking Ignorance Production in the Field of Reproductive Biomedicine: An Introduction.' *Reproductive Biomedicine & Society Online* 14 (2022): 216–21.

Tybjerg, Karin. 'From Bottled Babies to Biobanks: Medical Collections in the Twenty-First Century.' In *The Fate of Anatomical Collections*, edited by Rina Knoeff and Robert Zweinenberg, 263–78. Farnham: Ashgate, 2015.

Tydén, Mattias. 'The Scandinavian States: Reformed Eugenics Applied.' *The Oxford Handbook of the History of Eugenics*, edited by Alison Bashford and Philippa Levine, 363–76. New York: Oxford University Press, 2010.

Wadman, Meredith. *The Vaccine Race: Science, Politics, and the Human Costs of Defeating Disease*. New York: Viking, 2016.

Waldby, Catherine, and Melinda Cooper. 'The Biopolitics of Reproduction.' *Australian Feminist Studies* 23, no. 55 (2008): 57–73.

Waldby, Catherine, and Robert Mitchell. *Tissue Economies: Blood, Organs, and Cell Lines in Late Capitalism*. Durham, NC: Duke University Press, 2006.

Whiteley, Rebecca. *Birth Figures: Early Modern Prints and the Pregnant Body.* Chicago: University of Chicago Press, 2023.

Wiesner, Merry E. 'The Midwives of South Germany and the Public/Private Dichotomy.' In *The Art of Midwifery: Early Modern Midwives in Europe*, edited by Hilary Marland, 77–94. London and New York: Routledge, 1993.

Wilson, Duncan. *Tissue Culture in Science and Society: The Public Life of a Biological Technique in Twentieth Century Britain*. Basingstoke: Palgrave Macmillan, 2011.

Wilson, Emily K. 'Ex Utero: Live Human Fetal Research and the Films of Davenport Hooker.' *Bulletin of the History of Medicine* 88, no. 1 (2014): 132–60.

Wisselgren, Per. 'Reforming the Science-Policy Boundary: The Myrdals and the Swedish Tradition of Governmental Commissions.' In *Academics and Public Intellectuals*, edited by Sven Eliaeson and Ragnvald Kalleberg, 173–95. Newcastle: Cambridge Scholars, 2008.

Withycombe, Shannon. *Lost: Miscarriage in Nineteenth-Century America*. New Brunswick, NJ: Rutgers University Press, 2019.

Wolf, Jaqueline H. *Cesarean Section: An American History of Risk, Technology and Consequence*. Baltimore: Johns Hopkins University Press, 2018.

Woods, Robert. *Death before Birth: Fetal Health and Mortality in Historical Perspective*. Oxford: Oxford University Press, 2009.

Zuckerman, Phil. 'Why Are Danes and Swedes So Irreligious?' *Nordic Journal of Religion and Society* 22 (2009): 55–69.

Index

An italicized page number indicates a figure or table.

www.ingramcontent.com/pod-product-compliance
Lightning Source LLC
Chambersburg PA
CBHW071249230926
51849CB00001B/278